Qigong Massage

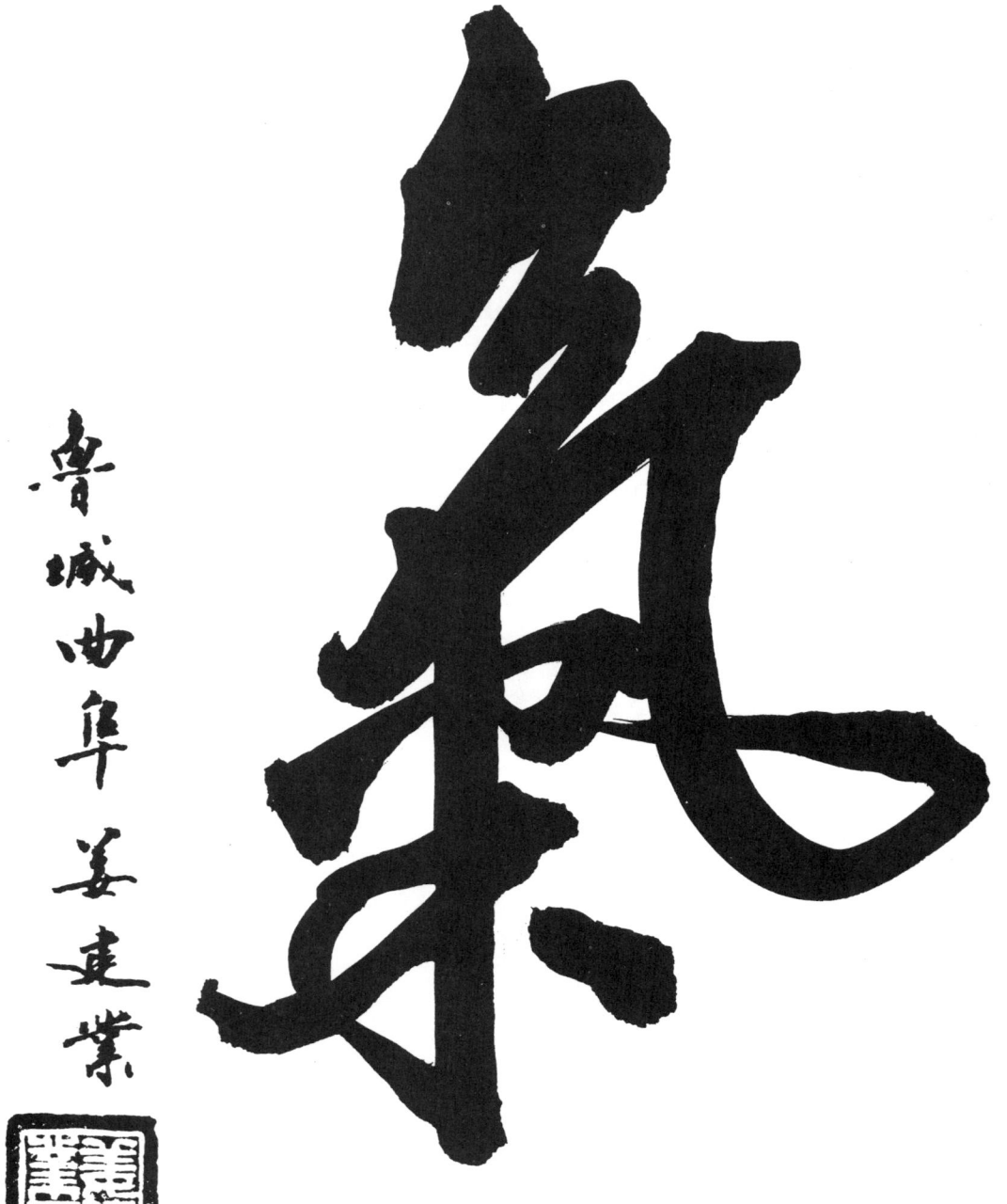

Qigong Massage

FUNDAMENTAL TECHNIQUES
FOR HEALTH AND RELAXATION

DR. YANG, JWING-MING

YMAA Publication Center
Boston, Mass. USA

YMAA Publication Center, Inc.
Main Office
4354 Washington Street
Boston, Massachusetts, 02131
1-800-669-8892 • www.ymaa.com • ymaa@aol.com

First Edition Copyright © 1992 by Yang, Jwing-Ming
Second Edition Copyright © 2005 by Yang, Jwing-Ming

All rights reserved including the right of
reproduction in whole or in part in any form.

Editor: James O'Leary
Cover Design: Vadim Goretsky

ISBN-10: 1-59439-048-7
ISBN-13: 978-1-59439-048-7

10 9 8 7 6 5 4 3 2

Publisher's Cataloging in Publication

Yang, Jwing-Ming, 1946-

Qigong massage : fundamental techniques for health and relaxation / Yang, Jwing-Ming. -- [2nd ed.] -- Boston, Mass. : YMAA Publication Center, 2005.

p. ; cm.

Includes glossary of Chinese terms and index.
ISBN: 1-59439-048-7
ISBN-13: 978-1-59439-048-7

1. Qi gong. 2. Massage therapy. 3. Medicine, Chinese. I. Title.

RM723.C5 Y36 2005   2005930891
615.8/22--dc22   0509

Disclaimer:
The author and publisher of this material are NOT RESPONSIBLE in any manner whatsoever for any injury which may occur through reading or following the instructions in this manual. The activities, physical or otherwise, described in this material may be too strenuous or dangerous for some people, and the reader(s) should consult a physician before engaging in them.

Figures 3-17 and 3-18 from the *LifeART Collection of Images* ©1989-1997 by Techpool Studios, Columbus, OH.

Printed in Canada.

Dedicated to my wife
Mei-Ling Yang (楊美玲)

and my children
James C. Yang (楊志堅)
Kathy K. Yang (楊愷怡)
Nicholas C. Yang (楊志豪)

Romanization of Chinese Words

This book uses the Pinyin romanization system of Chinese to English. Pinyin is standard in the People's Republic of China, and in several world organizations, including the United Nations. Pinyin, which was introduced in China in the 1950's, replaces the Wade-Giles and Yale systems. In some cases, the more popular spelling of a word may be used for clarity.

Some common conversions:

Pinyin	Also Spelled As	Pronunciation
Qi	Chi	chē
Qigong	Chi Kung	chē kŭng
Qin Na	Chin Na	chĭn nă
Jin	Jing	jĭn
Gongfu	Kung Fu	gōng foo
Taijiquan	Tai Chi Chuan	tī jē chüén

For more information, please refer to *The People's Republic of China: Administrative Atlas, The Reform of the Chinese Written Language,* or a contemporary manual of style.

Contents

About the Author ix
Foreword by Dr. Wu, Chengde xv
Preface (from the First Edition) xvii
Preface (for the New Edition) xxi
Acknowledgments xxiii

Part One. Introduction 介紹

Chapter 1. General Concepts 一般概念
1-1. Introduction 介紹 3
1-2. Qi, Qigong, and Man 氣、氣功與人 6
1-3. Definition and Categories of Qigong Massage 氣功按摩之定義與分類 ... 17
1-4. History of Qigong Massage 氣功按摩史 22
1-5. About This Book 關於這本書 29

Chapter 2. General Foundations 一般基礎
2-1. Introduction 介紹 33
2-2. Understanding the Physical Body 瞭解人身物體 34
2-3. Understanding the Qi Body 瞭解人身氣體 43
2-4. Understanding the Mental Body 瞭解人身心理體 90
2-5. Gates and Junctions in the Human Body 人身氣體之通門與結點 93
2-6. Important Points in Qigong Massage 氣功按摩之要點 101

Chapter 3. Qigong Practices for Massage 按摩之氣功練習
3-1. Introduction 介紹 103
3-2. Qigong Training Theory 氣功訓練之理論 105
3-3. Qigong Practices for Massage 按摩之氣功練習 124

Chapter 4. Massage Techniques 按摩技術
4-1. Introduction 介紹 143
4-2. The Tools of Massage 按摩施技位 143
4-3. Massage Techniques and Training 按摩技術與訓練 156

Part Two. General Massage 普通按摩

Chapter 5. General Concepts 一般概念
5-1. Introduction 介紹 191
5-2. Purposes of General Massage 普通按摩之目的 192
5-3. Theory of General Massage 普通按摩之理論 194
5-4. Rules of General Massage 普通按摩之原則 200

Chapter 6. General Massage 普通按摩
    6-1. Introduction 介紹 209
    6-2. Massaging the Mental Body 心理按摩 212
    6-3. Massaging the Head 頭部按摩 214
    6-4. Massaging the Back 背部按摩 242
    6-5. Massaging the Back of the Limbs 四肢背部之按摩 261
    6-6. Massaging the Chest and Abdomen 胸部與腹部之按摩 295
    6-7. Massaging the Front of the Limbs 四肢前部之按摩 310

Chapter 7. General Self-Massage 普通自我按摩
    7-1. General Concepts 一般概念 319
    7-2. Self-Massage 自我按摩 323
    7-3. Self-Massage of the Internal Organs 內臟自我按摩 346

Chapter 8. Conclusion 結論 363

Appendix A. Translation and Glossary of Chinese
    Terms 中文術語之翻譯與解釋 365

Index 索引 378

About the Author
Dr. Yang, Jwing-Ming, Ph.D. 楊俊敏博士

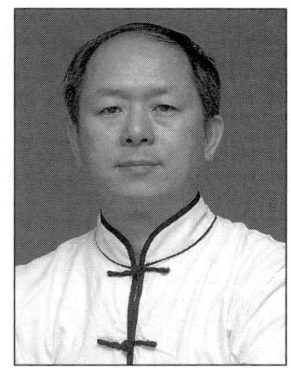

Dr. Yang, Jwing-Ming was born on August 11th, 1946, in Xinzhu Xian (新竹縣), Taiwan (台灣), Republic of China (中華民國). He started his Wushu (武術) (Gongfu or Kung Fu, 功夫) training at the age of fifteen under the Shaolin White Crane (Bai He, 少林白鶴) Master Cheng, Gin-Gsao (曾金灶) (1911-1976). Master Cheng originally learned Taizuquan (太祖拳) from his grandfather when he was a child. When Master Cheng was fifteen years old, he started learning White Crane from Master Jin, Shao-Feng (金紹峰), and followed him for twenty-three years until Master Jin's death.

In thirteen years of study (1961-1974) under Master Cheng, Dr. Yang became an expert in the White Crane Style of Chinese martial arts, which includes both the use of barehands and of various weapons such as saber, staff, spear, trident, two short rods, and many other weapons. With the same master he also studied White Crane Qigong (氣功), Qin Na (or Chin Na, 擒拿), Tui Na (推拿) and Dian Xue massages (點穴按摩), and herbal treatment.

At the age of sixteen, Dr. Yang began the study of Yang Style Taijiquan (楊氏太極拳) under Master Gao, Tao (高濤). After learning from Master Gao, Dr. Yang continued his study and research of Taijiquan with several masters and senior practitioners such as Master Li, Mao-Ching (李茂清) and Mr. Wilson Chen (陳威伸) in Taipei (台北). Master Li learned his Taijiquan from the well-known Master Han, Ching-Tang (韓慶堂), and Mr. Chen learned his Taijiquan from Master Zhang, Xiang-San (張祥三). Dr. Yang has mastered the Taiji barehand sequence, pushing hands, the two-man fighting sequence, Taiji sword, Taiji saber, and Taiji Qigong.

When Dr. Yang was eighteen years old he entered Tamkang College (淡江學院) in Taipei Xian (台北縣) to study Physics. In college he began the study of traditional Shaolin Long Fist (Changquan or Chang Chuan, 少林長拳) with Master Li, Mao-Ching at the Tamkang College Guoshu Club (淡江國術社) (1964-1968), and eventually became an assistant instructor under Master Li. In 1971 he completed his M.S. degree in Physics at the National Taiwan University (台灣大學), and then served in the Chinese Air Force from 1971 to 1972. In the service, Dr. Yang taught Physics at the Junior Academy of the Chinese Air Force (空軍幼校) while also teaching Wushu. After being honorably discharged in 1972, he returned to Tamkang College to teach Physics and resumed study under Master Li, Mao-Ching. From Master Li, Dr. Yang learned Northern Style Wushu, which includes both barehand (especially kicking) techniques and numerous weapons.

In 1974, Dr. Yang came to the United States to study Mechanical Engineering at Purdue University. At the request of a few students, Dr. Yang began to teach Gongfu

(Kung Fu), which resulted in the foundation of the Purdue University Chinese Kung Fu Research Club in the spring of 1975. While at Purdue, Dr. Yang also taught college-credited courses in Taijiquan. In May of 1978 he was awarded a Ph.D. in Mechanical Engineering by Purdue.

In 1980, Dr. Yang moved to Houston to work for Texas Instruments. While in Houston he founded Yang's Shaolin Kung Fu Academy, which was eventually taken over by his disciple Mr. Jeffery Bolt after moving to Boston in 1982. Dr. Yang founded Yang's Martial Arts Academy (YMAA) in Boston on October 1, 1982.

In January of 1984 he gave up his engineering career to devote more time to research, writing, and teaching. In March of 1986 he purchased property in the Jamaica Plain area of Boston to be used as the headquarters of the new organization, Yang's Martial Arts Association (YMAA). The organization has continued to expand, and, as of July 1st 1989, YMAA has become just one division of Yang's Oriental Arts Association, Inc. (YOAA, Inc.).

In summary, Dr. Yang has been involved in Chinese Wushu since 1961. During this time, he has spent thirteen years learning Shaolin White Crane (Bai He), Shaolin Long Fist (Changquan), and Taijiquan. Dr. Yang has more than thirty-three years of instructional experience: seven years in Taiwan, five years at Purdue University, two years in Houston, Texas, and nineteen years in Boston, Massachusetts.

In addition, Dr. Yang has also been invited to offer seminars around the world to share his knowledge of Chinese martial arts and Qigong. The countries he has visited include Argentina, Austria, Barbados, Botswana, Belgium, Bermuda, Canada, Chile, England, France, Germany, Holland, Hungary, Ireland, Italy, Latvia, Mexico, Poland, Portugal, Saudi Arabia, Spain, South Africa, Switzerland, and Venezuela.

Since 1986, YMAA has become an international organization, which currently includes 56 schools located in Argentina, Belgium, Canada, Chile, France, Holland, Hungary, Iran, Ireland, Italy, Poland, Portugal, South Africa, United Kingdom, Venezuela, and the United States. Many of Dr. Yang's books and videotapes have been translated into languages such as French, Italian, Spanish, Polish, Czech, Bulgarian, Russian, Hungarian, and Iranian.

Dr. Yang has published thirty-one other volumes on the martial arts and Qigong:

1. *Shaolin Chin Na;* Unique Publications, Inc., 1980.

2. *Shaolin Long Fist Kung Fu;* Unique Publications, Inc., 1981.

3. *Yang Style Tai Chi Chuan;* Unique Publications, Inc., 1981.

4. *Introduction to Ancient Chinese Weapons;* Unique Publications, Inc., 1985.

5. *Qigong for Health and Martial Arts;* YMAA Publication Center, 1985.

6. *Northern Shaolin Sword;* YMAA Publication Center, 1985.

7. *Tai Chi Theory and Martial Power;* YMAA Publication Center, 1986.

8. *Tai Chi Chuan Martial Applications;* YMAA Publication Center, 1986.

9. *Analysis of Shaolin Chin Na;* YMAA Publication Center, 1987; 2nd Edition, 2004.
10. *Eight Simple Qigong Exercises for Health;* YMAA Publication Center, 1988.
11. *The Root of Chinese Qigong—The Secrets of Qigong Training;* YMAA Publication Center, 1989.
12. *Qigong—The Secret of Youth;* YMAA Publication Center, 1989.
13. *Xingyiquan—Theory and Applications;* YMAA Publication Center, 1990.
14. *The Essence of Taiji Qigong—Health and Martial Arts;* YMAA Publication Center, 1990.
15. *Qigong for Arthritis;* YMAA Publication Center, 1991; 2nd Edition, 2005.
16. *Chinese Qigong Massage—General Massage;* YMAA Publication Center, 1992.
17. *How to Defend Yourself;* YMAA Publication Center, 1992.
18. *Baguazhang—Emei Baguazhang;* YMAA Publication Center, 1994.
19. *Comprehensive Applications of Shaolin Chin Na—The Practical Defense of Chinese Seizing Arts;* YMAA Publication Center, 1995.
20. *Taiji Chin Na—The Seizing Art of Taijiquan;* YMAA Publication Center, 1995.
21. *The Essence of Shaolin White Crane;* YMAA Publication Center, 1996.
22. *Back Pain—Chinese Qigong for Healing and Prevention;* YMAA Publication Center, 1997; 2nd Edition, 2004.
23. *Ancient Chinese Weapons;* YMAA Publication Center, 1999.
24. *Taijiquan—Classical Yang Style;* YMAA Publication Center, 1999.
25. *Tai Chi Secrets of Ancient Masters;* YMAA Publication Center, 1999.
26. *Taiji Sword—Classical Yang Style;* YMAA Publication Center, 1999.
27. *Tai Chi Secrets of Wǔ and Li Styles;* YMAA Publication Center, 2001.
28. *Tai Chi Secrets of Yang Style;* YMAA Publication Center, 2001.
29. *Tai Chi Secrets of Wu Style;* YMAA Publication Center, 2002.
30. *Taijiquan Theory of Dr. Yang, Jwing-Ming;* YMAA Publication Center, 2003.
31. *Qigong Meditation—Embryonic Breathing;* YMAA Publication Center, 2003.

Dr. Yang has also published the following videotapes and DVD:
Videotapes:
1. *Yang Style Tai Chi Chuan and Its Applications;* YMAA Publication Center, 1984.

2. *Shaolin Long Fist Kung Fu—Lien Bu Chuan and Its Applications;* YMAA Publication Center, 1985.

3. *Shaolin Long Fist Kung Fu—Gung Li Chuan and Its Applications;* YMAA Publication Center, 1986.

4. *Shaolin Chin Na;* YMAA Publication Center, 1987.

5. *Wai Dan Chi Kung, Vol. 1—The Eight Pieces of Brocade;* YMAA Publication Center, 1987.

6. *The Essence of Tai Chi Chi Kung;* YMAA Publication Center, 1990.

7. *Qigong for Arthritis;* YMAA Publication Center, 1991.

8. *Qigong Massage—Self Massage;* YMAA Publication Center, 1992.

9. *Qigong Massage—With a Partner;* YMAA Publication Center, 1992.

10. *Defend Yourself 1—Unarmed Attack;* YMAA Publication Center, 1992.

11. *Defend Yourself 2—Knife Attack;* YMAA Publication Center, 1992.

12. *Comprehensive Applications of Shaolin Chin Na 1;* YMAA Publication Center, 1995.

13. *Comprehensive Applications of Shaolin Chin Na 2;* YMAA Publication Center, 1995.

14. *Shaolin Long Fist Kung Fu—Yi Lu Mai Fu & Er Lu Mai Fu;* YMAA Publication Center, 1995.

15. *Shaolin Long Fist Kung Fu—Shi Zi Tang;* YMAA Publication Center, 1995.

16. *Taiji Chin Na;* YMAA Publication Center, 1995.

17. *Emei Baguazhang—1; Basic Training, Qigong, Eight Palms, and Applications;* YMAA Publication Center, 1995.

18. *Emei Baguazhang—2; Swimming Body Baguazhang and Its Applications;* YMAA Publication Center, 1995.

19. *Emei Baguazhang—3; Bagua Deer Hook Sword and Its Applications;* YMAA Publication Center, 1995.

20. *Xingyiquan—12 Animal Patterns and Their Applications;* YMAA Publication Center, 1995.

21. *24 and 48 Simplified Taijiquan;* YMAA Publication Center, 1995.

22. *White Crane Hard Qigong;* YMAA Publication Center, 1997.

23. *White Crane Soft Qigong;* YMAA Publication Center, 1997.

24. *Xiao Hu Yan—Intermediate Level Long Fist Sequence;* YMAA Publication Center, 1997.

25. *Back Pain—Chinese Qigong for Healing and Prevention;* YMAA Publication Center, 1997.
26. *Scientific Foundation of Chinese Qigong;* YMAA Publication Center, 1997.
27. *Taijiquan—Classical Yang Style;* YMAA Publication Center, 1999.
28. *Taiji Sword—Classical Yang Style;* YMAA Publication Center, 1999.
29. *Chin Na in Depth—1;* YMAA Publication Center, 2000.
30. *Chin Na in Depth—2;* YMAA Publication Center, 2000.
31. *San Cai Jian & Its Applications;* YMAA Publication Center, 2000.
32. *Kun Wu Jian & Its Applications;* YMAA Publication Center, 2000.
33. *Qi Men Jian & Its Applications;* YMAA Publication Center, 2000.
34. *Chin Na in Depth—3;* YMAA Publication Center, 2001.
35. Chin Na in Depth—4; YMAA Publication Center, 2001.
36. *Chin Na in Depth—5;* YMAA Publication Center, 2001.
37. *Chin Na in Depth—6;* YMAA Publication Center, 2001.
38. *12 Routines Tan Tui*; YMAA Publication Center, 2001.
39. *Chin Na in Depth—7;* YMAA Publication Center, 2002.
40. *Chin Na in Depth—8;* YMAA Publication Center, 2002.
41. *Chin Na in Depth—9;* YMAA Publication Center, 2002.
42. *Chin Na in Depth—10;* YMAA Publication Center, 2002.
43. *Chin Na in Depth—11;* YMAA Publication Center, 2002.
44. *Chin Na in Depth—12;* YMAA Publication Center, 2002.
45. *White Crane Gongfu—1;* YMAA Publication Center, 2002.
46. *White Crane Gongfu—2;* YMAA Publication Center, 2002.
47. *Taijiquan Pushing Hands—1;* YMAA Publication Center, 2003.
48. *Taijiquan Pushing Hands—2;* YMAA Publication Center, 2003.
49. *Taiji Saber and Its Applications;* YMAA Publication Center, 2003.
50. *Taiji Symbol Sticking Hands—1;* YMAA Publication Center, 2003.
51. *Taiji Ball Qigong—1;* YMAA Publication Center, 2003.
52. *Taiji Ball Qigong—2;* YMAA Publication Center, 2003.
53. *Taijiquan Pushing Hands—3;* YMAA Publication Center, 2004.
54. *Taijiquan Pushing Hands—4;* YMAA Publication Center, 2004.
55. *Taiji Symbol Sticking Hands—2;* YMAA Publication Center, 2003.
56. *Taiji Ball Qigong—3;* YMAA Publication Center, 2003.

57. *Taiji Ball Qigong—4;* YMAA Publication Center, 2003.
58. *Shaolin White Crane Gongfu 3—Basic Training;* YMAA Publication Center, 2004.
59. *Advanced Practical Chin Na—1;* YMAA Publication Center, 2004.
60. *Advanced Practical Chin Na—2;* YMAA Publication Center, 2004.
61. *Taiji Chin Na in Depth—1;* YMAA Publication Center, 2004.
62. *Taiji Chin Na in Depth—2;* YMAA Publication Center, 2004.
63. *Taiji Chin Na in Depth—3;* YMAA Publication Center, 2004.
64. *Taiji Chin Na in Depth—4;* YMAA Publication Center, 2004.
65. *Tai Chi Fighting Set;* YMAA Publication Center, 2004.

DVD:
1. *Chin Na in Depth—1, 2, 3, 4;* YMAA Publication Center, 2003.
2. *White Crane Qigong;* YMAA Publication Center, 2003.
3. *Taijiquan, Classical Yang Style;* YMAA Publication Center, 2003.
4. *Chin Na in Depth—5, 6, 7, 8;* YMAA Publication Center, 2003.
5. *Chin Na in Depth—9, 10, 11, 12;* YMAA Publication Center, 2003.
6. *Eight Simple Qigong Exercises for Health;* YMAA Publication Center, 2003.
7. *Shaolin Long Fist Kung Fu;* YMAA Publication Center, 2004.
8. *Shaolin White Crane Gong Fu 1, 2—Basic Training;* YMAA Publication Center, 2004.
9. Taiji Sword, Classical Yang Style, YMAA Publication Center, 2005.

Foreword
by Dr. Wu, Chengde (吳誠德醫師)
Houston Institute of Chinese Martial Arts and Medicine

Traditional Chinese medicine developed out of the experiences accumulated over thousands of years in the battle against disease. It has helped more than a billion Chinese to both maintain their health and prevent illness. Qigong massage has a long history, and has been an important part of Chinese medical system. Chinese Qigong massage, like other Chinese medical practices, is considered an important and effective method of treating and even preventing disease. For thousands of years it has had an important role in Chinese medicine.

The theory of Qigong massage, like other Chinese medical practices, has been built on the foundation of the concept of Qi. It especially emphasizes the smooth circulation of Qi, its proper level, the quality of its circulation, and also how to use it to prevent disease. In fact, compared with other forms of Chinese medicine, Qigong massage has its own unique effectiveness and benefits. It is therefore commonly used together with Chinese herbs and acupuncture to provide a treatment which is more effective than would be possible with any one form of treatment alone.

The advantages of practicing Qigong are that it does not require a large space or any equipment, and it is easy to learn and practice. Qigong massage can be used anywhere and anytime.

For the last several decades I have been engaged in study, research, and treatments related to the Chinese martial arts and traditional medicine. In addition to filling demanding jobs as a professor at the Shanghai Chinese Medical Institute and as Head Physician at Longhua Hospital, I was also appointed Bone Injury Category Educational Minister of the Chinese Medical Association in China, Administrator of the Shanghai Chinese Medical Study Society, Vice Minister of the Injury Category Study Society, member and Research Administrator of the Shanghai Recovery Medical Study Society, member of the Chinese Shanghai Athletic Medical Society, member of the Chinese Wushu Study Association, and also advisor of the Yangtze River Wugong Medical Treatment Research Institute. I have therefore had countless chances to work with many other medical experts.

In 1989, before I was invited to Houston and later took up residence here, I was already very interested in investigating the position of Chinese medicine in America. Because Chinese medicine is a treasure to human health and happiness, and has been built on the foundation of the relationship of Qi to man's physical and mental bodies, over the course of several thousand years of study and research its experiences and achievements are in some ways very different from those obtained by Western medicine.

In the last two years, I was very surprised to discover that almost every American praises and favors Chinese cooking and says, "Chinese food tastes good." However, only a very few of them know anything about Chinese medicine and its achievements.

Chinese medicine in America is still in its infancy. Because of the cultural differences between West and East, people can easily become confused about the concepts of Chinese medicine. This is especially true since science today still cannot understand and accept the concept of Qi, or study it objectively. Under these conditions, it is especially necessary and urgent for knowledgeable, experienced Qigong researchers, when they publish articles or books, to maintain a centered and neutral viewpoint in their discussions. Only then can confusion be avoided and the general public be encouraged to get involved.

After I came to the United States, I was very fortunate to meet Dr. Yang, Jwing-Ming and to learn that Dr. Yang has a deep understanding of both Chinese martial arts and Qigong. His publications are numerous and profound. His dream is to greatly increase the exchange of culture between East and West. He believes, therefore, that it is his responsibility to help introduce Chinese culture to the West, especially Wushu and medical Qigong.

In Dr. Yang's sincerely written works, the reader discovers clear explanations based on his scientific background. His approach of using the scientific method to explain the traditional experience is accurate and objective. Therefore, I am very happy to write the foreword for this book, *Chinese Qigong Massage* [title of first edition]. This will also fulfill part of my wish to help in the development of Chinese culture in Western society.

—Dr. Wu, Chengde
September, 1991

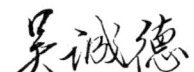

Preface (from the First Edition)

Although modern medicine has brought us healthier lives and has significantly extended the average lifespan, there are still many problems that it cannot solve. Modern medicine will often cure one symptom, only to create another. Many treatments seem to be designed only to provide relief from symptoms, rather than identifying and treating the root of the problem.

Even though today's medicine has reached a higher level of quality than ever before, if we compare it to the medicine that we will have in another hundred or a thousand years, it is clear that medicine is only in its infancy.

When looked at objectively, it is clear that there are still many problems with Western medicine. First, the research of the past 50 years has focused on curing, rather than prevention. The whole attention of the medical establishment has been focused on treating problems after they have manifested. Educating the public only becomes a priority when a situation has become serious. The medical knowledge or medical common sense of the general public is still at a childlike level.

Another problem with Western medicine is that it concentrates solely on the physical problem and ignores inner energy (bioelectricity or Qi). Few Western physicians understand that Qi (氣) is at the root of every sickness, and is the source of the failure of any physical organ or cell. If you wish to prevent sickness, your first concern must be the Qi that is circulating in the body. If there is a persistent abnormality in the supply or circulation of Qi, the physical body will be damaged and symptoms will manifest. If you wish to cure the root of a sickness, you must first resolve any problems with the Qi. If you regulate the Qi supply and circulation back to normal, you can repair the physical damage and regain health. In light of this, it would seem that one course for future medical research should be to determine the role Qi plays in our health.

Because Western medicine is unfamiliar with Qi, it has difficulty dealing with the mental illnesses which are related to energy imbalances in the brain. It is also totally unprepared to deal with the spiritual side of the human body. According to Chinese Qigong and medical science, the human spirit is closely related to the mind and the Qi which is circulating through the brain.

In less than a century, science has made great strides in physical medicine, but it has failed almost completely to investigate our internal energy. Because of this, modern medicine has been only half successful. However, in the last fifteen years, Qi theory has gradually been accepted by Western physicians. It is now believed that Qi is what has come to be called bioelectricity. It is the (Yin) energy which keeps the (Yang) machine of the body running properly.

Science has recently discovered that growth hormones can slow down the aging process. For many centuries, an important part of Chinese Qigong practice has been learning how to use the mind to lead Qi to the pituitary gland in the brain in order to reactivate and maintain the production of the growth hormone. Although it is not understood precisely how this occurred in the body, nourishing the brain with Qi proves to be an effective way to increase the lifespan.

I believe that if East and West can sincerely work at exchanging knowledge, humanity can have a bright and healthy future. During the next fifty years we must study the mental and spiritual sides of medicine which are related to Qi. Our understanding of medicine will be complete only when we understand this invisible side of our beings. The various institutions that are engaged in medical research should begin allocating money and effort to this field now. Those that do will be considered the pioneers of the medicine of the future.

The Chinese people have always believed that in order to have harmony, two universal forces must be in balance. These two forces are classified as Yin (陰) (negative) and Yang (陽) (positive). When these Yin and Yang forces interact, Qi (氣) (energy) is produced and life is generated. This close relationship between life and Yin and Yang is the way of Dao (or Tao) (道). The theory of Yin and Yang has given birth to a large part of Chinese culture, and has had a particularly great influence on Chinese medicine and Qigong.

It is believed that in order to have a long, healthy, and happy life, you have to balance the Yin and Yang in your body. Traditionally, the Qi body (internal energy body) is considered to be the Yin body, while the physical body is the Yang body. While the physical body can be seen, the Yin body cannot be seen, it can only be felt. Yin energy is the origin of life and makes possible the growth of Yang. Therefore, when Yin energy weakens or suddenly increases, the result will be manifested in the Yang (physical) body. If the imbalance persists, physical damage or even failure to function will occur in the body.

For this reason, practitioners of Chinese medicine and Qigong have always devoted a major part of their practice and research to maintaining the balance of Yin and Yang. In addition to developing physical exercises to maintain the health of the physical body, they have also been concerned with maintaining an abundant supply of Qi and keeping it circulating smoothly.

Massage is a very simple Qigong practice which can increase the Qi and blood circulation in the body. It is widely studied and practiced in Chinese medicine and martial arts. Because massage can regulate and adjust the Qi circulating in the body, it is used not only to maintain health and prevent illness, but also to heal injuries and cure many illnesses.

Chinese massage can be classified into four categories: relaxation massage for health (Pu Tong An Mo, 普通按摩), Tui Na (push-grab) massage for treating injury and some illnesses (Tui Na An Mo, 推拿按摩), Dian Xue (cavity press) massage for illnesses (Dian Xue An Mo, 點穴按摩), and external Qi healing (Wai Qi Liao Fa, 外氣療法). We will cover the discussion of these categories in three volumes. In the first volume, we will review the basic theory of Qigong and survey the history of massage in China. In addition, we will introduce the theory and the techniques of general massage and also some techniques for self-massage. In the second volume, we will discuss Tui Na (push-grab) and Dian Xue (cavity press) of massage separately. Finally, in the third volume, we will introduce the training and the healing methods of the external Qi healing (Wai Qi Liao Fa).

If you are not familiar with the theory and philosophy of Chinese Qigong, we recommend you read the YMAA book *The Root of Chinese Qigong* first. It will give you a clear understanding of general Qigong practices.

These three volumes are written for your reference, and are not meant to be the authority on massage. Do not hesitate to compare them with what you have learned from other sources about Chinese and other types of massage.

My knowledge of techniques and theory, which is primarily in the fields of relaxation massage, Tui Na, and some Dian Xue, comes from my White Crane martial arts master. My knowledge of the deeper aspects of Dian Xue massage, which is used for curing illness, is limited. Most of the information on this subject in this book was compiled from several Chinese publications. I hope that those who are more proficient in this field will come forth and share their understanding and experience.

Finally, in order to be consistent with international usage, we have started using the Pinyin system for spelling Chinese words. We hope that this will be more convenient for those readers who consult other Chinese books. However, in order to avoid confusion, commonly accepted spellings of names will not be changed, such as Tamkang College and Taipei. In addition, the spelling which individuals have chosen for their names will not be changed either, such as my name, Yang, Jwing-Ming, or Wen-Ching Wu, etc.

Preface (for the New Edition)

When the first edition of this book was published in 1992, it generated tremendous public interest in Chinese medicine. However, due to my busy schedule, I have never had a chance to get started on my second and third massage books: *Tui Na and Dian Xue Massage* and also *External Qi Healing Massage.* Now, due to public demand, I have decided to finish these two volumes before I retire from my writing career.

However, it is a difficult and challenging task. This is because there have been more Chinese documents and books published in the last twelve years. Now, in addition to my personal limited experience and few old personal collections, there is much more information available. To read them, understand them, compile them, and then covert it from Chinese into English language is more challenging than ever in my writing career.

In order to make all three volumes consistent, such as using Pinyin with original Chinese, updating to current understanding- especially about Qi and its relationship with massage, explanation of the treatments, etc. I decided to re-edit this earlier book. Furthermore, to make this new edition more complete, some important Qigong practices related to massage will be added. I hope that through this effort, you will find a better connection among these three volumes.

I cannot promise when I will complete the other two volumes. However, I will try to finish before I retire. The reasons that it will take so long to complete these two books are not only because the information is harder to interpret and compile, but also because of my busy schedule. Other than these two books, I still plan to write another 10 volumes related to spiritual cultivation, Taijiquan, and Qigong. In addition to this, in order to earn my living, I need to travel and offer seminars around the world.

I had a dream when I resigned my engineering job in 1984. I wanted to spend my life time to introduce Chinese traditional culture and spiritual science to the western world. However, the more I have accomplished, it seems the more should be done. Time has become more and more of a problem, especially when you are getting older and older. It seems every minute and second becomes shorter and shorter. How we value the rest of our life time has become a big issue.

I wish to see a non-profit organization established that can do the same task with as wide and deep a scale as I am attempting now. I sincerely believe through this effort, the east and west will be able to understand each other better through this cultural exchange. From this exchange, we can learn from each other and learn to live peacefully and harmoniously with each other. I believe all human beings are eager to see the great harmony and peace of this world.

In this new edition, all the original Chinese has been included in the text for those who understand it. The translations and the glossary of Chinese terms have been redone. Most important of all, an additional chapter, Chapter 3, has been added. In this chapter, Qigong practice for massage is introduced. I hope that through this chapter, those readers interested in massage will be able to develop their massage practice to a more profound level.

—Dr. Yang, Jwing-Ming

Acknowledgments
(from the First Edition)

Thanks to A. Reza Farman-Farmaian for the photography, Wen-Ching Wu for the drawings, Michael Wiederhold for the typesetting, and Douglas Goodman for his drawings and cover design. Thanks also to John Chris Beiskis for general help, to David Ripianzi, James O'Leary, Jeffrey Pratt, Jenifer Menefee, and many other YMAA members for proofing the manuscript and for contributing many valuable suggestions and discussions. Special thanks to Alan Dougall for his editing and to Mr. Jianye Jiang for his beautiful calligraphy. Again, deepest appreciation to Dr. Thomas G. Gutheil for his continued support.

Acknowledgments
(for the New Edition)

Thanks to Tim Comrie for his photography and typesetting. Thanks to Kyle McCauley for appearing in the photographs. Thanks to Erik Elsemans, Ciaran Harris, Joel Pittaway, Barry Morley, and Susan Bullowa for proofing the manuscript and contributing many valuable suggestions and discussions. Special thanks to Vadim Goretsky for the cover design and James O'Leary for editing.

PART ONE
Introduction 介紹

CHAPTER 1

General Concepts 一般概念

1-1. INTRODUCTION 介紹

Although health has always been one of mankind's main concerns, most people aren't very interested in learning how to keep themselves healthy. It seems that we don't really appreciate our health until we have lost it. The fact is, the best way to stay healthy is to prevent sickness from occurring. Your body is like a machine in that performing preventive maintenance is cheaper than waiting for something to go wrong and then fixing it. Furthermore, in many cases it is impossible to bring the body back to the state it was in before the sickness. Also, when you are sick your body tends to degenerate faster than it usually does in the normal process of aging.

You may have noticed that many illnesses do not pop up overnight. In fact, many of them are caused by our bad habits and the way we abuse our bodies. Often, unhealthy conditions are made worse by our ignoring what is going on in our own bodies. Too many people think that their health is their physician's concern and responsibility, and not their own. In fact, if you are willing to pay attention to your own state of health you can probably cut your health problems in half.

Since ancient times, Chinese medicine and Qigong (氣功) have been very much concerned with maintaining health and preventing illness. According to Chinese medicine, the human body has two components: the Qi body (inner energy body, or Yin body) and the physical body (manifestation body, or Yang body). Chinese medicine considers the Qi body to be the foundation of the Yang body, and the root of health and longevity. This means that Yin energy is the origin of life, and it makes the growth of Yang possible. When Yin energy weakens or suddenly increases, the change is manifested in the Yang (physical) body. If the imbalance persists, physical damage or even failure to function will occur in the body.

For example, if you are not feeling well and go to see a Western physician, he will examine you and perhaps take X-rays. If he cannot find any defect or damage in your physical body, he will probably tell you that you are perfectly healthy, or that what you feel is only in your mind. However, when you go to see a traditional Chinese physician, he will first gauge the Qi levels of the twelve primary Qi channels (Shi Er Jing, 十二經) which are related to your internal organs. If the physician finds any abnormality in your Qi circulation, he will use acupuncture, herbs, massage, Qigong, or other methods to adjust it. This will prevent physical damage from occurring. This concept is very different from that of Western physicians, who wait for visible, physical damage to actually occur before they consider you to be sick.

Another way in which traditional Chinese medicine differs from Western medicine is that Chinese medicine treats the entire body as a whole, rather than only treating that part of the body which is sick. For example, if there is a problem with the liver, the Western physician will treat it as a liver problem only. However, in Chinese medicine the treatment will be very different, for the physician will be concerned with how the problem in the liver arose. What is the root of the abnormal Qi circulation in the liver? Is it because the kidney Qi is too Yang, or is it because the heart Qi is too Yin? If you want to understand the roots of a problem with an organ, you need to know how it relates to all the other organs. According to Chinese medicine, all of the internal organs are related and connected through the Qi, and they affect each other's functioning. Therefore, in order to treat a problem, the physician must find the source of the sickness, and not just treat the symptoms. If the cause of the illness is not removed, the illness can return.

For these reasons, Chinese medicine and Qigong are greatly concerned with maintaining the Yin/Yang balance in the organs and maintaining and improving the Qi circulation in the body. For thousands of years, Qigong massage has proven to be one of the safest and most efficient ways of doing this, and thereby maintaining health and preventing sickness.

Massage is a natural human instinct. When you have pain in some part of your body, your first, natural reaction is to rub it with your hand to reduce the pain. In the beginning, people probably didn't pay much attention to how the pain was released. They simply recognized that massage could reduce pain, relax the patient, increase energy and vitality, and even cure many kinds of sickness.

No one country can claim to have invented the art of massage. Almost every culture in the world has developed or adopted massage techniques at some point in its history. Although the techniques may be somewhat different, and the depth of the theory varies widely, the major purpose of massage treatment to increase circulation of fluids and energy in the body and improve health is the same.

The Chinese people have been practicing and researching massage for more than four thousand years, and have developed a comprehensive and consistent theory of massage treatment which is closely integrated with the larger fields of Chinese medicine and Qigong theory. They have tried to answer such questions as: In what ways can massage benefit people? How is Qi (internal energy) related to massage? What is the best treatment in specific cases?

Over the years, many different schools of massage have sprung up, and countless techniques have been developed based on their experience in treatments. However, the differences in the techniques of each school do not matter, since the theory and approach remain the same. Therefore, it is extremely important for you to understand the *Why, What,* and *How.* If you simply learn the techniques of massage without knowing the root theory and principles, your knowledge will be restricted to the branches and flowers, and your development will be limited.

To understand Chinese massage, the first question you must ask is: How does Chinese massage differ from Western massage? Chinese massage is commonly called Qigong massage, because it is based on affecting the energetic (Qi) system, as well as the circulatory systems of blood and lymph. (Remember Chinese medicine holds that imbalances or blockages in the Qi circulation system are the root of the body's illnesses.) Therefore, in order to effectively use massage to help the patient recover from sickness, the physician must study Qi, understand the Qi circulatory system in the body, train their own Qi, and learn how to use their Qi while massaging in order to help the patient to regain Qi balance. Massage is classified as one of the major fields of Qigong in China, and requires a long period of concentrated study. You can see that Chinese Qigong massage was developed for healing, rather than just relaxation and enjoyment. If you wish to start learning basic Qigong theory, you can start with the YMAA book: *The Root of Chinese Qigong.*

The second question you need to ask is: How does Chinese massage differ from Japanese Shiatsu massage? If you investigate the Japanese culture, you will find that much of it originated in China. This is especially true with regard to medicine and religion. The study of Qi and Chinese medical practices such as acupuncture have been major influences on Japanese culture, and Shiatsu is one of the results of this. Once you have read this book you will realize that Japanese Shiatsu massage is actually part of Chinese cavity press or acupressure massage, which is discussed in the second volume of this book. Naturally, because of several hundred years of separate development, many techniques and theories of treatment are somewhat different. It may therefore be worthwhile to compare the two arts, so that you can choose the best techniques for your practice.

Qigong massage has proven to be effective in treating injuries and illnesses, although, in many cases, it does not get results as fast as Western medicine. However, it does have a number of advantages: 1. There are no side effects; 2. It can correct problems at their root and in a natural way; 3. Unlike Western medicine, it does not use chemicals, which all too often prove to be addictive and enslaving; and 4. Massage increases your awareness and understanding of your bodies (both the physical and the energy bodies). Knowing yourself better is the key to preventing illness.

Please remember, however, that Western medicine has many strong points, and you should take advantage of them. The wisest way is to coordinate the oriental and the Western ways. Of course, to do this you need to have some knowledge of both approaches.

At this point in human history we have the greatest opportunity so far to communicate with each other freely and openly. If we continue to adhere only to the knowledge which our own culture has developed, and ignore all that has been developed in different cultures, then our minds are sure to be stuck in the ancient past.

Next we will review the concepts of Qi and Qigong. In the third section we will summarize the different categories of Chinese Qigong massage. In the fourth section we will survey the history of Chinese Qigong massage, and in the last section we will discuss how to use this book.

1-2. Qi, Qigong, and Man 氣、氣功與人

Before we discuss the relationship of Qi to the human body, we should first define Qi and Qigong. We will first discuss the general concept of Qi, including both the traditional understanding and the modern scientific viewpoint, and then we will use the modern concepts to explain Qigong. If you would like to investigate these subjects in more detail, please refer to the YMAA book: *The Root of Chinese Qigong*.

A General Definition of Qi 氣的一般定義

Qi is the energy or natural force which fills the universe. The Chinese have traditionally believed that there are three major powers in the universe. These Three Powers (San Cai, 三才) are Heaven (Tian, 天), Earth (Di, 地), and Man (Ren, 人). Heaven (the sky or universe) has Heaven Qi (Tian Qi, 天氣), the most important of the three, which is made up of the forces which the heavenly bodies exert on the earth, such as sunshine, moonlight, the moon's gravity, and the energy from the stars. In ancient times, the Chinese believed that weather, climate, and natural disasters were governed by Heaven Qi. Chinese people still refer to the weather as Tian Qi (天氣) (Heaven Qi). Every energy field strives to stay in balance, so whenever the Heaven Qi loses its balance, it tries to rebalance itself. Then the wind must blow, rain must fall, even tornados or hurricanes must happen in order for the Heaven Qi to reach a new energy balance.

Under Heaven Qi, is Earth Qi (Di Qi, 地氣). It is influenced and controlled by Heaven Qi. For example, too much rain will force a river to flood or change its path. Without rain, the plants will die. The Chinese believe that Earth Qi is made up of lines and patterns of energy, as well as the earth's magnetic field and the heat concealed underground. These energies must also balance, otherwise disasters such as earthquakes will occur. When the Qi of the earth is balanced, plants will grow and animals thrive.

Finally, within the Earth Qi, each individual person, animal, and plant has its own Qi field, which always seeks to be balanced. When any individual thing loses its Qi balance, it will sicken, die, and decompose. All natural things, including mankind and our Human Qi (Ren Qi, 人氣), grow within and are influenced by the natural cycles of Heaven Qi and Earth Qi. Throughout the history of Qigong, people have been most interested in Human Qi and its relationship with Heaven Qi and Earth Qi.

In China, Qi is defined as any type of energy which is able to demonstrate power and strength. This energy can be electricity, magnetism, heat, or light. In China, electric power is called Dian Qi (電氣) (Electric Qi), and heat is called Re Qi (熱氣) (Heat Qi). When a person is alive, his body's energy is called Ren Qi (人氣) (Human Qi).

Qi is also commonly used to express the energy state of something, especially living things. As mentioned before, the weather is called Tian Qi (天氣) (Heaven Qi) because it indicates the energy state of the heavens. When a thing is alive it has Huo Qi (活氣) (Vital Qi), and when it is dead it has Si Qi (死氣) (Dead Qi) or Gui Qi (鬼氣) (Ghost Qi). When a person is righteous and has the spiritual strength to do good, he is said to have Zheng Qi (正氣) (Normal Qi or Righteous Qi). The spiritual state or morale of an army is called Qi Shi (氣勢) (energy state).

You can see that the word Qi has a wider and more general definition than most people think. It does not refer only to the energy circulating in the human body. Furthermore, the word "Qi" (氣) can represent the energy itself, and it can also be used to express the manner or state of the energy. It is important to understand this when you practice Qigong, so that your mind is not channeled into a narrow understanding of Qi, which would limit your future understanding and development.

A Narrow Definition of Qi 氣之狹義

Now that you understand the general definition of Qi, let us look at how Qi is defined in Qigong society today. As mentioned before, among the Three Powers (San Cai, 三才), the Chinese have been most concerned with the Qi which is related to our health and longevity. Therefore, after four thousand years of emphasizing Human Qi (Ren Qi, 人氣), when people mention Qi they usually mean the Qi circulating in our bodies.

If we look at the Chinese medical and Qigong documents that were written about two thousand years ago, the word "Qi" was written "炁." This character is constructed of two words, "旡" on the top, which means "nothing;" and "灬" on the bottom, which means "fire." This means that the word Qi was actually written as "no fire" in ancient times. If we go back through Chinese medical and Qigong history, it is not hard to understand this expression.

In ancient times, what the Chinese physicians or Qigong practitioners were looking for in their practice was actually the Yin-Yang balance of the Qi which was circulating in the body. When this goal was reached, there was 'no fire' in the internal organs. This concept is very simple. According to Chinese medicine, each of our internal organs needs to receive a specific amount of Qi to function properly. If an organ receives an improper amount of Qi (usually too much, i.e. too Yang), it will start to malfunction, and, in time, physical damage will occur. Therefore, the goal of the medical or Qigong practitioner was to attain a state of 'no fire,' which eventually became the word Qi.

However, in more recent publications, the Qi of 'no fire' has been replaced by the word "氣," which is again constructed of two words, "气" which means "air," and "米" which means "rice." This shows that later practitioners realized that the Qi circulating in our bodies is produced mainly by the inhalation of air and the consumption of food (rice). (Air is called Kong Qi (空氣), which means literally "space energy.")

For a long time, people were confused about just what type of energy was circulating in our bodies. Many people believed that it was heat, others considered it to be electricity, and many others assumed that it was a mixture of heat, electricity, and light.

This confusion lasted until about 1980's, when the concept of Qi gradually became clear. If we think carefully about what we know from science, we can see that (except possibly for gravity) there is actually only one type of energy in this universe, and that is electromagnetic energy. This means that light (electromagnetic waves) and heat (infrared waves) are also part of electromagnetic energy. This makes it very clear that the Qi circulating in our bodies is actually bioelectricity, and that our body is a living electromagnetic field.[1] This field is affected by our thoughts, feelings, activities, the food we eat, the quality of the air we breathe, our lifestyle, the natural energy that surrounds us, and also the unnatural energy which modern science inflicts upon us.

Next, let us define Qigong. Once you understand what Qigong is, you will be able to better understand the role that Qigong massage plays in Chinese medicine and Qigong society.

A General Definition of Qigong 氣功的一般定義

We have explained that Qi is energy, and that it is found in the heavens, in the earth, and in every living thing. In China, the word "Gong" (功) is often used instead of "Gongfu" (or Kung Fu) (功夫), which means "energy and time." Any study or training which requires a lot of energy and time to learn or to accomplish is called Gongfu. The term can be applied to any special skill or study as long as it requires time, energy, and patience. Therefore, *The correct definition of Qigong is any training or study dealing with Qi which takes a long time and a lot of effort.* You can see from this definition that Qigong is a science which studies the energy in nature. The main difference between this energy science and Western energy science is that Qigong focuses on the inner energy of human beings, while Western energy science pays more attention to the energy outside of the human body. When you study Qigong, it is worthwhile to also consider the modern, scientific point of view, and not restrict yourself to only the traditional beliefs.

The Chinese have studied Qi for thousands of years. Some of the information on the patterns and cycles of nature has been recorded in books, one of which is the *Yi Jing* (易經) (*Book of Changes*; 1122 B.C.). When the *Yi Jing* was written, the Chinese people, as mentioned earlier, believed that natural power included Tian (天) (Heaven), Di (地) (Earth), and Ren (人) (Man). These are called San Cai (三才) (The Three Powers) and are manifested by the three Qi's: Heaven Qi (Tian Qi, 天氣), Earth Qi (Di Qi, 地氣), and Human Qi (Ren Qi, 人氣). These three facets of nature have their definite rules and cycles. The rules never change, and the cycles repeat regularly. The Chinese people used an understanding of these natural principles and the *Yi Jing* to calculate the changes of natural Qi. This calculation is called Bagua (八卦) (The Eight Trigrams). From the Eight Trigrams are derived the 64 hexagrams. Therefore, the *Yi Jing* was probably the first book which taught the Chinese people about Qi and its variations in nature and man. The relationship of the Three Natural Powers and their Qi variations were later discussed extensively in the book *Qi Hua Lun* (氣化論) (*Theory of Qi's Variation*).

Understanding Heaven Qi is very difficult, and it was especially so in ancient times when the science was just developing. But since nature is always repeating itself, the experiences accumulated over the years have made it possible to trace the natural patterns. Understanding the rules and cycles of Tian Shi (天時) (Heavenly Timing) will help you to understand natural changes of the seasons, climate, weather, rain, snow, drought, and all other natural occurrences. If you observe carefully, you will be able to see many of these routine patterns and cycles caused by the rebalancing of the Qi fields. Among the natural cycles are those which repeat every day, month, or year, as well as cycles of twelve years and sixty years.

Earth Qi (Di Qi, 地氣) is a part of Heaven Qi (Tian Qi, 天氣). If you can understand the rules and the structure of the earth, you will be able to understand how mountains and rivers are formed, how plants grow, how rivers move, what part of the country is best for someone, where to build a house and which direction it should face so that it is a healthy place to live, and many other things related to the earth. In China today there are people, called Di Li Shi (地理師) (geomancy teachers) or Feng Shui Shi (風水師) (wind water teachers), who make their living this way. The term Feng Shui (風水) (wind water) is commonly used because the location and character of the wind and water in a landscape are the most important factors in evaluating a location. These experts use the accumulated body of geomantic knowledge and the *Yi Jing* (易經) to help people make important decisions such as where and how to build a house, where to bury their dead, and how to rearrange or redecorate homes and offices so that they are better places to live and work in. Many people even believe that setting up a store or business according to the guidance of Feng Shui can make it more prosperous.

Among the three Qi's, Human Qi (Ren Qi, 人氣) is probably the one studied most thoroughly. The study of Human Qi covers a large number of different subjects. The Chinese people believe that Human Qi is affected and controlled by Heaven Qi and Earth Qi, and that they in fact determine your destiny. Therefore, if you understand the relationship between nature and people, in addition to understanding human relations (Ren Shi, 人事), you will be able to predict wars, the destiny of a country, a person's desires and temperament, and even their future. The people who practice this profession are called Suan Ming Shi (算命師) (calculate life teachers).

However, the greatest achievement in the study of Human Qi is in regard to health and longevity. Since Qi is the source of life, if you understand how Qi functions and know how to regulate it correctly, you should be able to live a long and healthy life. Remember that you are part of nature, and you are channeled into the cycles of nature.

If you go against this natural cycle, you may become sick, so it is in your best interest to follow the way of nature. This is the meaning of Dao (道), which can be translated as "The Natural Way."

Many different aspects of Human Qi have been researched, including acupuncture, acupressure, herbal treatment, meditation, and Qigong exercises. The use of acupuncture, acupressure, and herbal treatment to adjust Human Qi flow has become the root of Chinese medical science. Meditation and moving Qigong exercises are used widely by the Chinese people to improve their health or even to cure certain illnesses. In addition, Daoists and Buddhists use meditation and Qigong exercises in their pursuit of enlightenment.

In conclusion, the study of any of the aspects of Qi including Heaven Qi, Earth Qi, and Human Qi should be called Qigong. However, since the term is usually used today only in reference to the cultivation of Human Qi through meditation and exercises, we will only use it in this narrower sense to avoid confusion.

A Narrow Definition of Qigong 氣功之狹義

As mentioned earlier, the narrow definition of Qi is "the energy circulating in the human body." Therefore, the narrow definition of Qigong is "the study of the Qi circulating in the human body." Because our bodies are part of nature, the narrow definition of Qigong should also include the study of how our bodies relate to Heaven Qi and Earth Qi. Chinese Qigong consists today of several different fields: acupuncture, herbs for regulating human Qi, martial arts Qigong, Qigong massage, Qigong exercises, Qigong healing, and religious enlightenment Qigong. Naturally, these fields are mutually related, and in many cases cannot be separated.

The Chinese have discovered that the human body has twelve major channels (Shi Er Jing, 十二經) and eight vessels (Ba Mai, 八脈) through which the Qi circulates. The twelve channels are like rivers which distribute Qi throughout the body, and also connect the extremities (fingers and toes) to the internal organs. Here you should understand that the 'internal organs' of Chinese medicine do not necessarily correspond to the physical organs as understood in the West, but rather to a set of clinical functions similar to each other, and related to the organ system. The eight vessels, which are often referred to as the extraordinary vessels, function like reservoirs and regulate the distribution and circulation of Qi in your body.

When the Qi in the eight reservoirs is full and strong, the Qi in the rivers is strong and will be regulated efficiently. When there is stagnation in any of these twelve channels or rivers, the Qi which flows to the body's extremities and to the internal organs will be abnormal, and illness may develop. You should understand that every channel has its particular Qi flow strength, and every channel is different. All of these different levels of Qi strength are affected by your mind, the weather, the time of day, the food you have eaten, and even your mood. For example, when the weather is dry the Qi in the lungs will tend to be more positive than when it is moist. When you are angry, the

Qi flow in your liver channel will be abnormal. The Qi strength in the different channels varies throughout the day in a regular cycle, and at any particular time one channel is strongest. For example, between 11 A.M. and 1 P.M. the Qi flow in the heart channel is the strongest. Furthermore, the Qi level of the same organ can be different from one person to another.

Whenever the Qi flow in the twelve rivers or channels is not normal, the eight reservoirs will regulate the Qi flow and bring it back to normal. For example, when you experience a sudden shock, the Qi flow in the bladder immediately becomes deficient. Normally, the reservoir will immediately regulate the Qi in this channel so that you recover from the shock. However, if the reservoir Qi is also deficient, or if the effect of the shock is too great and there is not enough time to regulate the Qi, the bladder will suddenly contract, causing unavoidable urination.

When a person is sick because of an injury, his Qi level tends to be either too positive (excessive, Yang) or too negative (deficient, Yin). A Chinese physician would either use a prescription of herbs to adjust the Qi, or else he would insert acupuncture needles at various spots on the channels to inhibit the flow in some channels and stimulate the flow in others, so that balance can be restored. However, there is another alternative, and that is to use certain physical and mental exercises to adjust the Qi. In other words, to use Qigong.

The above discussion is only to offer an idea of the narrow definition of Qigong. In fact, when people talk about Qigong today, most of the time they are referring to the mental and physical exercises that work with the Qi.

A Modern Definition of Qi 氣的近代定義

It is important that you know about the progress that has been made by modern science in the study of Qi. This will keep you from getting stuck in the ancient concepts and level of understanding.

In ancient China, people had very little knowledge of electricity. They only knew from acupuncture that when a needle was inserted into the acupuncture cavities, some kind of energy other than heat was produced which often caused a shock or a tickling sensation. It was not until the last few decades, when the Chinese people were more acquainted with electromagnetic science, that they began to recognize that this energy circulating in the body, which they called Qi, might be the same thing as what today's science calls bioelectricity.

It is understood now that the human body is constructed of many different electrically conductive materials, and that it forms a living electromagnetic field and circuit. Electromagnetic energy is continuously being generated in the human body through the biochemical reaction of food and air, and circulated by the electromotive forces (EMF) generated within the body.

In addition, you are also constantly being affected by external electromagnetic fields such as that of the earth, or the electrical fields generated by clouds. When you practice

Chinese medicine or Qigong, you need to be aware of these outside factors and take them into account.

Countless experiments have been conducted in China, Japan, and other countries to study how external magnetic or electrical fields can affect and adjust the body's Qi field. Many acupuncturists use magnets and electricity in their treatments. They attach a magnet to the skin over a cavity and leave it there for a period of time. The magnetic field gradually affects the Qi circulation in that channel. Alternatively, they insert needles into cavities and then run an electric current through the needle to reach the Qi channels directly. Although many experimenters have claimed a degree of success in their experiments, none has been able to publish any detailed and convincing proof of the results, or give a good explanation of the theory behind the experiment. As with many other attempts to explain the *How* and *Why* of acupuncture, conclusive proof is elusive, and many unanswered questions remain. Of course, this theory is quite new, and it will probably take a lot more study and research before it is verified and completely understood. At present, there are many conservative acupuncturists who are skeptical.

To untie this knot, we must look at what modern Western science has discovered about bioelectromagnetic energy. Many bioelectricity-related reports have been published, and frequently the results are closely related to what is experienced in Chinese Qigong training and medical science. For example, during the electrophysiological research of the 1960's, several investigators discovered that bones are piezoelectric; that is, when they are stressed, mechanical energy is converted to electrical energy in the form of electric current.[1] This might explain one of the practices of Marrow Washing Qigong in which the stress on the bones and muscles is increased in certain ways to increase the Qi circulation.

Dr. Robert O. Becker has done important work in this field. His book, *The Body Electric* reports on much of the research concerning the body's electric field.[2] It is presently believed that food and air are the fuels which generate the electricity in the body through biochemical reaction. This electricity, which is circulated throughout the entire body through electrically conductive tissue, is one of the main energy sources which keep the cells of the physical body alive.

Whenever you have an injury or are sick, your body's electrical circulation is affected. If this circulation of electricity stops, you die. But bioelectric energy not only maintains life, it is also responsible for repairing physical damage. Many researchers have sought ways of using external electrical or magnetic fields to speed up the body's recovery from physical injury. Richard Leviton reports that: "Researchers at Loma Linda University's School of Medicine in California have found, following studies in sixteen countries with over 1,000 patients, that low-frequency, low-intensity magnetic energy has been successful in treating chronic pain related to tissue ischemia, and also worked in clearing up slow-healing ulcers, and in 90 percent of patients tested, raised blood flow significantly."[3]

Mr. Leviton also reports that every cell of the body functions like an electric battery and is able to store electric charges. He reports that: "Other biomagnetic investigators take an even closer look to find out what is happening, right down to the level of the blood, the organs, and the individual cell, which they regard as 'a small electric battery'."[3] This has convinced me that our entire body is just like a big battery which is assembled from millions of small batteries. All of these batteries together form the human electromagnetic field.

Furthermore, much of the research on the body's electrical field relates to acupuncture. For example, Dr. Becker reports that the conductivity of the skin is much higher at acupuncture cavities, and that it is now possible to locate them precisely by measuring the skin's conductivity. Many of these reports prove that the acupuncture which has been done in China for thousands of years is reasonable and scientific.

Some researchers use the theory of the body's electricity to explain many of the ancient miracles which have been attributed to the practice of Qigong. A report by Albert L. Huebner states: "These demonstrations of body electricity in human beings may also offer a new explanation of an ancient healing practice. If weak external fields can produce powerful physiological effects, it may be that fields from human tissues in one person are capable of producing clinical improvements in another. In short, the method of healing known as the laying on of hands could be an especially subtle form of electrical stimulation."[1]

Another frequently reported phenomenon is that when a Qigong practitioner has reached a high level of development, a halo would appear behind and/or around their head during meditation. This is commonly seen in paintings of Jesus Christ, the Buddha, and various Oriental gods. Frequently the light is pictured as surrounding the whole body. This phenomenon may again be explained by the body electric theory. When a person has cultivated their Qi (electricity) to a high level, the Qi may be led to accumulate in the head. This Qi may then interact with the oxygen molecules in the air, and ionize them, causing them to glow.

Although the link between the theory of the body electric and the Chinese theory of Qi is becoming more accepted and better proven, there are still many questions to be answered. For example, how can the mind lead Qi (electricity)? How actually does the mind generate an EMF (electromotive force) to circulate the electricity in the body? How is the human electromagnetic field affected by the multitude of other electric fields which surround us, such as radio and television waves, or the fields generated by household electrical wiring or electrical appliances? How can we readjust our electromagnetic fields and survive in outer space or on other planets where the magnetic field is completely different from the earth's? You can see that the future of Qigong and bioelectric science is a challenging and exciting one. It is about time that we started to use modern technology to understand the inner energy world which has been for the most part ignored by Western society.

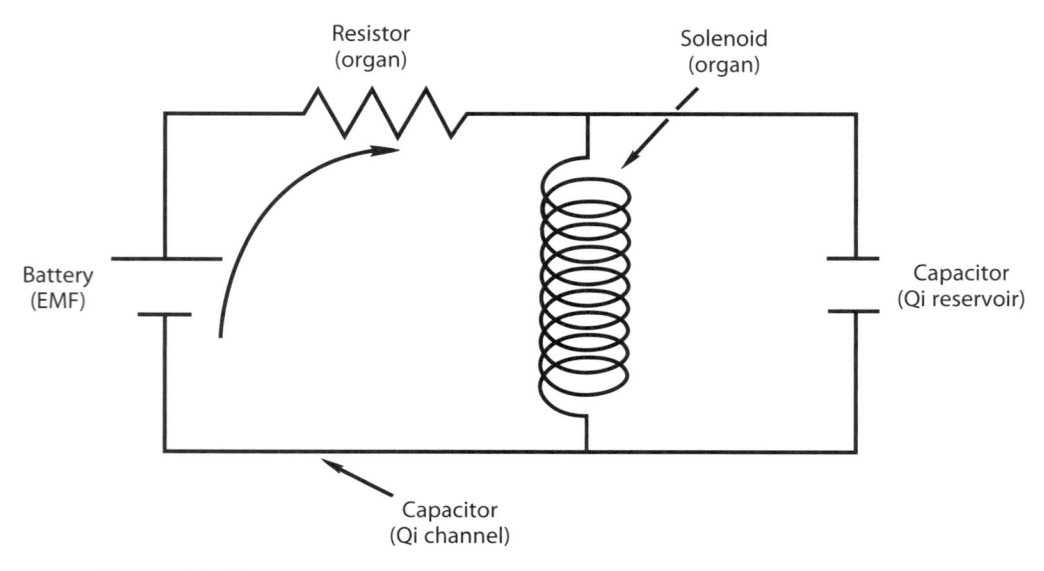

FIGURE 1-1. THE HUMAN BIOELECTRIC CIRCUIT IS SIMILAR TO AN ELECTRIC CIRCUIT.

A Modern Definition of Qigong 氣功之近代定義

If you now accept that the inner energy (Qi) circulating in our bodies is bioelectricity, then we can easily create a definition of Qigong based on the concept of electricity.

Let us assume that the circuit shown in Figure 1-1 is similar to the circuit in our bodies. Unfortunately, although we now have a certain degree of understanding of this circuit from acupuncture, we still do not know in detail exactly what the body's circuit looks like. We know that there are twelve primary Qi channels (Qi rivers) (Jing, 經) and eight vessels (Qi reservoirs) (Mai, 脈) in our body. There are also thousands of small Qi channels (Luo, 絡) which allow the Qi to reach the skin and the bone marrow. In this circuit, the twelve internal organs are connected and mutually related through these channels.

If you look at the electric circuit in the illustration, you will see that:

1. The Qi channels are like the wires which carry the electric current.
2. The internal organs are like the electrical components such as resistors and solenoids.
3. The Qi vessels are like a capacitor, which regulates the current in the circuit.

How do you keep this electrical circuit functioning most efficiently? Your first concern is with the resistance of the wire which carries the current. In a machine, you want to use a wire which has a high level of conductivity and low resistance, otherwise the current may melt the wire. Therefore, the wire should be of a material like copper or perhaps even gold. In your body, you want to keep the current flowing smoothly. This means that your first task is to remove anything which interferes with the flow and cause stagnation. Fat has low conductivity, so you should use diet and exercise to remove excess fat from your body. You should also learn how to relax your physical body, because this opens all of the Qi channels. This is why relaxation is the first goal in Taijiquan and many Qigong exercises.

Your next concern in maintaining a healthy electrical circuit is the components—your internal organs. If you do not have the correct level of current in your organs, they will either burn out from too much current (Yang, 陽) or malfunction because of a deficient level of current (Yin, 陰). In order to avoid these problems in a machine, you use a capacitor to regulate the current. Whenever there is too much current, the capacitor absorbs and stores the excess, and whenever the current is weak, the capacitor supplies current to raise the level. The eight Qi vessels are your body's capacitors. Qigong is concerned with learning how to increase the level of Qi in these vessels so that they will be able to supply current when needed and keep the internal organs functioning smoothly. This is especially important as you get older and your Qi level is generally lower.

Finally, in order to have a healthy circuit, you have to be concerned with the components themselves. If any of them are not strong and of good quality, the entire circuit will have problems. This means that the final concern in Qigong practice is how to maintain or even rebuild the health of your internal organs. Before we go any further, we should point out that there is an important difference between the circuit shown in the diagram and the Qi circuit in our bodies. This difference is that the human body is alive, and, with the proper Qi nourishment, all of the cells can be regrown and the state of health improved. For example, if you are able to jog about three miles today, and if you keep jogging regularly and gradually increase the distance, eventually you will be able to easily jog five miles. This is because your body rebuilds and readjusts itself to fit the circumstances.

This means that, if we are able to increase the Qi flow through our internal organs, they can become stronger and healthier. Naturally, the increase in Qi must be slow and gradual so that the organs can readjust to it. In order to increase the Qi flow in your body, you need to work with the EMF (electromotive force) in your body. If you do not know what EMF is, please imagine two containers filled with water and connected by a tube. If both containers have the same water level, then the water will not flow. However, if one side is higher than the other, the water will flow from that container to the other. In electricity, this potential difference is called electromotive force. Naturally, the higher the EMF is, the stronger the current will flow.

You can see from this discussion that the key to effective Qigong practice is, in addition to removing resistance from the Qi channels, learning how to increase the EMF in your body. Now let us see what the sources of EMF in the body are, so that we may use them to increase the flow of bioelectricity. Generally speaking, there are six major sources:

1. **Natural Energy.** Since your body is constructed of electrically conductive material, its electromagnetic field is always affected by the sun, the moon, clouds, the earth's magnetic field, and by the other energies around you. The major influences are the radiation of the sun and moon, the moon's gravity, and the earth's magnetic field. These affect your Qi circulation significantly, and are responsible for the pattern of your Qi circulation since you were formed. We are now also being greatly affected by the energy pollution generated by modern technology, such as electromagnetic waves generated by radio, TV, microwave ovens, computers, and many other devices.

2. **Food and Air.** In order to maintain life, we take in food and air essence through our mouths and noses. These essences are then converted into Qi through biochemical reaction in the chest and digestive system (called the Triple Burner in Chinese medicine). When Qi is converted from the essence, an EMF is generated that circulates the Qi throughout the body. Consequently, a major part of Qigong is devoted to getting the proper kinds of food and fresh air.

3. **Thinking.** The human mind is the most important and efficient source of bioelectric EMF. Any time you move to do something you must first generate an idea (Yi, 意). This idea generates the EMF and leads the Qi through the nervous system to energize the appropriate muscles to carry out the desired motion. The more you can concentrate, the stronger the EMF you can generate, and the stronger the flow of Qi you can lead. Naturally, the stronger the flow of Qi you lead to the muscles, the more they will be energized. Because of this, the mind is considered the most important factor in Qigong training.

4. **Exercise.** Exercise converts the food essence (fat) stored in your body into Qi, and therefore builds up the EMF. Many Qigong styles have been created which utilize movement for this purpose.

5. **Converting Pre-Birth Essence into Qi.** The hormones produced by our endocrine glands are referred to as Pre-Birth Essence or Original Essence (Yuan Jing, 元精) in Chinese medicine. They can be used to regulate the biochemical reaction which converts the food or fat into Qi. Hormones acts as catalysts in our body's biochemical reaction process (metabolism). Thus, hormones are able to stimulate the functioning of our physical body, thereby increasing our vitality. Balancing hormone production when you are young and increasing its production when you are old are important subjects in Chinese Qigong.

6. **Artificial Stimulation.** The enhancement or the adjustment of the Qi circulation can also be done artificially. This is the basic theory of Chinese medi-

cine such as acupuncture and Qigong massage. From external artificial Qi stimulation, the Qi can be brought to a state of balance, thus preventing or curing sickness.

In this section we have attempted to explain the general concepts behind Qi and Qigong. The same principles also apply to Qigong massage, whose goal is also to maintain and improve Qi circulation so that you can stay healthy, heal injuries, and fight illness. Since Qigong massage is only a branch of Chinese Qigong, it would be very helpful for you to also study other types of Qigong which have grown from the same root; you would then have a better overview of the whole field of Qigong.

1-3. Definition and Categories of Qigong Massage
氣功按摩之定義與分類

Because there are so many categories of Chinese Qigong massage, and it is very easy to become confused, we will first define each one of them and explain its scope, boundaries, and purposes.

Chinese massage is commonly called An Mo (按摩). "An" (按) means "press" and "Mo" (摩) means "rub." Chinese massage is constructed around the two major techniques press and rub, though, of course, many other techniques are also used. Chinese massage can be broken down into four major categories, depending upon the specialized techniques which it uses for its particular purposes. They are Pu Tong An Mo (普通按摩) (General Massage), Tui Na An Mo (推拿按摩) (Push Grab Massage, Dian Xue An Mo (點穴按摩) (Cavity Press Massage), and Qi An Mo (氣按摩) (Qi Massage).

In this section, we will define each category, briefly review its basic theory, and point out how it differs from the other categories. However, I would like to point out here that, because the basic theories and principles are the same for all the categories, many masseurs are familiar with more than one category.

1. Pu Tong An Mo (General Massage) 普通按摩

The most common and popular category of massage in China is called Pu Tong An Mo (普通按摩) (General Massage). In the West it is sometimes translated as "Relaxation Massage." The goals of general or relaxation massage are probably the simplest, as are the techniques. Because this kind of massage does not deal with injuries or illness, no in-depth knowledge of the Qi channels and Chinese medical theory is required. This category is also the safest.

In all of the larger cities throughout the Orient are many masseurs whom people patronize to relax and recover from fatigue. Many of these masseurs are blind. There are several reasons for this: 1. Blind people have a more acute sense of touch, and can usually massage better than sighted people; 2. Since blind people cannot see your body, there was less shame in being massaged by them in the older, puritanical societies; 3. Massage was the easiest way for a blind person to earn a living. In Oriental cities, it used to be very common to hear the sound of a flute in the evening. That was how blind masseurs advertised that they were looking for customers. These people usually were not skilled in Tui Na (推拿) or Dian Xue (點穴). They simply massaged the muscles to help the customer relax. This 'Muscle Grabbing Massage' is called Zhua Long (抓龍), which means "Grabbing the Dragon." "Dragon" here refers to the muscles or tendons.

The purposes of this kind of massage are:

- **A. Relaxation.** This includes both physical and mental relaxation. Even if you aren't involved in strenuous physical activity, worry, stress, and responsibility can cause mental tension. Physical tension can be caused by incorrect posture, worry, or even intense thinking. Tension causes your Qi and blood circulation to become stagnant. When this condition persists it can lead to insomnia, nervous breakdown, and even physical damage because of insufficient Qi and blood nourishment. Relaxation or general massage can calm your agitated mind, relax your physical body, and allow the Qi and blood to circulate smoothly.

- **B. Recovery from Fatigue.** Recovery from fatigue refers primarily to physical fatigue from hard labor or exercise. Acid accumulates in the muscles, and causes aches and muscular soreness. General massage is very effective in improving Qi and blood circulation, which helps to remove the accumulated acid.

- **C. Preventing Illness.** One of the main purposes of relaxation massage is the prevention of illness by smoothing out the Qi and blood circulation before any physical damage can occur. Smooth Qi and blood circulation is essential to maintaining the normal functioning of our thinking and our physical body. This is the primary difference between relaxation massage and the other three categories of massage, which are used to treat injuries and illness.

- **D. Slowing Down Aging.** Maintaining smooth Qi and blood circulation is the key to slowing down the aging process. As we grow older, our Qi and blood circulation slows down and becomes more stagnant. General massage helps to overcome this.

- **E. Speeding Recovery from Sudden Environmental Qi Disturbances.** When our environment changes suddenly, the Qi in our bodies will often not be able to change as quickly. For example, when the weather changes suddenly, our bodies cannot adjust quickly enough, and we may get sick. This problem is especially serious today when modern transportation can bring you from one part of the world to another in a very short time. The sudden changes in the time of day, weather, and altitude can cause problems such as jet lag. General or relaxation massage helps the body to adjust itself to these changes.

F. Enjoyment. The last purpose of relaxation or general massage is enjoyment. Many people get massaged even when they do not have any unhealthy symptoms. Their reason is very simple: massage makes you feel good. This feeling comes mostly from the mind and the relaxation of the physical body. However, there is another reason, and that is the emotional comfort which one obtains from massage. Many people massage each other looking for the emotional balance that comes from touching and being touched by another human being. Most of the time the people involved know each other. This is similar to why we hug lovers and friends.

2. Tui Na An Mo (Push Grab Massage) 推拿按摩

Tui Na An Mo (推拿按摩) is also often simply called 'Tui Na' (推拿). The two words mean "push" and "grab to control," and refer to the two main techniques. Tui Na has two main purposes. The first is for treating injuries, and the second is for treating illnesses, especially of small children. People are often confused about the differences between general massage and Tui Na massage, especially since most practitioners of Tui Na massage are also experts in general massage. However, if you look at the differences in the purposes of these two arts, they are quite easy to distinguish.

The first type of Tui Na is widely practiced by Chinese martial artists because they emphasize techniques for treating injuries which commonly occur during training. This kind of Tui Na is often called Die Da (跌打), which means "Fall Strike," to reflect the fact that it specializes in treating injuries caused by falling and being struck. This art treats primarily external injuries such as bruises, ligament damage, Qi stagnation due to old injuries, broken bones, joint dislocations, and so on.

Traditional physicians were also trained in the treatment of injuries. For example, during the Song dynasty (960-1280 A.D.) (宋朝) part of the training of a physician involved bone realignment, and was called Zheng Gu Ke (正骨科), or "Align the Bone Category," and in the Ming dynasty (1368-1644 A.D.) (明朝) the training was called Jie Gu Ke (接骨科), which means "Connect Bone Category." You might assume from the names that Zheng Gu and Jie Gu dealt with bone problems exclusively, but this is not the case. Since bone problems are among the most serious external injuries, these two terms were often used to represent Tui Na. This is simply because the physician who knows how to correct bone injuries usually is an expert in all other external injuries. In southern China, Taiwan (臺灣) and Fujian province (福建), Tui Na or Zheng Gu is also commonly called Cao Jie (操接), which means "Manipulate to Connect." This gives some indication of how difficult it is to determine precisely what a name refers to, and also to the overlap in coverage among the various types of massage.

Ancient documents tell us that Tui Na has been used since the Ming dynasty (1368 A.D.) to cure some illnesses of small children and occasionally adults. The reason for this is very simple. Treatment by acupuncture requires the willing cooperation of the patient as the physician inserts needles, and the patient needs to remain still for a while. This is almost impossible with small children. It is much easier for the physician to use Tui Na techniques to stimulate or sedate the Qi and achieve the same goal as acupuncture. Naturally, the Tui Na masseur must know how to diagnose diseases and evaluate the Qi of the patient, so this type of Tui Na is done mostly by physicians. This does not mean that masters of martial Tui Na do not know how to cure illnesses with Tui Na. In fact, many martial artists were knowledgeable physicians.

3. Dian Xue An Mo (Cavity Press Massage) 點穴按摩

The next category of Chinese massage is Dian Xue An Mo (點穴按摩) or simply Dian Xue (點穴), which means literally "point cavity." Dian Xue is commonly translated "acupressure" in the West. This category uses mainly Press and Rub techniques on cavities and certain non-cavity points. According to Chinese medicine, there are more than seven hundred cavities which can be used for acupuncture treatment. Needles are inserted into these cavities to access the channels and adjust the Qi circulation. It was discovered that there are about 108 cavities where finger pressure can access Qi channels. That was the beginning of acupressure. It was also learned that stimulating one of these cavities vigorously would damage the internal organ related to it, a fact which greatly interested the martial artists.

Like acupuncture, cavity press techniques adjust Qi in the channels to make the related organs either more positive or negative. Therefore, Dian Xue An Mo specializes in curing sicknesses caused by Qi imbalance. As you can imagine, physicians contributed greatly to the development of this art. Dian Xue An Mo is the root of Japanese Shiatsu massage.

To use Dian Xue, a physician or a martial artist must have a thorough knowledge of Qi channels and acupuncture, and must be experienced in working directly with Qi. They need to know precisely what treatments are needed for which ailments, and they need to be skilled in applying the correct pressure to the right cavity at the appropriate time of day.

Since both Tui Na and Dian Xue utilize the Qi channels, just what is the difference between them? Tui Na works mainly on the channels while Dian Xue works on the cavities. The pressure used in Dian Xue massage is more penetrating than that used in Tui Na massage, and so, in adults, Dian Xue massage is quicker and more effective. However, Dian Xue is not used much in the treatment of infants, since its potent power can easily injure their internal organs. Also, few physicians possess the required depth of knowledge to effectively use Dian Xue.

According to the available documents, very few martial artists were involved in training Qi before 500 A.D. Since then, however, many have taken it up in order to learn how to disturb an opponent's Qi. The Southern and internal Chinese martial styles are especially known for this. Some of the higher level martial artists also became experts in using the art for healing as well as killing. Because martial artists had to be skilled in Tui Na to cure the external injuries caused by training or combat, high level martial priests or artists were recognized as the real experts in Chinese massage society.

Nowadays, however, acupressure physicians are more popular and easier to find than martial artists who are skilled in healing, and they are usually much more experienced in curing sickness. In addition, many physicians who specialize in Dian Xue massage are also familiar with the Tui Na techniques, and those who use mainly the Tui Na are often experienced in Dian Xue, so the combination term Dian Xue Tui Na (點穴推拿) (Point Cavity Push Grab) is often heard.

4. Qi An Mo (Qi Massage) 氣按摩

The last category of massage is Qi massage. Qi massage is commonly called Wai Qi Liao Fa (外氣療法) which means "Curing with External Qi," and is commonly translated "Qigong Healing" in the West today. This term implies that the massage is done through Qi correspondence rather than touch. Because it does not use "press" (An) and "rub" (Mo), it is often not considered to be massage. However, since the goal of Wai Qi Liao Fa is to smooth out the Qi and improve the Qi and blood circulation, which is the same as all other forms of massage, I would like to include it in our discussion.

To understand Qi massage, you must recognize that Qi is the bioelectricity circulating in the body. Because it is electricity, it can be conducted or led through electrical correspondence. Actually, everybody has the ability to do Qi healing. To give an example, when people are sad, their Qi is Yin (陰) (deficient). If you hold their hands or hug them, your Qi will nourish them and they will immediately feel better. We have been doing this instinctively for a long time. The only difference between the average person and a Qigong master is that the latter has trained in Qi healing, and can therefore be more effective.

There are two kinds of Qi massage, one which involves touching the skin, and one which does not. Qi massage which uses skin contact is further subdivided into two categories. In the first one, the Qigong master or physician uses Dian Xue massage, but also uses their own Qi to nourish the patient through the cavities if the patient's Qi is too deficient (Yin), or to remove excess Qi through skin contact if there is an excess of Qi (Yang). The practitioner must be sure to get rid of the Qi they have absorbed, or they might be harmed by it. It is therefore important to be highly skilled in Qigong before practicing Qi healing.

The second kind of Qi massage using skin contact is when the practitioner lightly touches the patient's skin and has their Qi correspond with the patient's Qi. This mutual correspondence allows the healer to lead the disordered Qi back into the proper pattern. Again, the practitioner must also know how to keep their own Qi from being unbalanced by the patient's. It is essential in this kind of healing that the healer and the patient cooperate closely with each other.

In the Qi massage which does not use skin contact, the practitioner uses the fingertips or the Laogong (P-8) (勞宮) cavity in the palm (which is the gate through which one's Qi communicates with the outside world) to focus Qi in a cavity or area of the patient's body. They are able to use their Qi to affect the Qi in the patient, without even touching them. Another method is to move their hands over the patient's body to help them to smooth a disordered pattern of Qi. Theoretically, massage which doesn't use skin contact is safer for the practitioner, since one does not absorb Qi from the patient, which may threaten the health of the practitioner.

You can see that there is some ambiguity as to just what should be included under the term "massage." If your definition of massage depends upon its purpose, then any technique which helps to smooth and improve the Qi and blood circulation should be considered massage. However, if you define massage as using the techniques of Press (An, 按) and Rub (Mo, 摩), then there needs to be actual skin contact, and Wai Qi Liao Fa (外氣療法) would not be included.

1-4. History of Qigong Massage 氣功按摩史

Since massage is a natural, instinctive human reaction to pain, injury, and even sickness, we cannot determine when massage really started in any culture. However, every country has its own history of massage. In this section we will only cover the history of massage in China, according to the records and documents which are available today.

When you study the history of massage in China, you need to recognize the various groups which have contributed the most over the past several thousand years. You then need to understand how and why they became involved in massage. Finally, you need to be aware of how much each group has contributed to massage as it is practiced today. With this understanding, you will be able to avoid confusion over the many different categories of massage.

There were four main groups which significantly influenced massage in China: physicians, martial artists, the clergy, and laymen masseurs. Let us first look briefly at each of these groups.

1. Physicians 醫師

When people are injured, they will usually seek out a physician. Massage has always been one of the main methods of treating injuries. It can lessen pain, improve Qi and blood circulation, and release mental tension. All of these can help to effect a rapid recovery. As mentioned earlier, this type of injury treatment is called Tui Na massage. Later, Tui Na massage eventually developed into a way of treating illnesses in small children.

Acupuncture has also been developing since the beginning of Chinese culture. Out of the principles of acupuncture was developed acupressure or Dian Xue massage (cavity press), which was widely used by physicians. Most of the documents available on this subject were written by physicians. Frequently, massage was discussed together with other methods of treatment such as acupuncture or herbs. The pre-eminence of the physicians was probably attributable to the fact that they were usually the best educated and the most open-minded of the four groups that contributed to the development of massage. In addition, they probably had the most experience. Furthermore, new discoveries and ideas were put into writing, and books spread the new knowledge far and wide. This communication and exchange of techniques brought medical massage to the highest level. In fact, many Chinese physicians were also experts in all categories of Qigong massage.

In the last fifty years, Qi massage, also commonly called Qi healing, has become more popular among physicians in China. It used to be kept secret, and practiced only by Qigong practitioners and physicians who were also expert in Qigong. Since this healing technique has been revealed to the general public, we can confidently predict that it will become more popular and widely accepted during the next fifty years.

2. Martial Artists 武術家

The second largest group of contributors to the development of Chinese massage was the martial artists. Although the history of martial arts massage is not as long as that of medical massage, and there are not as many documents available, it has probably reached a higher level than medical massage in certain areas. This is especially true in the treatment of both internal and external injuries.

How can this have happened? If you look at how and why martial artists developed massage techniques, you will understand why most Chinese people will go to a martial artist to get an injury treated, rather than to a general physician. First, you should understand that martial artists had more experience with injuries than most people, and it was absolutely necessary for them to know how to treat themselves and each other. Tui Na massage was one of the main methods of treatment, and used to be a required course of study for all Chinese martial artists.

Next, you should know that after training long and hard, massage was the best way to get rid of fatigue and eliminate the acid accumulated in the muscles. Massaging each other helped martial artists recover from fatigue, but it also helped them understand the structure of the body and the Qi distribution system. This was very necessary in combat. Therefore, martial artists were often also experts in general and relaxation massage.

The third point which will help you to understand the development of massage in martial society is that massage taught the martial artist precisely where the cavities (vital points) were located. Because most massage points are also used as striking points, massage training was the best way for the student to learn the cavities and experience their depth. When you strike these cavities with power you will cause injury or even death by disturbing the Qi. But you can use the same cavities in healing by applying gentle pressure or rubbing in order to adjust disturbed Qi. Massage was a necessity for any martial artist who wanted to reach the higher levels. Because of this, martial artists who had reached a high level of skill were also experts in cavity press massage for healing. Of course, much of the knowledge of healing could have been obtained from the books available at that time, and many of the martial artists were also physicians. This re-emphasizes the fact that, regardless of how Chinese medicine was developed, it was always based on the same Qi theory, and an understanding of this theory was necessary for reaching the higher levels of the martial arts.

The final point I would like to make is that almost all Chinese martial styles train Qigong. It is necessary for reaching the higher levels of power generation, which is critical for the effective use of techniques in combat. As a result, many martial artists in China become experts in Qigong. One of the best ways to understand Qi and its relationship with the physical body is through massage. Massage helps you to train your Qi, and improves your concentration, which is important for cavity strike techniques.

Countless martial styles have been developed in China over the last five thousand years. Traditionally, each style kept its training theory and fighting techniques secret, and the information was passed down to only a few, trusted students. It was only in the last fifty years that a limited number of books or documents were revealed to the public.

3. Clergy 僧侶與道士

The third group that contributed to the development of massage in China was the religious community, mostly Buddhist and Daoist monks. Qigong was part of their training for attaining Buddhahood or enlightenment, and it also included massage. For example, massage is an integral part of the training of Muscle/Tendon Changing (Yi Jin Jing, 易筋經) and Brain/Marrow Washing (Xi Sui Jing, 洗髓經). This school of massage was restricted to those within the monastic society. However, some of the massage techniques were revealed to the public in this century by martial artists within the society (e.g., Shaolin and Wudang monks.)

4. Laymen 俗家

The last group which contributed to the development of massage is probably the largest, although the level of their practice was the most superficial. The people who gave general, relaxation massages to the general public can be found all over the Orient. They give enjoyable, relaxing massages, and help their clients to release the stress and tension which builds up in daily life. They usually do not pay much attention to using Qi for healing. There are a few books available on this type of massage, but they do not go into the subject of healing very deeply.

Next, we will survey the general history of Chinese massage. Because massage in China is a part of medical treatment and shares the same foundation of Qi theory, it is necessary to understand the development of Chinese medicine when you look at the history of massage. Most of the documents in this section have come from physicians.

In the Xia dynasty (2205-1766 B.C.) (夏朝), when most tools were made of stone, acupuncturists manipulated their patients' Qi with stone probes ((Shi Zhen, 石針) or (Bian Shi, 砭石)) and bone (Gu Zhen, 骨針), or even thorns.[4] It was recorded in *Shan Hai Jing, Dong Shan Jing* (山海經·東山經) (*Mountain Ocean Classic, East Mountain*

Classic) that: "On the mountain of Gao (高), there is much jade on the top and many Zhen Shi (箴石) underneath."[5] Zhen Shi was later explained by Dr. Shi, Guo-Pu (世郭璞): "Zhen Shi is used as a probing needle for curing pain and swelling."[6] Stone probes (needles), were again explained by Xu, Shen (許慎) in his book *Shuo Wen Jie Zi* (說文解字) (*Analysis of Documents with Explanation of Terms*) during Han dynasty (206 B.C.-221 A.D.) (漢朝): "Bian (砭) (stone probe), use the stone to pierce the sickness."[7]

During the Shang dynasty (1766-1122 B.C.) (商朝), stone tools, including acupuncture needles, were widely replaced by bronze ones. An archeological dig at a late Shang dynasty burial ground called Yin Xu (殷墟) discovered more than 160,000 pieces of turtle shell and animal bone which were covered with written characters. This writing, called Jia Gu Wen (甲骨文) (Oracle-Bone Scripture), was the earliest evidence of the Chinese use of the written word. These inscriptions revealed that different sicknesses were already named from the problems generated from organs. It was also discovered that wine was already being used externally for medical treatments.[4]

In the Zhou dynasty (1122-255 B.C.) (周朝) there was record of a clear classification of four different categories of disorders, which included injuries. The book *Li Ji, Yue Ling Meng Qiu* (禮記・月令孟秋) records treatments for cuts in the skin, muscular swelling, and broken bones, and discussed using both internal and external treatments.

Then, during the Spring and Autumn period (722-484 B.C.) (Chun Qiu, 春秋), the famous medical book *Nei Jing* (內經) discussed in detail the treatment of external injuries and the use of herbs in healing. Massage was the most important part of the treatment.

It was recorded in the *Shi Ji* (史記) (*Historical Record*) that in the Qin dynasty (255-206 B.C.) (秦朝), the famous doctor Bian Que (扁鵲) asked his assistant Zi You (子游) to massage Crown Prince Guo (虢太子), who suffered from epilepsy.

During the Han dynasty (206 B.C.-221 A.D.) (漢朝), the famous doctor Hua Tuo (華佗) used acupuncture, herbs, and manual therapies (i.e. massage and alignment techniques for dislocated and broken bones). Hua Tuo was the first doctor to emphasize combining acupuncture and massage. Also, Dr. Zhang, Ji-Zuo (張機作) in his book *Shang Han Ran Bing Lun* (傷寒染病論) (*The Theory of Typhus Contamination*) not only summarized a theoretical and systematic discussion of medical theory, treatments, and diagnosis, but also recorded many methods of massage treatment.

It was recorded in *Han Shu Yi Wen Zhi* (漢書藝文志) (*Han's Book of Arts and Scholarship*) (206 B.C.-221 A.D.) that "during the reign of the Yellow Emperor, Qi Bo (歧伯) has written ten classics of An Mo ……"[8,9] Unfortunately, these have been lost. However, we can see from this mention that An Mo was already being comprehensively studied and practiced. Also in the same period, Dr. Zhang, Zhong-Jing (張仲景) in his book *Jin Kui Yao Lue* (金匱要略) (*Prescriptions from the Golden Chamber*) mentioned first aid techniques for someone who had been hanged. He says, "Use the hand to press on the chest, and move frequently."[10,11] This is the earliest record of using massage for emergency care.

The oldest Chinese medical book, *Huang Di Nei Jing* (黃帝內經) (*Internal Classic of* the Yellow Emperor) mentions massage. For example, in the *Su Wen* (素問) section, the Xue Qi Xing Zhi Pian (血氣形志篇) (Chapter on Blood, Qi, Shape, and Spirit), it says: "The pattern frequently gets shocked, and the Jing (經) (i.e. primary Qi channels) and Luo (絡) (i.e. smaller channels) are not communicating. Sickness is generated from this lack of feeling. Then cure with An Mo (按摩) and herbs."[9,12] When the systems of the body get shocked often, a pattern of tension builds up and interferes with the Qi and blood circulation. There may be poor communication between the Jing and Luo, or between different Jing channels. When this happens, a part of the body may feel numb. This can be cured with massage and herbs.

Again, in *Yi Fa Fang Yi Lun* (異法方宜論) (*Treatise on Different Methods of Proper Treatment*) it says: "In the central area (of China), because the ground is flat and wet, there are therefore millions of living things in the heaven and earth, the food eaten by the people is varied, and the people do not like to work. For this reason, the sicknesses are mostly paralysis and withering, cold and hot. They should be cured by leading (the Qi) with An (按) and Qiao (蹻)."[9,13] When people are inactive, their bodies become insensitive and weak. They are therefore subject to illness caused by rapid changes is the weather. Their condition can be improved by enhancing their Qi circulation through An (按) (i.e. An Mo) and Qiao (蹻) (i.e. using the feet to massage).

During the Jin dynasty (265-420 A.D.) (晉朝), Dr. Ge, Hong (葛洪) in his book: *Shi Hou Jiu Zu Fang* (時后救卒方) (*The Methods of Preparing for Emergencies; Reviving from Unconsciousness*) recorded many methods of correcting dislocations, such as of the jaws, and setting broken bones.[4] This book also says, "To revive from a sudden faint, ..., use the fingers to grab Renzhong (Gv-26) (人中) cavity, which will immediately revive the patient."[11,14] Also, in his book *Bao Pu Zi* (抱朴子) (*Embrace Simplicity*) Dr. Ge, Hong says, "Where there is swelling and pain, using the hands to massage can cure."[11,15]

In the Sui dynasty (605-618 A.D.) (隋朝), the book *Sui Shu Bai Guan Zhi* (隋書百官志) (*The Record of Hundreds of Officers in the Sui Dynasty*) recorded that in the Imperial Hospital there was a division of An Mo, and there were two An Mo physicians. It was also recorded in Dr. Chao, Yuan-Fang's (巢元方) book, *Zhu Bing Yuan Hou Lun* (諸病源後論) (*Thesis on the Origins and Symptoms of Various Diseases*) that self-massage for healing was taught in several places.[9]

By the Tang dynasty (618-907 A.D.) (唐朝), An Mo had become very popular. Old editions of *Tang Shu Zhi Guan Zhi* (唐書職官志) (*Record of Official Positions in the Tang Dynasty*) recorded the names of men who were "Masters of An Mo." The new edition of *Record of Official Positions in the Tang Dynasty* had a record of a medical division which had one Doctor of An Mo and four Masters of An Mo.

Tang Liu Dian (唐六典) (*Tang's Six Records*) recorded even more details. It records that there were 56 An Mo technicians and 15 An Mo students in the Imperial Hospital. This was more than the number of acupuncturists and herbalists at that time. This indicates the importance of An Mo in the medical system of that time.

Also in this period, Dr. Wang, Tao (王燾) in his book *Wai Tai Mi Yao* (外臺秘要) (*The Extra Important Secret*) mentioned how to use massage to cure stomach pain, saying: "Rub both hands to make them warm, use them to massage the stomach; (this is) able to lead Qi downward."[11,16] In addition, Dr. Sun, Si-Miao (孫思邈) in his book *Qian Jin Fang* (千金方) (*Thousand Gold Prescriptions*) introduced a massage system called Lao Zi's 49 Massage Techniques. In addition, Dr. Lin, Dao-Ren's (藺道人) book: *Xian Shou Li Shang Xu Duan Mi Fang* (仙授理傷續斷秘方) (*The Secret Prescriptions for Connecting Broken Bones*) further contributed an in-depth theory and methods of treatment for injuries.[4] In the period of Tang Tian Bao (742-756 A.D.) (唐天寶), massage techniques were exported into Japan.[9] They were the ancestors of today's Japanese massage.

During the Song dynasty (960-1280 AD.) (宋朝), Dr. Zhang, Gao (張杲) in his book *Yi Shuo* (醫說) (*Talks on Medicine*) introduced massage techniques using the feet to increase Qi and blood circulation to expedite the healing of broken bones.[4] Dr. Pang, An-Shi (龐安時) taught how to use massage to help in childbirth.[11] The fourth volume of *Jing Ji Zong Lun* (經濟總論) (*The Total Record of Economics*) talks about healing, and includes a detailed analysis of how to use An Mo for healing. It says, "(For some sicknesses) you can use An, (for others) use Mo, sometimes use both, all called An Mo. When An (press), do not Mo (rub), (when) Mo (rub), do not An (press). Press with hands, when rubbing, use herbs sometimes. These are An and Mo. Fit (them) to the right purpose."[11,17] The book *Ru Men Shi Shi* (儒門視事) (*The Confucian Point of View*) also mentions how massage can increase perspiration, which gave the people a clear idea of how to cure sickness with An Mo.[11]

In the Yuan dynasty (1206-1368 A.D.) (元朝), "bone correction" was established as the thirteenth category in the medical system, and became an important part of medical expertise. Tui Na An Mo was a part of bone correction technique. A famous document from this period was Dr. Wei, Yi-Lin's (危亦林) *Shi Yi De Xiao Fang* (世醫得效方) (*Effective Prescriptions of Well-known Doctors*), which systematically compiled effective prescriptions discovered before the Yuan dynasty. Dr. Li, Zhong-Nan's (李仲南) *Yong Lei Qian Fang* (永類鈐方) (*Permanent Seal Techniques*) was another well-known book which discussed bone setting, especially how to correct the bones.[4]

In the Ming dynasty (1368-1644 A.D.) (明朝), An Mo was one of the thirteen specialties in the imperial examination. During this period, many more books were published about the treatment of injuries. For example, Dr. Zhu, Su's (朱橚) *Pu Ji Fang, Zhe Shang Men* (普濟方・折傷門) (*General Saving Methods, Category for Broken Bones and Injuries*), Dr. Wang, Ken-Tang's (王肯堂) *Yang Yi Zhun Sheng* (瘍醫準繩) (*The Rules of Healing Injuries*) are two of the many publications dealing with the treatment of injuries.[4] In addition, the book *Xiao Er An Mo Jing* (小兒按摩經) (*Massage Classic for Small Children*) and the book *Xiao Er Tui Na Mi Jue* (小兒推拿秘訣) (*The Secret of Tui Na for Small Children*) were also published during this period.[11] You can see that Tui Na massage had gradually come to be used for treating children's illnesses.

During the Ming and Qing dynasties (1368-1911 A.D.) (明朝；清朝), Tui Na massage became more popular for treating sickness in small children. Acupuncture needs the cooperation of the patient, who must remain still during the treatment. Small children cannot be relied upon to lie still for any length of time, and their movements can break or bend the needles. Tui Na massage requires no needles, and although it is not quite as effective as acupuncture in many cases, it has proven to be safer and easier.

The available documents show that *Xiao Er Tui Na* (小兒推拿) (*Small Children Tui Na*) had become one of the main courses of study during this period. For example, during the Ming dynasty (明朝), the appendix of Dr. Yang, Ji-Zhou's (楊繼洲) book *Zhen Jiu Da Cheng* (針灸大成) (*The Great Compendium of Acupuncture and Moxibustion*) contained a section entitled "Bao Ying Shen Shu An Mo Jing" (保嬰神術按摩經) ("The Classic of Marvelous Massage Techniques for Protecting Babies") which discussed the use of massage to cure sickness of small babies. Also in the same period, Dr. Hu, Lian-Bi's (胡璉璧) book *Xiao Er Tui Na Fang Mai Huo Ying Mi Zhi Quan Shu* (小兒推拿方脈活嬰秘旨全書) (*The Complete Book of Secret Keys to Massaging Small Children*) and Dr. Zhou, Yue-Fu's (周嶽甫) book *Xiao Er Tui Na Mi Jue* (小兒推拿秘訣) (*The Secret of Tui Na for Small Children*) also contributed a great deal of knowledge.[9]

During the Qing dynasty (1644-1911 A.D.) (清朝), Dr. Cheng, Qian's (呈謙) book *Yi Zong Jin Jian; Zheng Gu Xin Fa Yao Zhi* (醫宗金鑒・正骨心法要旨) (*The Gold Study of Medicine, The Important Keys to Correcting Bones*) systematically compiled all of the publications on the subject, and became the most systematic and thorough book on the treatment of injuries. In this book, Dr. Cheng divided all of the treatment techniques into eight categories. They are Mo (摸) (touch), Jie (接) (connect), Duan (端) (hold up), Ti (提) (lift), Tui (推) (push), Na (拿) (grab), An (按) (press), and Mo (摩) (rub). In addition to Dr. Cheng's book, Dr. Qian, Xiu-Chang's (錢秀昌) *Shang Ke Bu Yao* (傷科補要) (*The Complementary Important Keys to Treating Injuries*), Dr. Gu, Shi-Cheng's (顧世澄) *Yang Yi Da Quan* (瘍醫大全) (*The Great Achievement of Treating Injuries*), Hu, Ting-Guang's (胡廷光) *Shang Ke Hui Cuan* (傷科匯篆) (*The Compilation of Injury Categories*), Yue, Zhu-Quan's (越竹泉) *Shang Ke Da Cheng* (傷科大成) (*The Great Achievement of Injury Categories*), all had very systematic and detailed methods for the treatment of injuries.[4]

During the late Qing dynasty (晚清), the use of Tui Na to treat small children had developed even further, and the techniques had even spread to lay society. This is indicated by the countless numbers of books published at this time. Some of the famous ones are Dr. Xiong, Ying-Xiong's (熊應雄) *Tui Na Guang Yi* (推拿廣義) (*The Wide Definition of Tui Na*), Xia, Yu-Zhu's (夏禹鑄) *You Ke Tie Jing* (幼科鐵鏡) (*The Iron Mirror for Small Children*), and Dr. Luo, Qian-An's (駱潛庵) *You Ke Tui Na Mi Shu* (幼科推拿秘術) (*The Secret Book of Tui Na for Small Children*).[9]

From the Qing dynasty until now, in addition to continuing to practice the massage techniques which had already been developed, a great emphasis began to be placed on Qi massage (also called Qigong healing). Interest in Qi massage has steadily grown, as modern communication speeds word of its effectiveness around the world. This is an exciting period in which traditional medicine must accept the scrutiny of modern science. People today are not satisfied with just getting good results, they also want to know how and why something works.

You can see from this brief account that most of the contributions came from within the medical community. It was not until the beginning of this century that the massage techniques used by martial artists were revealed to lay society. Among the many martial styles of massage, Shaolin Massage (少林按摩) was the best known. Shaolin massage focused on physical massage until the practitioner had achieved a high level of understanding of Qi, and then he was introduced to Qi massage. This was very different from the massage which was passed down on Wudang mountain (武當山), wherein Qi was always the first concern. On Wudang mountain, the concept of Qi was taught in the very beginning of the training. The Shaolin and the Wudang schools of massage were best known in China for cavity press massage, which is related to the cavity press striking used in the martial arts.

There are other martial styles which have revealed their massage techniques, including Ying Zhua Men (鷹爪門) (Eagle Claw Style), Qian Long Men (乾龍門) (Heavenly Dragon Style), Feng Yang Men (鳳陽門) (Phoenix Sun Style), Mi Zong (秘宗) (Tibetan Secret Style), Shen Long (神龍) (Spiritual Dragon Style), and Yun Zhan (雲斬) (Cloud Cutting Style). Some of these styles are derived from Shaolin and Wudang styles. Many of the techniques passed down in these martial styles have been compiled and published, and are now widely available.

1-5. About This Book

This chapter should have given you a basic understanding of the general concepts of Chinese Qigong massage, and of the important role it has played in the history of Chinese medicine. It is important that we now investigate how much of this treasure of knowledge and experience can be borrowed and applied to contemporary and even future medical science. This is the reason I wrote this book. Hopefully, this work will build a bridge to facilitate communication between the East and the West.

Before you read any further, I would like to stress a few points. First, I do not consider that I am an expert in all forms of Chinese Qigong massage. In fact, since the field is so wide and so deep, there are very few people today who can claim to be experts in all aspects of Chinese massage. Therefore, you should not treat this book as an authority. This book is just like many other massage books which can contribute some oriental concepts, and which you can use for reference and to stimulate your thinking. As I explained in the preface, this book is based on my limited knowledge and experience, and on a dozen printed books which discuss Qigong massage in depth. I sincerely hope that those who are masters of Qigong massage will open their minds and hearts, and share their knowledge and experience. This is the only way that Qigong massage can grow and progress today, and it is the only way that this art can gain the widespread respect it deserves.

The second point I would like to emphasize is that in order to learn from the past, we must first remain humble and appreciate the treasure which has been passed to us. Only then will we have the correct attitude for evaluating its value today and in the future.

The science of Chinese Qigong sprang from the natural human reaction to the threat of disease. Like acupuncture, Qigong massage developed out of the basic theory of Qi and its relationship to our health. It is based upon more than five thousand years of practice, as well as a solid theoretical foundation.

If we look at today's medical science, on the one hand, we understand the physical body extremely well. On the other hand, our understanding of Qi or bioelectricity is still in its infancy. It is now beginning to be understood that, if we can thoroughly understand both the physical side and the inner energy side of the human body, medicine can advance to a new stage. It is therefore especially crucial to understand that the information which has been passed down to us may be the gate which leads us to this new field of understanding.

The third point which I would like to make is that when you practice any Qigong, you must first ask: *What, Why,* and *How.* "What" means: "What am I looking for?" "What do I expect?" and "What should I do?" Then you must ask, "Why do I need it?" "Why does it work?" "Why must I do it this way instead of that way?." Finally, you must determine, "How does it work?" "How much have I advanced toward my goal?" And "How will I be able to advance further?"

It is very important to understand what you are practicing, not just automatically to repeat what you have learned. Understanding is the root of any work. With understanding you will be able to know your goal. Once you know your goal, your mind can be firm and steady. With this understanding, you will be able to see why something has happened, and what the principles and theories behind it are. Without all of this, your work will be done blindly, and it will be a long and painful process. Only when you are sure what your target is and why you need to reach it should you raise the question of how you are going to accomplish it. The answers to all of these questions form the root of your practice, and will help you to avoid the doubt and confusion that uncertainty brings. If you keep this root, you will be able to apply the theory and make it grow—you will know how to create. Without this root, what you learn will be only branches and flowers, and in time they will wither.

Finally, I would like to make a very important point: The best way to reach a high level of ability and understanding of massage is by doing a great deal of massage. While this book will offer you a general guideline, massaging people is what will give you experience, encourage you to ponder, to continue studying, and to develop yourself. The more you massage yourself and others, the more you will be able to understand. If you wish to advance to the higher levels of ability, it is also advisable to study the basic theory of Chinese medicine. Studying Qigong is also necessary if you wish to understand Qi massage and Qi healing.

Again, I would like to remind you to keep your mind open. If you can do this, you will be more able to see and more willing to accept knowledge from a wide variety of sources. A wise man never stops learning.

References

1. "Life's Invisible Current," by Albert L. Huebner, *East West Journal,* June 1986.
2. *The Body Electric,* by Robert O. Becker, M.D. and Gary Selden, Quill, William Morrow, New York, 1985.
3. "Healing with Nature's Energy by Richard Leviton," *East West Journal,* June 1986.
4. 〝中醫骨傷科基礎〞，丁繼華，吳誠德。(*The Foundation of the Chinese Medicine in Category of Bone Injury*), by Ding, Ji-Hua and Wu, Chengde, Taipei, Taiwan, 1986.
5. 《山海經·東山經》：〝高氏之山，其上多玉，其下多箴石。〞
6. 世郭璞：〝箴石，可以為砭針治痛腫者。〞
7. 許慎，《說文解字》：〝砭，以石刺病也。〞
8. 《漢書藝文志》：〝黃帝時，歧伯著按摩十卷。〞
9. 〝按摩大全〞，蕭文忠等編。(*The Completeness of An Mo*), by Xiao, Wen-Zhong, etc., Taipei, Taiwan, 1986.
10. 張仲景，《金匱要略》：〝以手按據胸上，數動之。〞
11. 〝按摩推拿手法萃錦〞，李茂林。(*The Refined Collection of An Mo Tui Na Techniques*), by Li, Mao-Lin, Peiking, China, 1985.
12. 《素問血氣形志篇》：〝形數驚恐，經絡不通，病生於不仁，治之以按摩醪藥。〞
13. 《異法方宜論》：〝中央者，其地平以濕，天地所以生萬物也眾，其民食雜而不勞，其病多痿厥寒熱，其治宜導引按蹻。〞
14. 《時後備急方》：〝救卒中惡死，…，令爪其病人人中，取醒。〞
15. 葛洪，《抱朴子》：〝其腫痛所在，以摩之皆手下即愈。〞

16. 王燾，《外臺秘要》：〝兩手相摩令熱，以摩腹，令氣下。〞

17. 《經濟總論》：〝可按可摩，時兼而用，通謂之按摩；按之弗摩，按之以手，摩或兼以藥，曰按曰摩，適所用也。〞

CHAPTER 2
General Foundations 一般基礎

2-1. Introduction 介紹

In the last chapter, we briefly introduced the general theory of massage. However, in order to massage effectively, you need to have a much deeper understanding of the theory. This, plus the experience you have accumulated, will greatly increase your ability to accurately analyze the needs of the patient. Remember, knowledge is the Yin side of massage, and it forms the foundation for the Yang side, which is practicing massage.

Although the basic theory remains the same in all four categories of Chinese Qigong massage, the goals of each category and the theory of how to approach the goals are often very different. For example, while Tui Na (推拿) and Dian Xue (點穴) massage both regulate the Qi levels in the channels, they each go about it in quite different ways. In order to avoid confusion, we will discuss how each category applies the theory when we introduce that category.

In this chapter, we will discuss some of the important concepts which form the foundation for all four categories. However, the most important thing you need to know is the structure of the human body. Lacking this, you will be like a blind man walking in the street.

The first thing you need to know about the physical body is that it is only a part of your entire being. According to Chinese medicine and religion, a living human body consists of three parts: 1. A Yang part, the physical body, which manifests the activities (life) of the body; 2. A Yin part, the inner energy (Qi or bioelectricity) part of the body, which nourishes the physical body and keeps it alive; and 3. The refined product of the Yin and Yang parts: the spiritual or mental body.

Western medicine usually devotes all of its attention to problems in the physical body, and usually ignores problems in the energy body. Because of this, there is a wealth of publications about the structure of the physical body, and the level of understanding is quite profound. It cannot be denied that in the understanding of the physical human body, Western science is the world leader. However, in regards to the structure of the inner energy body, it is still in the beginning stage. In fact, it was not until the last two decades that the concept of bioelectricity was even recognized by Western medicine.

As mentioned in the first chapter, Yin (Qi) is the root of the life while Yang (physical action) is the manifestation of life. Yin and Yang must be balanced. Whenever there is a deficiency or excess in either the Yin side or the Yang side, the body will become sick. Most illnesses are caused by the abnormal distribution and circulation of Qi, i.e., by the Yin side of the body. Therefore, when you study the structure of the human body, you must not limit yourself by studying only the physical side. Both sides are mutually related and cannot be separated. However, you must also beware of going to the other extreme and mixing or confusing the two concepts.

Many people still confuse the Qi distribution system with the nervous system. We know from Western science that physically there are three major networks in the human body: the circulatory system, the nervous system, and the lymphatic system. All three are physical, visible systems. However, in order to keep functioning properly, these three systems need energy, which the Chinese call Qi, and Western science calls bioelectricity. Naturally, in order to supply Qi to these systems efficiently, the Qi system must be organized and structured similarly to the other three systems. Because of this, it is not really surprising that many people still believe that the Qi system is just the Chinese name for the nervous system.

To clear up this confusion, in the next section we will briefly review the physical structure of the human body. If you would like to know about this subject in more detail, there are many anatomy books available. In the third section, we will summarize the structure of the human Qi body. If you would like to know more about this subject, many books on Chinese medicine are now available in English. Then, in the fourth section, we will explain the refined product of the physical and Qi bodies, the spirit or the mental body.

Once you have a clear understanding of the structure of the human body, the fifth section will discuss the gates (Tong Men, 通門) or junctions (Jiao Hui Dian, 交會點) in the body. Understanding the gates or junctions is a crucial key to performing a successful massage. Finally, in the last section, we will list a number of important points to remember that apply to all categories of massage. Naturally, there are also many other rules which apply to one category or the other, but we will bring these up when those categories are discussed.

2-2. UNDERSTANDING THE PHYSICAL BODY 瞭解人身物體

First, let us take a look at the general structure of the body. When you look at a portion of your body, for example, an arm, the first thing you see is the skin (Figure 2-1). On the skin are hairs and thousands of pores. The pores are like gates through which waste is eliminated from your body, and through which Qi is exchanged with the environment. According to Chinese Qigong, if your Qi is able to reach the skin and abundantly nourish every cell and the circulatory systems there (i.e. if your Guardian Qi (Wei Qi, 衛氣) is strong), the skin and hair will stay youthful and healthy. However, when the Qi is weak or the supply is abnormal, which happens, for example, when you grow older, the symptoms appear first in the hair and skin. Therefore, one of the purposes of

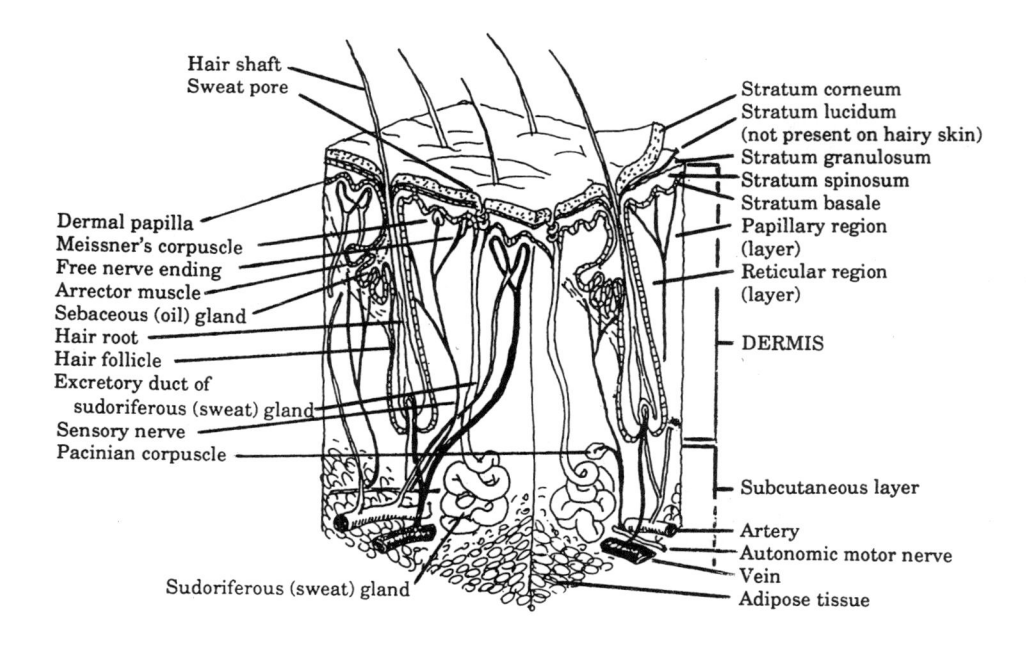

FIGURE 2-1. ANATOMICAL STRUCTURE OF THE SKIN.

general massage is to lead Qi to the skin, to improve the smooth circulation of the blood, and to maintain the sensitivity of the nerves.

Right under the surface of the skin is a thick layer of fat. Fat is the stored essence of food. In other words, when we eat more than we need, the excess which is not excreted is stored in the body as fat. This fat is usually carried by the blood cells to every part of the body. The more fat there is in the blood stream, the more sluggish the circulation is. Fat can be stored under the skin, in the fasciae, and in the bone marrow. The more fat you have stored in your body, the poorer your Qi and blood circulation will be.

Underneath the layer of fat, but before the muscles, is a layer of fascia. Fasciae are found in many places in the body. The first place is between the skin and the muscles, the second place is between the layers of muscle, the third place is between the muscles and the bones, and the last place is around the internal organs. Next time you buy a chicken, if you cut it open and examine it you should be able to locate these fasciae, which are thin layers of transparent membrane. Fat is stored in the fasciae. It is also known that the fat and the fascia are not conductors of Qi. This means whenever the Qi is passing through fasciae, the resistance will be higher and affect the Qi circulation. Therefore, one of the purposes of general massage is to remove the fat accumulated in the fasciae. Physical exercise can also accomplish this.

Between the fasciae and the muscles are found the veins, nerves, and sometimes lymph vessels (Figure 2-2). If you remove some of the muscles, you will see the main

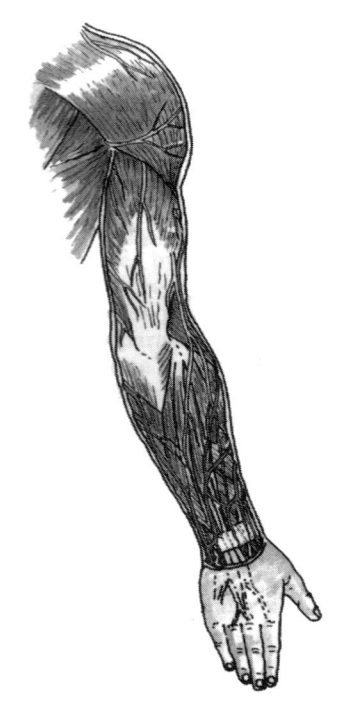

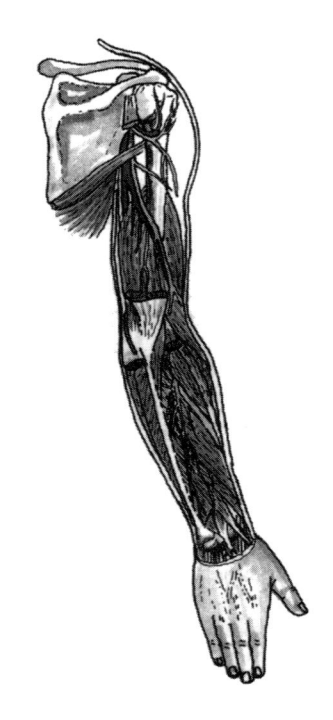

FIGURE 2-2. SUPERFICIAL ANATOMICAL STRUCTURE OF THE POSTERIOR ASPECT OF THE ARM.

FIGURE 2-3. ANATOMICAL STRUCTURE OF THE MIDDLE LAYER OF THE POSTERIOR ASPECT OF THE ARM.

arteries, and the main nerves (Figure 2-3). Beneath the muscle is the bone (Figure 2-4), and inside the bone is the marrow (Figure 2-5).

Now let us first look at the body's two physical circulatory systems: the blood vascular system and the lymph vascular system. Then we will review another important system, the nervous system.

1. Blood System 血液循環系統

Blood is considered to be the "elixir of life" in the West. Blood is mainly composed of red cells, white cells, platelets and plasma. The red cells carry nourishment (including oxygen and Qi) to the organs and tissues through the arteries. Waste materials are also carried away from the tissues by the blood to the eliminative organs. The blood finally returns to the heart through the veins. The blood acts as a conduit for essential products made by various organs, carrying these products to other organs which need them to function properly and survive. Each blood cell has properties not unlike that of a small battery, allowing them to store electrical charges and carry them throughout the body. Because of this, blood may also help to equalize the energy level throughout the body, facilitating harmonious interaction between all the diverse bodily components that it supplies.

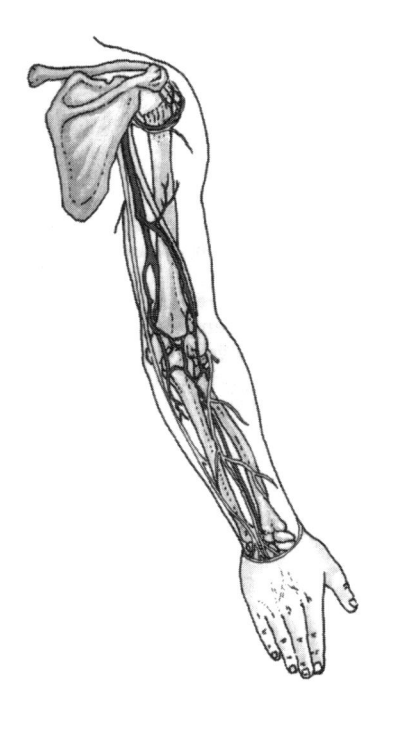

1. Epiphysis
2. Spongy bone
3. Medullary cavity
4. Compact bone
5. Nutrient foramen
6. Diaphysis

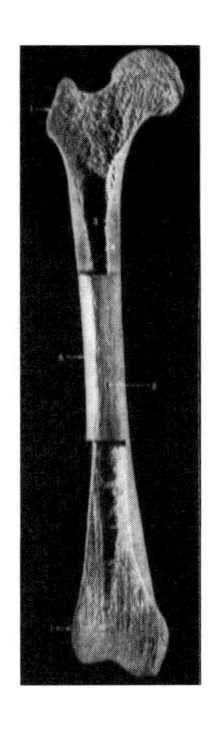

FIGURE 2-4. DEEP ANATOMICAL STRUCTURE OF THE ANTERIOR ASPECT OF THE ARM.

FIGURE 2-5. BONE AND BONE MARROW.

The main function of white blood cells is to seek out, identify and destroy germs by literally eating them alive. The white cells are not alone, however, in their germ hunting mission. Other parts of the blood, including its fluid portion (i.e. plasma), carry germ-killing substances. There are proteins in the plasma which play an integral role in this endeavor. Finally, platelets, along with other substances, help to enable the blood to coagulate (i.e. solidify). This avoids major loss of blood from minor cuts or wounds.

There are a number of important points here. The first is that the blood cells are the nourishment conveyors of the body. Any defect in the smooth flow of blood in the blood vessels will be reflected in a failure of the other cells of the body to receive the proper amount of oxygen, nutrition, and Qi. New, fresh blood cells are constantly being produced in the bone marrow to replace the old cells. When the bone marrow is not functioning properly or has been damaged through neglect or old age, the blood cells produced will be of inferior quality. According to Chinese Qigong, if you want the marrow to keep producing healthy blood cells, you have to keep the marrow well-supplied with Qi. This has become a very important part of Chinese Qigong, and is called Bone Marrow Washing Qigong (Xi Sui Qigong, 洗髓氣功). If you are interested in more on this subject, please refer to the YMAA book, *Qigong—Secret of Youth*.

The second important point is that, in order to keep the blood cells supplying the

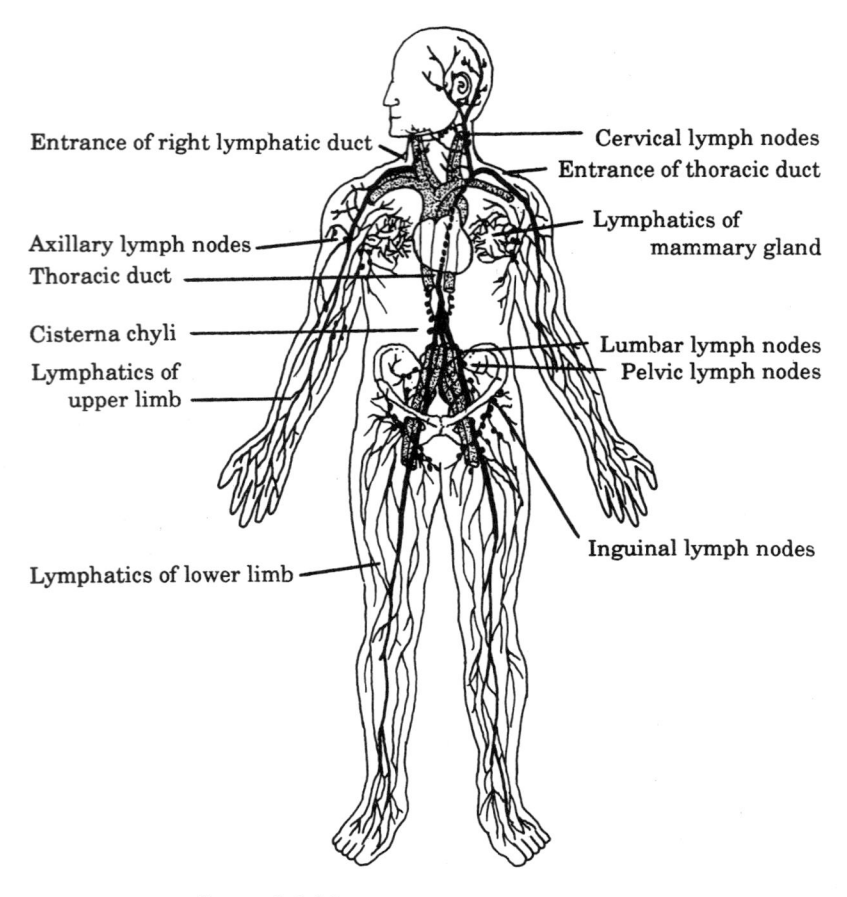

FIGURE 2-6. MAJOR LYMPH VESSELS OF THE BODY.

body with nourishment and removing waste, the circulatory system must be healthy. While it is very difficult to use massage to improve the Qi supply to the bone marrow, it is very easy to use general massage to improve blood circulation. The main blood vessels are located under the muscles, between the muscles, and on the surface of the muscles. Since tensing the muscles constricts the blood vessels, massaging the muscles will relieve tension on the vessels and improve circulation. In addition, general massage can help to reduce stored fat, thereby increasing the responsiveness of this vital circulatory system.

2. Lymphatic System 淋巴循環系統

Lymph is a transparent, watery, colorless or sometimes slightly yellow fluid. The lymphatic system consists of this fluid, the vessels that carry it into the blood—the lymph vessels or lymphatics, and a series of lymph organs including the lymph nodes, tonsils, spleen, and thymus (Figure 2-6).

Lymph vessels of the lymph-capillary type arise in nearly all parts of the body.

Lymph-capillaries take up any blood-plasma which has been discharged for nourishment purposes from the blood-capillaries into the tissue-spaces, and returns it into veins near the heart. Most of these lymphatics empty themselves into one main reservoir called the thoracic duct, which runs upward along the anterior of the spine, opening into large veins on the left side of the neck, at its base. The rest of the lymphatics empty into a smaller reservoir which runs into corresponding veins on the right side of the neck base. Lymph's primary function is to remove bacteria and certain proteins from the tissues, to transport fat from the intestines, and to supply lymphocytes to the blood.

Lymph nodes, which are also commonly referred to as lymph glands, are oval or round bodies which are found adjacent to the lymphatic vessels. They supply lymphocytes to the circulatory system and cleanse the lymph by removing bacteria and foreign particles. One commonly known example of these glands are the tonsils.

One of the largest lymphoid structures in the human body is the spleen. The spleen, which filters and stores blood, is located on the left side of the torso below the diaphragm. Finally, the thymus is a ductless glandlike body, positioned just behind the top of the sternum. The thymus reaches its maximum development in childhood, and plays some part in building resistance to disease. However, by adulthood this organ is usually vestigial, having no further known use.

3. The Nervous System 神經循環系統

A nerve is a bundle of fibers uniting the central nervous system with the organs and other parts of the body. Nerves relay sensory stimuli as well as motor impulses from different parts of the body to one another.

All multicellular animals except sponges possess nervous systems. They are essentially regulatory mechanisms, controlling internal bodily functions and responses to external stimuli. The human nervous system is made up of two component sub-systems: the central nervous system (CNS) and the peripheral nervous system (PNS) (Figure 2-7).

Making up the central nervous system (CNS) are the brain and the spinal cord, which are contained and protected within the skull and the spine respectively. The CNS integrates, interprets, and transmits messages to and from the brain and the periphery of the body.

Making up the peripheral nervous system (PNS) is all nervous tissue found outside of the skull and spinal column, including not only the nerve fibers that carry impulses, but also groupings of fibers (plexuses) and nerve cell bodies (ganglions) that are found in the periphery. The PNS registers changes in the internal and external environments of the body, transmitting this information to the CNS for action, and then delivering the orders of the CNS to muscles and glands for response.

The PNS includes 12 pairs of cranial nerves which attach to the brain and their associated ganglions, as well as 31 pairs of spinal nerves and their ganglions. Finally, the PNS also includes specialized receptors and endings on muscles.

In terms of the function and interaction of all these constituent components, the

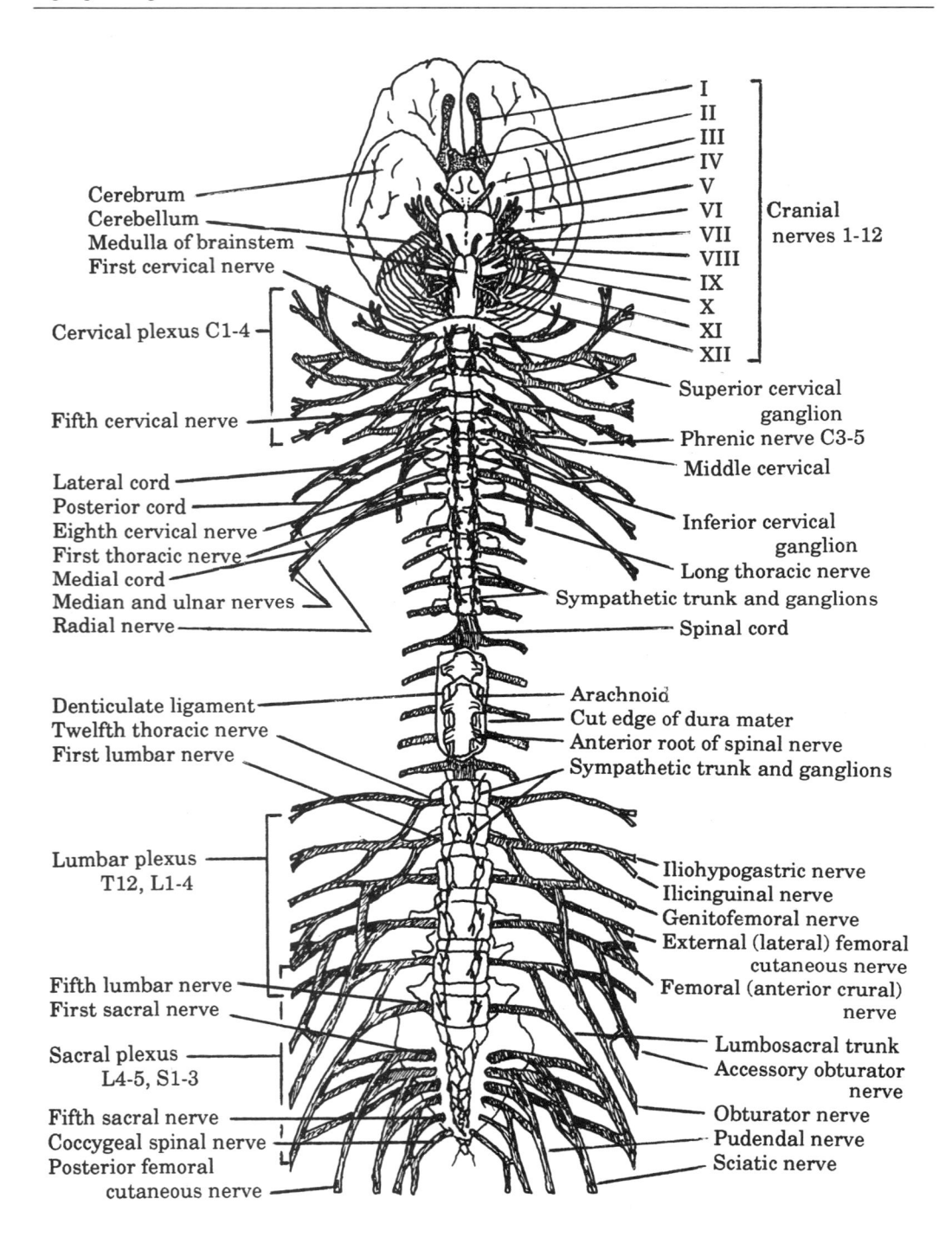

FIGURE 2-7. BASIC ORGANIZATION OF THE NERVOUS SYSTEM.

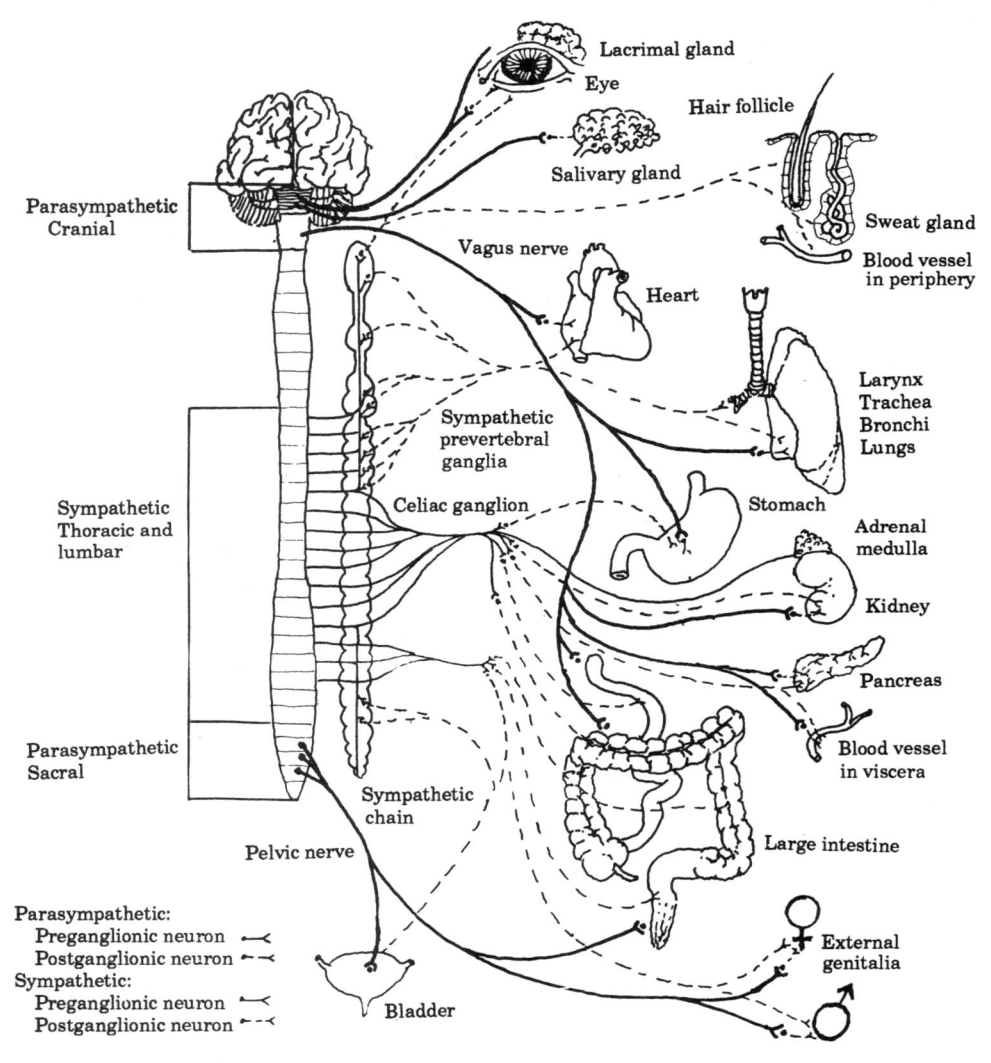

FIGURE 2-8. A SCHEMATIC REPRESENTATION OF THE AUTONOMIC NERVOUS SYSTEM AND THE ORGANS IT SERVES.

PNS is simple yet efficient. It is 'built' out of somatic fibers (somatic nervous system) that provide the nerves for the skeletal muscles as well as the skin's special receptors (for touch, pressure, heat, cold), and autonomic fibers (autonomic nervous system). The autonomic fibers carry impulses from the heart, vessels, lungs, gastrointestinal tract, genitourinary tract, and other vascular and visceral structures (Figure 2-8). These fibers make possible the reflexes which control breathing, heart rate, blood pressure, and other bodily functions in an involuntary and unbroken manner. Most organs receive fibers from two subdivisions of the autonomic nervous system. The parasympathetic (craniosacral) division, which is comprised of certain cranial nerves and several of the sacral spinal nerves, furnishes nervous influences for the purpose of conservation of body sources and maintenance of nominal function levels. The sympathetic (thoracolumbar) division, which is comprised of the thoracic and lumber spinal nerves, furnishes impulses for the purpose of elevating body activity in order to tolerate or resist stressful or hazardous situations. In this way an organ may have its operation intensified or diminished according to the demands of the situation for survival.

This brief anatomic discussion of the nervous system shows us that the brain and spinal cord are the center of our feeling and functioning. We have seen that nerves from the spinal cord extend out and connect to the entire body, including the limbs and also the internal organs.

There are a number of other facts about the nervous system that are also important. First, our state of mind is linked to the condition of our physical body through our nervous system. This means that if we are mentally tense or relaxed, our physical body will react accordingly. Second, the nervous system is constructed of tissue fibers, which are part of the material side of our body. In order to function properly, in fact, even to stay alive, this material needs Qi. Third, if we compare the system of Qi distribution with the nervous system we see that, although they are related, they are not the same system. The Qi circulatory system does not supply Qi only to the nervous system exclusively, it supplies it to all of the body's cells.

The nervous system plays a critical role in the practice of Qigong. The nervous system enables us to *feel* what is going on everywhere in our body. Since the mind leads the Qi, if we want to lead Qi somewhere we have to be able to feel that place. If we cannot feel that place, then the mind cannot lead the Qi there, since it does not know where it is.

The nervous system is responsible for our ability to feel, and it is our ability to feel that governs the Qi. This means that the condition of the nervous system is directly related to the Qi circulation in our body. In Qigong massage therefore, while we should pay particular attention to the Qi system, the nervous system should be second in our priorities.

To massage the nervous system, you start with the central nervous system, which includes the brain and the spinal cord, and then you loosen up the places where the peripheral nervous system extends out from the spinal cord to the limbs and internal organs. All of these junctions are located on the sides of the vertebrae.

After the head, the spine is the most important place to massage. The spine consists of seven cervical vertebrae (the neck area), twelve thoracic vertebrae (the rib area), five lumbar vertebrae (the waist area), the sacrum (which consists of five pieces), and the coccyx or tailbone (four pieces) (Figure 2-9).

It is important to know how the central nervous system relates to the internal organs, which was illustrated in Figure 2-8. Massaging the nervous system in and around the spine stimulates the corresponding internal organs and improves their func-

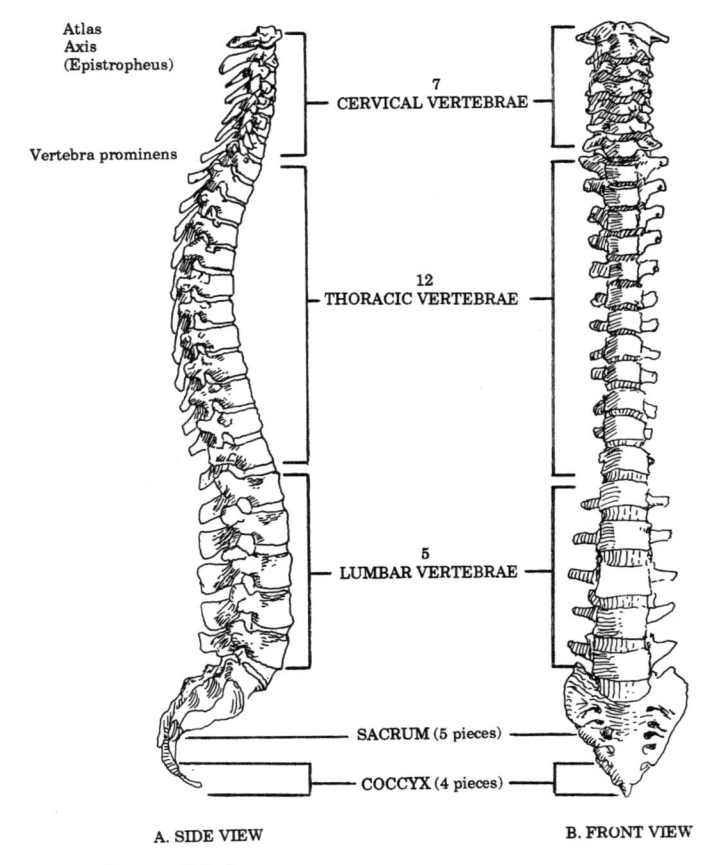

FIGURE 2-9. SIDE AND FRONT VIEWS OF THE VERTEBRAL COLUMN.

tioning. This means that when you massage the spine, you indirectly massage the internal organs.

Finally, you also need to know how the central nervous system is related to the skin on the limbs. Since you touch a person's skin when you do general massage, and since sections of the skin are related to sections of the central nervous system, you can smooth out the Qi and relieve nervous tension from the spine to the ends of the limbs. An area of the skin with sensory fibers from a single spinal nerve is called a dermatome. Figure 2-10 shows the dermatomes of the arms and legs.

2-3. UNDERSTANDING THE QI BODY 瞭解人身氣體

Before discussing the Qi body, I would first like you to understand that you cannot actually see the Qi circulatory system. This is because we cannot see the difference between regular muscle tissue and the electrically conductive fascial tissue with the naked eye. At present, it seems reasonable to conclude that all of the Qi channels are

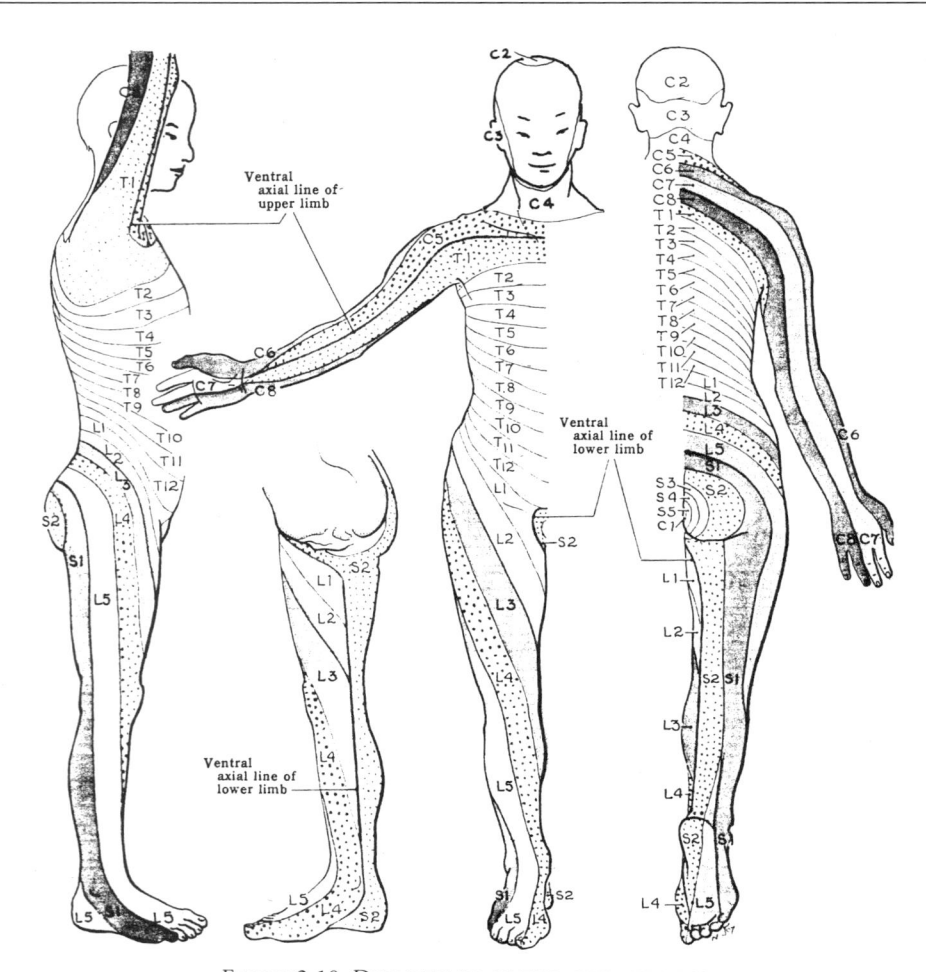

FIGURE 2-10. DERMATOMES OF THE ARMS AND LEGS.

hidden in these tissues. Exactly how these channels are formed is a mystery that is still awaiting further study with modern equipment. Next, in order to help you understand the Qi circulatory system, I would like to review some of the important concepts in Chinese medicine. This will help you to understand the rest of this section.

Qi 氣. Although we discussed the definition of Qi in the last chapter, it is so important that it is worth going over again. Qi is the energy which circulates within the body. Your entire body is like a factory and your organs are like the many machines operating inside the factory. Your brain is like management, directing the entire operation. In order to keep the factory functioning properly, you need a power supply. The power supply is connected to each machine with many wires and cables. Each machine must receive the appropriate level of power; too much power will damage the machine and shorten its life, and too little power will not enable the machine to function properly. You can see that without a proper power supply in the factory, production will be off, and if the power supply stops, the entire factory is dead. It is the same with your body. When your body does not have a normal energy (Qi) supply, the organs will not function properly, and you will become sick; and if the Qi circulation stops, you will die.

You should realize that your entire body is alive, including every blood cell, every nerve tissue, and every muscle fiber. All of these physical, fundamental structures of the body need Qi to maintain their existence and their ability to function. The system which distributes Qi throughout your body is much like the wiring system in a factory, connecting the power source to the machines.

From the viewpoint of function, Chinese medical science classifies Qi in the following ways:

1. Original Qi (Yuan Qi, 元氣): This Qi is converted from Original Essence (Yuan Jing, 元精) which you inherented from your parents. Original Essence is stored in the kidneys.

2. Organ Qi (Zan Fu Zhi Qi, 臟腑之氣): This Qi is responsible for the functioning of the organs.

3. Channel Qi (Jing Qi, 經氣): This Qi is responsible for the transportive and moving functions of the channels.

4. Nourishing Qi (Ying Qi, 營氣): The main responsibilities of this Qi are transforming and creating blood. Nourishing Qi also moves with the blood and helps the blood to nourish the tissues of the body.

5. Guardian Qi (Wei Qi, 衛氣): (Also commonly translated as Protective Qi). This Qi circulates outside the channels and the organs. Guardian Qi's responsibilities are to warm the organs, to travel between the skin and the flesh to regulate the opening and closing of the pores, and to protect and moisten the skin, hair, and nails. This Qi is able to provide the body with a defense against external negative influences such as cold weather.

6. Ancestral Qi (Zong Qi, 宗氣): This Qi gathers (resides) in the chest with its center at the Shanzhong (Co-l7) (膻中) cavity (Figure 2-11). Ancestral Qi is able to travel up to the throat and down to the abdomen. It is responsible for breathing and speaking, regulating heart beat, and, when cultivated through meditation, Ancestral Qi can strengthen the body.

Blood 血. The Western concept of blood is only part of the Chinese conception of blood. Although blood is seen as a red fluid, in Chinese medical science it is also regarded as a force which is involved with the sensitivity of the sense organs and the inner vitality of the body. Since the main responsibility of blood is to carry nourishment to every part of the body, it is closely related to Nourishing Qi.

Qi and Blood 氣、血. In Chinese medicine, Qi is considered Yang (陽) and blood is considered Yin (陰). Qi is said to be the 'commander' of blood because blood relies on Qi for its generation (out of food and air), and for its power to move through and

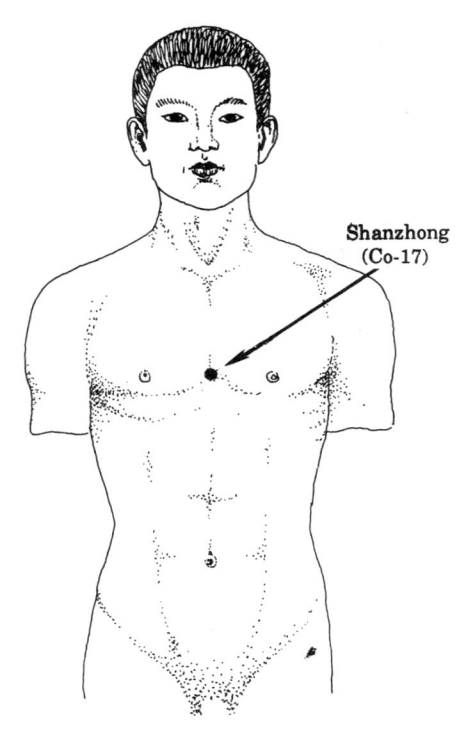

FIGURE 2-11. THE SHANZHONG CAVITY (Co-17).

remain in the blood vessels. It is also said that blood is the 'mother' of Qi because the strength of Qi depends upon the nutrition and moisture carried in the blood. Therefore, Qi and blood are believed to complement each other.

Organs (Viscera) and Bowels 臟、腑. The concept of the organs in Chinese medicine differs significantly from that of Western medicine. In Chinese medicine *the organs are systems of functions, and not mere physical objects.* Generally, this means that within the description of the organs, almost all of the body's functions can be defined and explained.

In Chinese medical science, the organs are divided into two main groups: the Yin (inner) organs and Yang (outer) organs. There are six Yin organs and six Yang organs. Five of the Yin organs (excluding the pericardium) are called Zang (臟), which means viscera. These five (liver, heart, spleen, lungs, and kidneys) are considered the core of the entire system. Usually, when a discussion involves the channels and all the organs, the pericardium is added; otherwise it is treated as an adjunct of the heart. According to Chinese medicine, *the Yin organs 'store and do not drain.'* That means that their functions are directed toward sustaining homeostasis, both physically and mentally.

The six Yang organs are called Fu (腑), which means 'bowels,' and include the gall bladder, small intestine, large intestine, stomach, bladder, and triple burner. According to Chinese medicine, these *Yang organs 'drain and do not store.'* This refers to their

	WOOD 木	FIRE 火	EARTH 土	METAL 金	WATER 水
Direction	East	South	Center	West	North
Season	Spring	Summer	Long Summer	Autumn	Winter
Climactic Condition	Wind	Summer Heat	Dampness	Dryness	Cold
Process	Birth	Growth	Transformation	Harvest	Storage
Color	Green	Red	Yellow	White	Black
Taste	Sour	Bitter	Sweet	Pungent	Salty
Smell	Goatish	Burning	Fragrant	Rank	Rotten
Yin Organ	Liver	Heart	Spleen	Lungs	Kidneys
Yang Organ	Gall Bladder	Small Intestine	Stomach	Large Intestine	Bladder
Opening	Eyes	Tongue	Mouth	Nose	Ears
Tissue	Sinews	Blood Vessels	Flesh	Skin/Hair	Bones
Emotion	Anger	Happiness	Pensiveness	Sadness	Fear
Human Sound	Shout	Laughter	Song	Weeping	Groan

TABLE 2-1. TABLE OF CORRESPONDENCES ASSOCIATED WITH THE FIVE PHASES.

responsibility in the transformation and the disposal of food and waste. All the Yang organs receive food or a product of food, and then pass it along.

In Table 2-1, you will notice that each Yang organ is associated with a Yin organ by a special Yin/Yang relationship (or Inner/Outer relationship). Pairs of related Yin and Yang organs belong to the same Phase, and their Qi channels are sequential to each other in Qi circulation. They are so closely linked that a disease in one will usually affect the other.

Yin and Yang 陰、陽. Yin and Yang are not contradictory. Nor is one considered 'good,' and the other 'bad.' To obtain health, a harmony is sought between them and any imbalance is avoided. Yin and Yang are relative, not absolute.

Five Phases (Five Elements) 五行. The Five Phases are (Wu Xing, 五行): Wood (Mu, 木), Fire (Huo, 火), Earth (Tu, 土), Metal (Jin, 金), and Water (Shui, 水). They are also commonly translated as the 'Five Elements.' In Chinese, Xing (行) means "to walk or to move"; probably more pertinent, it means "a process." The Five Phases are thought of as the five properties inherent in all things. Each phase symbolizes a category of related functions and qualities. For example, Wood is linked with active functions that are in phase with growth or with increasing. Fire expresses that the functions have reached a maximum state and are ready to decline. Metal represents declining functions. Water symbolizes that the functions have declined and are ready to grow. And finally, Earth is associated with balance or neutrality. Therefore, Earth is the center point of the five phases.

The relationships between the five phases are shown in Figure 2-12.

Qi Channels and Vessels 經、脈. Jing (經) is commonly translated "meridians" or "primary Qi channels." Your body has twelve channels, which Chinese medicine considers to be like rivers of Qi. Each channel, although referred to in the singular, is actually a pair of mirror-image channels, one on either side of the body. One end of each of

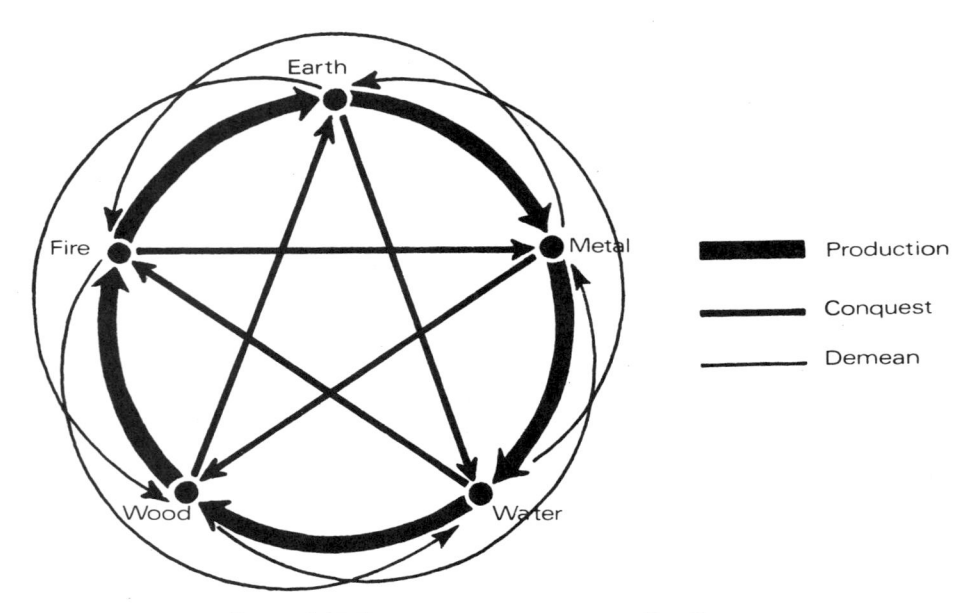

FIGURE 2-12. RELATIONSHIPS BETWEEN THE FIVE PHASES.

these twelve channels is associated with one of the twelve organs, while the other end is connected to a toe or finger (six channels are connected to the fingers and the other six are connected to the toes).

There are eight Qi Mai (氣脈) or "Qi vessels" in your body. They are often compared to *reservoirs* because they store Qi for your system. They can also be compared to batteries and capacitors in an electrical system. Batteries store and then release electrical current, and capacitors regulate the electrical current in the same way that the vessels regulate the Qi in your channels and organs.

There are other Qi channels called Luo (絡) or "Qi branches." They are often compared to *streams* because they spread Qi from rivers. There are millions of Luo spreading out from the channels to distribute Qi to every cell in the body. The Luo carry Qi from the channels outward to nourish the skin, hair, eyes, nails, etc., and also inward to the bone marrow to maintain the production of blood cells. Luo also connect the organs, enabling them to communicate and cooperate with each other.

The next term you must know is Xue (穴), which is translated as "cavity." Your body has more than seven hundred of these cavities, through which acupuncturists access the Qi channels with needles or other methods.

In order for you to be healthy, the Qi must flow smoothly and continuously in the channels. However, sometimes there are blockages, and the flow becomes stagnant. Blockages can be caused by eating poor quality food, by injuries, or by the physical degeneration that occurs as you age. Another problem occurs when the Qi is not flowing at the proper level. Acupuncturists have several ways of treating these problems, including the insertion of needles in certain cavities to adjust the flow of Qi.

The Twelve Primary Qi Channels (Shi Er Jing, 十二經)

In this subsection we will briefly review the twelve primary Qi channels. As a Qigong masseur you need to know how the Qi in each channel and related organ can be affected by the seasons, the weather, emotions, and food. Table 2-1 offers you a guideline to these relationships.

You should also know the organ's Yin and Yang. In our body, as mentioned, there are six Yang organs and six Yin organs. Each Yang organ is associated with a Yin organ by a special Yin/Yang relationship. Paired Yin and Yang organs belong to the same phase in the Five Phases. Their channels are sequential to each other in the circulation of Qi, their functions are closely related, and disease in one usually affects the other. In Chinese medicine, the channel corresponding to the Yang organ is often used to treat disorders of its related Yin organ.

In the limbs, the Yang channels are on the external side of the limbs while the Yin channels are on the internal side. Generally speaking, the external sides of the limbs are more Yang and are more resistant and prepared for an attack, while the internal sides are more Yin and weaker.

The organs are further subdivided in order to distinguish the different levels of the Yin/Yang characteristics. The Yang organs are divided into Greater Yang (Taiyang, 太陽), Lesser Yang (Shaoyang, 少陽), and Yang Brightness (Yangming, 陽明). The Yin organs are divided into Greater Yin (Taiyin, 太陰), Lesser Yin (Shaoyin, 少陰), and Absolute Yin (Jueyin, 厥陰). In the following discussion, all of the classifications will be shown in the title, for example: the Lung Channel of Hand—Greater Yin.

1. The Lung Channel of Hand—Greater Yin (Figure 2-13)
(*Shou Taiyin Fei Jing,* 手太陰肺經)

Course:

Course #1:

(1). Stomach (Zhong Jiao, 中焦; middle triple burner)—(2). Large intestine—(3). Diaphragm—(4). Lung—(5). Throat—(6). Upper Arm—(7). Mid-Elbow—(8). Forearm—(9). Wrist—(10). Thenar—(11). Pollex (Shaoshang, L-11, 少商).

Course #2:

(12). Above the styloid process at the wrist—(13). Index Finger (Shangyang, LI-1, 商陽).

Related Viscera:

Lung (Pertaining Organ), large intestine, stomach, and kidney.

Cavities:

Zhongfu (L-1) (中府), Yunmen (L-2) (雲門), Tianfu (L-3) (天府), Xiabai (L-4) (俠白), Chize (L-5) (尺澤), Kongzui (L-6) (孔最), Lieque (L-7) (列缺), Jingqu (L-8) (經渠), Taiyuan (L-9) (太淵), Yuji (L-10) (魚際), and Shaoshang (L-11) (少商).

- Points Belonging to Channels
△ Points of Intersection
----- Connecting Lines
———— Primary Channels on Which There are Points
------ Primary Channels and Branches without Points

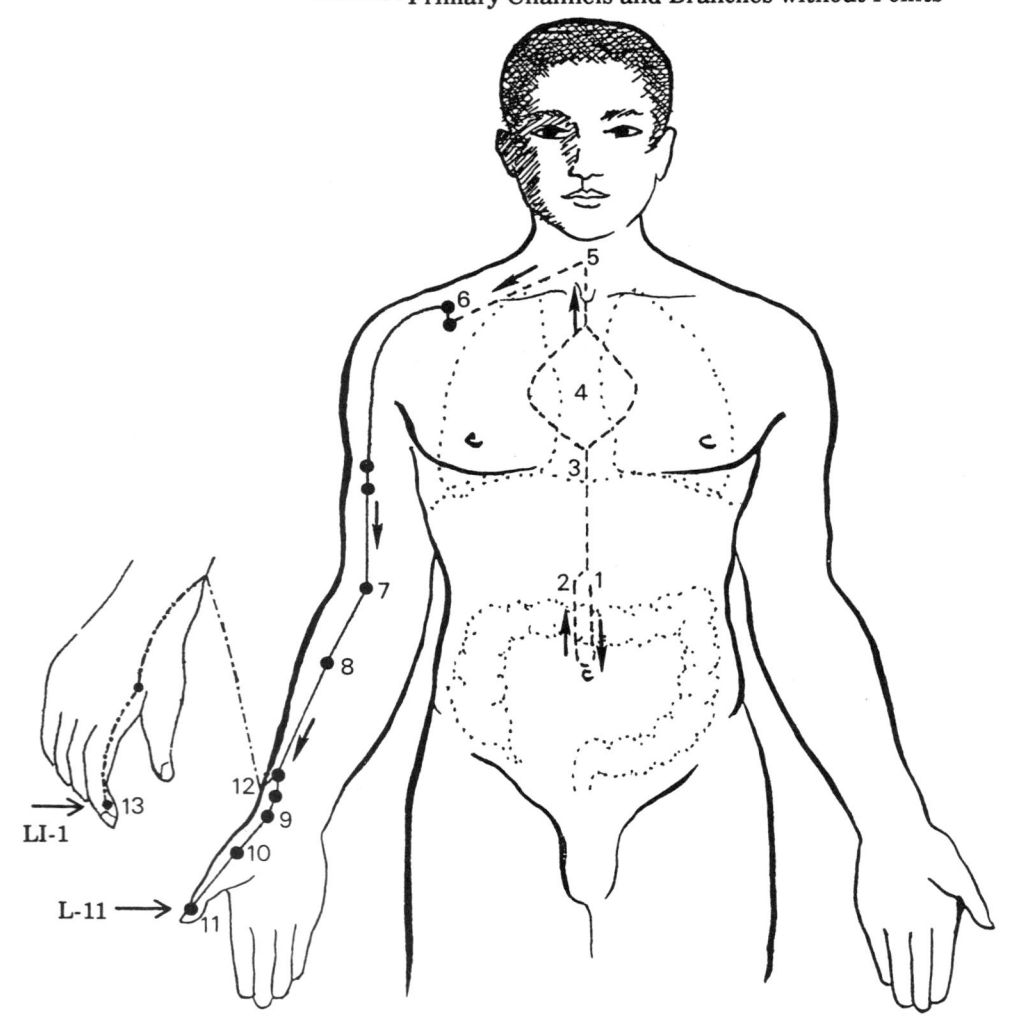

FIGURE 2-13. THE LUNG CHANNEL OF THE HAND-GREATER YIN.

Discussion:

The lungs (Yin) and the large intestine (Yang) are considered paired organs. From Table 2-1 you can see that they belong to Metal (Jin, 金) in the Five Phases (Wu Xing, 五行), the westerly direction, the season of autumn, the dry climatic condition, the color white, the pungent taste, the rank odor, the emotion of sadness, and the sound of weeping. Their opening is the nose, and they govern skin and hair.

In Qigong practice, since the lungs belong to Metal, they are able to regulate heartburn. The heart belongs to Fire (Huo, 火). Whenever the heart has excess Qi, deep breathing is able to lead the heart's fire to the lungs, and therefore cool the heartburn. When the weather is changing from damp, hot summer into dry and cool autumn, lungs are the first organ to sense the change. If your lungs are not able to readjust themselves to fit the new situation smoothly, you will catch a cold. The lungs access the outside world through your nose. The lungs are responsible for taking Qi from the air, and for the energy (Qi) state of the body.

Breathing is considered a strategy for leading Qi to the extremities such as skin and hair. When your breathing is regulated properly, you are able to strengthen your body's Guardian Qi (Wei Qi, 衛氣) and generate an expansive Qi shield to protect your body. You are also able to raise or lower your Qi state through your breathing. For example, when you are angry, deep breathing is able to calm your excited Qi state.

The lungs are sensitive to emotional changes, especially when you are sad or angry. They also control that part of the liquid metabolism which distributes liquid to the skin.

Because the lungs are usually the first to be attacked by exogenous diseases, they are called the Delicate Organ. These diseases can also cause what is called the Non-Spreading of the Lung Qi. The main symptom of a problem with the lungs is coughing, which is a form of Rebellious Qi (since the lung Qi normally flows downward). If coughing is also accompanied by lassitude, shortness of breath, light foamy phlegm, and weakness in the voice, it is called Deficient Lung Qi. However, if the cough is a dry one, with little phlegm, a parched throat and mouth, and Deficient Yin symptoms (such as night sweating, low grade fever, red cheeks, etc.), the condition is referred as Deficient Lung Yin.

2. The Large Intestine Channel of Hand—Yang Brightness (Figure 2-14) (Shou Yangming Da Chang Jing, 手陽明大腸經)

Course:

Course #1:

(1). Index finger (Shangyang, LI-1, 商陽)—(2). Wrist—(3). Elbow—(4). Shoulder Joint—(5). Governing vessel at Dazhui (Gv-14) (大椎)—(6). Supraclavicular Fossa (Quepen, S-12, 缺盆)—(7). Lung—(8). Diaphragm—(9). Large intestine.

Course #2:

(6). Supraclavicular Fossa—(10). Neck—(11). Cheek—(12). Lower Gum—(13). Renzhong (Gv-26) (人中)—(14). Side of the nose (Yingxiang. LI-20, 迎香).

Related Viscera:

Large intestine (Pertaining Organ), lung, and stomach.

Cavities:

Shangyang (LI-1) (商陽), Erjian (LI-2) (二間), Sanjian (LI-3) (三間), Hegu (LI-4) (合谷), Yangxi (LI-5) (陽溪), Pianli (LI-6) (偏歷), Wenliu (LI-7) (溫溜), Xialian (LI-8) (下廉), Shanglian (LI-9) (上廉), Shousanli (LI-10) (手三里), Quchi (LI-11) (曲池),

Qigong Massage

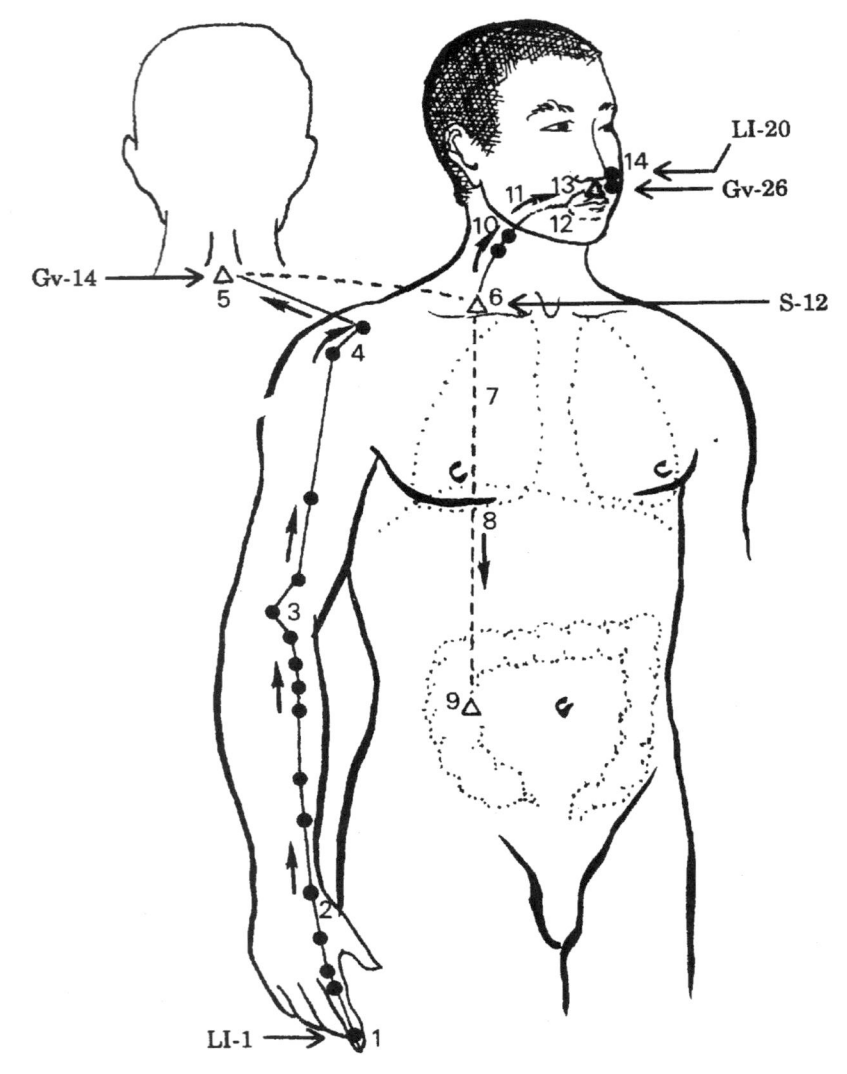

FIGURE 2-14. THE LARGE INTESTINE CHANNEL OF THE HAND-YANG BRIGHTNESS.

Zhouliao (LI-12) (肘髎), Hand-Wuli (LI-13) (手五里), Binao (LI-14) (臂臑), Jianyu (LI-15) (肩髃), Jugu (LI-16) (巨骨), Tianding (LI-17) (天鼎), Futu (LI-18) (扶突), Heliao (LI-19) (禾髎), and Yingxiang (LI-20) (迎香).

Discussion:

The lungs (Yin) and the large intestine (Yang) are considered paired organs. From Table 2-1 you can see that they belong to Metal (Jin, 金) in the Five Phases (Wu Xing, 五行), the westerly direction, the season of autumn, the dry climatic condition, the color white, the pungent taste, the rank odor, the emotion of sadness, and the sound of weeping. Their opening is the nose, and they govern skin and hair.

The main function of the large intestine is the metabolism of water and the passing of water. It extracts water from the waste material received from the small intestine, sends it on to the urinary bladder, and excretes the solid material as stool. Many disorders affecting this organ are categorized as spleen and stomach patterns. Certain abdominal pains are considered manifestations of a blockage of Qi or blood in the large intestine.

In Qigong, the Dan Tian in the lower abdomen is considered the residence of Original Qi (Yuan Qi, 元氣). In order to keep this Qi at its residence, this area must be strong and healthy. The Qi circulating around the intestines must not be stagnant. When you practice Qigong you must learn how to regulate your breathing to smooth the Qi flow in the large intestine and the lungs. This will allow you to relax the front of your body and regulate the Qi flow in the other organs.

3. The Stomach Channel of Foot—Yang Brightness (Figure 2-15)
(Zu Yangming Wei Jing, 足陽明胃經)

Course:

Course #1:

(1). Sides of the nose (Yingxiang, LI-20, 迎香)—(2). Root of the nose—(3). Lateral side of the nose—(4). Upper gum—(5). Renzhong (Gv-26) (人中)—(6). Chengjiang (Co-24) (承漿)—(7). Daying (S-5) (大迎)—(8). Jiache (S-6) (頰車)—(9). Ear—(10). Hair line—(ii). Shenting (Gv-24) (神庭).

Course #2:

(7). Daying (S-5) (大迎)—(12). Renying (S-9) (人迎)—(13). Throat—(14). Into the chest—(15). Through the diaphragm to Zhongwan (Co-12) (中脘).

Course #3:

(16). Infraclavicular Fossa—(17). Along the sides of the umbilicus—(18). Qichong (S-30) (氣沖)—(19). Biguan (S-31) (髀關)—(20). Futu (S-32) (伏兔)—(21). Dubi (S-35) (犢鼻)—(22). Lateral side of tibia—(23). Dorsal aspect of the foot—(24). Lateral side of the tip of the second toe (Lidui, S-45) (厲兌).

Course #4:

(25). Below the knee—(26). Lateral side of the middle toe.

Course #5:

(27). Dorsum of the foot (Chongyang, S-42, 沖陽)—(28). Along the medial margin of the hallus and emerges out at its tip (Yinbai, Sp-1, 隱白).

Related Viscera:

Stomach (Pertaining Organ), spleen, heart, small intestine, and large intestine.

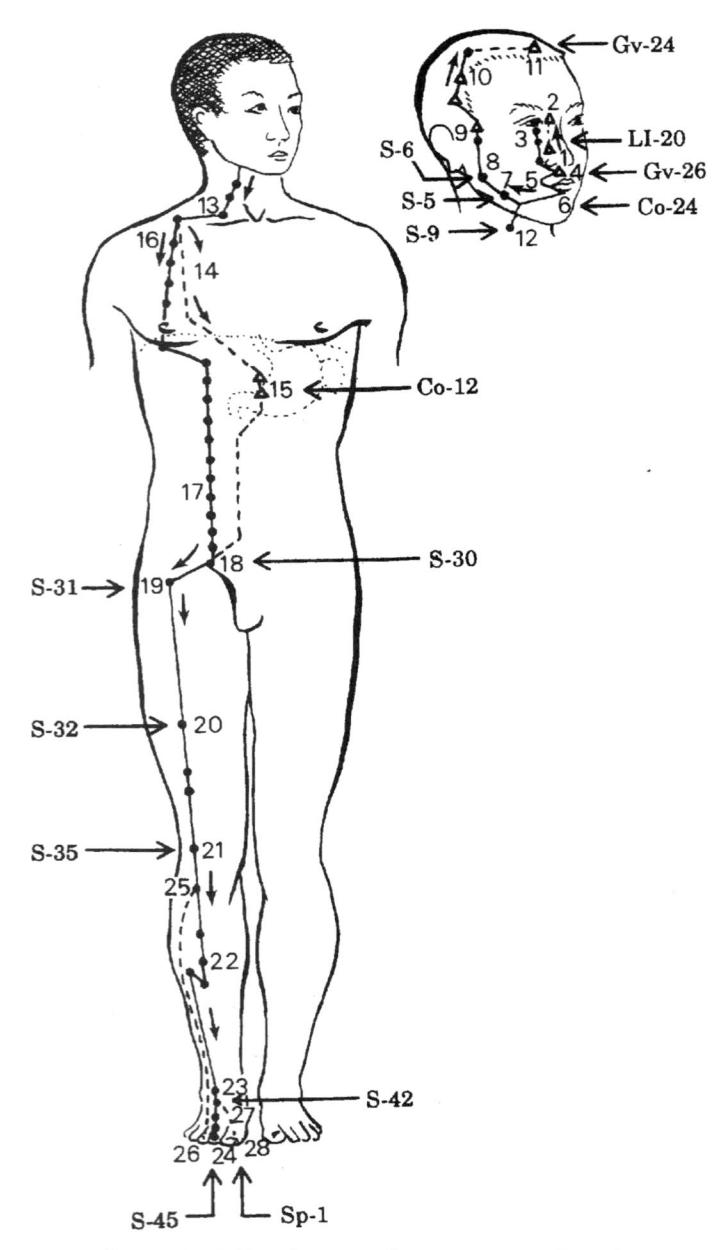

FIGURE 2-15. THE STOMACH CHANNEL OF THE FOOT-YANG BRIGHTNESS.

Cavities:

Chengqi (S-1) (承泣), Sibai (S-2) (四白), Juliao (S-3) (巨髎), Dicang (S-4) (地倉), Daying (S-5) (大迎), Jiache (S-6) (頰車), Xiaguan (S-7) (下關), Touwei (S-8) (頭維), Renying (S-9) (人迎), Shuitu (S-10) (水突), Qishe (S-11) (氣舍), Quepen (S-12) (缺盆), Qihu (S-13) (氣戶), Kufang (S-14) (庫房), Wuyi (S-15) (屋翳), Yingchuang (S-16) (膺窗), Ruzhong (S-17) (乳中), Rugen (S-18) (乳根), Burong (S-19) (不容), Chengman (S-20) (承滿), Liangmen (S-21) (梁門), Guanmen (S-22) (關門), Taiyi (S-23) (太乙), Huaroumen (S-24) (滑肉門), Tianshu (S-25) (天樞), Wailing (S-26) (外陵), Daju (S-27) (大巨), Shuidao (S-28) (水道), Guilai (S-29) (歸來), Qichong (S-30) (氣沖), Biguan (S-31) (髀關), Futu (S-32) (伏兔), Yinshi (S-33) (陰市), Liangqiu (S-34) (梁丘), Dubi (S-35) (犢鼻), Zusanli (S-36) (足三里), Shangjuxu (S-37) (上巨虛), Tiaokou (S-38) (條口), Xiajuxu (S-39) (下巨虛), Fenglong (S-40) (豐隆), Jiexi (S-41) (解溪), Chongyang (S-42) (沖陽), Xiangu (S-43) (陷谷), Neiting (S-44) (內庭), Lidui (S-45) (歷兌).

Discussion:

The spleen (Yin) and the stomach (Yang) are paired organs. They belong to Earth (Tu, 土) in the Five Phases (Wu Xing, 五行), the center, the season of long summer (the end of summer), the climatic condition of dampness, the color yellow, the emotion of pensiveness, the taste of sweetness, fragrant odor, and the sound of singing. Their opening is the mouth and they control the flesh and the limbs.

The Yin/Yang relationship between the spleen and the stomach is a particularly strong example of the relationship between organs. The stomach receives food while the spleen transports nutrients. The stomach moves things downward while the spleen moves things upward. The stomach likes dampness while the spleen likes dryness.

Though there are some patterns relating to deficiency of the stomach (many of these originate in the spleen), most stomach disorders are caused from excess. Stomach Fire gives a painful, burning sensation in the stomach, unusual hunger, bleeding of the gums, constipation, and halitosis.

Once saliva has begun the process of digestion, food passes to the stomach, located in the Middle Sanjiao (Zhongjiao, 中焦) (middle triple burner) area. The stomach breaks down the food, and then passes it on to the intestines, where the essence is absorbed and converted into Qi, and circulated through the entire body.

The stomach is related to the emotion of pensiveness. When you are upset, the stomach will not function normally. In Qigong, regulating the mind is the first step to maintaining the stomach in a healthy condition. The type of food you eat is the second consideration. The proper amount and quality of food will help you to obtain high quality Qi to circulate in your body.

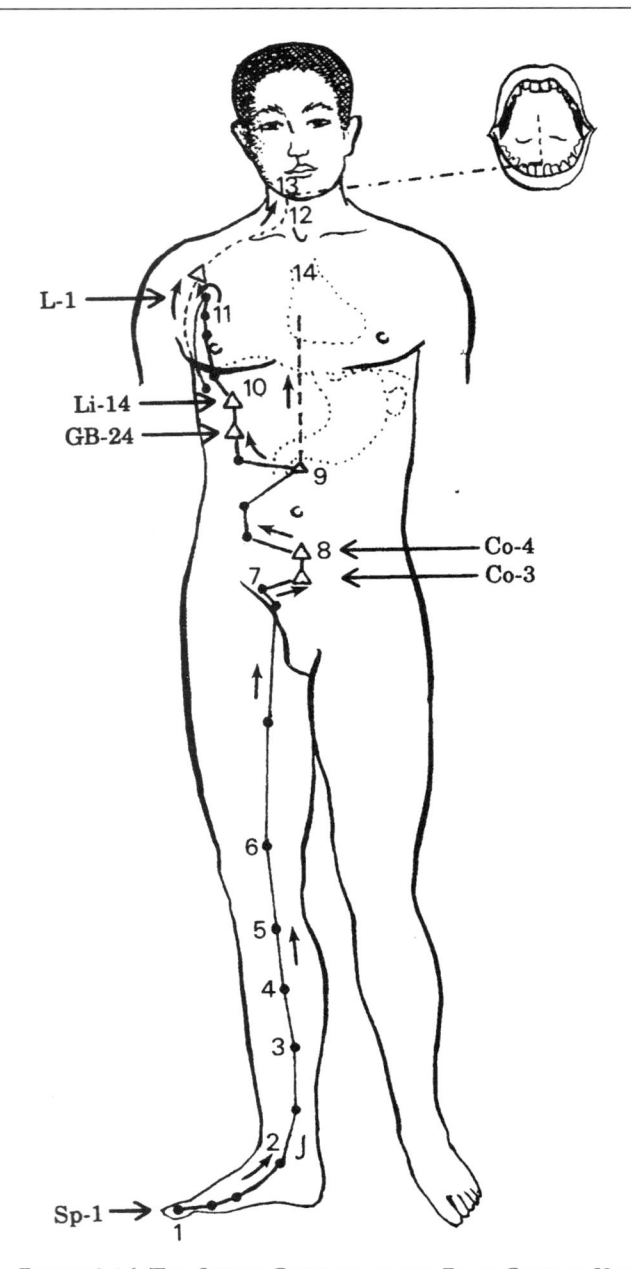

FIGURE 2-16. THE SPLEEN CHANNEL OF THE FOOT-GREATER YIN.

4. The Spleen Channel of Foot—Greater Yin (Figure 2-16) (Zu Taiyin Pi Jing, 足太陰脾經)

Course:

Course #1:
(1). Medial tip of the big toe (Yinbai, Sp-1) (隱白)—(2). Anterior border of the

medial malleolus—(3). Along the posterior border of the tibia—(4). Medial aspect of the leg—(5). Medial aspect of the art. genus—(6). Anterior medial aspect of the thigh—(7). Enter the abdomen—(8). Zhongji (Co-3) (中極) and Guanyuan (Co-4) (關元)—(9). Pertains to the spleen and communicates with the stomach—(10). Riyue (GB-24) (日月) and Qimen (Li-14) (期門)—(11). Penetrates the diaphragm through Zhongfu (L-1) (中府)—(12). Throat—(13). Root of the tongue.

Course #2:

(9). Stomach—(14). Through the diaphragm and disperses into the heart.

Related Viscera:

Spleen (Pertaining Organ), stomach, heart, lung, and intestines.

Cavities:

Yinbai (Sp-1) (隱白), Dadu (Sp-2) (大都), Taibai (Sp-3) (太白), Gongsun (Sp-4) (公孫), Shangqiu (Sp-5) (商丘), Sanyinjiao (Sp-6) (三陰交), Lougu (Sp-7) (漏谷), Diji (Sp-8) (地機), Yinlingquan (Sp-9) (陰陵泉), Xuehai (Sp-10) (血海), Jimen (Sp-11) (箕門), Chongmen (Sp-12) (沖門), Fushe (Sp-l3) (府舍), Fujie (Sp-14) (腹結), Daheng (Sp-15) (大橫), Fuai (Sp-16) (腹哀), Shidou (Sp-17) (食竇), Tianxi (Sp-18) (天溪), Xiongxiang (Sp-19) (胸鄉), Zhourong (Sp-20) (周榮), Dabao (Sp-21) (大包).

Discussion:

The spleen (Yin) and the stomach (Yang) are paired organs. They belong to Earth (Tu, 土) in the Five Phases (Wu Xing, 五行), the central direction, the season of long summer (the end of summer), the climatic condition of dampness, the color yellow, the emotion of pensiveness, the taste of sweetness, fragrant odor, and the sound of singing. Their opening is the mouth and they control the flesh and the limbs.

The spleen is the main organ of digestion. Its function is to transport nutrients and regulate the blood (regulate means to keep it within the channels). It is responsible for the transformation of food into nourishment.

When the spleen is weak, the body will not be able to use the nourishment available in food. This will cause general lassitude, fatigue, and a pasty complexion. The upper abdomen is considered the province of the spleen. Deficient spleen Qi is shown by a sense of malaise or fullness in that area. Because it is required that the transportive function of the spleen distribute its Qi upward, weakness in the spleen will usually cause diarrhea. Spleen Qi is also regarded as the Middle Qi, and it is responsible for holding the viscera in place. Insufficiency of the Middle Qi will presage prolapsed stomach, kidneys, etc. In more serious cases, the spleen Yang Qi will be deficient, which is manifested in diarrhea, cold limbs, and abdominal pain that can be soothed by the warmth of frequent hot drinks.

If any of the above symptoms are accompanied by bleeding, especially from the digestive tract or uterus, it is called 'Spleen Not Controlling the Blood.'

Qigong Massage

Cold and Dampness Harassing the Spleen is a manifestation characterized by a pent-up feeling in the chest and a bloated sensation in the abdomen, lassitude, lack of appetite and taste, a feeling of cold in the limbs, a dark yellowish hue to the skin, some edema and diarrhea or watery stool. The cold and dampness prevent the spleen from performing its transforming and transporting functions. This leads to a great disturbance in water metabolism and is one of the origins of Phlegm.

In Qigong training, one of the final goals is to regulate the Qi flow to its original (normal) level in the five Yin organs. Among them, the spleen is the last and the hardest organ to regulate. It is believed that if you are able to regulate the Qi in your spleen to a normal and healthy level, you will have grasped the key to health and longevity.

5. The Heart Channel of Hand—Lesser Yin (Figure 2-17)
(Shou Shaoyin Xin Jing, 手少陰心經)

Course:

Course #1:

(1). Heart—(2). Lung—(3). Below the axilla—(4). Upper arm—(5). Antecubital fossa—(6). Between ossa metacarpal IV and V—(7). Tip of the little finger (Shaochong, H-9, 少沖).

Course #2:

(1). Heart—(8). Diaphragm—(9). Small intestine.

Course #3:

(1). Heart—(10). Throat—(11). Tissues surrounding the eye (orbital system).

Related Viscera:

Heart (Pertaining Organ), small intestine, lung, and kidney.

Cavities:

Jiquan (H-1) (極泉), Qingling (H-2) (青靈), Shaohai (H-3) (少海), Lingdao (H-4) (靈道), Tongli (H-5) (通里), Yinxi (H-6) 陰郄), Shenmen (H-7) (神門), Shaofu (H-8) (少府), Shaochong (H-9) (少沖).

Discussion:

The heart and the small intestine are paired organs. The heart is considered Yin, and the small intestine is considered Yang, balancing this paired channel. These two organs correspond to Fire (Huo, 火) in the Five Phases (Wu Xing, 五行), the southerly direction, the summer season, the climatic condition of heat, the color red, the emotion of happiness, the sound of laughter, the taste of bitterness, and the odor of burning. Their point of entry is the tongue, they control the blood vessels and are reflected in the face.

Almost all of the problems and disorders of the heart are associated with weakness. The four major types of heart weakness are Deficient Heart Qi, Deficient Heart Yang, Deficient Heart Blood, and Deficient Heart Yin.

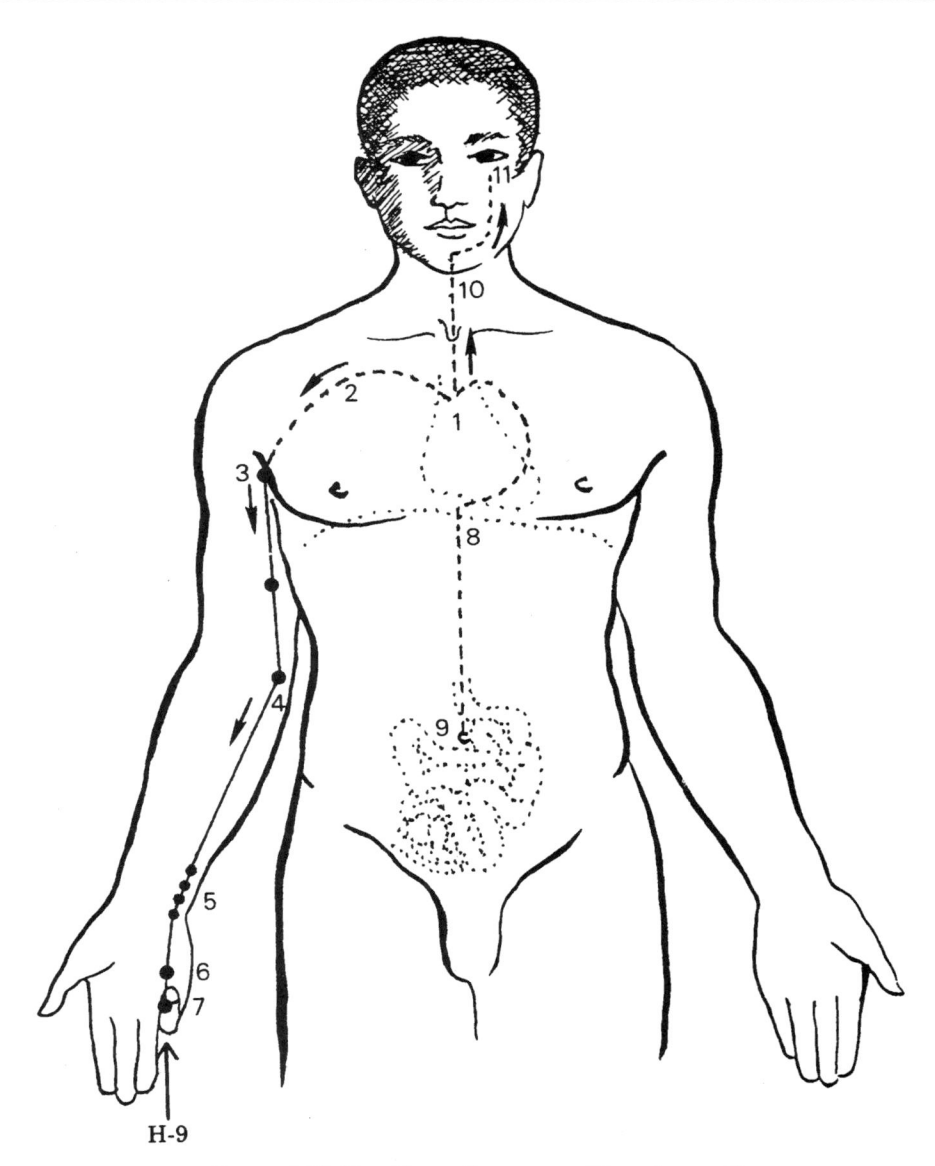

FIGURE 2-17. THE HEART CHANNEL OF HAND LESSER YIN.

The main functions of the heart are associated with the spirit and the blood vessels. The heart governs the blood vessels and is responsible for moving blood through them. It also stores the spirit, and is the organ usually associated with mental processes. Therefore, some forms of emotional distress, dizziness, palpitations, shortness of breath, and lack of vitality are common symptoms of heart ailments. Deficient Heart Qi is symbolized by general lassitude, panting and shallow breathing, and frequent sweating. If the face is swollen and ashen gray or bluish-green, and the limbs are cold, it is called

Deficient Heart Yang. The symptoms of restlessness, irritability, dizziness, absentmindedness, and insomnia are typical signs of Deficient Heart Blood. In Deficient Heart Yin cases, developments with a flushed feeling in the palms and face, low grade fever, and night sweating will occur.

The symptom of Heart Excess arises from an excess of Heart Fire. This is manifested by fever, occasionally accompanied by delirium, a racking pulse, intense restlessness, insomnia or frequent nightmares, a bright red face, a red or blistered and painful tongue, and often a burning sensation during urination. The latter symptom is the result of Heat being transferred from the heart to the small intestine, which interferes with the small intestine's role in metabolism and the body's management of water.

In Qigong society, it is believed that the mind is associated with the heart, and that it is also directly related to the spirit. The term heart (Xin, 心) is usually used to represent the emotional mind or ideas. The Middle Dan Tian (Zhong Dan Tian, 中丹田) at the solar plexus is considered the residence of the Fire Qi. This Fire is used to nourish the brain and the spirit (Shen, 神) at its residence, the Upper Dan Tian (Shang Dan Tian, 上丹田) or third eye. In Chinese medicine it is said that the heart is the temple of the spirit because it supplies Fire Qi and can nourish the spirit without limit.

Generally speaking, the heart is very sensitive during the summertime. The heart is a Yin channel, and when the summer Yang comes it can increase the heart's Qi level and cause problems. Emotional disturbances, such as excitement from happiness, are considered harmful to the heart as well, especially during the summertime. Qigong emphasizes regulating the heart in the summer.

6. The Small Intestine Channel of Hand—Greater Yang (Figure 2-18) (Shou Taiyang Xiao Chang Jing, 手太陽小腸經)

Course:

Course #1:

(1). Tip of the digitus minimus (Shaoze, SI-1, 少澤)—(2). Wrist—(3). Top of elbow—(4). Dorsal surface of the upper arm—(5). Shoulder—(6). Circle around the superior and inferior fossa of the scapula—(7). Meets Dazhui (Gv-14) (大椎)—(8). Enters the supraclavicular fossa—(9). Heart—(10). Passes along the esophagus—(11). Diaphragm—(12). Stomach—(13). Small intestine.

Course #2:

(8). Supraclavicular fossa—(14). Neck—(15). Cheek—(16). Tongziliao (GB-1) (瞳子髎)—(17). Into the ear.

Course #3:

(18). Cheek—(19). Jingming (B-1)—(20). Distributes over zygoma obliquely.

Related Viscera:

Small intestine (Pertaining Organ), heart, and stomach.

Chapter 2: General Foundations

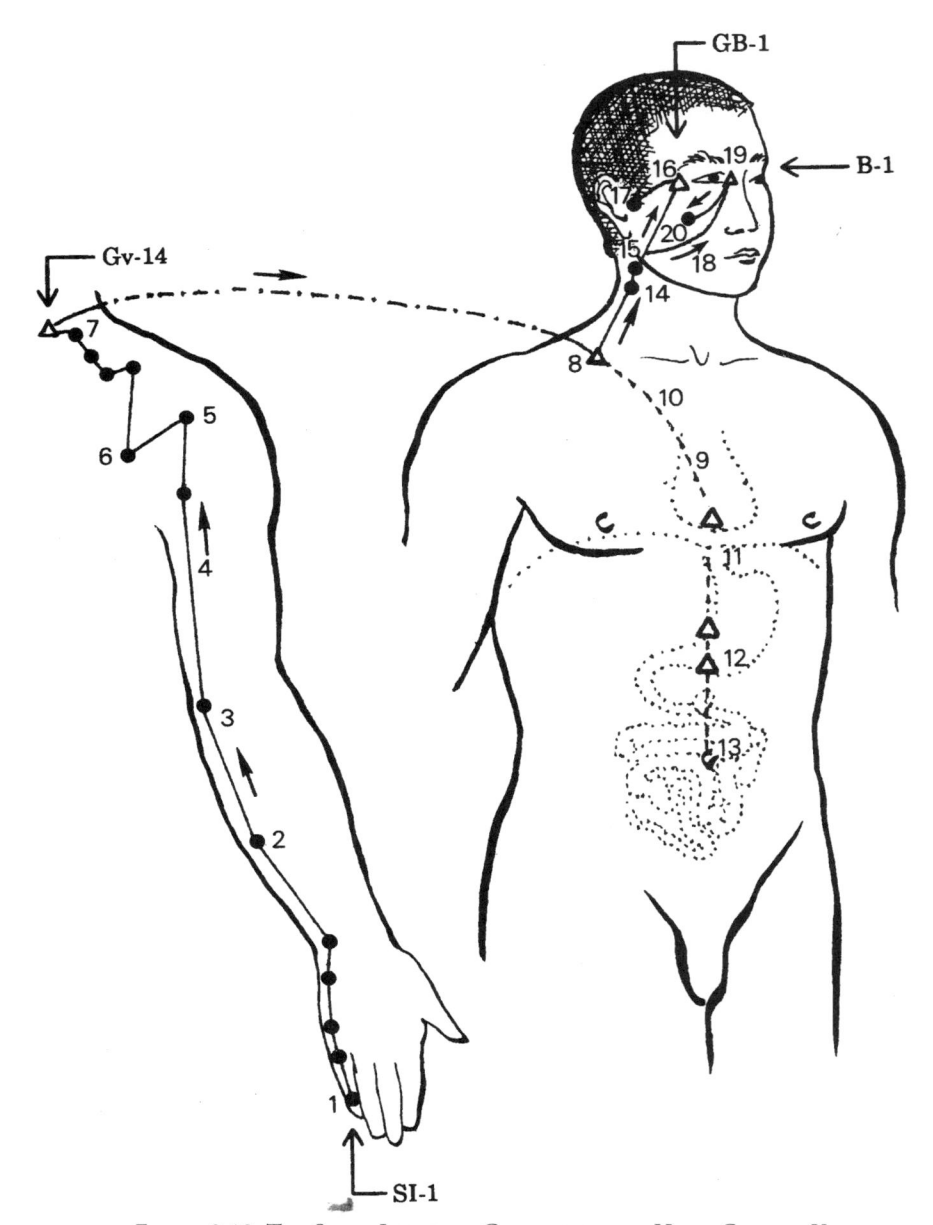

FIGURE 2-18. THE SMALL INTESTINE CHANNEL OF THE HAND-GREATER YANG.

Cavities:

Shaoze (SI-1) (少澤), Qiangu (SI-2) (前谷), Houxi (SI-3) (后溪), Hand-Wangu (SI-4) (腕骨), Yanggu (SI-5) (陽谷), Yanglao (SI-6) (養老), Zhizheng (SI-7) (支正), Xiaohai (SI-8) (小海), Jianzhen (SI-9) (肩貞), Naoshu (SI-10) (臑俞), Tianzong (SI-11) (天宗), Bingfeng (SI-12) (秉風), Quyuan (SI-13) (曲垣), Jianwaishu (SI-14) (肩外俞),

Jianzhongshu (SI-15) (肩中俞), Tianchuang (SI-16) (天窗), Tianrong (SI-17) (天容), Quanliao (SI-18) (顴髎), Tinggong (SI-19) (聽宮).

Discussion:

The heart and the small intestine are paired organs. The heart is considered Yin, and the small intestine is considered Yang, balancing this paired channel. These two organs correspond to Fire (Huo, 火) in the Five Phases (Wu Xing, 五行), the southerly direction, the summer season, the climatic condition of heat, the color red, the emotion of happiness, the sound of laughter, the taste of bitterness, and the odor of burning. Their point of entry is the tongue. They control the blood vessels and are reflected in the face.

The major function of the small intestine is to separate waste material from the nutritious elements in food. The nutritious elements are then distributed throughout the body and the waste is sent on to the large intestine.

The small and large intestines are located in the Lower Dan Tian (Xia Dan Tian, 下丹田). In order to store the Original Qi (Yuan Qi, 元氣) converted from Original Essence (Yuan Jing, 元精), the abdomen must be healthy and the Qi circulation in the area of the intestines must be smooth and natural. The best way to reach this goal is through abdominal breathing exercises. One such exercise is to lead the Original Qi upward following the heart and small intestine Qi channels to cool down the heart fire.

7. The Urinary Bladder Channel of Foot—Greater Yang (Figure 2-19) (Zu Taiyang Pang Guang Jing, 足太陽膀胱經)

Course:

Course #1:
(1). Canthus medial—(2). Shenting (Gv-24) (神庭)—(3). Baihui (Gv-20) (百會).
Course #2:
(3). Baihui (Gv-20) (百會)—(4). Fubai (GB-10) (浮白), Head-Qiaoyin (GB-11) (頭竅陰), and Wangu (Head-Wangu, GB-12) (完骨), etc.
Course #3:
(3). Baihui (Gv-20) (百會)—(5). Naohu (Gv-17) (腦戶)—(6). Neck—(7). Dazhui (Gv-14) (大椎) and Taodao (Gv-13) (陶道)—(8). Lumber region—(9). Kidney—(10). Urinary bladder.
Course #4:
(8). Lumbar region—(11). Crosses the buttock—(12). Popliteal fossa.
Course #5:
(6). Neck—(13). Medial side of the scapula—(14). Lumber region—(15). Lateral side of the thigh—(16). Popliteal fossa—(17). M. gastrocnemius—(18). Pushen (B-61) (仆參)—(19). The lateral side of the tip of the small toe (Zhiyin, B-67) (至陰).

Related Viscera:

Urinary bladder (Pertaining Organ), kidney, brain, and heart.

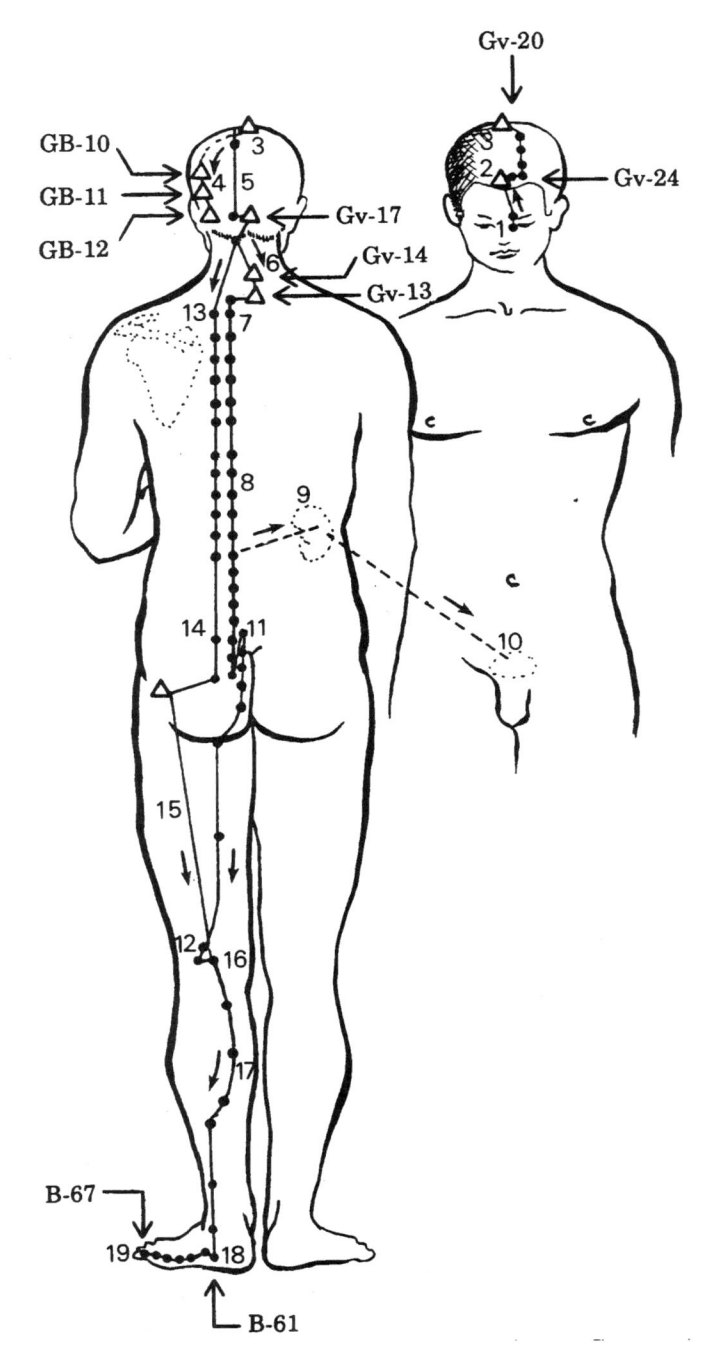

FIGURE 2-19. THE URINARY BLADDER CHANNEL OF THE FOOT-GREATER YANG.

Cavities:

Jingming (B-1) (睛明), Zanzhu (B-2) (攢竹), Meichong (B-3) (眉沖), Quchai (B-4) (曲差), Wuchu (B-5) (五處), Chengguang (B-6) (承光), Tongtian (B-7) (通天), Luoque (B-8) (絡卻), Yuzhen (B-9) (玉枕), Tianzhu (B-10) (天柱), Dazhu (B-11) (大杼), Fengmen (B-12) (風門), Feishu (B-13) (肺俞), Jueyinshu (B-14) (厥陰俞), Xinshu (B-15) (心俞), Dushu (B-16) (督俞), Geshu (B-17) (膈俞), Ganshu (B-18) (肝俞), Danshu (B-19) (膽俞), Pishu (B-20) (脾俞), Weishu (B-21) (胃俞), Sanjiaoshu (B-22) (三焦俞), Shenshu (B-23) (腎俞), Qihaishu (B-24) (氣海俞), Dachangshu (B-25) (大腸俞), Guanyuanshu (B-26) (關元俞), Xiaochangshu (B-27) (小腸俞), Pangguanshu (B-28) (膀胱俞), Zhonglushu (B-29) (中膂俞), Baihuanshu (B-30) (白環俞), Shangliao (B-31) (上髎), Ciliao (B-32) (次髎), Zhongliao (B-33) (中髎), Xialiao (B-34) (下髎), Huiyang (B-35) (會陽), Fufen (B-36) (附分), Pohu (B-37) (魄戶), Gaohuangshu (B-38) (膏肓俞), Shentang (B-39) (神堂), Yixi (B-40) (譩譆), Geguan (B-41) (膈關), Hunmen (B-42) (魂門), Yanggang (B-43) (陽綱), Yishe (B-44) (意舍), Weicang (B-45) (胃倉), Huangmen (B-46) (肓門), Zhishi (B-47) (志室), Baohuang (B-48) (胞肓), Zhibian (B-49) (秩邊), Chengfu (B-50) (承扶), Yinmen (B-51) (殷門), Fuxi (B-52) (浮郄), Weiyang (B-53) (委陽), Weizhong (B-54) (委中), Heyang (B-55) (合陽), Chengjin (B-56) (承筋), Chengshan (B-57) (承山), Feiyang (B-58) (飛揚), Fuyang (B-59) (附陽), Kunlun (B-60) (昆侖), Pushen (B-61) (仆參), Shenmai (B-62) (申脈), Jinmen (B-63) (金門), Jinggu (B-64) (京骨), Shugu (B-65) (束骨), Foot-Tonggu (B-66) (足通谷), and Zhiyin (B-67) (至陰).

Discussion:

The kidneys (Yin) and the urinary bladder (Yang) are paired organs. They correspond to Water (Shui, 水) in the Five Phases (Wu Xing, 五行), the winter season, the cold climatic condition, the northerly direction, the color black, the emotion of fear, the taste of salt, the smell of decay, and the sound of groaning. Their sensory organ is the ear. Their opening is the urethra. They control the bones, marrow, and brain, and their health is reflected in the hair of the head.

The main function of the urinary bladder is to transform fluids into urine and excrete it from the body.

In Qigong, the urinary bladder has never enjoyed serious attention. However, its pairing partner the kidney is one of the most important organs—one with which all Qigong practitioners are concerned and train most often. The reason for this is simply that the kidneys are the residence of the Original Essence (Yuan Jing, 元精).

8. The Kidney Channel of Foot—Lesser Yin (Figure 2-20)
(Zu Shaoyin Shen Jing, 足少陰腎經*)*

Course:

Course #1:

(1). Small toe—(2). Inferior aspect of the navicular tuberosity (Rangu, K-2, 然谷)—(3). Behind the malleolus medialis—(4). Spreads to the heel—(5). M. gastrocnemius—(6). Medial side of the popliteal fossa—(7). Posterior aspect of the thigh—(8). Enters kidney—(9). Communicates with the urinary bladder—(10). Guanyuan (Co-4) (關元) and Zhongji (Co-3) (中極).

Course #2:

(9). Kidney—(11). Liver and diaphragm—(12). Enters the lung—(13). Along the throat—(14). Root of the tongue.

Course #3:

(12). Lung—(15). Heart and spreads to the chest.

Related Viscera:

Kidney (Pertaining Organ), urinary bladder, liver, lung, heart, and other organs.

Cavities:

Yongquan (K-1) (湧泉), Rangu (K-2) (然谷), Taixi (K-3) (太溪), Dazhong (K-4) (大鐘), Shuiquan (K-5) (水泉), Zhaohai (K-6) (照海), Fuliu (K-7) (復溜), Jiaoxin (K-8) (交信), Zhubin (K-9) (築賓), Yingu (K-10) (陰谷), Henggu (K-11) (橫骨), Dahe (K-12) (大赫), Qixue (K-13) (氣穴), Siman (K-14) (四滿), Abdomen-Zhongzhu (K-15) (中注), Huangshu (K-16) (肓俞), Shangqu (K-17) (商曲), Shiguan (K-18) (石關), Yindu (K-19) (陰都), Abdomen-Tonggu (K-20) (腹通谷), Youmen (K-21) (幽門), Bulang (K-22) (步廊), Shenfeng (K-23) (神封), Lingxu (K-24) (靈墟), Shencang (K-25) (神藏), Yuzhong (K-26) (彧中), and Shufu (K-27) (俞府).

Discussion:

The kidneys (Yin) and the urinary bladder (Yang) are paired organs. They correspond to Water (Shui, 水) in the Five Phases (Wu Xing, 五行), the winter season, the cold climatic condition, the northerly direction, the color black, the emotion of fear, the taste of salt, a rotten smell, and the sound of groaning. Their sensory organ is the ear. Their opening is the urethra. They control the bones, marrow, and brain, and their health is reflected in the hair of the head.

The kidneys store Original Essence (Yuan Jing, 元精) and are therefore responsible for growth, development, and reproductive functions. They play the primary role in water metabolism and control the body's liquids, and also hold the body's most fundamental Yin and Yang.

Because the kidneys are the repositories of the basal Yin and Yang of the body, any disorder, if sufficiently chronic, will involve the kidneys. More significantly, a disease of the

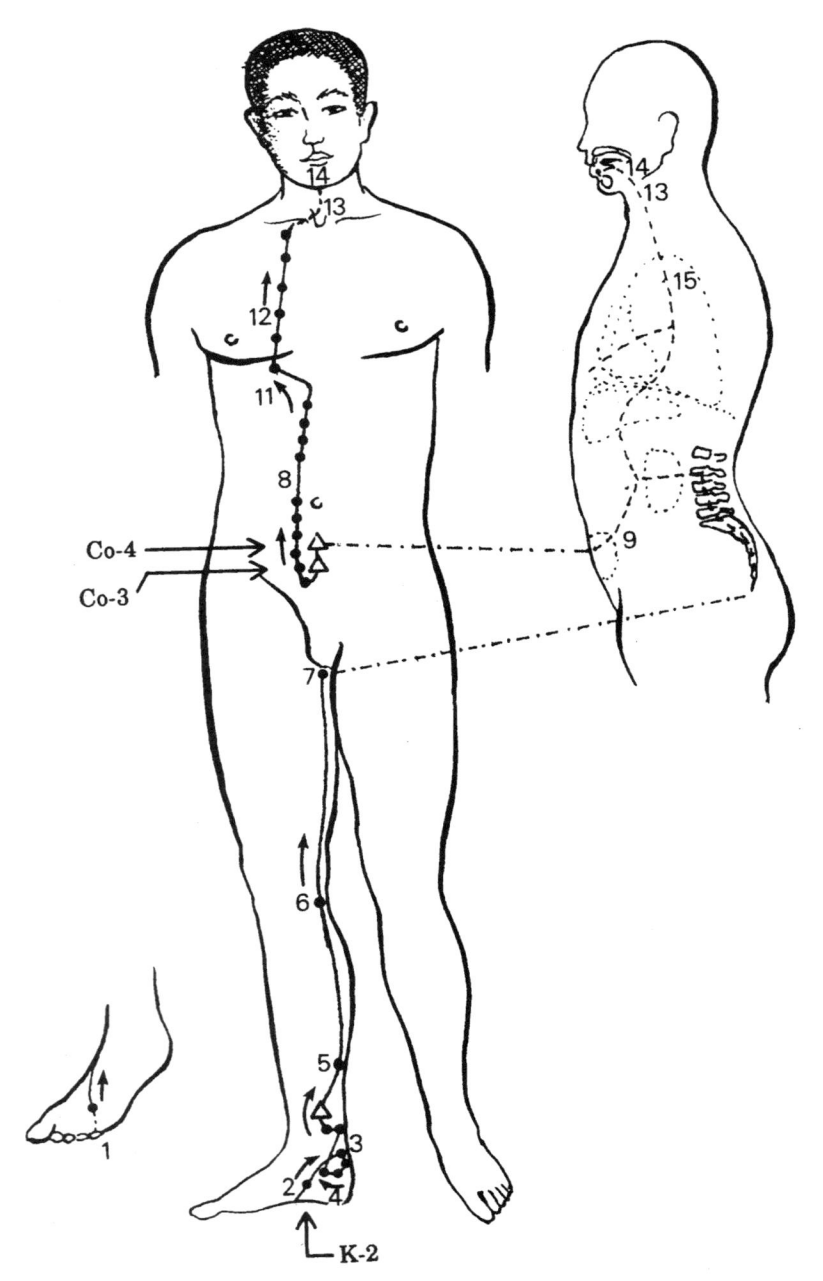

FIGURE 2-20. THE KINDEY CHANNEL OF THE FOOT-LESSER YIN.

kidneys will usually lead to problems in other organs. Methods of strengthening the kidneys are therefore used by both medical and Qigong societies to increase or maintain vitality and health. The symptoms of Deficient Kidney Yang or Yin are typical symptoms of the disorder, and will appear to a certain extent as Deficient Yang or Yin patterns in any organ.

It is easy to understand and memorize the symptoms of Deficient Kidney Yin if one learns the correspondences of the kidneys and remembers that Yin represents the constructive, nourishing, and fluid aspects of the body. Usually, the lower back is weak and sore, there is ringing in the ears and loss of hearing acuity, the face is ashen or dark, especially under the eyes. It is common to feel dizziness and thirst, and to experience night sweats and low grade fevers. In addition, men have little semen and tend toward premature ejaculation, while women have little or no menstruation.

Deficient Kidney Yang symptoms are significantly associated with loss of energy or warmth. Similar to Deficient Kidney Yin, there is commonly ringing in the ears, dizziness, and soreness in the lower back. However, the soreness is characterized by a feeling of coldness, lassitude, and fatigue. Weakness in the legs can be noticed. In men, there is a tendency toward impotence, and in both sexes, clear and voluminous urine or incontinence.

Usually, Deficient Kidney Yin generates similar disorders in the heart and liver, while Deficient Kidney Yang disturbs the functions of the spleen and lungs. The progression could be in the opposite direction. When this pattern is associated with the lungs, it is called 'Kidney Not Receiving Qi,' a type of wheezing characterized by difficult breathing, mainly during inhalation. In addition to the Deficient Kidney Yang symptoms, this condition is also manifested by a faint voice, coughing, puffiness in the face, and spontaneous sweating.

The kidneys perform an important role in the metabolism of water. If these functions are disrupted, the condition of Deficient Kidneys will lead to Spreading Water.

In Qigong practice, essence (Jing, 精) is considered the most original source of human vitality. Qi is converted from essence, and this Qi supplies the entire body and nourishes the brain and spirit. It is believed by both Chinese medical and Qigong societies that the kidneys are the residence of Original Essence (Yuan Jing, 元精). In order to protect your inherent essence, you must strengthen your kidneys. Only when your kidneys are strong will you be able to keep your essence at its residence. Therefore, keeping the kidneys healthy has become one of the most important subjects in Qigong.

Maintaining the kidneys in a healthy state includes protecting the physical kidneys from degeneration, and maintaining a smooth and correct level of Qi flow. In order to reach this goal, the diet must be considered. For example, too much salt is harmful to the kidneys, and eating too much eggplant will weaken the kidneys. In addition, the condition of the body is also important. Such things as overworking without proper rest will increase tension on the kidneys and make the Qi flow stagnant. In winter, the kidneys will have more tension than in summer. Due to this, the Qi flow is more stagnant in the wintertime than in the summertime. Consequently, back pain problems increase in the winter.

In order to protect the kidneys, Qigong practitioners have studied the relationship of the kidneys to nature, food, and even to emotional states. They have developed massage techniques and specific exercises to increase Qi circulation in the kidneys during the winter. Since the health of the kidneys is related to the emotions as well, learning how to regulate the mind in order to regulate the Qi has become one of the major training goals in Qigong.

9. The Pericardium Channel of Hand—Absolute Yin (Figure 2-21) (Shou Jueyin Xin Bao Jing, 手厥陰心包經)

Course:

Course #1:
(1). Pericardium—(2). Below the armpit—(3). Axilla—(4). Forearm—(5). Wrist—(6). Palm—(7). Tip of middle finger (Zhongchong, P-9, 中沖).

Course #2:
(1). Pericardium—(8). Diaphragm—(9). Connects triple burner (Sanjiao, 三焦)

Course #3:
(6). Palm (Laogong, P-8, 勞宮)—(10). Tip of ring finger (Guanchong, TB-1, 關沖).

Related Viscera:

Pericardium (Pertaining Organ) and triple burner (Sanjiao, 三焦).

Cavities:

Tianchi (P-1) (天池), Tianquan (P-2) (天泉), Quze (P-3) (曲澤), Ximen (P-4) (郄門), Jianshi (P-5) (間使), Neiguan (P-6) (內關), Daling (P-7) (大陵), Laogong (P-8) (勞宮), and Zhongchong (P-9) (中沖).

Discussion:

The pericardium (Yin) and the triple burner (Yang) are paired organs. They are said to correspond to the 'Ministerial Fire,' as opposed to the 'Sovereign Fire' of the heart and small intestine. Though the pericardium has no separate physiological functions, it is generally mentioned with regard to the delirium induced by high fevers.

The regulation of Qi in the pericardium is considered a very important subject in Qigong. It is believed that the heart, the most vital organ in your body, must have a proper level of Qi circulation in order to function normally. The Qi level of the heart can be raised easily to an abnormal state by illness, emotional disturbance, exercise, or injury. The function of the pericardium is to dissipate the excess Qi from the heart and direct it to the Laogong (P-8) (勞宮) cavity, located in the center of the palm. From Laogong, the excess Qi will be released naturally and hence, regulate the heart's Qi level. The Laogong cavity is used in Qigong massage to reduce the body's temperature during a fever. You can see that the purpose of the pericardium is to regulate the Qi in the heart through the Laogong cavity.

You should understand that in Qigong it is believed that there are five centers (called gates) where the Qi of the body is able to communicate with the surrounding

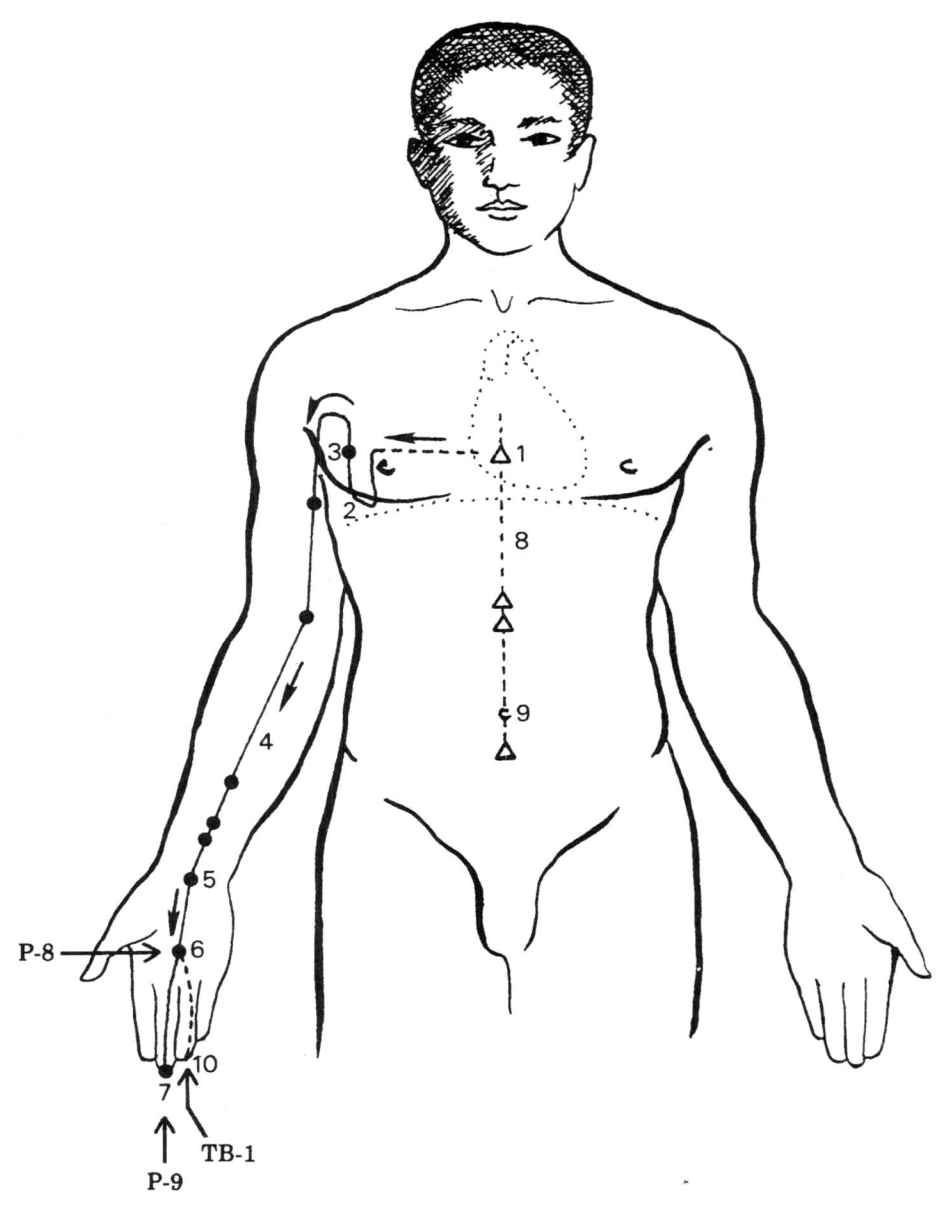

FIGURE 2-21. THE PERICARDIUM CHANNEL OF THE HAND-ABSOLUTE YIN.

environment, and, consequently, regulate the Qi level in your body. Two of these five centers are the Laogong cavities, and two others are the Yongquan (K-1) (湧泉) cavities, used to regulate the Qi in the kidneys. The fifth one is your face or crown. The face is connected and related to many of your organs. Whenever any of your organ Qi is not normal, it shows on your face.

10. The Triple Burner Channel of Hand- Lesser Yang (Figure 2-22) (Shou Shaoyang San Jiao Jing, 手少陽三焦經)

Course:

Course #1:

(1). Tip of the ring finger (Guanchong, TB-1, 關沖)—(2). Between the ossa metacarpal IV and V—(3). Wrist—(4). Dorsal side of the forearm—(5). Passing the olecranon—(6). Lateral aspect of the upper arm—(7). Shoulder—(8). Jianjing (GB-21) (肩井)—(9). Enters the supraclavicular fossa—(10). Branches out in the chest, communicating with the pencardium—(11). Diaphragm—(12). Links successively the upper, middle, and lower portions of the body cavity.

Course #2:

(10). Shanzhong (Co-17) (膻中)—(13). Supraclavicular fossa—(14). Neck—(15). Dazhui (Gv-14) (大椎)—(16). Posterior border of the ear—(17). Xuanli (GB-6) (懸厘) and Hanyan (GB-4) (頷厭)—(18). Quanliao (SI-18) (顴髎).

Course #3:

(19). Retro-auricular region where it enters the ear (20). Emerges in front of the ear—(21). Lateral canthus.

Related Viscera:

It pertains to the upper, middle and lower portions of the body cavity (Sanjiao) and communicates with the pericardium.

Cavities:

Guanchong (TB-1) (關沖), Yemen (TB-2) (液門), Hand-Zhongzhu (TB-3) (手中渚), Yangchi (TB-4) (陽池), Waiguan (TB-5) (外關), Zhigou (TB-6) (支溝), Huizong (TB-7) (會宗), Sanyangluo (TB-8) (三陽絡), Sidu (TB-9) (四瀆), Tianjing (TB-10) (天井), Qinglengyuan (TB-l1) (清冷淵), Xiaoluo (TB-12) (消濼), Naohui (TB-13) (臑會), Jianliao (TB-14) (肩髎), Tianliao (TB-15) (天髎), Tianyou (TB-16) (天牖), Yifeng (TB-17) (翳風), Qimai (TB-18) (瘈脈), Luxi (TB-19) (顱息), Jiaosun (TB-20) (角孫), Ermen (TB-21) (耳門), Ear-Heliao (TB-22) (和髎), and Sizhukong (TB-23) (絲竹空).

Discussion:

At least as far back as the 3rd century A.D., in the *Classic of Difficulties* (*Nan Jing*, 難經) the triple burner was regarded as "having a name but no form." In the *Inner Classic* (*Nei Jing*, 內經), the triple burner was considered an organ that coordinated all the functions of water metabolism. In other traditional documents, the burners were considered three regions of the body that were used to group the organs. The upper burner includes the chest, neck, and head as well as the functions of the heart and lungs. The middle burner is the region between the chest and the navel, and includes the functions of the stomach, liver, and spleen. The lower burner spans the lower abdomen, and

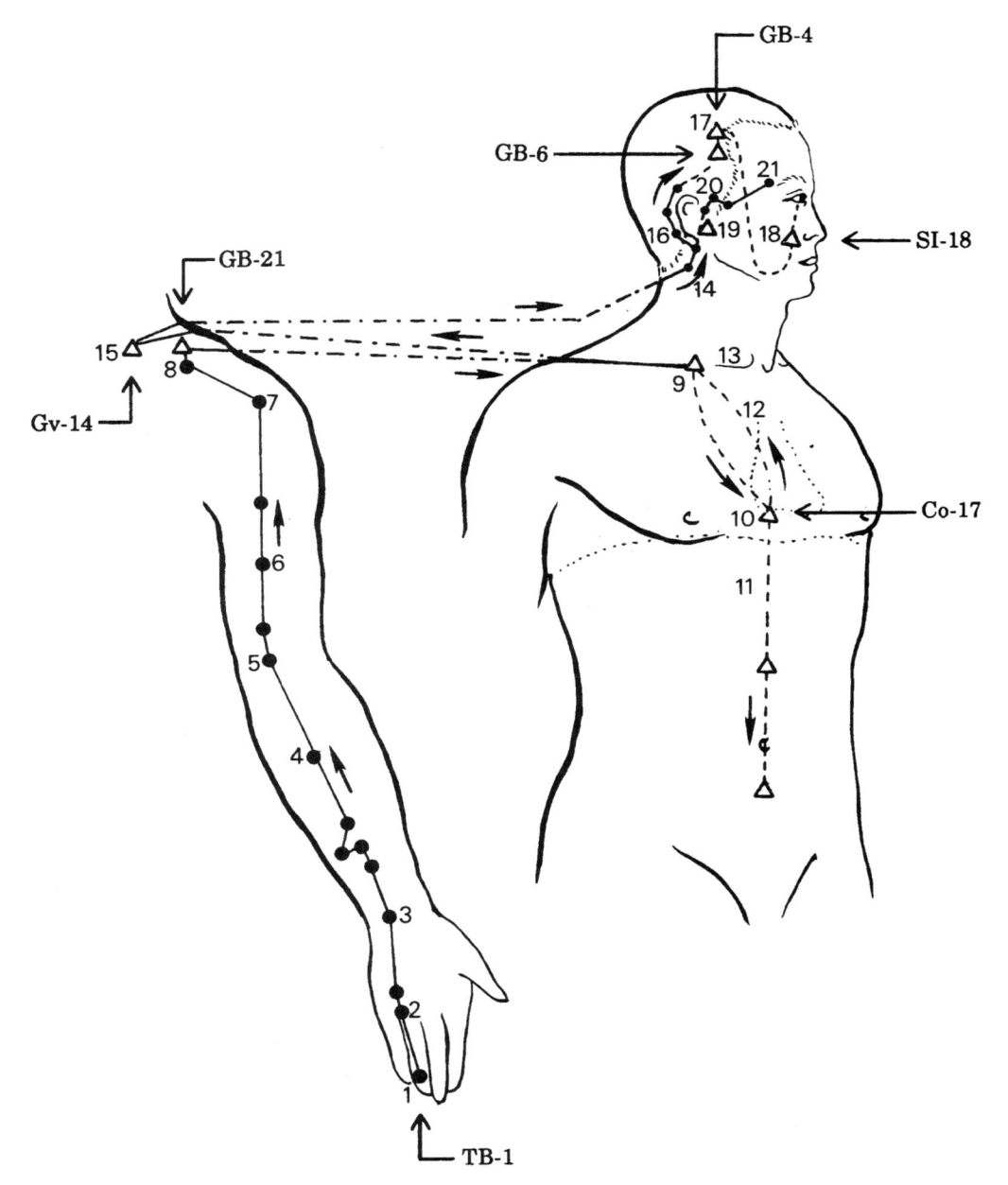

FIGURE 2-22. THE TRIPLE BURNER CHANNEL OF THE HAND-LESSER YANG.

the functions of the kidneys and urinary bladder. Therefore, the upper burner has been compared to a mist which spreads the blood and Qi, the middle burner is like a foam which churns up food in the process of digestion, and the lower burner resembles a swamp where all the impure substances are excreted.

Regulating the Qi to a normally 'smooth-flow' state is one of the main Qigong training methods for maintaining health. It is normally done through Wai Dan (外丹) (i.e. External Elixir) exercises, and it is believed that the Qi must flow around internal organs smoothly in order for them to maintain their normal functions. This means that in order to keep Qi flow smooth and the organs healthy, you must first learn how to regulate and relax muscles that are holding and related to a given organ. External movements also exercise internal muscles. One of the most common external exercises is regulating the triple burner by lifting your hands up above your head and then moving them down slowly. These up and down arm movements extend and relax the internal muscles and thereby increase Qi flow.

11. The Gall Bladder Channel of Foot—Lesser Yang (Figure 2-23) (Zu Shaoyang Dan Jing, 足少陽膽經)

Course:

Course #1:

(1). Outer canthus of the eye (Tongziliao, GB-1, 瞳子髎)—(2). Nose-Heliao (TB-22) (和髎)—(3). Jiaosun (TB-20) (角孫)—(4). Dazhui (Gv-14) (大椎)—(5). Enters the supraclavicular fossa.

Course #2:

(6). Retro-auricular region, passes through Yifeng (TB-17) (翳風)—(7). Tinggong (SI-19) (聽宮) and Xiaguan (S-7) (下關).

Course #3:

(1). Outer canthus of the eye—(8). Daying (S-5) (大迎)—(9). Infraorbital region—(10). Jiache (S-6) (頰車)—(11), Supraclavicular fossa—(12). Into the chest—(13). Tianchi (P-1) (天池)—(14). Communicates with the liver—(15). Pertains to the gall bladder—(16). Inside of the hypochondrium—(17). Around the genitals—(18). Hip (Huantiao, GB-30, 環跳).

Course #4:

(19). Supraclavicular fossa—(20). Axilla—(21). Lateral aspect of the chest—(22). Through the hypochondrium—(23), Zhangmen (Li-13) (章門)—(24) Along the lateral aspect of thigh—(25). Knee—(26). Anterior aspect of the fibula—(27), Anterior aspect of the malleolus—(28) Lateral side of the tip of the 4th toe or Zuqiaoyin (GB-44) (足竅陰).

Course #5:

(29) Dorsum of the foot (Linqi, GB-41, 臨泣)—(30). Big toe (Dadun, Li-1, 大敦).

Related Viscera:

Gall bladder (Pertaining Organ), liven, and heart.

Chapter 2: General Foundations

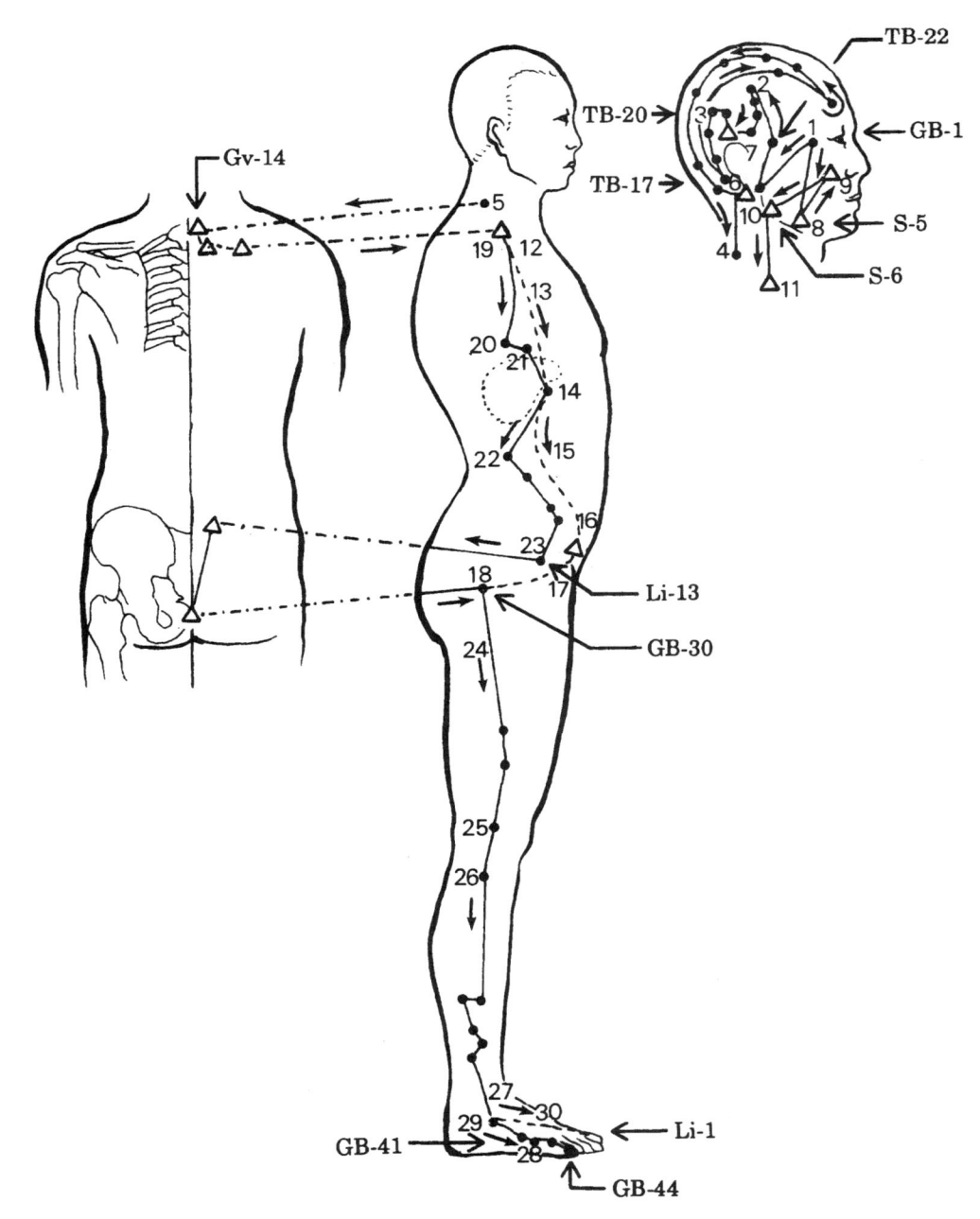

FIGURE 2-23. THE GALL BLADDER CHANNEL OF THE FOOT-LESSER YANG.

Cavities:

Tongziliao (GB-1) (瞳子髎), Tinghui (GB-2) (聽會), Shangguan (GB-3) (上關), Hanyan (GB-4) (頷厭), Xuanlu (GB-5) (懸顱), Xuanli (GB-6) (懸厘), Qubin (GB-7)

73

(曲鬢), Shuaigu (GB-8) (率谷), Tianchong (GB-9) (天沖), Fubai (GB-10) (浮白), Head-Qiaoyin (GB-11) (頭竅陰), Head-Wangu (GB-12) (頭完骨), Benshen (GB-13) (本神), Yangbai (GB-14) (陽白), Head-Linqi (GB-15) (頭臨泣), Muchuang (GB-16) (目窗), Zhengying (GB-17) (正營), Chengling (GB-18) (承靈), Naokong (GB-19) (腦空), Fengchi (GB-20) (風池), Jianjing (GB-21) (肩井), Yuanye (GB-22) (淵液), Zhejin (GB-23) (輒筋), Riyue (GB-24) (日月), Jingmen (GB-25) (京門), Daimai (GB-26) (帶脈), Wushu (GB-27) (五樞), Weidao (GB-28) (維道), Femur-Juliao (GB-29) (居髎), Huantiao (GB-30) (環跳), Fengshi (GB-31) (風市), Femur-Zhongdu (GB-32) (中瀆), Xiyangguan (GB-33) (膝陽關), Yanglingquan (GB-34) (陽陵泉), Yangjiao (GB-35) (陽交), Waiqiu (GB-36) (外丘), Guangming (GB-37) (光明), Yangfu (GB-38) (陽輔), Xuanzhong (GB-39) (懸鐘), Qiuxu (GB-40) (丘墟), Foot-Linqi (GB-41) (足臨泣), Diwuhui (GB-42) (地五會), Xiaxi (GB-43) (俠溪), Foot-Qiaoyin (GB-44) (足竅陰).

Discussion:

The liver (Yin) and the gall bladder (Yang) are paired organs. They correspond to Wood (Mu, 木) in the Five Phases (Wu Xing, 五行), the direction east, the spring season, the climatic wind, the color green, the emotion of anger, the taste of sourness, the goatish odor, and the sound of shouting. Their point of entry is the eyes. They control the sinews (muscles and joints), and their health is reflected in the finger and toe nails.

The main function of the gall bladder is storing and excreting the bile produced by the liver. Together with the heart, the gall bladder is responsible for decision-making.

The main disease related to the gall bladder is a disorder affecting the flow of bile, usually caused by Dampness and Heat. This is commonly manifested by pain in the region of the liver, an oppressive sensation of fullness in the abdomen, and yellowish eyes, skin, urine, and tongue.

The gall bladder has never enjoyed serious attention during Qigong training. Its paired partner the liver however, has received much more attention.

12. The Liver Channel of Foot—Absolute Yin (Figure 2-24) (Zu Jueyin Gan Jing, 足厥陰肝經)

Course:

Course #1:

(1). Behind the nail of the big toe—(2). Malleolus medialis—(3). Sanyinjiao (Sp-6) (三陰交)—(4). Side of shin—(5). Side of knee—(6). Medial aspect of the thigh—(7). Chongmen (Sp-12) (沖門) and Fushe (Sp-13) (府舍)—(8). Pubic region—(9). Lower abdomen—(10). Qugu (Co-2) (曲骨), Zhongji (Co-3) (中極), and Guanyuan (Co-4) (關元)—(11). Liver—(12). Lower chest—(13). Neck posterior—(14). Upper palate—(15). Tissues of the eye—(16). Forehead—(17). Vertex.

Course #2:

(15). Eye—(18). Cheek—(19), Curves around the inner surface of the lips.

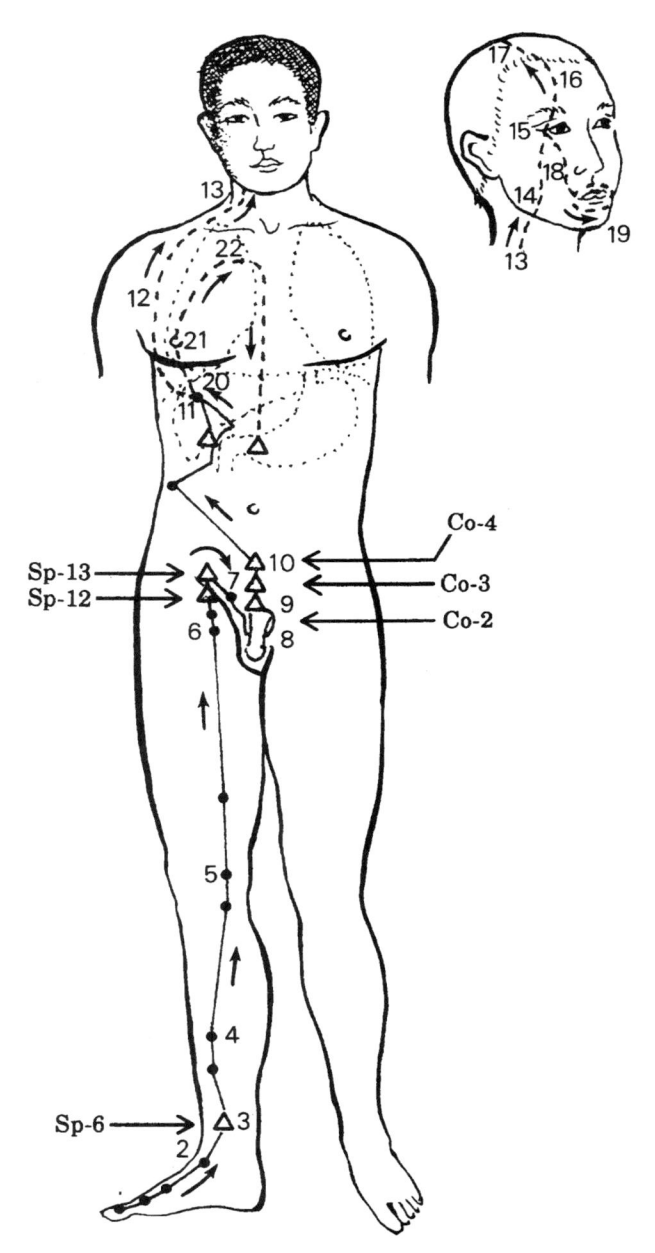

FIGURE 2-24. THE LIVER CHANNEL OF THE FOOT-ABSOLUTE YIN.

Course #3:
(20). Liver—(21). Through diaphragm—(22). Lung.

Related Viscera:

Liver (Pertaining Organ), gall bladder, lung, stomach, and brain.

Cavities:

Dadun (Li-1) (大敦), Xingjian (Li-2) (行間), Taichong (Li-3) (太沖), Zhongfeng (Li-4) (中封), Ligou (Li-5) (蠡溝), Tibia-Zhongdu (Li-6) (中都), Xiguan (Li-7) (膝關), Ququan (Li-8) (曲泉), Yinbao (Li-9) (陰包), Femur-Wuli (Li-10) (足五里), Yinlian (Li-11) (陰廉), Jimai (Li-12) (急脈), Zhangmen (Li-13) (章門), and Qimen (Li-14) (期門).

Discussion:

The liver (Yin) and the gall bladder (Yang) are considered paired organs. They correspond to Wood (Mu, 木) in the Five Phases (Wu Xing, 五行), the direction east, the spring season, the climatic condition of wind, the color green, the emotion of anger, the taste of sourness, the goatish odor, and the sound of shouting. Their point of entry is the eyes. They control the sinews (muscles and joints), and their health is reflected in the finger and toe nails.

The main task of the liver is spreading and regulating Qi throughout the entire body. Its unique character is flowing and free. Therefore, depression or frustration can disturb the functioning of the liver. In addition, the liver is also responsible for storing blood when the body is at rest. This characteristic, together with its control over the lower abdomen, makes it the most critical organ in regards to women's menstrual cycle and sexuality.

Depression or long-term frustration can stagnate the liver's spreading function and result in continuing depression, a bad temper, and a painful, swollen feeling in the chest and sides. If this condition worsens, it may cause disharmony between the liver and the stomach and/or spleen. This disorder is symbolized by the 'rebellion' of Qi in the latter organs, whereby Qi moves in the opposite direction than is normal. For example, the stomach Qi normally descends, so rebellious Qi means hiccoughing, vomiting, etc. In the case of the spleen, the Qi ordinarily moves upward, so rebellious Qi in this organ means diarrhea.

Depression of the liver Qi is the main cause of many women's disorders, including menstrual irregularities, swollen and painful breasts, etc.

One of the most important responsibilities of the liver is the storage of blood with intended emphasis upon nourishing and moistening. Whenever the liver blood is deficient, the liver will not be able to handle the function of moistening. This is generally shown as dry and painful eyes with blurred or weak vision, lack of suppleness or pain in moving the joints, dry skin, dizziness, and infrequent or spotty menstruation. If the Deficient Liver Yin has become serious, the conditions Rising Liver Fire or Hyper Liver Yang Ascending occur. These occurrences are evidenced in ill-temper, restlessness, headache, vertigo, red face and eyes, and a parched mouth. If the liver Yin is so deficient that it is incapable of securing the liver Yang, many of the symptoms appear as disorders of the head. Weakness in the lower joints may also be manifested.

The liver is one of the five Yin organs whose Qi level the Qigong practitioner wants to regulate. Since the liver and the gall bladder are directly connected, when the liver's

Qi is regulated, the Qi circulating in the gall bladder will also be regulated. Many methods have been developed for regulating the liver Qi. Wai Dan Qigong (外丹氣功) works through the limbs. For example, when the arms are moved up and down, the internal muscles surrounding the liver will be moved and the Qi around the liver will be circulated smoothly. In Nei Dan Qigong (內丹氣功), it is believed that the liver is closely related to your mind. It is also believed that when your mind is regulated, the Qi circulation in the liver will be normal and therefore the liver will function properly.

Important Points

1. The spleen, liver, and heart are the organs with the most direct relationship with the blood. The spleen filters the blood (modifying the blood's structure), the liver stores the blood, and the heart moves it. Any problem associated with the blood will involve at least one of these organs.

2. The liver and the kidney are closely related. Their channels cross in many places. The liver stores blood; the kidney stores essence. These substances, both of which are Yin, have a considerable influence on the reproductive functions.

3. The heart (upper burner. Fire) and the kidney (lower burner, Water) keep each other in check and are dependent upon one another. The spirit of the heart and the essence of the kidneys cooperate in establishing and maintaining human consciousness.

4. The spleen's digestive function is associated with the distributive functions of the liver. Disharmony between these two results in various digestive troubles. The transportive and digestive functions of the spleen (also called the Middle Qi) depend upon the strength of the kidney Yang.

5. Although the lungs govern Qi, Qi from the lungs must mix with essence from the kidneys before Original Qi can be produced. The lungs govern Qi, the liver spreads Qi, and the kidneys provide its basis.

The Eight Extraordinary Qi Vessels (Ba Mai, 八脈)

The eight extraordinary Qi vessels and the twelve primary Qi channels (meridians) comprise the main part of the channel system. Most of the eight vessels branch out from the twelve primary channels and share the function of circulating Qi throughout the body. These vessels form a web of complex interconnections with the channels. At the same time, each has its own functional characteristics and clinical utility independent of the channels.

Traditional Chinese medicine emphasizes the twelve primary organ-related channels and only two of the eight vessels (the Governing and the Conception vessels) (Du Mai, Ren Mai; 督脈、任脈). The other six vessels are not used very often simply because they are not understood as well as the other channels, and there is still a lot of research being conducted on them. Although they were discovered two thousand years ago, little has been written about them. There is a lot of research on the extraordinary vessels being conducted today, especially in Japan, but the results of one researcher often contradict the results that another has achieved.

In this subsection we would like to compile and summarize the important points from the limited number of available documents. Since references from original Chinese sources are very scarce, and references from Western textbooks are tentative, esoteric, or in disagreement with one another, I have used my own judgement in selecting ideas and details. Before reviewing these eight vessels, we will first define them and then summarize their functions.

What are the Eight Vessels? The eight vessels are called Qi Jing Ba Mai (奇經八脈). "Qi" (奇) means "odd, strange, or mysterious." "Jing" (經) means "meridian or channels." "Ba" (八) means "eight" and "Mai" (脈) means "vessels." "Qi Jing Ba Mai" is then translated as "Odd Meridians and Eight Vessels" or "Extraordinary Meridians (EM)." "Odd" has a meaning of strange in Chinese. It is used simply because these eight vessels are not well understood yet. Many Chinese doctors explain that they are called "Odd" simply because there are four vessels that are not paired. Since these eight vessels also contribute to the maintenance of homeostasis, sometimes they are called Homeostatic Meridians. French acupuncturists call them 'Miraculous Meridians' because they were able to create therapeutic effects when all other techniques had failed. In addition, because each of these channels exerts a strong effect upon psychic functioning and individuality, the command points are among the most important psychological points in the body. For this reason, they are occasionally called 'The Eight Psychic Channels.'

These vessels are: 1. Governing Vessel (Du Mai, 督脈); 2. Conception Vessel (Ren Mai, 任脈); 3. Thrusting Vessel (Chong Mai, 衝脈); 4. Girdle Vessel (Dai Mai, 帶脈); 5. Yang Heel Vessel (Yangqiao Mai, 陽蹻脈); 6. Yin Heel Vessel (Yinqiao Mai, 陰蹻脈); 7. Yang Linking Vessel (Yangwei Mai, 陽維脈); and 8. Yin Linking Vessel (Yinwei Mai, 陰維脈).

General Functions of the Eight Vessels

1. **Serve as Qi Reservoirs:** Because the eight vessels are so different from each other, it is difficult to generalize their characteristics and functions. However, one of the most common characteristics of the eight vessels was specified by Bian Que (扁鵲) in his *Nan Jing* (難經) (*The Classic of Difficulties*). He reported that "the twelve organ-related Qi channels constitute rivers, and the eight extraordinary vessels constitute reservoirs." These reservoirs, especially the Conception and Governing vessels, absorb excess Qi from the main channels, and then return it when they are deficient.

You should understand however, that because of the limited number of traditional documents, as well as the lack of modern, scientific methods of Qi research, it is difficult to determine the precise behavior and characteristics of these eight vessels. They can be understood on a number of different levels, and they perform different functions and contain every kind of Qi such as Ying Qi (營氣), Wei Qi (衛氣), Jing Qi (精氣), and even blood.

When the twelve primary channels are deficient in Qi, the eight vessels will supply it. This store of Qi can easily be tapped into with acupuncture needles through those cavities connecting the eight vessels to the twelve channels. The connection cavities behave like the gates of a reservoir, which can be used to adjust the strength of the Qi flow in the rivers and the level of Qi in the reservoir. Sometimes, when it is necessary, the reservoir will release Qi by itself. For example, when a person has had a shock, either physically or mentally, the Qi in some of the main channels will be deficient. This will cause particular organs to be stressed, and Qi will accumulate rapidly around these organs. When this happens, the reservoir must release Qi to increase the deficient circulation and prevent further damage.

2. **Guard Specific Areas Against 'Evil Qi' (Xie Qi, 邪氣):** The Qi which protects the body from outside intruders is called Wei Qi (衛氣) (Guardian Qi). Among the eight vessels, the Thrusting vessel, the Governing vessel, and the Conception vessel play major roles in guarding the abdomen, thorax, and the back.

3. **Regulate the Changes of Life Cycles:** According to Chapter 1 of *Su Wen* (素問), the Thrusting vessel and the Conception vessel also regulate the changes of the life cycles which occur at seven year intervals for women and eight year intervals for men.

4. **Circulate Jing Qi to the Entire Body, Particularly the Five 'Ancestral Organs':** One of the most important functions of the eight vessels is to deliver Jing Qi (精氣) (Essence Qi, which has been converted from Original Essence and sexual essence) to the entire body, including the skin and hair. They must also deliver Jing Qi to the five ancestral organs: the brain and spinal cord, the liver and gall bladder, the bone marrow, the uterus, and the blood system.

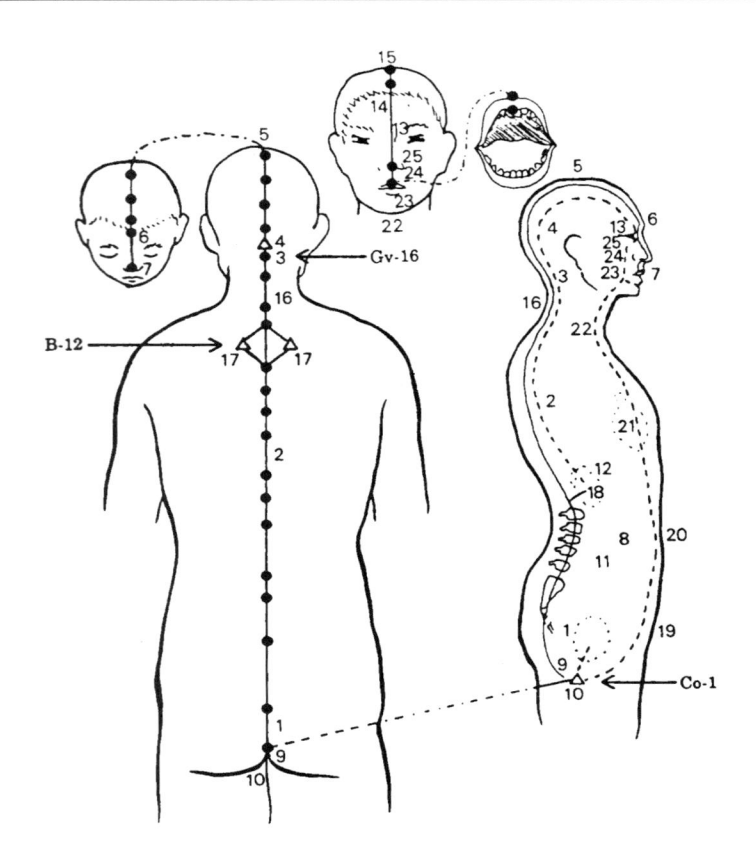

FIGURE 2-25. THE GOVERNING VESSEL (DU MAI).

1. The Governing Vessel (Figure 2-25) (Du Mai, 督脈)

Course:

Course #1:

(1). Perineum—(2). Along the middle of the spine—(3). Fengfu (Gv-16) (風府)—(4). Enters the brain—(5). To the top of the head—(6). Midline of the forehead across the bridge of the nose—(7). Upper lip.

Course #2:

(8). Pelvic region—(9). Descends to the genitals and perineum—(10). Tip of the coccyx—(11). Gluteal region (intersects the kidney and urinary bladder channels)—(12). Returns to the spinal column and then joins with the kidneys.

Course #3:

(13). Inner canthus of the eye—(14). Two (bilateral) branches, ascend across the forehead—(15). Converge at the vertex (enters the brain)—(16). Emerges at the lower end of the nape of the neck—(17). Divides into two branches which descend along opposite sides of the spine to the waist—(18). Kidneys.

Course #4.

(19). Lower abdomen—(20). Across the navel—(21). Passes through the heart—(22). Enters the trachea—(23). Crosses the cheek and encircles the mouth—(24). Terminates at a point below the middle of the eye.

***This vessel intersects Fengmen (B-12) (風門) and Huiyin (Co-1) (會陰).

Cavities:

Changqiang (Gv-1) (長強), Yaoshu (Gv-2) (腰俞), Yaoyangguan (Gv-3) (腰陽關), Mingmen (Gv-4) (命門), Xuanshu (Gv-5) (懸樞), Jizhong (Gv-6) (脊中), Zhongshu (Gv-7) (中樞), Jinsuo (Gv-8) (筋縮), Zhiyang (Gv-9) (至陽), Lingtai (Gv-10) (靈臺), Shendao (Gv-11) (神道), Shenzhu (Gv-12) (身柱), Taodao (Gv-13) (陶道), Dazhui (Gv-14) (大椎), Yamen (Gv-15) (啞門), Fengfu (Gv-16) (風府), Naohu (Gv-17) (腦戶), Qiangjian (Gv-18) (強間), Houding (Gv-19) (后頂), Baihui (Gv-20) (百會), Qianding (Gv-21) (前頂), Xinhui (Gv-22) (囟會), Shangxing (Gv-23) (上星), Shenting (Gv-24) (神庭), Suliao (Gv-25) (素髎), Renzhong (Gv-26) (人中), Duiduan (Gv-27) (兌端), and Yinjiao (Gv-28) (齦交).

Discussion:

The Governing Vessel is the confluence of all the Yang channels, over which it is said to 'govern.' Because it controls all the Yang channels, it is called the Sea of Yang Meridians. This is apparent from its pathway because it flows up the midline of the back, a Yang area, and in the center of all Yang channels (except the stomach channel which flows in the front). The Governing Vessel governs all the Yang channels, which means that it can be used to increase the Yang energy of the body.

Since the Governing Vessel is the Sea of Yang Meridians and it controls or governs the back, the area richest in Guardian Qi (Wei Qi, 衛氣), it is also responsible for the circulation of the body's Guardian Qi to guard against external evil intruders. The circulation of Guardian Qi starts from Fengfu (Gv-16) (風府), and moves down the Governing Vessel to Huiyin (Co-1) (會陰). It is said that it takes 21 days for the Guardian Qi to flow from Fengfu to Huiyin, and 9 days from Huiyin to the throat, making it a monthly cycle.

According to Chinese medical science, Guardian Qi is Yang Qi and therefore represents the 'Fire' of the body. Its quick and ubiquitous circulation keeps the fire going in the body and controls the loss of body heat. Guardian Qi is also inextricably linked with the fluids that flow outside the channels, in the skin and flesh. Consequently, through the breathing (under control of the lungs), Guardian Qi is responsible for the opening and the closing of the pores, and also controls sweating.

The Governing vessel is also responsible for nourishing the five ancestral organs, which include the brain and spinal cord. This is one of the ways in which the kidneys 'control' the brain, as is said in Chinese medicine.

Because of their importance to health, the Governing vessel and the Conception vessel are considered the two most important Qi channels to be trained in Qigong, especially in Nei Dan (內丹). Training related to these two vessels includes: 1. How to fill them with Qi so that you have enough to regulate the twelve channels, 2. How to open up stagnant areas in these two vessels so that the Qi flows smoothly and strongly, 3. How to effectively direct the Qi to nourish the brain and raise up the Shen (神) (spirit), 4. How to effectively govern the Qi in the twelve channels, and nourish the organs, 5. How to use your raised Shen to lead the Guardian Qi to the skin and strengthen the Guardian Qi shield covering your body.

In Nei Dan Qigong training, when you have filled up the Qi in these two vessels and can effectively circulate the Qi in them, you have achieved the Small Circulation (Xiao Zhou Tian, 小周天). In order to do this, you must know how to convert the essence stored in the kidneys into Qi, circulate this Qi in the Governing and Conception vessels, and finally lead this Qi to the head to nourish the brain and Shen.

2. The Conception Vessel (Figure 2-26) (Ren Mai, 任脈)

Course:

Course #1:

(1). Lower abdomen below Qugu (Co-2) (曲骨)—(2). Ascends along the Midline of the abdomen and chest—(3). Crosses the throat and jaw—(4). winds around the mouth—(5). Terminates in the region of the eye.

Course #2:

(6). Pelvic cavity—(7). Enters the spine and ascends along the back.

***This vessel intersects Chengqi (S-1) (承泣) and Yinjiao (Gv-28) (齦交).

Cavities:

Huiyin (Co-1) (會陰), Qugu (Co-2) (曲骨), Zhongli (Co-3) (中極), Guanyuan (Co-4) (關元), Shimen (Co-5) (石門), Qihai (Co-6) (氣海), Abdomen-Yinjiao (Co-7) (陰交), Shenjue (Co-8) (神闕), Shuifen (Co-9) (水分), Xiawan (Co-10) (下脘), Jianli (Co-11) (建里), Zhongwan (Co-12) (中脘), Shangwan (Co-13) (上脘), Juque (Co-14) (巨闕), Jiuwei (Co-15) (鳩尾), Zhongting (Co-16) (中庭), Shanzhong (Co-17) (膻中), Yutang (Co-18) (玉堂), Chest-Zigong (Co-19) (紫宮), Huagai (Co-20) (華蓋), Xuanji (Co-21) (璇璣), Tiantu (Co-22) (天突), Lianquan (Co-23) (廉泉), and Chengjiang (Co-24) (承漿).

Discussion:

Ren (任) in Chinese means "direction, responsibility." Ren Mai (任脈), the "Conception Vessel," has a major role in Qi circulation, monitoring and directing all of

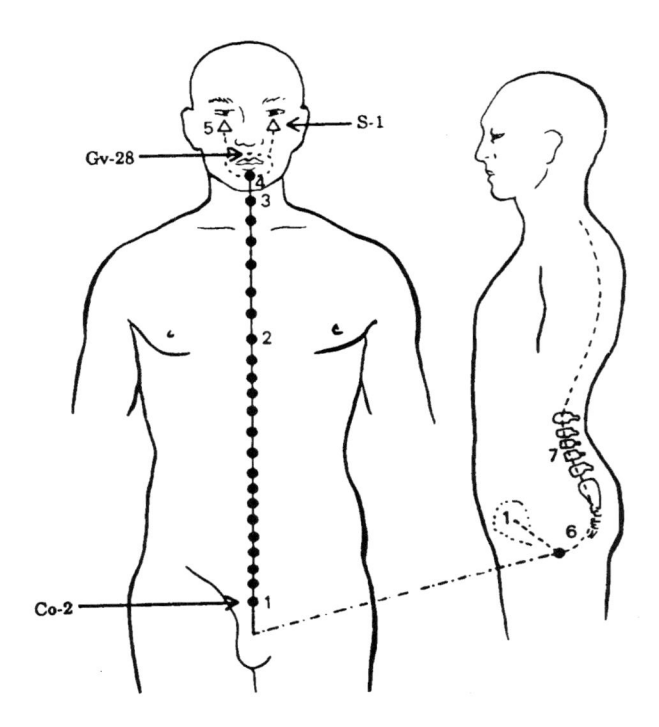

FIGURE 2-26. THE CONCEPTION VESSEL. (REN MAI).

the Yin channels (plus the stomach channel). The Conception Vessel is connected to the Thrusting (Chong Mai, 衝脈) and Yin Linking (Yinwei Mai, 陰維脈) vessels, and is able to increase the Yin energy of the body.

This vessel nourishes the uterus (one of the five ancestral organs) and the whole genital system. It is said in the *Nei Jing* (內經) (*Inner Classic*) that the Conception and Thrusting vessels contain both blood and essence Jing (精), and both flow up to the face and around the mouth. They contain more blood than essence in men, and thus promote the growth of the beard and body hair. Because women lose blood with their menstruation, they contain proportionately less blood and hence, no beard or body hair.

It was described in the *Su Wen* (素問) that both the Conception and Thrusting vessels control the life cycles every seven years for women and every eight years for men. It is the changes taking place in these vessels at those intervals that promote the major alterations in our lives.

In addition, the Conception vessel also controls the distribution and "dispersion" of Guardian Qi all over the abdomen and thorax via numerous small Qi branches (Luo, 絡). This vessel also plays an important role in the distribution of body fluids in the abdomen.

In Qigong society, this vessel and the Governing vessel are considered the most important among the Qi channels and vessels, and must be trained first. It is believed

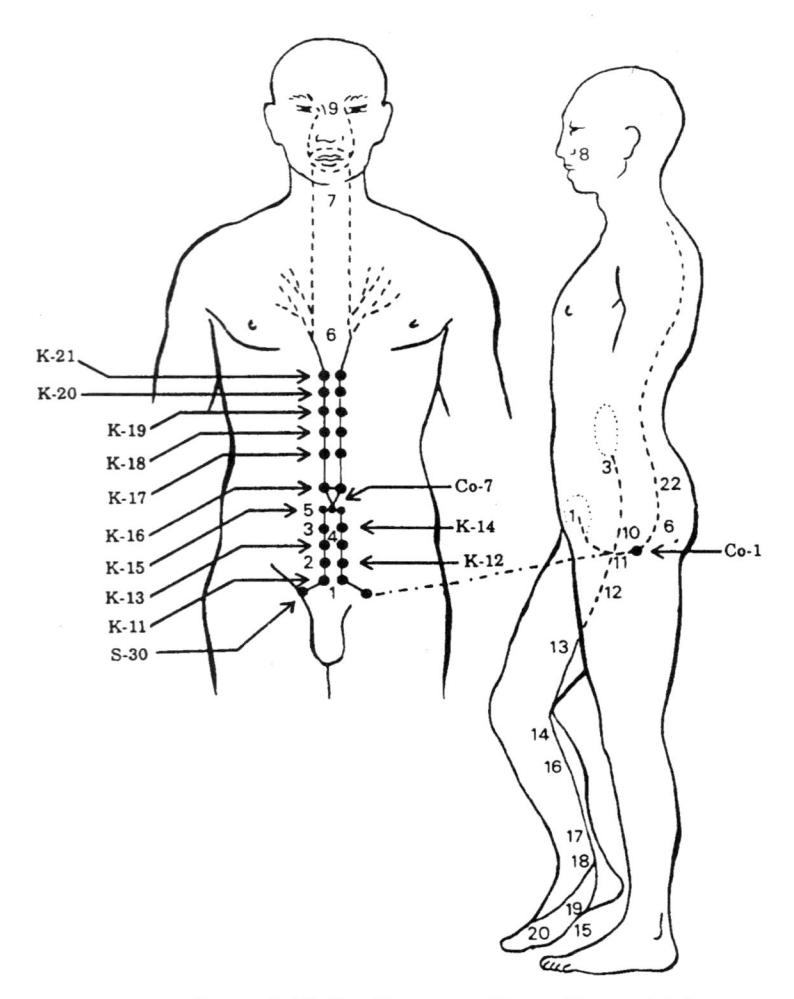

FIGURE 2-27. THE THRUSTING VESSEL (CHONG MAI).

that there is usually no significant Qi stagnation in the Conception vessel. However, it is important to increase the amount of Qi you are able to store, which also increases your ability to regulate the Yin channels.

3. The Thrusting Vessel (Figure 2-27) (Chong Mai, 衝脈)

Course:

Course #1:

(1). Lower abdomen—(2). Emerges along the Path of Qi—(3). Tracks the course of the kidney channel—(4). Ascends through the abdomen—(5). Skirts the navel—(6). Disperses in the chest.

Course #2:

(6). Chest—(7). Ascends across the throat—(8). Face—(9). Nasal cavity.

Course #3:

(1). Lower abdomen—(10). Below the kidney—(11). Emerges along the Path of Qi—(12). Descends along the medial aspect of the thigh—(13). Popliteal fossa—(14). Medial margin of the tibia and the posterior aspect of the medial malleolus—(15). Bottom of the foot.

Course #4:

(16). Tibia—(17). Toward the lateral margin of the bone—(18). enters the heel—(19). Crosses the tarsal bones of the foot—(20). Big toe.

Course #5:

(21). Pelvic cavity—(22). Enter the spine and circulates through the back.

***This vessel intersects Huiyin (Co-1) (會陰), Yinjiao (Co-7) (陰交), Qichong (S-30) (氣沖), Henggu (K-11) (橫骨), Dahe (K-12) (大赫), Qixue (K-l3) (氣穴), Siman (K-14) (四滿), Zhongzhu (K-15) (中注), Huangshu (K-16) (肓俞), Shangqu (K-17) (商曲), Shiguan (K-18) (石關), Yindu (K-19) (陰都), Tonggu (K-20) (腹通谷), and Youmen (K-21) (幽門).

Discussion:

One of the major purposes of the Thrusting vessel (Chong Mai, 衝脈) is to connect, to communicate, and to mutually support the Conception vessel (Ren Mai, 任脈). Because of this mutual Qi support, both can effectively regulate the Qi in the kidney channel. The kidneys are the residence of Original Qi (Yuan Qi, 元氣) and are considered one of the most vital Yin organs.

The Thrusting vessel is considered one of the most important and decisive vessels in successful Qigong training, especially in Marrow Washing. There are many reason for this. The first reason is that this vessel intersects two cavities on the Conception vessel: Huiyin (Co-1) (會陰) and Yinjiao (Co-7) (陰交). Huiyin means "meeting Yin" and is the cavity where the Yang and Yin Qi are transferred. Yinjiao means "Yin Junction" and is the cavity where the Original Qi (Water Qi or Yin Qi) interfaces with the Fire Qi created from food and air. The Thrusting Vessel also connects with eleven cavities on the kidney channel. The kidney is considered the residence of Original Essence (Yuan Jing, 元氣), which is converted into Original Qi (Yuan Qi, 元氣).

The second reason for the importance of the Thrusting Vessel in Qigong training is that this vessel is connected directly to the spinal cord and reaches up to the brain. The major goal of Marrow Washing Qigong (Xi Sui Qigong, 洗髓氣功) is to lead the Qi into the marrow and then further on to the head, nourishing the brain and spirit (Shen, 神).

And finally, the third reason is found in actual Qigong practice. There are three common training paths: Fire, Wind, and Water. In Fire path Qigong, the emphasis is on the Fire or Yang Qi circulating in the Governing vessel and therefore strengthening the muscles and organs. The Fire path is the main Qi training in Muscle/Tendon Changing (Yi Jin Jing, 易筋) Qigong. However, the Fire path can also cause the body to become too Yang, and therefore speed up the process of degeneration. In order to adjust the Fire to a proper level, Marrow Washing Qigong is also trained. This uses the Water path, in which Qi separates from the route of the Fire path at the Huiyin (Co-1) (會陰) cavity, enters the spinal cord, and finally reaches up to the head. The Water path teaches how to use Original Qi to cool down the body, and then to use this Qi to nourish the brain and train the spirit. Learning to adjust the Fire and Water Qi circulation in the body is called Kan-Li (坎離), which means Water-Fire. You can see from this that the Thrusting vessel plays a very important role in Qigong training.

4. The Girdle Vessel (Figure 2-28) (Dai Mai, 帶脈)

Course:

(1). Below the hypochondrium at the level of the 2nd lumbar vertebra—(2). Turns downward and encircles the body at the waist like a girdle.

***This vessel intersects Daimai (GB-26) (帶脈), Wushu (GB-27) (五樞), and Weidao (GB-28) (維道).

Discussion:

The major purpose of the Girdle vessel is to regulate the Qi of the gall bladder. It is also responsible for the Qi's horizontal balance. If you have lost this balance, you will have lost your center and balance both mentally and physically.

From the point of view of Qigong, the Girdle vessel is also responsible for the strength of the waist area. When Qi is full and circulating smoothly back pain will be avoided. In addition, because the kidneys are located nearby, this vessel is also responsible for Qi circulation around the kidneys, maintaining the kidneys' health. Most important of all for the Girdle vessel is the fact that the Lower Tian is located in its area. In order to lead Original Qi from the kidneys to the Lower Dan Tian, the waist area must be healthy and relaxed. This means that the Qi flow in the waist area must be smooth. The training of the Girdle vessel has been highly developed, and will be discussed in a later YMAA Book.

5. The Yang Heel Vessel (Figure 2-29) (Yangqiao Mai, 陽蹻脈)

Course:

(1). Below the lateral malleolus at Shenmai (B-62) (申脈)—(2). Ascends along the lateral aspect of the leg—(3). Posterior aspect of the hypochondrium 3. Lateral side of the shoulder—(4). Traverses the neck—(5). Passes beside the mouth—(6). Inner canthus (joins the Yin Heel vessel and the urinary bladder channel)—(7). Ascends across the forehead—(8). Winds behind the ear to Fengchi (GB-20) (風池)—(9). Enters the brain at Fengfu (Gv-16) (風府).

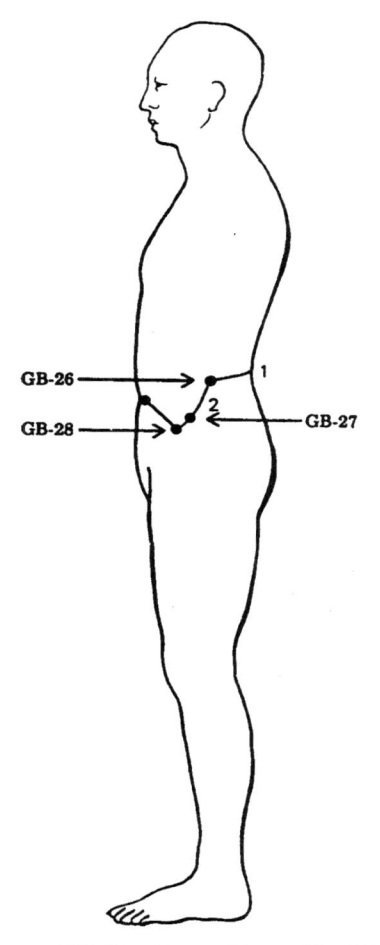

FIGURE 2-28. THE GIRDLE VESSEL (DAI MAI).

***This vessel intersects Shenmai (B-62) (申脈), Pushen (B-61) (仆參), Fuyang (B-59) (附陽), Jingming (B-l) (睛明), Juliao (GB-29) (居髎), Fengchi (GB-20) (風池), Naoshu (SI-10) (臑俞), Jugu (LI-16) (巨骨), Jianyu (LI-15) (肩髃), Dicang (S-4) (地倉), Juliao (S-3) (巨髎), Chengqi (S-1) (承泣), and Fengfu (Gv-16) (風府).

Discussion:

While the preceding four vessels (Governing, Conception, Thrusting, and Girdle) are located in the trunk, the Yang Heel Vessel and the next three are located in the trunk and legs. (In addition, each of these four vessels is paired.) For millions of years, man has been walking on his legs, which preform much more strenuous work than the arms. I believe that it was because of this that, as evolution proceeded, the legs gradually developed these vessels to supply Qi support and regulate the channels. If this is true, it may be that, as time goes on and man uses his legs less and less, in a few million years these vessels will gradually disappear.

You can see from the way that the Yang Heel vessel intersects with other Qi channels that it regulates the Yang channels, such as the urinary bladder, the gall bladder, the small intestine, and the large intestine. The Yang Heel vessel is also connected with the Governing vessel. The Qi filling this vessel is supplied mainly through exercising the legs, which converts the food essence or fat stored in the legs. This Qi is then led upward to nourish the Yang channels. It is believed in Qigong that, since this vessel is also connected with your brain, certain leg exercises can be used to cure headaches. Since a headache is caused by excess Qi in the head, exercising the legs will draw this Qi downward to the leg muscles and relieve the pressure in the head.

Most of the training that relates to this vessel is Wai Dan (外丹). Wai Dan Qigong is considered Yang, and specializes in training the Yang channels, while Nei Dan (內丹) Qigong is considered relatively Yin and emphasizes the Yin channels more.

6. The Yin Heel Vessel (Figure 2-29) (Yinqiao Mai, 陰蹻脈)

Course:

(1). Zhaohai (K-6) (照海) below the medial malleolus—(2). Extends upward along the medial aspect of the leg—(3). Crossing the perineum and chest entering the supraclavicular fossa—(4), Ascends through the throat and emerges in front of Renying (S-9) (人迎)—(5), Traverses the medial aspect of the cheek—(6). Inner canthus (joins the urinary bladder channel and Yang Heel vessels)—(7). Ascends over the head and into the brain.

***This vessel intersects Zhaohai (K-6) (照海), Jiaoxin (K-8) (交信), and Jingming (B-1) (睛明).

Discussion:

The Yin Heel vessel is connected with two cavities of the kidney channel. Therefore, one of the major sources of Qi for this vessel is the conversion of the kidney essence into Qi. It is believed in Qigong society that the other major Qi source is the essence of the external kidneys (testicles or ovaries). In Marrow Washing Qigong (Xi Sui Qigong, 洗髓氣功), one of the training processes is to stimulate the testicles in order to increase the hormone production and increase the conversion of the essence into Qi. At the same time, you would learn how to lead the Qi in this vessel up to the head to nourish the brain and spirit (Shen, 神). With this nourishment, you would be able to reach Buddhahood or enlightenment. From a health and longevity point of view, the raised spirit will be able to efficiently direct the Qi of the entire body and maintain your health.

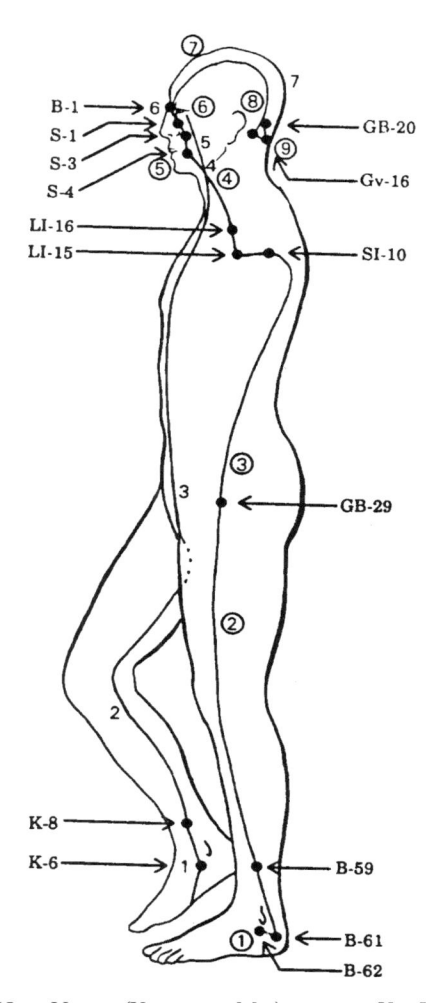

FIGURE 2-29. THE YANG HEEL VESSEL (YANGQIAO MAI) AND THE YIN HEEL VESSEL (YINQIAO MAI).

7. The Yang Linking Vessel (Figure 2-30) (Yangwei Mai, 陽維脈)

Course:

(1). Jinmen (B-63) (金門) on the heel—(2). Ascends along the lateral aspect of the leg—(3). Lower abdomen—(4). Slants upward across the posterior aspect of the hypochondrium—(5). Across the posterior axillary fold to the shoulder—(6). Ascends the neck and crosses behind the ear—(7). Proceeds to the forehead—(8). Doubles back over the head—(9). Fengfu (Gv-16) (風府).

***This vessel intersects Jinmen (B-63) (金門), Yangjiao (GB-35) (陽交), Jianjing (GB-21) (肩井), Fengchi (GB-20) (風池), Naokong (GB-19) (腦空), Chengling (GB-18) (承靈), Zhengying (GB-17) (正營), Muchuang (GB-16) (目窗), Head-Linqi (GB-

15) (頭臨泣), Yangbai (GB-14) (陽白), Benshen (GB-13) (本神), Tianliao (TB-15) (天髎), Naoshu (SI-10) (臑俞), Yamen (Gv-15) (啞門), Fengfu (Gv-16) (風府), and Touwei (S-8) (頭維).

Discussion:

The Yang Linking vessel regulates the Qi mainly in the Yang channels: the urinary bladder, gall bladder, triple burner, small intestine, and stomach channels. It is also connected with the Governing vessel at Yamen (Gv-15) (啞門) and Fengfu (Gv-16) (風府). This vessel and the Yang Heel vessel have not been emphasized much in Qigong, except in Iron Shirt (Tie Bu Shan, 鐵布衫) training where these two and the Governing vessel are trained.

8. The Yin Linking Vessel (Figure 2-30) (Yinwei Mai, 陰維脈)

Course:

(1). Lower leg at Zhubin (K-9) (築賓)—(2). Ascending along the medial aspect of the leg—(3), Enters the lower abdomen—(4). Upward across the chest—(5). Throat (meets Tiantu (Co-22) (天突) and Lianquan (Co-23) (廉泉)),

***This vessel intersects Zhubin (K-9) (築賓), Chongmen (Sp-12) (沖門), Fushe (Sp-13) (府舍), Daheng (Sp-15) (大橫), Fuai (Sp-16) (腹哀), Qimen (Li-14) (期門), Tiantu (Co-22) (天突), and Lianquan (Co-23) (廉泉).

Discussion:

The Yin Linking vessel has connections with the kidney, spleen, and liver Yin channels. The Yin Linking vessel also communicates with the Conception vessel at two cavities. This vessel is not trained much in Qigong except marrow/brain washing Qigong (Xi Sui Qigong, 洗髓氣功).

2-4. UNDERSTANDING THE MENTAL BODY 瞭解人身心理體

Let us now discuss the third part of the human body, the mental or spiritual body. First, let us consider the difference between the mental and the spiritual. Even with today's science, it is very difficult to define these two aspects of our nature, so we must look to the experiences gained in the past. According to Chinese understanding, the mental part of us includes both the physical and the Qi aspects of our being which are related to thinking. The physical parts are the nervous system and the brain, which need Qi to exist and function. If the physical brain and nervous system receive the right amount of Qi and stay healthy, the mind will be able to think clearly and judge wisely. However, if the Qi supply is not normal, the brain and nervous system will not function properly, and mental problems may occur. Naturally, if the Qi supply stops, these physical systems will die. Therefore, in order to keep the mental system functioning properly, Chinese Qigong places heavy emphasis on learning how to lead Qi to the brain

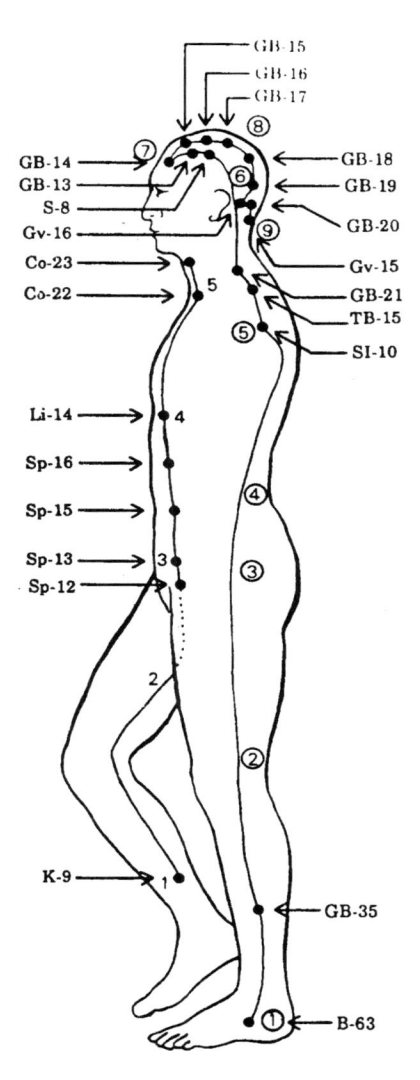

FIGURE 2-30. THE YANG LINKING VESSEL (YANGWEI MAI) AND THE YIN LINKING VESSEL (YINWEI MAI).

to nourish it, and also how to maintain the entire nervous system.

Only when the mental aspect of your being is healthy are you able to build up the spiritual part of your body. It is very difficult to understand and define this spiritual part. The various religions were created to search for the truth of this matter. Asian religions believe that when the human spirit has been cultivated to a very high level, we will be able to leave the cycle of reincarnation and gain eternal life. Religions in the West have similar beliefs.

The mental part of our being can be considered a lower level of our spirit which has not yet been well cultivated. The Chinese religions believe that when this lower level of spirit is cultivated, the Qi in the body will be able to combine and communicate with the Qi of nature. This enables us to better understand the patterns of natural Qi, and ultimately learn how to avoid reincarnation and gain spiritual independence. This level of growth is called "enlightenment" (Shen Tong, 神通) in Daoism and "Buddhahood" (Cheng Fo, 成佛) in Buddhism.

The mental part of our being is actually our thinking, which can be manifested externally. When manifestation occurs, the process is completed through the Qi circulatory and nervous systems. This means that the mind, Qi, and physical body cannot be separated. In order to calm down the physical body, we must first calm down the Qi body through the nervous system. In order to calm down the Qi body, we must first regulate the mind.

Because of the closeness of the mind, Qi, and physical body, regulating the mind (Tiao Xin, 調心) is an important part of Qigong training. Chinese medicine and Qigong teach that there are two minds, one is called Xin (心) and the other is called Yi (意). The mind which is generated by emotional disturbances is called Xin. Xin means "heart" in Chinese. Any occurrence which is able to touch your heart and disturb your neutral mind is called Xin. For example, if you are upset because someone has said something bad about you, the thoughts or intentions that you have are considered to be Xin. Or when your regular Qigong practice time comes by, but you are lazy and decide not to practice, the thinking which led to this decision is called Xin. Xin can therefore be translated "emotional mind."

However, when the thoughts come from wise thinking and clear judgement, then this kind of mind is called Yi, which can be translated as "intention" or "wisdom mind." What the wisdom mind has conceived, you can usually accomplish.

Unfortunately, the emotional mind usually dominates the wisdom mind. When people react to events, it is usually according to their emotional feelings rather than their calm judgement. One of the main goals of Chinese Qigong is developing the wisdom mind so that it can 'govern' the emotional mind. When this happens, emotional disturbances will not occur, and the mind can be peaceful and calm. The emotional mind is considered to be Yang while the wisdom mind is Yin. The training works to balance Yin and Yang.

You can see that the mental body actually is constructed of two "minds." When either mind is too strong and causes your actions to deviate from the neutral, balanced state, you then lose your mental balance. This will also affect how your physical body functions. According to Chinese religious Qigong, when the Yin and Yang minds are in mutual balance, the human spirit can be raised to a supernatural state and reach the stage of enlightenment or Buddhahood.

In general massage, to relax the physical body you must first remove emotional disturbances from the mind. This means that the first thing you should do is to massage the mental body so that the mind can be calm and relaxed. Only when the patient's mind is relaxed can their physical body be relaxed. Only when the physical body is relaxed can the Qi move easily and smoothly in the body. This is the key to successful massage.

2-5. Gates and Junctions in the Human Body 人身氣體之通門與結點

In this section, we would like to explain two terms which are used frequently in Qigong. The first term is "Men" (門), which can be translated "gate" or "door;" the second term is "Jie" (結), which can be translated "knot" or "junction."

A 'gate' usually means a door through which the Qi can enter or exit a place. They are therefore commonly called "Qi gates." Actually, in Chinese medicine, these gates are called Qi Xue (氣穴) (Qi cavities) or simply Xue (穴) (cavities). According to Chinese medicine and Qigong, many of these Qi gates are crucial in maintaining health, curing sicknesses, and even practicing Qigong. These gates are usually called Qiao Men (竅門) (tricky gates) in order to distinguish them from the other gates. Most of these gates are used in Qigong massage. Since obstructions in these gates can affect the smooth circulation of Qi, treating them properly can improve the Qi circulation.

Many of these tricky gates have several different names which are used by the various groups that utilize them. Names may vary between the physicians, martial artists, Qigong practitioners, and the religious communities. For example, the cavity between the thumb and the second finger is called Hegu (合谷) in medicine, while it is called Hukou (虎口) in martial arts society. The cavity on the top of the head is called Baihui (百會) in medicine, Tianlingai (天靈蓋) in the martial arts, and Niwangon (泥丸宮) in Daoist Qigong. Therefore, do not be confused if you hear someone call a cavity by a different name.

There are two types of gates. One is the 'external Qi gate,' through which Qi can enter or leave the body. You can use these gates to adjust the body's energy level. For example, when you are excited or nervous, your heart has an excess of 'fire,' which may damage it. The excess heat in the heart can be moved to the pericardium, and then brought through the Qi channels to the center of the palms where it can be released into the air through the Laogong (P-8) (勞宮) cavities (Figure 2-31). When this happens, your palms feel warm and perspire.

The communication of Qi between your body and the air does not happen only through the acupuncture cavities. There are many non-cavity gates, such as the nose and anus, which handle a great deal of the work.

The second type of Qi gate is the 'internal Qi gate,' which enables the Qi to communicate between the different parts of the body. Many of these gates are cavities, while many others are not. For example, the neck is the Qi gate through which the head and the body communicate. The joints in the arms and legs are also considered gates.

The second term you need to understand is "Jie" (結), which means "knot" or "junction." Usually the term refers to physical knots or junctions, such as where a large

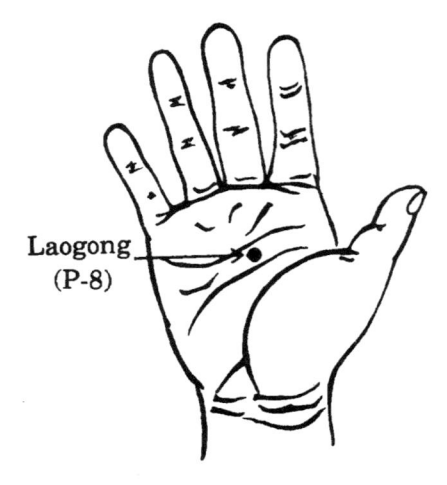

FIGURE 2-31. THE LAOGONG CAVITY (P-8).

nerve or blood vessel branches out into many smaller nerves or vessels. When these areas are tense, they can interfere with smooth Qi and blood circulation. Most of these places are also Qi gates, which is not surprising, since it is the Qi which controls the nervous system.

In this section, we will first discuss the gates on the surface of the body, and then we will identify others which are inside the body. We will only mention the more important gates here. Others will be discussed in the appropriate sections when we discuss general massage in Part Two.

Gates on the Surface of the Body

Eyes, Mouth, Ears, and Nose. These four organs are the most important gates which allow you to communicate with the outside world. Whenever you look at something, your eyes receive energy (Qi) from it, and this energy is passed to your brain for recognition. The eyes are usually considered to only receive Qi, although many Qigong masters believe that the eyes can also emit it.

The mouth takes in food, which Chinese medicine and Qigong consider to be Post-birth essence. It is this essence, when it is converted into Qi, which nourishes the body. Therefore, the main purpose of the mouth is to receive this essence. However, when you are sick, the mouth is also used to release extra heat or waste from the body. For example, when you have a cold, coughing releases heat. The sounds which come out of the mouth can also release Qi from the body, and different sounds can release the excess Qi from different organs. For example, when you are happy your heart has an excess of 'fire' or heat. When you laugh you make the sound "Ha" (哈), which releases the heat. The mouth plays an important part in Qigong, and a great deal of study has been devoted to how different sounds can be used to balance the Qi in the internal organs.

The ears receive sound energy, and the brain responds to the different wavelengths of the energy. Like the eyes, the ears are not normally used to release or emit energy.

Finally, the nose brings air into and out of the body. When you inhale, you take in oxygen, another form of Post-birth essence, which is converted into Qi. The nose also releases carbon-dioxide which we do not need in the body. Chemically, when the oxygen is taken into the body, a chemical reaction begins. The final product of this reaction is carbon-dioxide, which contains the body's waste carbon (from the biochemical reaction). This is eliminated from your body when you exhale.

Anus and Urethra. The anus and urethra are also gates which release waste from the body, and, at the same time, release excess Qi. When waste elimination is irregular, your body can be in a state of either excess or deficiency. For instance, when you have diarrhea your body becomes deficient because of the too frequent elimination, but when you are constipated, there will be an excess of Qi in your body, and you will feel heat accumulating internally. Because of this, both Western and oriental physicians will check their patient's regularity as a part of their diagnosis. The same theory also applies to the urethra.

Pores. The millions of pores in your skin are probably responsible for releasing the greatest amount of Qi from your body. When you are too hot, the heat is released through the pores. In the summertime, when the Qi in your internal organs is normally sufficient, and the Qi in the surrounding air is also sufficient, your pores will be wide open to release any excess heat from your body. However, in the wintertime, the Qi in the surrounding air is deficient. In order to protect your internal Qi, most of your pores will stay closed to seal the Qi inside. You can see that your pores are designed to adjust the Qi in the body.

An important part of Chinese Qigong is the practice of skin breathing. This makes it possible for the Qi to reach all the pores smoothly so that they can keep functioning properly. Naturally, the activity of the pores is controlled by the sensations you receive from the nerves in your skin. You can keep the nervous system functioning properly if you keep it supplied with a steady amount of Qi. It is believed that the most effective way of preventing colds is to practice skin breathing (Fu Xi, 膚息) Qigong. This technique is discussed in the YMAA book: *The Root of Chinese Qigong.*

There is another Qigong practice in which Qi can be stored in the bone marrow instead of being released into the air and wasted. This practice is called Brain/Marrow Washing Qigong (Xi Sui Qigong, 洗髓氣功). Normally, aging is caused by deficient Qi nourishment of the brain and of the bone marrow, which manufactures blood cells. If Qi can be led inward to the brain and bone marrow, they can keep functioning significantly longer than usual. In addition, the excess Qi produced in the body can be efficiently used, instead of released into the air. Conserving Qi is especially important as you get older: in fact, it is the key to longevity. If you would like to know more about brain/marrow washing Qigong, please refer to the YMAA book: *Qigong—The Secret of Youth.*

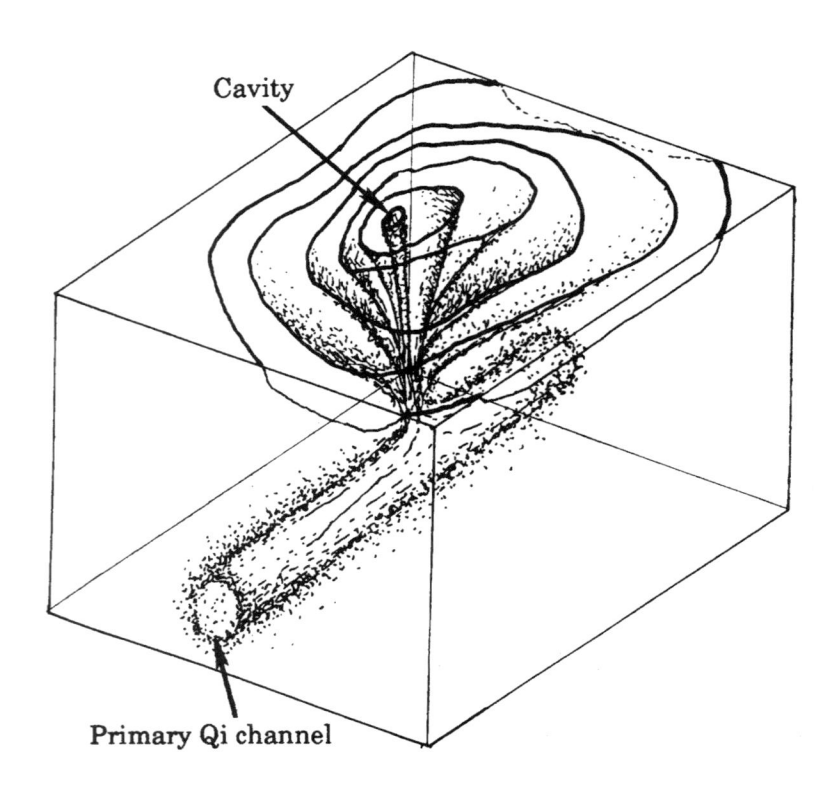

FIGURE 2-32. ELECTRICAL CONDUCTIVITY MAP OF SKIN AT AN ACUPUNCTURE POINT.

Tips of Fingers and Toes. According to Chinese medicine, there are six primary Qi channels connected to the tips of the fingers, and another six connected to the tips of the toes. It is believed that because we are continually using the fingers for working and the toes for walking, the Qi has to reach smoothly to the tips of the fingers and toes to maintain their sensitivity. This is the reason for the gates in the ends of the toes and fingers. These gates are the reason that, when you massage someone with your fingers, you can exchange Qi effectively with them.

Cavities. It has recently been discovered that what Chinese acupuncture calls "cavities" (Xue, 穴) are actually tiny spots of higher electrical conductivity than the surrounding skin.[1] This higher conductivity creates a tunnel or path from the surface to the primary Qi channels under the skin and muscles (Figure 2-32). The cavities bring the excess Qi circulating in the primary Qi channels out to the surface of the skin and release it to the air. All of these cavities can be used in Qigong massage to release excess Qi.

Of the more than 700 acupuncture cavities, about 108 can be reached by the fingers. Acupressure and Dian Xue (點穴) are systems of treatment which use the hands or fingers to press and rub the cavities in order to regulate the Qi circulation in the channels. Some of the Dian Xue techniques are well known and used frequently by

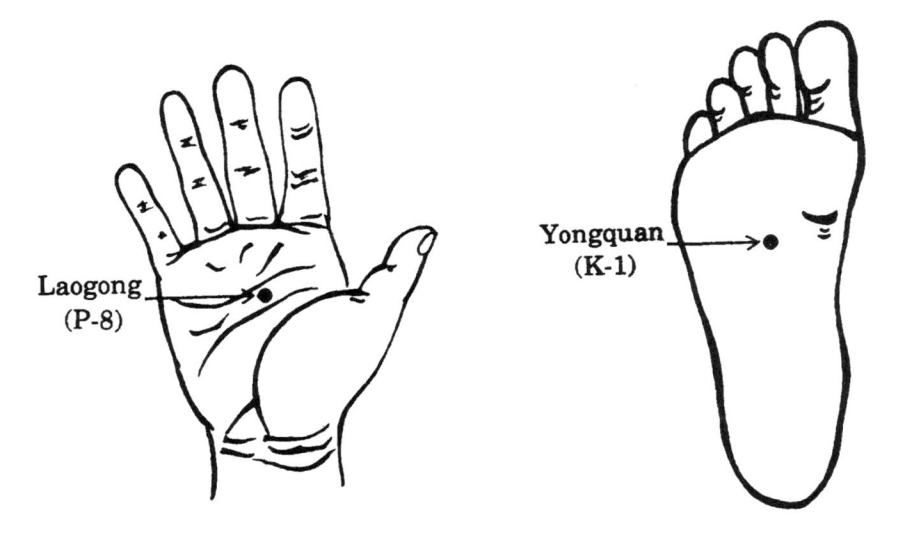

FIGURE 2-33. THE LAOGONG CAVITY.

FIGURE 2-34. THE YONGQUAN CAVITY.

practitioners of general massage.

A number of the cavities are larger than the others, and it is easier to establish communication with the Qi through them. These cavities play an important role in Qigong massage. These gates are the Baihui (Gv-20) (百會), Naohu (Gv-17) (腦戶), Yintang (M-HN-3, 印堂), Mingmen (Gv-4) (命門), Laogong (P-8) (勞宮), and Yongquan (K-1) (湧泉) cavities. The most important of these are the two Laogong cavities located in the centers of the palms (Figure 2-33), and the two Yongquan cavities located on the bottom of the feet (Figure 2-34). These four gates are used to regulate the condition of the Qi in the heart and the kidneys. Massaging these four gates keeps them open and exchanging Qi with the environment.

There are a few other gates or areas through which the Qi can communicate easily inside and outside of the body. For example, the nipples are considered Qi gates, although they have not been studied very extensively. Also, the pores around the joints are more open than elsewhere, and so the Qi exchange occurs there more easily.

Gates or Junctions Inside the Body

Joint Junctions. Joints are the junctions or passages where the Qi and blood communicate between one section of the body and another. If the Qi and blood circulation is blocked at a joint, a part of the body will not obtain the proper nourishment, and will malfunction or suffer some damage as a consequence.

In Qigong massage, the joints are separated into three categories. The first category consists of the central joints (i.e. spinal joints) which are the passageway for Qi and neural messages between the brain and every part of the body. Since these joints are related to our thinking and feeling, they are considered to be the most important in Qigong massage. The second most important set of joints are those which connect the six major parts of the body. These six parts are the head, the two arms, the two legs, and the torso. These six main parts are connected by the neck, the shoulder joints, and the hip joints. The third kind of junction includes all the other joints of the body. Although some are more important than others, they are all junctions of Qi and blood. These joints include the jaw, elbows, wrists, finger joints, knees, ankles, toe joints, and a number of other, minor ones.

Whenever you are tense, the Qi and the blood circulation in the joints can be affected. Blockages of the joint junctions can also have many other causes, such as injuries, joint diseases such as arthritis, degeneration due to aging, etc. In massage, when you have loosened the joints, you are already one third of the way to your goal.

Junctions of the Arteries and Nerves. The body contains many nerve and artery junctions, usually where a main artery or nerve branches out into many smaller arteries or nerves. An example is the place under the ear where the main artery and nerves branch upward from the neck (Figure 2-35). Whenever this place is blocked, the brain will not obtain enough oxygen, and brain cells will wither or even die. You therefore need to learn how to massage this area to keep the junction open. Although many Junctions are located around the joints, many other are not related to the joints (e.g., the temple).

Gates to the Main Nerves. We have already explained how, in Qigong, the nervous system, mind, and Qi cannot be separated. Since the nerves are the bridge between the mind and the Qi, Qigong massage devotes a great deal of attention to massaging the nerves.

In addition to massaging the nerve endings such as are found in the skin, general massage also has ways to massage the major nerves. There are many places in the body where you can reach them. These gates are usually found on the Yin sides of the joints, such as on the inside of the elbows (Figure 2-36), the back of the knees, and in the armpits. Since these gates access the central nervous system, it is important to use the correct techniques and the proper amount of power. Too much stimulation will only cause more tension, and increase Qi and blood stagnation.

Qi Junctions. There are twelve primary Qi channels in the body. The Qi circulating in them can be affected by our thinking, tension, sickness, or by the food and air we take in. There are a number of places where the Qi is most likely to become stagnant. Most of these places are also where the acupuncture cavities are located. Physicians can insert a needle through the cavity to reach the stagnation and release it, or else they can massage the area and release the stagnation. In fact, this is how Dian Xue (點穴) massage treats illness.

Chapter 2: General Foundations

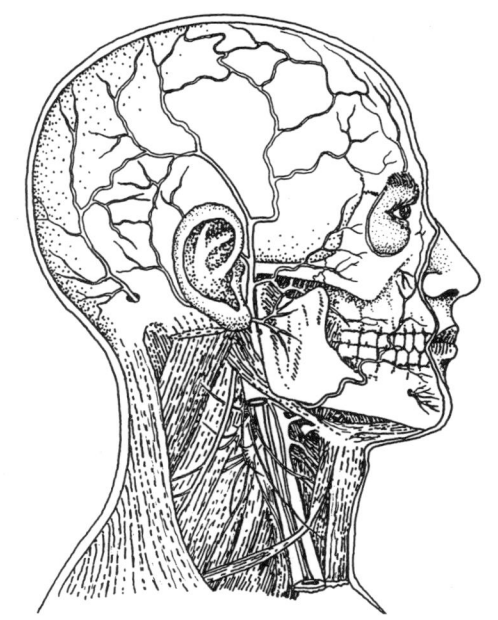

FIGURE 2-35. ANATOMICAL STRUCTURE OF THE HEAD.

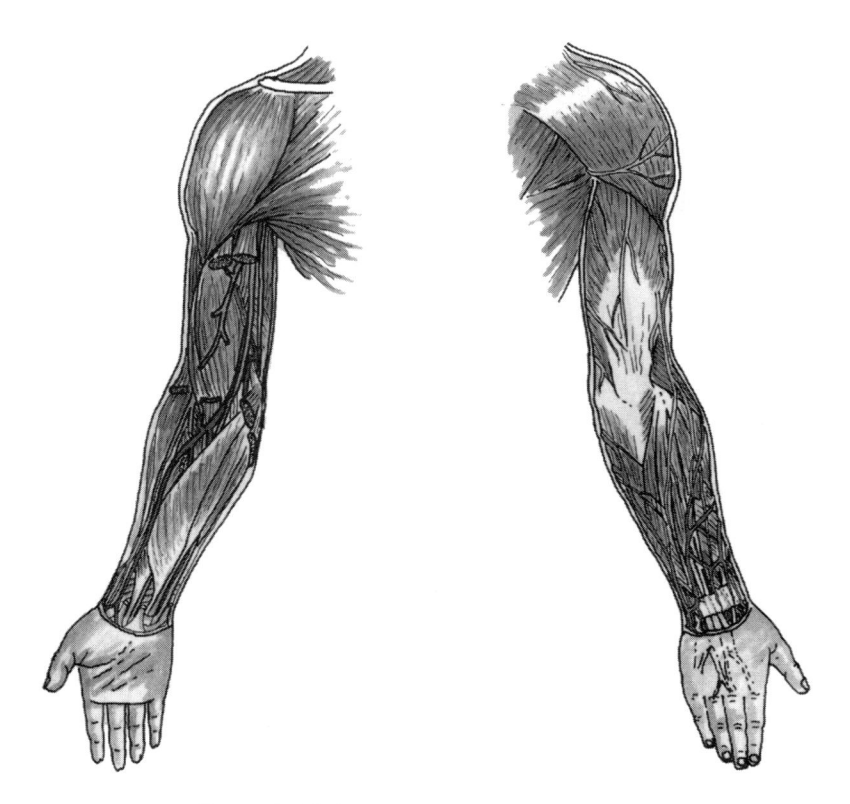

FIGURE 2-36. ANATOMICAL STRUCTURE OF THE ARM.

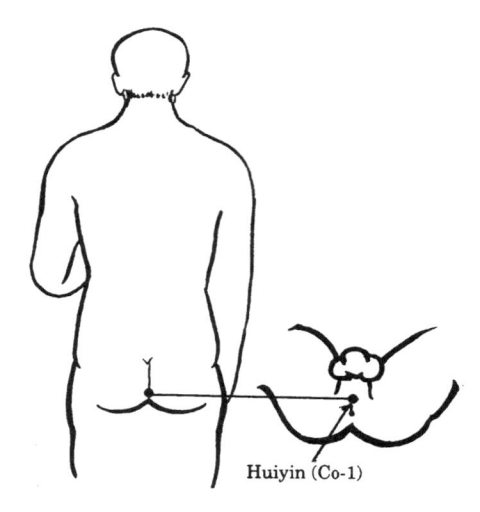

FIGURE 2-37. THE HUIYIN CAVITY (CO-1).

When you study Qigong massage, you must learn the paths of the twelve channels, as well as which places are likely to become stagnant, and how to remove the stagnation by stimulating the cavities.

Chinese medicine and Qigong consider the junctions where a channel or vessel with Yin Qi joins a channel or vessel with Yang Qi (or vice versa) to be extremely important for your health. It is believed that when the Qi cannot transmit smoothly from one phase to another, you may become sick. Usually, these transmissions or changes happen according to natural timing, such as the transition between day and night, the lunar month, the seasons, or the year. For example, the Qi is circulating more strongly in the front (Yin) side of your body during the daytime, and in the back (Yang) side of your body during the night.

In general Qigong massage, there are two cavities which are considered the most important for the exchange of Yin and Yang. The first one is the Huiyin (Co-1) (會陰) cavity, located in the perineum between the genitals and anus (Figure 2-37). The Huiyin cavity is the place where the Yin Conception Vessel (Ren Mai, 任脈) joins the Yang Governing Vessel (Du Mai, 督脈).

The second cavity is called Renzhong (Gv-26) (人中), and is located under the nose (Figure 2-38). Although this cavity is not the exact location where the Yin-Yang exchange takes place (which is actually in the roof of the mouth), stimulating this cavity will improve the exchange.

In addition to regulating the transmission of Qi, these two cavities can also be used to raise up the spirit of vitality, for example, in reviving someone who has fainted.

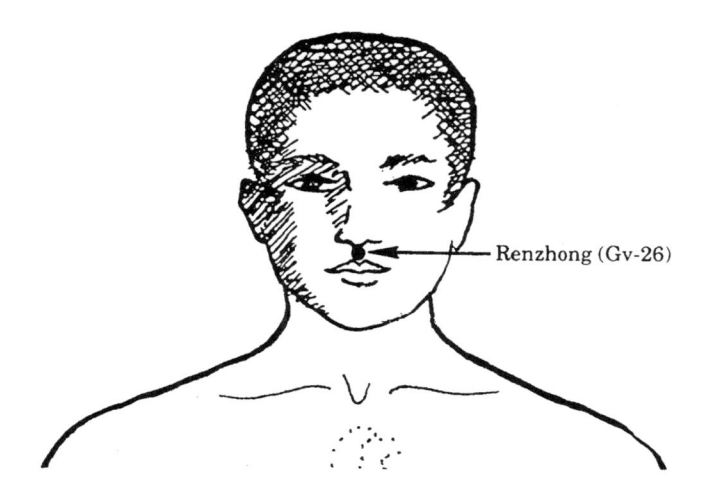

FIGURE 2-38. THE RENZHONG CAVITY (GV-26).

2-6. IMPORTANT POINTS IN QIGONG MASSAGE 氣功按摩之要點

Whichever type of Qigong massage you are practicing, there are a number of important points which you should keep in mind:

1. The temperature in the room should be warm enough so that the patient is comfortable. During the massage, their body will be wholly or partially exposed to the air. If it is too cold, they may be tense, and they may even catch a cold. Needless to say, this would prevent you from gaining their whole-hearted cooperation.

2. You should use a massage table which is comfortable for the patient, and of a height which is comfortable for you. If the table is too high or too low, it will feel awkward to you, and your concentration will be disturbed.

3. The patient should dress comfortably, with loose clothing. Also, whatever they are lying on should be made of natural material. For example, if they are lying on polyester sheet, a great mass of Qi (static charges) can accumulate in the material and affect the treatment.

4. The air should be circulating gently. If the air is stagnant, both you and the patient will feel uncomfortable.

5. Do not massage a person who has just eaten, or who is hungry, since the massage might be uncomfortable, especially when you work on their stomach.

6. Don't have a light directly over the patient, since this would make them uncomfortable.

7. The room should be as quiet as possible. Noise is always disturbing during massage, though sometimes soft music might help them to relax.
8. The patient's body should be clean, and your hands should also be clean and warm. Many masseurs will place a silk handkerchief on the area they are massaging to avoid directly touching the skin. However, this reduces the sensitivity of their touch, and limits the Qi communication between them and the patient.
9. Before starting, always ask yourself the following questions. What is the purpose of the massage? What does the patient expect? Is the massage for relaxation and enjoyment, or is it to treat an illness? Am I confident that I have enough experience to give this massage? Remember, understanding yourself and the patient is the key to a successful treatment.
10. Always understand the patient's body. Different levels of power should be used for different patients, and for different purposes. You will also vary the techniques you use, depending upon the patient. The better you understand the patient's body, the more you will know about the battlefield upon which you are fighting sickness.
11. Always diagnose the case carefully, and determine how serious the problem is. For example, if the injury involves a cracked bone, then you should not massage the area with power, since that would hinder the healing of the bone. Wrong treatments only make matters worse.
12. When you massage a patient, do not cause pain or tickle them, since this will cause them to tense.
13. If you are treating the patient externally with herbs, do not apply them anywhere where there are cuts or breaks in the skin, since this may cause an infection.
14. Keep your fingernails short! Long nails will limit how you can use your hands, and they will make your patient nervous.
15. You must reach an understanding with your patient if you are to massage any area about which they are shy.
16. Ask the patient for permission before using massage oil. Some people don't like it.
17. Always explain to the patient or massage partner what you are going to do. This will allow them to prepare themselves mentally, and will increase their confidence in you.

Reference

1. *The Body Electric* by Robert O. Becker, M.D. and Gary Selden, Quill, William Morrow, New York, 1985.

CHAPTER 3
Qigong Practices for Massage 按摩之氣功練習

3-1. INTRODUCTION 介紹

In Chinese healing massage society, to become a proficient masseur, almost all aspirants train special Qigong that allows them to achieve a profound level of feeling, concentration, and effective treatment. The reason is very simple. Massage is considered to be a kind of meditation that brings your feeling and concentrated mind to a profound state. While in this state, you and your patient's feelings and Qi are united and harmonized with each other. Consequently, your patient can be successfully treated.

Through more than two thousand years of massage practice, many various schools developed. Among these schools, not only are the specialities and techniques of treatment different, but also the training methods. Qigong trainings which serve different purposes of each individual school are also different. For example, among those schools which focus on the treatment of sickness, Dian Xue techniques are trained and practiced more than in those schools which specialize in injuries in which Tui Na is the main focus of training. Therefore, the strength of the fingers and mental concentration are emphasized than in Tui Na massage, in which the conditioning of the wrists and palms are taken more seriously.

However, it does not matter what training a school stresses, the theory and training principles remain the same. Once you understand these training theories and principles, you can create any special training which may serve the purpose better.

Generally speaking, there are several purposes of Qigong training in massage:

1. To condition the physical body of the masseur. To a proficient masseur, good physical conditioning is always the first concern. Very often, after a masseur treats few patients, he/she will experience bodily injury, especially in the joints area such as on the fingers, wrists, or even the lower back. These injuries can be caused by over use in these joints. Therefore, in order to become a proficient masseur, you must first condition those joints and muscles, which are used most often for strength and endurance. Strength will offer you the power to reach deep and endurance will allow you to last long.

2. To be able to concentrate and focus. Mind is considered to be the general in a battle. When you treat a patient, it is your mind that makes the diagnosis, and it is also your mind that feels the patient and your body. Through this communication and understanding, you can treat your patient effectively. Therefore, concentrating your mind in the treatment and focusing it in a special treating area—or even a tiny cavity—has always been a crucial key in successful massage treatment. Qigong practice will allow you to bring your mind to a profoundly calm and concentrated state.

3. To establish a higher level of feeling and sensitivity. Once you have a concentrated and focused mind, you can establish a high level of feeling and sensitivity. In Chinese medicine, 'feeling' is a language which allows your mind to communicate with your body and your patient's body. If you have a high level of feeling or sensitivity, then this communication will be easily recognized and understood. Under this condition, the treatments you have applied to your patient will be effective.

4. To use the mind to lead the Qi more efficiently. In order to execute your techniques effectively and skillfully, you must know how to use your mind to lead the Qi to your physical body so it can be manifested effectively. In addition, in Dian Xue and Qi massages, it is crucial that you are able to use your mind to lead the Qi for either nourishment (Bu, 補) or releasing (Xie, 洩). Naturally, how effective you are at leading the Qi depends on the level of concentration you are able to reach.

5. To build up a higher level of Qi storage in the body. Qi is the energetic aspect of your life. When the Qi is abundant and strongly circulating, your physical body will be healthy and strong. In massage, especially in Dian Xue and Qi massages, you are using your Qi to manipulate the patient's Qi and help him/her to recover. If you don't have abundant Qi storage, then not only will the treatment be ineffective, but also you may get sick yourself afterward. Remember, only if you have strong and abundant Qi should you manipulate it and use it for treatment, otherwise, you may obtain the negative affect to yourself.

6. To have a fast and effective recovery after massage. One of the crucial trainings in Dian Xue and Qi massages is learning how to achieve fast recovery both in your physical body and Qi body. Naturally, if you have a strong physical body and an abundant level of Qi storage, you already have an advantage for this recovery. Other than physical conditioning, you must also learn how to build up your Qi level to an abundant level. Finally, you must learn how to conserve your Qi so you will not abuse it or waste it.

In this chapter, we will first discuss the general Qigong training theory. Then, some of the most common Qigong practice in massage will be introduced section 3-3.

3-2. QIGONG TRAINING THEORY 氣功訓練之理論

Many people think that Qigong is a difficult subject to comprehend. In some ways, this is true. However, you must understand one thing. Regardless of how difficult the Qigong theory and practice of a particular style is, the basic theory and principles are very simple and remain the same for all Qigong styles. The basic theory and principles are the root of the entire Qigong practice. If you understand these roots, you will be able to grasp the key to the practice and grow. All of the Qigong styles originated from these roots, but each one has blossomed differently.

In this section we will discuss these basic Qigong training theories and principles. With this knowledge as a foundation, you will be able to understand not only what you should be doing, but also why you are doing it. Naturally, it is impossible to discuss all of the basic Qigong ideas in such a short section. However, it will offer you the key to open the gate into the spacious, four thousand year old garden of Chinese Qigong. If you wish to know more about the theory of Qigong, please refer to *The Root of Chinese Qigong*, by YMAA.

The Concept of Yin and Yang, Kan and Li

The concept of Yin (陰) and Yang (陽) is the foundation of Chinese philosophy. From this philosophy, Chinese culture was developed. Naturally, this includes Chinese medicine and Qigong practice. Therefore, in order to understand Qigong, first you should study the concept of Yin and Yang. In addition, you should also understand the concept of Kan (坎) and Li (離) which, unfortunately, has been commonly confused with the concept of Yin and Yang even in China.

The Chinese have long believed that the universe is made up of two opposite forces—Yin (陰) and Yang (陽)—which must balance each other. When these two forces begin to lose their balance, nature finds a way to re-balance them. If the imbalance is significant, disaster will occur. However, when these two forces interact with each other smoothly and harmoniously, they manifest power and generate the millions of living things.

As mentioned earlier, Yin and Yang theory is also applied to the three great natural powers: heaven (Tian, 天), earth (Di, 地), and man (Ren, 人). For example, if the Yin and Yang forces of heaven (i.e. energy which comes to us from the sky) lose their balance, there can be tornadoes, hurricanes, or other natural disasters. When the Yin and Yang forces lose their balance on earth, rivers can change their paths and earthquakes can occur. When the Yin and Yang forces in the human body lose their balance, sickness and even death can occur. Experience has shown that the Yin and Yang balance in man is affected by the Yin and Yang balances of the earth and heaven. Similarly, the Yin and Yang balance of the earth is influenced by the heaven's Yin and Yang. Therefore, if you wish to have a healthy body and live a long life, you need to know how to adjust your body's Yin and Yang, and how to coordinate your Qi with the Yin and Yang energy of heaven and earth. The study of Yin and Yang in the human body is the root of Chinese medicine and Qigong.

Furthermore, the Chinese have also classified everything in the universe according to Yin and Yang. Even feelings, thoughts, strategy and the spirit are covered. For example, female is Yin and male is Yang, night is Yin and day is Yang, weak is Yin and strong is Yang, backward is Yin and forward is Yang, sad is Yin and happy is Yang, defense is Yin and offense is Yang, and so on.

Practitioners of Chinese medicine and Qigong believe that they must seek to understand the Yin and Yang of nature and the human body before they can adjust and regulate the body's energy balance into a more harmonious state. Only then can health be maintained and the causes of sicknesses be corrected.

Another thing which you should understand is that the concept of Yin and Yang is relative instead of absolute. For example, the number seven is Yang compared with three. However, if seven is compared with ten, then it is Yin. That means in order to decide Yin or Yang, a reference point must first be chosen. Therefore, if five is the Yin and Yang balance number, then seven is Yang and three is Yin. If we choose zero as the Yin and Yang balance number, then any positive is Yang and any negative number is Yin.

However, if what we are interested in is the most negative number, then we may choose the negative number as Yang and positive number as Yin with zero as the central number. For example, generally speaking in Qigong, techniques that can be seen physically and are the manifestation of Qi are considered Yang, and the techniques that cannot be seen but felt are treated as Yin. When the Yin and Yang concept is applied in Chinese medicine, since the Qi is the major concern and plays the main role in medicine, it is considered Yang, while the blood (physical) is considered Yin.

Now let us discuss how the concept of Yin and Yang is applied to the Qi circulating in the human body. Many people, even some Qigong practitioners, are still confused by this. When it is said that Qi can be either Yin or Yang, it does not mean that there are two different kinds of Qi like male and female, fire and water, or positive and negative charges. Qi is energy, and energy itself does not have Yin and Yang. It is like the energy which is generated from the sparking of negative and positive charges. Charges have the potential for generating energy, but are not the energy itself.

When it is said that Qi is Yin or Yang, it means that the Qi is too strong or too weak for a particular circumstance. Again, it is relative and not absolute. Naturally, this implies that the potential which generates the Qi is strong or weak. For example, the Qi from the sun is Yang Qi, and Qi from the moon is Yin Qi. This is because the sun's energy is Yang in comparison to Human Qi, while the moon's is Yin. In any discussion of energy where people are involved, Human Qi is used as the standard. People are always especially interested in what concerns them directly, so it is natural that we are interested primarily in Human Qi and tend to view all Qi from the perspective of human Qi. This is not unlike looking at the universe from the physical perspective of the Earth.

When we look at the Yin and Yang of Qi within the human body, however, we must redefine our point of reference. For example, when a person is dead, his residual human Qi (Gui Qi or ghost Qi, 鬼氣) is weak compared to a living person's. Therefore, the ghost Qi is Yin as it dissipates, while the living person's Qi is Yang. When discussing Qi within the body, in the Lung Channel for example, the reference point is the normal, healthy status of the Qi there. If the Qi is stronger than it is in the normal state, it is Yang, and, naturally, if it is weaker than this, it is Yin. There are twelve parts of the human body that are considered organs in Chinese medicine, six of them are Yin and six are Yang. The Yin organs are the Heart, Lungs, Kidneys, Liver, Spleen, and Pericardium, and the Yang organs are Small Intestine, Large Intestine, Urinary Bladder, Gall Bladder, Stomach, and Triple Burner. Generally speaking, the Qi level of the Yin organs is lower than that of the Yang organs. The Yin organs store Original Essence and process the Essence obtained from food and air, while the Yang organs handle digestion and excretion.

When the Qi in any of your organs is not in its normal state, you feel uncomfortable. If it is very much off from the normal state, the organ will start to malfunction and you may become sick. When this happens, the Qi in your entire body will also be affected and you will feel too Yang, perhaps feverish, or too Yin, such as the weakness after diarrhea.

Your body's Qi level is also affected by your natural environment, such as the weather, climate, and seasonal changes. Therefore, when the body's Qi level is classified, the reference point is the level which feels most comfortable for those particular circumstances. Naturally, each of us is a little bit different, and what feels best and most natural for one person may be a bit different for another person. That is why the doctor will usually ask "how do you feel?" It is according to your own standard that you are judged.

Breathing is closely related to the state of your Qi, and is therefore also considered Yin or Yang. When you exhale you expel air from your lungs, your mind moves outward, and the Qi around the body expands. In the Chinese martial arts, the exhale is generally used to expand the Qi to energize the muscles during an attack. Therefore, you can see that the exhale is Yang—it is expanding, offensive, and strong. Naturally, based on the same theory, the inhale is considered Yin.

Your breathing is closely related to your emotions. When you lose your temper, your breathing is short and fast, i.e. Yang. When you are sad, your body is more Yin, and you inhale more than you exhale in order to absorb Qi from the air to balance the body's Yin and bring the body back into balance. When you are excited and happy your body is Yang, and your exhale is longer than your inhale to get rid of the excess Yang which is caused by the excitement.

As mentioned before, your mind is also closely related to your Qi. Therefore, when your Qi is Yang, your mind is usually also Yang (excited) and vice versa. The mind can also be classified according to the Qi which generated it. The mind (Yi, 意) which is generated from the calm and peaceful Qi obtained from the Original Essence (Yuan Jing, 元精) is considered Yin. The mind (Xin, 心) which originates with the food and air essence is emotional, scattered, and excited, and it is considered Yang. The spirit, which is related to the Qi, can also be classified as Yang or Yin based on its origin.

Do not confuse Yin Qi and Yang Qi with Fire Qi (Huo Qi, 火氣) and Water Qi (Shui Qi, 水氣). When the Yin and Yang of Qi are mentioned, it refers to the level of Qi according to some reference point. However, when Water and Fire Qi are mentioned, it refers to the quality of the Qi. If you are interested in reading more about the Yin and Yang of Qi, please refer to the Book: *The Root of Chinese Qigong* and *Qigong— The Secret of Youth,* by YMAA.

The terms Kan (坎) and Li (離) occur frequently in Qigong documents. In the Eight Trigrams (Bagua, 八卦), Kan represents "Water" while Li represents "Fire." However, the everyday terms for water and fire are also often used. Kan and Li training has long been of major importance to Qigong practitioners. In order to understand why, you must understand these two words, and the theory behind them.

First you should understand that though Kan-Li and Yin-Yang are related, Kan and Li are not Yin and Yang. Kan is Water, which is able to cool your body down and make it more Yin, while Li is Fire, which warms your body and makes it more Yang. *Kan and Li are the methods or causes, while Yin and Yang are the results.* When Kan and Li are adjusted and regulated correctly, Yin and Yang will be balanced and interact harmoniously.

Qigong practitioners believe that your body is always too Yang, unless you are sick or have not eaten for a long time, in which case your body may be more Yin. Since your body is always Yang, it is degenerating and burning out. It is believed that this is the cause of aging. If you can use Water to cool down your body, you will be able to slow down the degeneration process and thereby lengthen your life. This is the main reason why Chinese Qigong practitioners have been studying ways of improving the quality of the Water in their bodies, and of reducing the quantity of the Fire. I believe that as a Qigong practitioner you should always keep this subject at the top of your list for study and research. If you earnestly ponder and experiment, you will be able to grasp the trick of adjusting them.

If you want to learn how to adjust them, you must understand that Water and Fire mean many things in your body. The first concerns your Qi. As mentioned earlier, Qi is classified as Fire and Water. When your Qi is not pure and causes your physical body to heat up and your mental/spiritual body to become unstable (Yang), it is classified as Fire Qi. The Qi which is pure and is able to cool both your physical and spiritual bodies (make them more Yin) is considered Water Qi. However, you body can never be purely Water. Water can cool down the Fire, but it must never totally quench it, because then you would be dead. It is also said that Fire Qi is able to agitate and stimulate the emotions, and from these emotions generate a 'mind.' This mind is called Xin (心) (i.e. heart), and is considered the Fire mind, Yang mind, or emotional mind. On the other hand, the mind that Water Qi generates is calm, steady, and wise. This mind is called Yi (意), and is considered to be the Water mind or wisdom mind. If your spirit is nourished by the Fire Qi, although your spirit may be high, it will be scattered and confused (a Yang spirit). Naturally, if the spirit is nourished and raised up by Water Qi, it will be firm and steady (a Yin mind). When your Yi is able to govern your emotional Xin effectively, your will (strong emotional intention) can be firm.

You can see from this discussion that your Qi is the main cause of the Yin and Yang of your physical body, your mind, and your spirit. To regulate your body's Yin and Yang, you must learn how to regulate your body's Water and Fire Qi, but in order to do this efficiently you must know their sources.

Once you have grasped the concepts of Yin-Yang and Kan-Li, then you have to think about how to adjust Kan and Li so that you can balance the Yin and Yang in your body.

Theoretically, a Qigong practitioner would like to keep his body in a state of Yin-Yang balance, which means the center point of the Yin and Yang forces. This center point is commonly called Wuji (無極) (no extremities). It is believed that Wuji is the original, natural state where Yin and Yang are not distinguished. In the Wuji state, nature is peaceful and calm. In the Wuji state, all of the Yin and Yang forces have gradually combined harmoniously and disappeared. When this Wuji theory is applied to human beings, it is the final goal of Qigong practice where your mind is neutral and absolutely calm. The Wuji state makes it possible for you to find the origin of your life, and to combine your Qi with the Qi of nature.

The ultimate goal and purpose of Qigong practice is to find this peaceful and natural state. In order to reach this goal, you must first understand your body's Yin and Yang so that you can balance them by adjusting your Kan and Li. Only when your Yin and Yang are balanced will you be able to find the center balance point, the Wuji state.

Theoretically, between the two extremes of Yin and Yang are millions of paths (i.e. different Kan and Li methods) which can lead you to the neutral center. This accounts for the hundreds of different styles of Qigong which have been created over the years. You can see that the theory of Yin and Yang and the methods of Kan and Li are the root of training all Chinese Qigong styles. Without this root, the essence of Qigong practice would be lost.

Three Treasures—Jing, Qi, and Shen (三寶 - 精、氣、神)

Before you start any Qigong training you must also understand the three treasures of your body (San Bao, 三寶): Jing (Essence, 精), Qi (Internal Energy, 氣), and Shen (Spirit, 神). They are also called the "three origins" or the "three roots" (San Yuan, 三元),

because they are considered the origins and roots of your life. Jing means Essence, the most original and refined part. Jing is the original source and most basic part of every living thing, and determines your nature and characteristics. It is the root of life. Sperm is called Jing Zi (精子), which means "Essence of the Son," because it contains the Jing of the father which is passed on to his son (or daughter) and becomes the son's Jing.

Qi, known as bioelectricity today, is the internal energy of your body. It is like the electricity which passes through a machine to keep it running. Qi comes either from the conversion of the Jing which you have received from your parents, or from the food you eat and the air you breathe.

Shen (Spirit) is the center of your mind and being. It is what makes you human, because animals do not have a Shen. The Shen in your body must be nourished by your Qi or energy. When your Qi is full, your Shen will be enlivened.

Chinese meditators and Qigong practitioners believe that the body contains two general types of Qi. The first type is called Pre-Birth Qi or Pre-Heaven Qi (Xian Tian Qi, 先天氣), and it comes from converted Original Jing (Yuan Jing, 元精), which you get from your parents at conception. The second type, which is called Post-Birth Qi or Post-Heaven Qi (Hou Tian Qi, 後天氣), is drawn from the Jing of the food and air we take in. When this Qi flows or is led to the brain, it can energize the Shen and soul. This energized and raised Shen is able to govern and lead the Qi to the entire body.

Each one of these three elements or treasures has its own root. You must know the roots so that you can strengthen and protect your three treasures.

1. Your body requires many kinds of Jing. Except for the Jing which you inherit from your parents, which is called Original Jing (Yuan Jing, 元精), all other Jings must be obtained from food and air. Among all of these Jings, Original Jing is the most important one. It is the root and the seed of your life, and your basic strength. If your parents were strong and healthy, your Original Jing will be strong and healthy, you will have a strong foundation on which to grow. The Chinese people believe that in order to stay healthy and live a long life, you must protect and maintain this Jing.

    According to Chinese medicine, the root of Original Jing before your birth was in your parents. After birth this Original Jing stays in its residence—the kidneys, which are considered the root of your Jing. When you keep this root strong, you will have sufficient Original Jing to supply to your body. Although you cannot increase the amount of Original Jing you have, Qigong training can improve the quality of your Jing. Qigong can also teach you how to convert your Jing into Original Qi more efficiently, and how to use this Qi effectively.

    If we analyze the concept of Jing from a modern physical scientific point of view, we might postulate that Jing is in the genetic material which we inherited from our parents. From this material, the structure and health of one person is different from all others. From different genes, the different levels of hormones in different people is controlled. When Chinese medicine says that the Original Jing is stored in the kidneys, it implies the hormones which are produced in the adrenal glands. According to Chinese medicine, there is no record of the endocrine glands. This implies that Chinese medicine has never understood the function of the endocrine. In my opinion, the Jing (essence) is stored in all of the endocrine glands. I believe that the most significant gland which stores the essence and affects the level of the entire body's Jing (hormone production) is the pituitary gland (corresponding to the Upper Dan Tian).

2. According to Chinese medicine and Qigong, Qi is converted both from the Jing which you have inherited from your parents and from the Jing which you draw from the food and air you breathe. Qi that is converted from the Original Jing which you inherited is called Original Qi (Yuan Qi, 元氣).[1] Just as Original Jing is the most important type of Jing, Original Qi is the most important type of Qi. It is pure and of high quality, while the Qi from food and air may make your body too positive or too negative, depending on how and where you absorb it. When you retain and protect your Original Jing, you will be able to generate Original Qi in a pure, continuous stream. As a Qigong practitioner, you must know how to convert your Original Jing into Original Qi in a smooth, steady stream.

Since your Original Qi comes from your Original Jing, they both have the kidneys for their root. When your kidneys are strong, the Original Jing is strong, and the Original Qi converted from this Original Jing will also be full and strong. This Qi resides in the Lower Dan Tian in your abdomen. Once you learn how to convert your Original Jing, you will be able to supply your body with all the Qi it needs.

Again, if we analyze the above concepts, we can see that the essence here means the hormone level which is produced from the adrenal glands on the top of your kidneys. In fact, we have already seen that the pituitary gland is considered the master of the glands, and when the hormone production in this gland is high, the hormone production of all other Endocrine Glands will also be high. When the hormone level of the body is high, the Qi is abundant and the circulation is smooth. When the hormone production level is high in the pituitary gland, the spirit (Shen, 神) residing in the center of your brain will be high. When the spirit is high, it is able to strongly and smoothly direct the Qi circulating in the body for function, repair and healing. This results in the development of spiritual healing science.

3. Shen (i.e. spirit, 神) is the force which keeps you alive. It has no substance, but it gives expression and appearance to your Jing. Shen is also the control

tower for the Qi. When your Shen is strong, your Qi is strong and you can lead it efficiently. The root of Shen (Spirit) is your mind (Yi, or intention). When your brain is energized and stimulated, your mind will be more aware and you will be able to concentrate more intensely. Also, your Shen will be raised. Advanced Qigong practitioners believe that your brain must always be sufficiently nourished by your Qi. It is the Qi which keeps your mind clear and concentrated. With an abundant Qi supply, the mind can be energized, and can raise the Shen and enhance your vitality.

The deeper levels of Qigong training include the conversion of Jing into Qi (Lian Jing Hua Qi, 練精化氣), which is then led to the brain to raise the Shen (Lian Qi Hua Shen, 練氣化神). This process is called Huan Jing Bu Nao (還精補腦) and means "return the Jing to nourish the brain." When Qi is led to the head, it stays at the Upper Dan Tian (at the center of the head), which is the residence of your Shen. Qi and Shen are mutually related. When your Shen is weak, your Qi is weak, and your body will degenerate rapidly. Shen is the headquarters of Qi. Likewise, Qi supports the Shen, energizing it and keeping it sharp, clear, and strong. If the Qi in your body is weak, your Shen will also be weak.

Scientifically, in order to maintain a high hormone production level, you must continue to supply bioelectricity to the pituitary gland. Without this basic energy, the gland will function inadequately. Therefore, one of the main Qigong practices is learning, through meditation, how to lead the Qi to the brain and nourish the pituitary gland.

From the above discussion, you can see that in order to have a healthy and strong body, you must first learn how to keep the Yin and Yang balance in your body. In addition, you should also learn how to adjust or regulate your body, allowing you to fit in the natural environment more harmoniously. Furthermore, you should learn how to retain and generate your Jing, strengthen and smooth your Qi flow, and enlighten your Shen. That means you should learn how to maintain the hormone production of your body, how to store the Qi in your Lower Dan Tian (battery) and smoothly circulate it in your body, and how to lead the Qi to the brain to nourish your Spirit. If you are interested in the further pursuit of enlightenment, then you must learn how to regulate your mind to a neutral state and build up a Spiritual Embryo (Sheng Tai, 聖胎). From the cultivation of this spiritual embryo, you will be able to separate your spiritual body and your physical body. If you are interested in this subject, please refer to *Qigong—The Secret of Youth* and *Qigong Meditation—Embryonic Breathing*, by YMAA.

Qigong Training Theory

Every Qigong form or practice has its special training purpose and theory. If you do not know the purpose and theory, you have lost the root (meaning) of the practice.

Therefore, as a Qigong practitioner, you must continue to ponder and practice until you understand the root of every set or form.

Now that you have learned the basic theory of the Qigong practice, let us discuss the general training principles. In Chinese Qigong society, it is commonly known that in order to reach the goal of Qigong practice, you must learn how to regulate the body (Tiao Shen, 調身), regulate the breathing (Tiao Xi, 調息), regulate the emotional mind (Tiao Xin, 調心), regulate the Qi (Tiao Qi, 調氣), and regulate the spirit (Tiao Shen, 調神). Tiao in Chinese is constructed from two words, "言" (Yan, means speaking or talking) and "周" (Zhou, means round or complete). That means the roundness (i.e. harmony) or the completeness is accomplished by negotiation. Like an out of tune in piano, you must adjust it and make it harmonize with its environment. This implies that, when you are regulating one of the above five processes, you must also coordinate and harmonize the other four regulating elements.

Regulating the body includes understanding how to find and build the root of the body, as well as the root of the individual forms you are practicing. To build a firm root, you must know how to keep your center, how to balance your body, and most important of all, how to relax so that the Qi can flow.

To regulate your breathing, you must learn how to breathe so that your respiration and your mind mutually correspond and cooperate. When you breathe this way, your mind will be able to attain peace more quickly, and therefore concentrate more easily on leading the Qi.

Regulating the mind involves learning how to keep your mind calm, peaceful, and centered, so that you can judge situations objectively and lead Qi to the desired places. The mind is the main key to success in Qigong practice.

Regulating the Qi is one of the ultimate goals of Qigong practice. In order to regulate your Qi effectively you must first have regulated your body, breathing, and mind. Only then will your mind be clear enough to sense how the Qi is distributed in your body, and understand how to adjust it.

For Buddhist and Daoist priests, who seek enlightenment or Buddhahood, regulating the spirit (Shen) is the final goal of Qigong. This enables them to maintain a neutral, objective perspective of life, and this perspective is the eternal life of the Buddha. The average Qigong practitioner has lower goals. He raises his spirit in order to increase his concentration and enhance his vitality. This makes it possible for him to lead Qi effectively throughout his entire body so that it carries out the managing and guarding duties. This maintains health and slows the aging process.

If you understand these few things you will be able to quickly enter into the field of Qigong. Without all of these important elements, your training will be ineffective and your time will be wasted.

Before you start training, you must first understand that all of the training originates in your mind. You must have a clear idea of what you are doing, and your mind must be calm, centered, and balanced. This also implies that your feeling, sensing, and judgment must be objective and accurate. This requires emotional balance and a clear mind. This takes a lot of hard work, but once you have reached this level you will have built the root of your physical training, and your Yi (mind) will be able to lead your Qi throughout your physical body.

Regulating the Body (Tiao Shen, 調身). When you learn any Qigong, either moving or still, the first step is to learn the correct postures or movements. After you have learned the postures and movements, learn how to improve them until you can perform the forms accurately. Then, you start to regulate your body until it has reached the stage which could provide the best condition for the Qi to build up or to circulate.

In Still Qigong practice or Soft Qigong movement, this means to adjust your body until it is in the most comfortable and relaxed state. This implies that your body must be centered and balanced. If it is not, you will be tense and uneasy, and this will affect the judgment of your Yi and the circulation of your Qi. In Chinese medical society it is said: "(When) shape (body's posture) is not correct, then the Qi will not be smooth. (When) the Qi is not smooth, the Yi (wisdom mind) will not be peaceful. (When) the Yi is not peaceful, then the Qi is disordered."[2] You should understand that the relaxation of your body originates with your Yi. Therefore, before you can relax your body, you must first relax or regulate your mind (Yi). This is called Shen Xin Ping Heng (身心平衡), which means "Body and heart (i.e. mind) balanced." The body and the mind are mutually related. A relaxed and balanced body helps your Yi to relax and concentrate. When your Yi is at peace and can judge things accurately, your body will be relaxed, balanced, centered, and rooted. Only when you are rooted, then you will be able to raise up your spirit of vitality.

Relaxation. Relaxation is one of the major keys to success in Qigong. You should remember that only when you are relaxed will all your Qi channels be open. In order to be relaxed, your Yi must first be relaxed and calm. When the Yi coordinates with your breathing, your body will be able to relax.

In Qigong practice there are three levels of relaxation. The first level is the external physical relaxation, or postural relaxation. This is a very superficial level, and almost anyone can reach it. It consists of adopting a comfortable stance and avoiding unnecessary strain in how you stand and move. The second level is the relaxation of the muscles and tendons. To do this your Yi must be directed deep into the muscles and tendons. This relaxation will help open your Qi channels, and will allow the Qi to sink and accumulate in the Dan Tian.

The final stage is the relaxation which reaches the internal organs and the bone marrow. Remember, only if you can relax deep into your body will your mind be able to lead the Qi there. Only at this stage will the Qi be able to reach everywhere. Then you will feel transparent—as if your whole body had disappeared. If you can reach this level of relaxation, you will be able to communicate with your organs and use Qigong to adjust or regulate the Qi disorders which are giving you problems. You will also be able to protect your organs more effectively, and therefore slow down their degeneration.

Rooting. In all Qigong practice it is very important to be rooted. Being rooted means to be stable and in firm contact with the ground. If you want to push a car, you have to be rooted so the force you exert into the car will be balanced by a force into the ground. If you are not rooted, when you push the car you will only push yourself away, and not move the car. Your root is made up of your body's root, center, and balance.

Before you can develop your root, you must first relax and let your body 'settle.' As you relax, the tension in the various parts of your body will dissolve, and you will find a comfortable way to stand. You will stop fighting the ground to keep your body up, and will learn to rely on your body's structure to support itself. This lets the muscles relax even more. Since your body isn't struggling to stand up, your Yi won't be pushing upward, and your body, mind, and Qi will all be able to sink. If you let dirty water sit quietly, the impurities will gradually settle down to the bottom, leaving the water above it clear. In the same way, if you relax your body enough to let it settle, your Qi will sink to your Dan Tian and the Bubbling Wells (Yongquan, K-1, 湧泉) in your feet, and your mind will become clear. Then you can begin to develop your root.

To root your body you must imitate a tree and grow an invisible root under your feet. This will give you a firm root to keep you stable in your training. Your root must be wide as well as deep. Naturally, your Yi must grow first, because it is the Yi which leads the Qi. Your Yi must be able to lead the Qi to your feet, and be able to communicate with the ground. Only when your Yi can communicate with the ground will your Qi be able to grow beyond your feet and enter the ground to build the root. The Bubbling Well cavity is the gate which enables your Qi to communicate with the ground.

After you have gained your root, you must learn how to keep your center. A stable center will make your Qi develop evenly and uniformly. If you lose this center, your Qi will not be led evenly. In order to keep your body centered, you must first center your Yi, and then match your body to it. Only under these conditions will the Qigong forms you practice have their root. Your mental and physical centers are the keys which enable you to lead your Qi beyond your body.

Balance is the product of rooting and centering. Balance includes balancing the Qi and the physical body. It does not matter which aspect of balance you are dealing with, first you must balance your Yi, and only then can you balance your Qi and your physical body. If your Yi is balanced, it can help you to make accurate judgments, and therefore to correct the path of the Qi flow.

Rooting includes not just rooting the body, but also the form or movement. The root of any form or movement is found in its purpose or principle. For example, in certain Qigong exercises you want to lead the Qi to your palms. In order to do this you may imagine that you are pushing an object forward while keeping your muscles relaxed.

In this exercise, your elbows must be down to build the sense of root for the push. If you raise the elbows, you lose the sense of intention of the movement, because the push would be ineffective if you were pushing something for real. Since the intention or purpose of the movement is its reason for being, you now have a purposeless movement, and you have no reason to lead Qi in any particular way. Therefore, in this case, the elbow is the root of the movement.

Regulating the Breath (Tiao Xi, 調息). Regulating the breath means to regulate your breathing until it is calm, smooth, and peaceful. Only when you have reached this point will you be able to make the breathing deep, slender, long, and soft, which is required for successful Qigong practice.

Breathing is affected by your emotions. For example, when you are angry or excited you exhale more strongly than you inhale. When you are sad, you inhale more strongly than you exhale. When your mind is peaceful and calm, your inhalation and exhalation are relatively equal. In order to keep your breathing calm, peaceful, and steady, your mind and emotions must first be calm and neutral. Therefore, in order to regulate your breathing, you must first regulate your mind.

The other side of the coin is that you can use your breathing to control your Yi. When your breathing is uniform, it is as if you were hypnotizing your Yi, which helps to calm it. You can see that Yi and breathing are interdependent, and that they cooperate with each other. Deep and calm breathing relaxes you and keeps your mind clear. It fills your lungs with plenty of air, so that your brain and entire body have an adequate supply of oxygen. In addition, deep and complete breathing enables the diaphragm to move up and down, which massages and stimulates the internal organs. For this reason, deep breathing exercises are also called "internal organ exercises."

Deep and complete breathing does not mean that you inhale and exhale to the maximum. This would cause the lungs and the surrounding muscles to tense up, which in turn would keep the air from circulating freely, and hinder the absorption of oxygen. Without enough oxygen, your mind becomes scattered, and the rest of your body tenses up. In correct breathing, you inhale and exhale to about 70% or 80% of capacity, so that your lungs stay relaxed.

You can conduct an easy experiment. Inhale deeply so that your lungs are completely full, and time how long you can hold your breath. Then try inhaling to only about 70% of your capacity, and see how long you can hold your breath. You will find that with the latter method you can last much longer than the first one. This is simply because the lungs and the surrounding muscles are relaxed. When they are relaxed, the rest of your body and your mind can also relax, which significantly decreases your need for oxygen. Therefore, when you regulate your breathing, the first priority is to keep your lungs relaxed and calm.

When training, your mind must first be calm so that your breathing can be regulated. When the breathing is regulated, your mind is able to reach a higher level of calmness. This calmness can again help you to regulate the breathing, until your mind is deep. After you have trained for a long time, your breathing will be full and slender, and your mind will be very clear. It is said: "Xin Xi Xiang Yi" (心息相依), which means "Heart (Mind) and breathing (are) mutually dependent." When you reach this meditative state, your heartbeat slows down, and your mind is very clear: you have entered the sphere of real meditation.

An ancient Daoist named Li, Qing-An (李清庵) said: "Regulating breathing means to regulate the real breathing until (you) stop."[3] This means that correct regulating means regulating is no longer necessary. Real regulating is no longer a conscious process, but has become so natural that it can be accomplished without conscious effort. In other words, although you start by consciously regulating your breath, you must get to the point where the regulating happens naturally, and you no longer have to think about it. When you breathe, if you concentrate your mind on your breathing, then it is not true regulating, because the Qi in your lungs will become stagnant. When you reach the level of true regulating, you don't have to pay attention to it, and you can use your mind efficiently to lead the Qi. Remember, wherever the Yi is, there is the Qi. If the Yi stops in one spot, the Qi will be stagnant. It is the Yi which leads the Qi and makes it move. Therefore, when you are in a state of correct breath regulation, your mind is free. There is no sound stagnation, urgency, or hesitation, and you can finally be calm and peaceful.

You can see that when the breath is regulated correctly, the Qi will also be regulated. They are mutually related and cannot be separated. This idea is explained frequently in the Daoist literature. The Daoist Guang Cheng Zi (廣成子) said: "One exhale, the Earth Qi rises; one inhale, the Heaven Qi descends; real man's (meaning one who has attained the real Dao) repeated breathing at the navel, then my real Qi is naturally connected."[4] This says that when you breathe you should move your abdomen, as if you were breathing from your navel. The earth Qi is the negative (Yin) energy from your kidneys, and the sky Qi is the positive (Yang) energy which comes from the food you eat and the air you breathe. When you breathe from the navel, these two Qi's will connect and combine. Some people think that they know what Qi is, but they really don't. Once you connect the two Qi's, you will know what the 'real' Qi is, and you may become a 'real' man, which means to attain the Dao.

The Daoist book *Chang Dao Zhen Yan* (唱道真言) (*Sing (of the) Dao (with) Real Words*) says: "One exhale one inhale to communicate Qi's function, one movement one calmness is the same as (i.e. is the source of) creation and variation."[5] The first part of this statement again implies that the functioning of Qi is connected with the breathing. The second part of this sentence means that all creation and variation come from the interaction of movement (Yang) and calmness (Yin). *Huang Ting Jing* (黃庭經) (*Yellow Yard Classic*) says: "Breathe Original Qi to seek immortality."[6] In China, the traditional Daoists wore yellow robes, and they meditated in a 'yard' or hall. This sentence means that in order to reach the goal of immortality, you must seek to find and understand the Original Qi which comes from the Dan Tian through correct breathing.

Moreover, the Daoist Wu Zhen Ren (伍真人) said: "Use the Post-Birth breathing to look for the real person's (i.e. the immortal's) breathing place."[7] In this sentence it is clear that in order to locate the immortal breathing place (the Dan Tian), you must rely on and know how to regulate your Post-Birth, or natural, breathing. Through regulating your Post-Birth breathing you will gradually be able to locate the residence of the Qi (the Dan Tian), and eventually you will be able to use your Dan Tian to breath like the immortal Daoists. Finally, in the Daoist song *Ling Yuan Da Dao Ge* (靈源大道歌) (*The Great Daoist Song of the Spirit's Origin*) it is said: "The Originals (Original Jing, Qi, and Shen) are internally transported peacefully, so that you can become real (immortal); (if you) depend (only) on external breathing (you) will not reach the end (goal)."[8] From this song, you can see the internal breathing (breathing at the Dan Tian) is the key to training your three treasures and finally reaching immortality. However, you must first know how to regulate your external breathing correctly.

All of these emphasize the importance of breathing. There are eight key words for air breathing which a Qigong practitioner should follow during his practice. Once you understand them you will be able to substantially shorten the time needed to reach your Qigong goals. These eight key words are: 1. Calm (Jing, 靜); 2. Slender (Xi, 細); 3. Deep (Shen, 深); 4. Long (Chang, 長); 5. Continuous (You, 悠); 6. Uniform (Yun, 勻); 7. Slow (Huan, 緩), and 8. Soft (Mian, 綿). These key words are self-explanatory, and with a little thought you should be able to understand them.

Regulating the Mind (Tiao Xin, 調心). It is said in Daoist society that: "(When) large Dao is taught, first stop thought; when thought is not stopped, (the lessons are) in vain."[9] This means that when you first practice Qigong, the most difficult training is to stop your thinking. The final goal for your mind is 'the thought of no thought' (無念之念). Your mind does not think of the past, the present, or the future. Your mind is completely separated from influences of the present such as worry, happiness, and sadness. Then your mind can be calm and steady, and can finally gain peace. Only when you are in the state of 'the thought of no thought' will you be relaxed and able to sense calmly and accurately.

Regulating your mind means using your consciousness to stop the activity in your mind in order to set it free from the bondage of ideas, emotion, and conscious thought. When you reach this level your mind will be calm, peaceful, empty, and light. Then your mind has really reached the goal of relaxation. Only when you reach this stage will you be able to relax deep into your marrow and internal organs. Only then will your mind be clear enough to see (feel) the internal Qi circulation and to communicate with your Qi and organs. In Daoist society it is called, Nei Shi Gongfu (內視功夫), which means the Gongfu of internal vision.

When you reach this real relaxation you may be able to sense the different elements which make up your body: solid matter, liquids, gases, energy, and spirit. You may even be able to see or feel the different colors that are associated with your five organs—green (liver), white (lungs), black (kidneys), yellow (spleen), and red (heart).

Once your mind is relaxed and regulated and you can sense your internal organs, you may decide to study the five element theory. This is a very profound subject, and it is sometimes interpreted differently by Oriental physicians and Qigong practitioners. When understood properly, it can give you a method of analyzing the interrelationships between your organs and help you devise ways to correct imbalances.

For example, the lungs correspond to the element Metal, and the heart to the element Fire. Metal (the lungs) can be used to adjust the heat of the Fire (the heart), because metal can take a large quantity of heat away from fire, (and thus cool down the heart). When you feel uneasy or have heartburn (excess fire in the heart), you may use deep breathing to calm down the uneasy emotions or cool off the heartburn.

Naturally, it will take a lot of practice to reach this level. In the beginning, you should not have any ideas or intentions, because they will make it harder for your mind to relax and empty itself of thoughts. Once you are in a state of "no thought," place your attention on your Lower Dan Tian (Xia Dan Tian, 下丹田). It is said "Yi Shou Dan Tian" (意守丹田), which means "The Mind is kept on the Dan Tian." The Dan Tian is the origin and residence of your Qi. Your mind can build up the Qi here (start the fire, Qi Huo, 起火), then lead the Qi anywhere you wish, and finally lead the Qi back to its residence. When your mind is on the Dan Tian, your Qi will always have a root. When you keep this root, your Qi will be strong and full, and it will go where you want it to go. You can see that when you practice Qigong, your mind cannot be completely empty and relaxed. You must find the firmness within the relaxation, then you can reach your goal.

In Qigong training, it is said: "Use your Yi (Mind) to lead your Qi" (Yi Yi Yin Qi) (以意引氣). Notice the word lead. Qi behaves like water—it cannot be pushed, but it can be led. When Qi is led, it will flow smoothly and without stagnation. When it is pushed, it will flood and enter the wrong paths. Remember wherever your Yi goes first, the Qi will naturally follow. For example, if you intend to lift an object, this intention is your Yi. This Yi will lead the Qi to the arms to energize the physical muscles, and then the object can be lifted.

It is said: "Your Yi cannot be on your Qi. Once your Yi is on your Qi, the Qi is stagnant."[10] When you want to walk from one spot to another, you must first mobilize your intention and direct it to the goal, then your body will follow. The mind must always be ahead of the body. If your mind stays on your body, you will not be able to move.

In Qigong training, the first thing is to know what Qi is. If you do not know what Qi is, how will you be able to lead it? Once you know what Qi is and experience it, then your Yi will have something to lead. The next thing in Qigong training is knowing how your Yi communicates with your Qi. That means that your Yi should be able to sense and feel the Qi flow and understand how strong and smooth it is. In Taiji Qigong society, it is commonly said that your Yi must 'listen' to your Qi and "understand" it. Listen means to pay careful attention to what you sense and feel. The more you pay attention, the better you will be able to understand. Only after you understand the Qi situation will your Yi be able to set up the strategy. In Qigong your mind or Yi must generate the idea (visualize your intention), which is like an order to your Qi to complete a certain mission.

The more your Yi communicates with your Qi, the more efficiently the Qi can be led. For this reason, as a Qigong beginner you must first learn about Yi and Qi, and also learn how to help them communicate efficiently. Yi is the key in Qigong practice. Without this Yi you would not be able to lead your Qi, let alone build up the strength of the Qi or circulate it throughout your entire body.

Remember when the Yi is strong, the Qi is strong, and when the Yi is weak, the Qi is weak. Therefore, the first step of Qigong training is to develop your Yi. The first secret of a strong Yi is calmness. When you are calm, you can see things clearly and not be disturbed by surrounding distractions. With your mind calm, you will be able to concentrate.

Confucius (Kong Zi, 孔子) said: "First you must be calm, then your mind can be steady. Once your mind is steady, then you are at peace. Only when you are at peace are you able to think and finally gain."[11] This procedure is also applied in meditation or Qigong exercise: First Calm, then Steady, Peace, Think, and finally Gain. When you practice Qigong, first you must learn to be emotionally calm. Once calm, you will be able to see what you want and firm your mind (steady). This firm and steady mind is your intention or Yi (it is how your Yi is generated). Only after you know what you really want will your mind gain peace and be able to relax emotionally and physically. Once you have reached this step, you must then concentrate or think in order to execute your intention. Under this thoughtful and concentrated mind, your Qi will follow and you will be able to gain what you wish.

However, the most difficult part of regulating the mind is learning how to neutralize the thoughts which keep coming back to bother you. This is especially true in still meditation practice. In still meditation, once you have entered a deep, profound meditative state, new thoughts, fantasies, your imagination, or any guilt from what you have done in the past that is hidden behind your mask will emerge and bother you. Normally, the first step of the regulating process is to stop new fantasies and images. Then, you must deal with your conscious mind. That means you must learn how to remove the mask from your face. Only then will you see yourself clearly. Therefore, the first step is to know yourself. Next, you must learn how to handle the problem instead of continuing to avoid it.

There are many ways of regulating your mind. However, the most important key to success is to use your wisdom mind to analyze the situation and find the solution. Do not let your emotional mind govern your thinking. Here, I would like to share with you a few stories about regulating the mind. Hopefully these stories can provide you with a guideline for your own regulation.

In China many centuries ago, two monks were walking side by side down a muddy road when they came upon a large puddle which completely blocked the road. A very beautiful lady in a lovely gown stood at the edge of the puddle, unable to go further without spoiling her clothes.

Without hesitation, one of the monks picked her up and carried her across the puddle, set her down on the other side, and continued on his way. Many hours later when the two monks were preparing to camp for the night, the second monk turned to the first and said, "I can no longer hold this back, I'm quite angry at you! We are not supposed to look at women, particularly pretty ones, never mind touch them. Why did you do that?" The first monk replied, "Brother, I left the woman at the mud puddle; why are you still carrying her?"

From this story, you can see that often, the thought which bothers you is created by nobody but yourself. If you can use your wisdom mind to govern yourself, many times you can set your mind free from emotional bondage regardless of the situation.

It is true that frequently the mind bothers or enslaves you to the desire for material enjoyment or money. From this desire, you misunderstand the meaning of life. A really happy life comes from satisfaction of both material and spiritual needs.

Have you ever thought about what the real meaning of your life is? What is the real goal for your life? Are you enslaved by money, power or love? What will make you truly happy?

I remember a story one of my professors at Taiwan University told me: "There was a jail with a prisoner in it," he said, "who was surrounded by mountains of money. He kept counting the money and feeling so happy about his life, thinking that he was the richest man in the whole world. A man passing by saw him and said through the tiny window: 'Why are you so happy, you are in prison?' Do you know that? The prisoner laughed: "No! No! It is not that I am inside the jail, it is that you are outside of the jail!"

How do you feel about this story? Do you want to be a prisoner and a slave to money, or do you want to be the real you and feel free internally? Think and be happy.

There is another story which was told to me by one of my students. Since I heard this story, it has always offered me a new guideline for my life. This new guideline is to appreciate what you have; only then will you have a peaceful mind. This does not mean you should not be aggressive in pursuing a better life. Keep pursuing by creating a new target and a new path for your life. It is Yang. However, often you will be depressed and discouraged from obstacles on this path. Therefore, you must also learn how to comfort yourself and appreciate what you already have. This is Yin. Only if you have both Yin and Yang can your life be happy and meaningful.

Long ago, there was a servant who served a bad tempered and impatient master. It did not matter how he tried, he was always blamed and beaten by this master. However, it was the strange truth that the servant was always happy, and his master was always sad and depressed.

One day, there was a kind man who could not understand this phenomena, and finally decided to ask this servant why he was always happy even though he was treated so badly. The servant replied: "Everyone has one day of life each day; half of the day is spent awake and the other half is spent sleeping. Although in the daytime, I am a servant and my master treats me badly, in the nighttime, I always dream that I am a king and there are thousands of servants serving me luxuriously. Look at my master: In the daytime, he is mad, depressed, greedy, and unhappy. In the nighttime, he has nightmares and cannot even have one night of nice rest. I really feel sorry for my master. Comparing me to him, I am surely happier than he is."

Friends, what do you think about this story? You are the only one responsible for your happiness. If you are not satisfied, and always complain about what you have obtained, you will be on the course of forever unhappiness. It is said in the western society: "If you smile, the whole world smiles with you, but if you cry, you cry alone." What an accurate saying!

Regulating the Qi (Tiao Qi, 調氣). Before you can regulate your Qi you must first regulate your body, breath, and mind. If you compare your body to a battlefield, then your mind is like the general who generates ideas and controls the situation, and your breathing is the strategy. Your Qi is like the soldiers who are led to the most advantageous places on the battlefield. All four elements are necessary and all four must be coordinated with each other if you are to win the war against sickness and aging.

If you want to arrange your soldiers most effectively for battle, you must know which area of the battlefield is most important, and where you are weakest (where your Qi is deficient) and need to send reinforcements. If you have more soldiers than you need in one area (excessive Qi), then you can send them somewhere else where the ranks are thin. As a general, you must also know how many soldiers are available for the battle, and how many you will need for protecting yourself and your headquarters. To be successful, not only do you need good strategy (breathing), but you also need to communicate and understand the situation effectively with your troops, or all of your strategy will be in vain. When your Yi (the general) knows how to regulate the body (knows the battlefield), how to regulate breathing (set up the strategy), and how to effectively regulate Qi (direct your soldiers), you will be able to reach the final goal of Qigong training.

In order to regulate your Qi so that it moves smoothly in the correct paths, you need more than just efficient Yi-Qi communication. You also need to know how to generate Qi. If you do not have enough Qi in your body, how can you regulate it? In a battle, if you do not have enough soldiers to set up your strategy, you have already lost.

When you practice Qigong, you must first train to make you Qi flow naturally and smoothly. There are some Qigong exercises in which you intentionally hold your Yi, and thus hold your Qi, in a specific area. As a beginner, however, you should first learn how to make the Qi flow smoothly instead of building a Qi dam, which is commonly done in external martial Qigong training.

In order to make Qi flow naturally and smoothly, your Yi must first be relaxed. Only when your Yi is relaxed will your body be relaxed and the Qi channels open for the Qi to circulate. Then you must coordinate your Qi flow with your breathing. Breathing regularly and calmly will make your Yi calm, and allow your body to relax even more.

Regulating Spirit (Tiao Shen, 調神). There is one thing that is more important than anything else in a battle, and that is fighting spirit. You may have the best general, who knows the battlefield well and is also an expert strategist, but if his soldiers do not have a high fighting spirit (morale), he might still lose. Remember, spirit is the center and root of a fight. When you keep this center, one soldier can be equal to ten soldiers. When his spirit is high, a soldier will obey his orders accurately and willingly, and his general will be able to control the situation efficiently. In a battle, in order for a soldier to have this kind of morale, he must know why he is fighting, how to fight, and what he can expect after the fight. Under these conditions, he will know what he is doing and why, and this understanding will raise up his spirit, strengthen his will, and increase his patience and endurance.

Shen, which is the Chinese term for spirit, originates from the Yi (the general). When the Shen is strong, the Yi is firm. When the Yi is firm, the Shen will be steady and calm. The Shen is the mental part of a soldier. When the Shen is high, the Qi is strong and easily directed. When the Qi is strong, the Shen is also strong.

To the religious Qigong practitioners, the goal of regulating the spirit is to set the spirit free from the bondage of the physical body, and thus reach the stage of Buddhahood or enlightenment. To the layman practitioners, the goal of regulating the spirit is to keep the spirit of living high to prevent the body from getting sick and degenerating. It is often seen that, before a person retires, he has good health. However, once retired, he will get sick easily and his physical condition will deteriorate quickly. When you are working, your spirit remains high and alert. This keeps the Qi circulating smoothly in the body.

All of these training concepts and procedures are common to all Chinese Qigong. To reach a deep level of understanding and penetrate to the essence of any Qigong practice, you should always keep these five training criteria in mind and examine them for deeper levels of meaning. This is the only way to gain the real mental and physical health benefits from your training. Always remember that Qigong training is not just the forms. Your feelings and comprehension are the essential roots of the entire training. This Yin side of the training has no limit, and the deeper you understand, the better you will see how much more there is to know.

3-3. Qigong Practices for Massage 按摩之氣功練習

In this section, I would like to introduce some Qigong practices for general massage. Naturally, all of these Qigong trainings are also commonly used to train Tui Na, Dian Xue, and Qi massage. The difference is the level of Qigong training in general massage is not as deep as that of those massages which require more concentration and power focusing. The main purposes of Qigong training in massage is to improve the strength and also to increase the endurance of the muscles, tendons, and ligaments at the joint areas.

Condition the Body (Regulating the Body)

The first and most basic Qigong training in massage is conditioning your own physical fitness. Without this training, you can injure yourself easily especially in joints such as the wrists, fingers, and lower back.

Wrists. For masseurs, the wrists are often the first place that gets injured in general massage. To strengthen the wrists, first inhale and then use one hand to press the other hand's four fingers (except the thumb) backward while exhaling (Figure 3-1). While you are doing this, first relax the wrist area while pressing, so the tendons at the inner side of the wrist can be stretched. Stretch it for a minute while breathing normally. Next, tense up the wrist while pressing for another minute. In this second pressing process, inhale and relax the wrist, then exhale and tense it up. In this second training, since the mind is more involved, reverse abdominal breathing is better (Please refer to the next subsection for a discussion of reversed abdominal breathing.). Finally, switch hands and condition the other hand with the same procedures.

Next, inhale and then use one hand to press the other hand's fingers (except the thumb) forward while exhaling (Figure 3-2). Again, first stretch the wrist for one minute and then tense up the wrist while pressing so the tendons can be conditioned for another minute. Again, switch hands and condition the other hand.

Use this same stretching and tensing idea to repeat the conditioning process with different angles.

- Hand bends backward and twisted clockwise (Figure 3-3).
- Hand bends backward and twisted counterclockwise (Figure 3-4).

Chapter 3: Qigong Practices for Massage

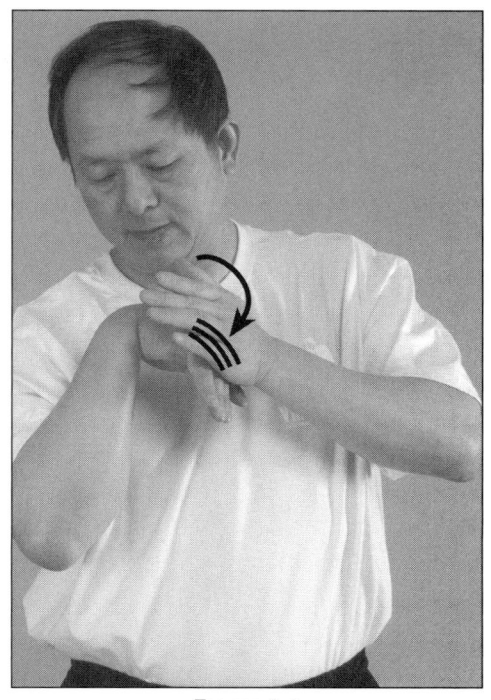

FIGURE 3-1

FIGURE 3-2

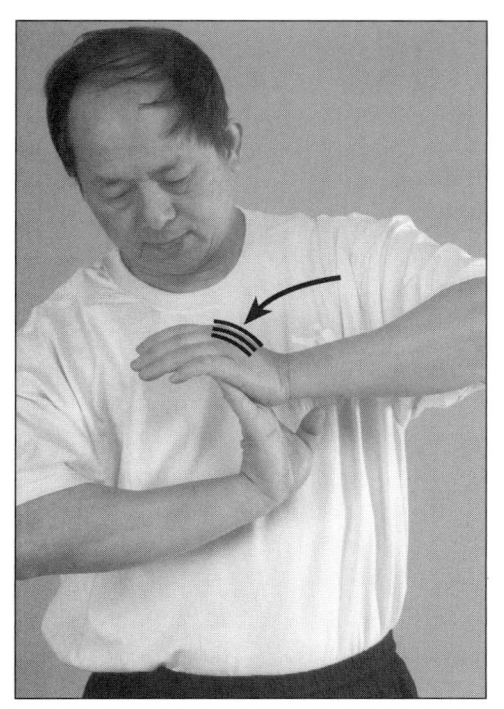

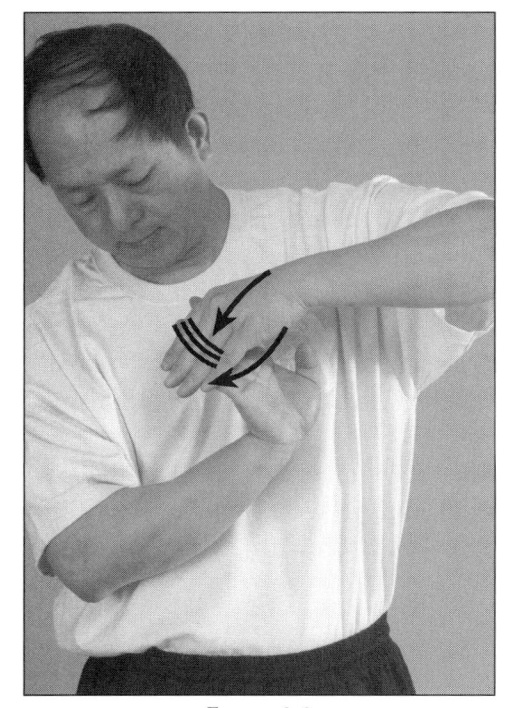

FIGURE 3-3

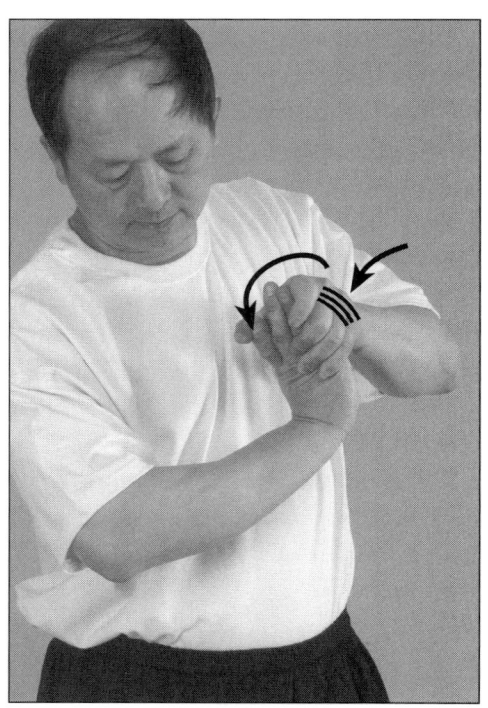

FIGURE 3-4

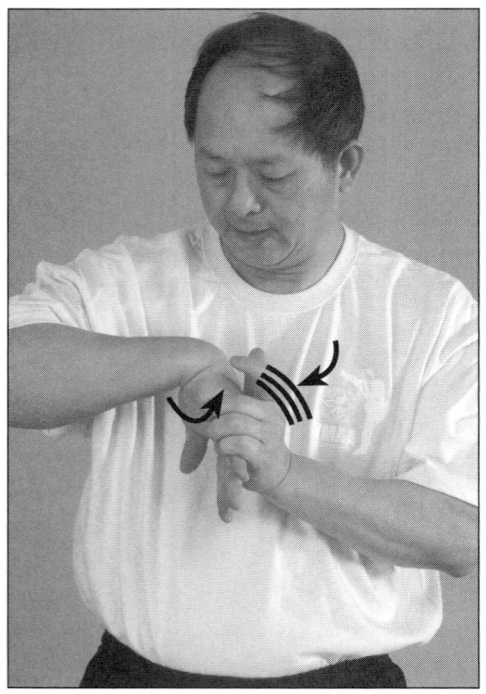

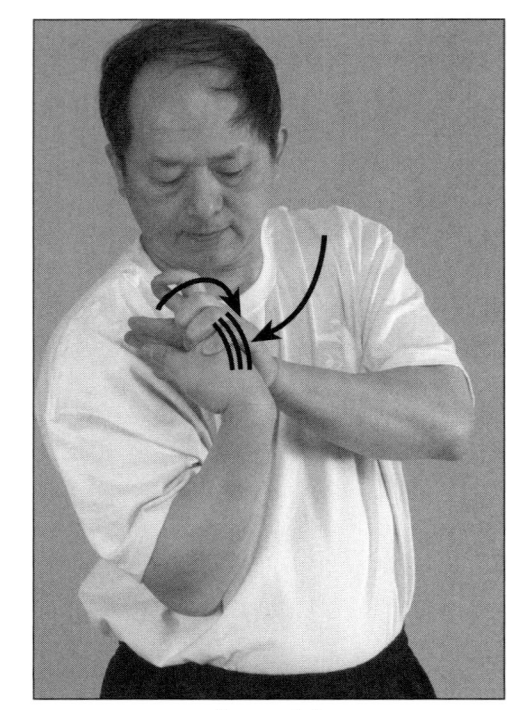

FIGURE 3-5

FIGURE 3-6

- Hand bends forward and twisted clockwise (Figure 3-5).
- Hand bends forward and twisted counterclockwise (Figure 3-6).

Fingers. The first method for training finger strength and endurance is to put yourself in a push-up position on the fingers. At the beginning, you should not use the finger tips to do the job; instead, you should use the pads of the last section of the fingers (Figure 3-7). Training this angle is very important for Tui Na masseurs. After you are able to stay in this position for a minute or more, gradually shift the touching point to the finger tips (Figure 3-8). When you are in this training position, whenever you exhale you should imagine that you are pushing your fingers against the floor. This is important for Dian Xue masseurs, since they commonly use the tips of their fingers to manipulate the stimulation of the cavities.

After you have built up a good level of strength and endurance, you should then use only four fingers to support yourself (lift the pinky), three fingers (thumb, index, and middle) (Figure 3-9), two fingers (thumb and index), and finally the thumb only (Figure 3-10).

Chapter 3: Qigong Practices for Massage

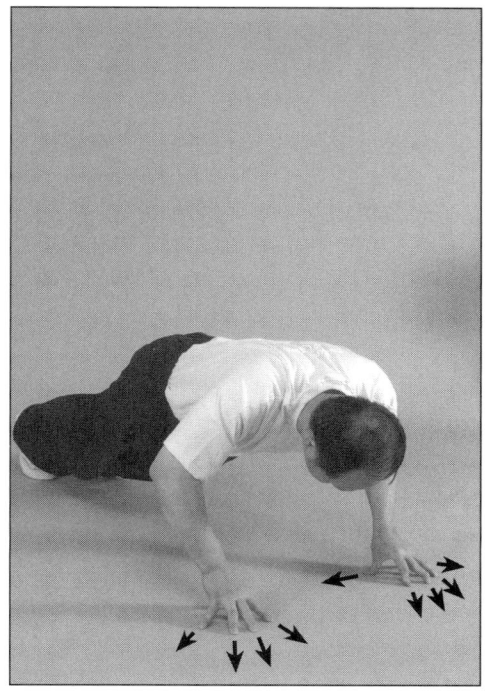

FIGURE 3-7

FIGURE 3-8

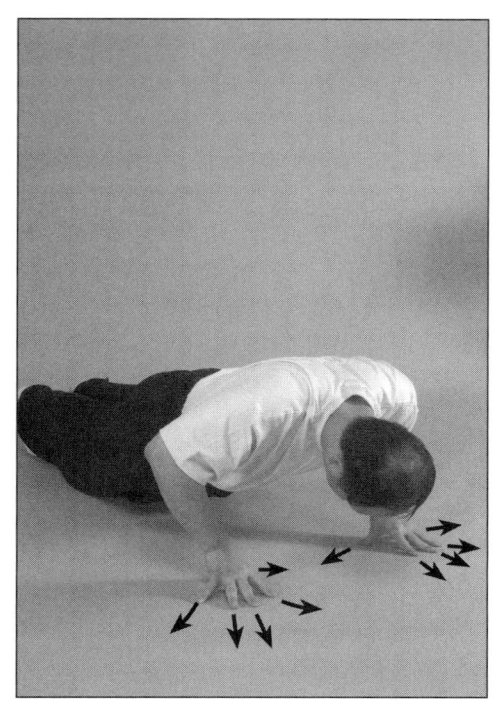

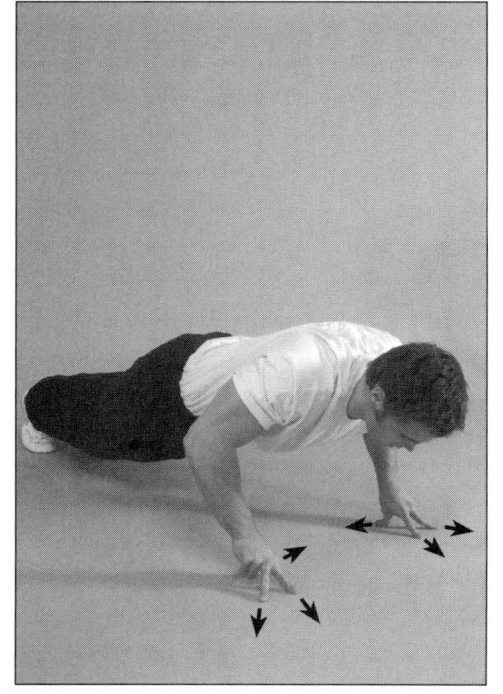

FIGURE 3-9

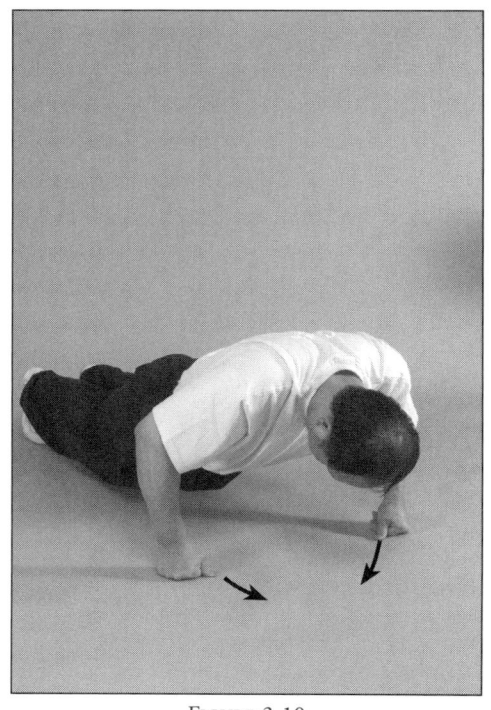

FIGURE 3-10

127

In addition, you should also condition the tendon and ligament tissues surrounding the finger joints. The way of reaching this goal is to press your fingers into a surface and then wave or circle your wrist (Figure 3-11). Remember, practicing more times is more important than applying more pressure. If you circle your wrist, you should practice both clockwise and counterclockwise. When you circle clockwise, you should exhale when you project your power forward and when you circle counterclockwise, you should inhale when you imagine you are drawing the Qi toward your wrist.

Finally, when you practice, you should align your elbows and shoulders correctly so that the pushing action has a good foundation and support.

Lower Back. It is also common for a masseur to be injured in his/her lower back or spine after treating multiple patients.

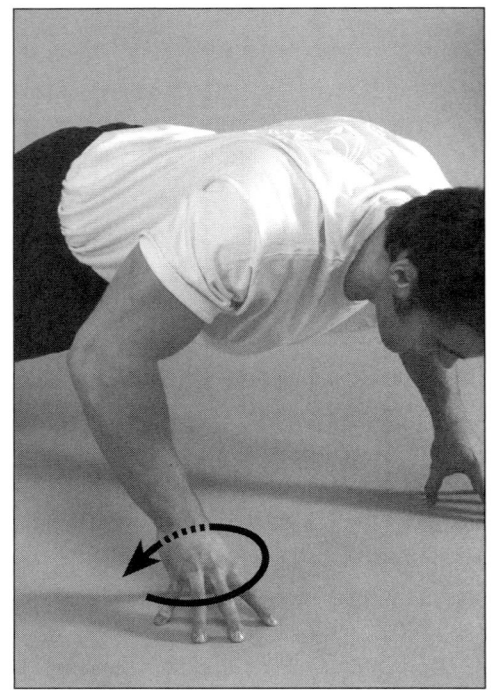

FIGURE 3-11

The reason for this is that to a proficient masseur, the waist area is very important in manipulating the massage process. Normally, if you know how to use your waist (i.e. center of gravity) to direct or to govern power, you will be centered. You must use the waist area to manipulate the process, but you must also maintain your relaxation in this area so the Qi can be led out and in to your Lower Dan Tian without stagnation.

However, it is common that a masseur will injure himself/herself due to long periods of massage. In this case, you must know how to loosen up the waist area and spine when it is tight. The appropriate exercises are exactly the same as those used to massage the internal organs through movements, which will be introduced in section 7-3. Please refer to this section for details of the movements.

Alignment of Joints. When you massage someone, the most important element is probably your postures. If your massage postures are correct, both the massaging power can be manipulated easily, and you can avoid unnecessary injuries to yourself. During massage, not only must your partner or patient feel comfortable, but you must also feel secure and easeful as well.

The key to reaching this goal is to have a good alignment of the entire body's joints when you massage. In addition, in every massage position, you must find good leverage for the power's balance. The first step of this training is to define all possible heights where your patient or partner is positioned. For example, your posture and body struc-

Chapter 3: Qigong Practices for Massage

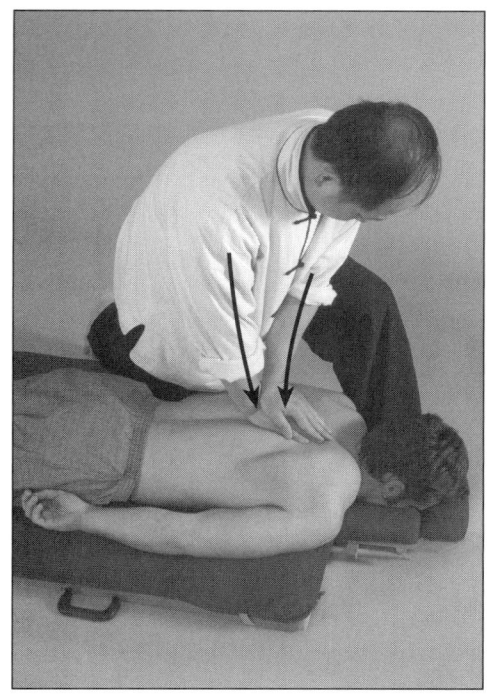

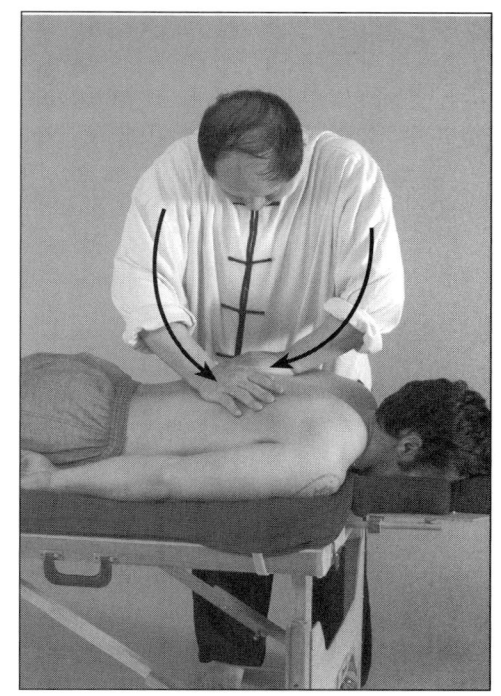

FIGURE 3-12

FIGURE 3-13

ture will be different when you massage a patient or a partner who is lying down on the floor in comparison to a patient who is on the massaging table. In addition, your position, massaging angle, and angles for leverage will also be different when your patient is sitting rather than lying down.

There are only a few common comfortable positions in which your patients can be situated. The most common position is lying down with the face looking downward or upward. The second position is sitting down on a chair or the floor. It is seldom that your patient is standing.

Once you have defined the patients height and position, then you must learn how to align your body's structure so you can manifest your massage power comfortably. For example, if a patient is lying down facing downward on the floor, then you should take advantage of your body's weight to increase your massage power (Figure 3-12). If you have become skillful, your patient will feel relaxed and comfortable and you will get tired easily. However, if your patient is on massage table, you will not have the advantage of using your body's weight in your massage. Therefore, you must build up firm structure and strength in your wrists, elbows, and shoulders (Figure 3-13). In addition, you must also learn how to connect your body with your arms and search for the leverage of power, so that when you massage, you are using your entire body instead of relying only on your arms. Since there are so many possible massage techniques and each one of them requires a specific position and posture, you must research all possibilities and practice. The key to success in this training relies on the level of your awareness. If you have a high level of awareness, you will be able to see and realize the wrong alignment and posture in your massage. Through time and experience, you will learn how to direct and correct yourself. This high level of feeling can only be obtained from Qigong practice with the coordination of breathing.

Relaxation (Joints and Muscles) (Centered and Balanced). When you are relaxed, you will find your center and balance easily. Once you have a center and balance, you will able to align your entire body into a good massage position. In addition, when you are relaxed, centered, and balanced, your mind will be calm and the feeling will be more accurate and alert. This will allow Qi to circulate smoothly in your body.

Relaxation includes both mental relaxation and physical relaxation. Remember-only if your mind is relaxed can your physical body be relaxed. When you have reached a deep level of relaxation, you

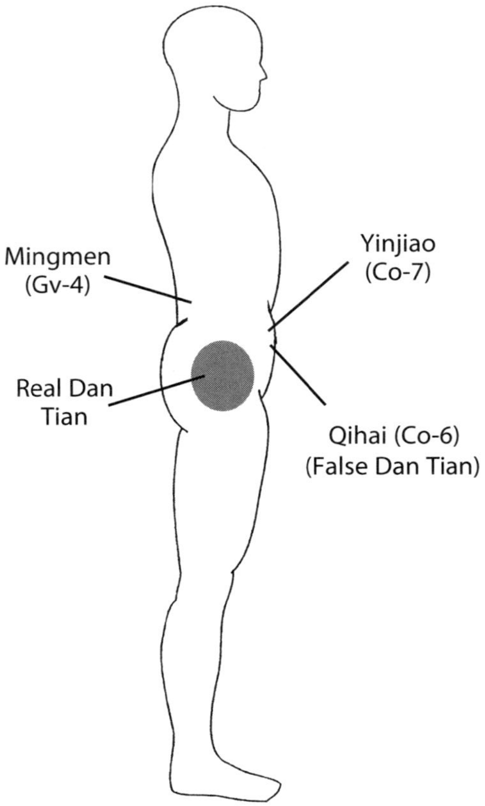

FIGURE 3-14. THE REAL LOWER DAN TIAN AND THE FALSE LOWER DAN TIAN

must learn how to keep your mind at the Real Lower Dan Tian (Zhen Xia Dan Tian, 真下丹田) at the center of gravity (Figure 3-14). This place is a human bio-battery. Once you can recognize and feel this center, you will be able to lead the Qi out and in from this center. This is a crucial key to healing and self-recovery.

Once you can register this center, you should learn how to lead the Qi to your muscles, tendons, and ligaments with the coordination of breathing. Remember, when your joints are relaxed, your muscles will be relaxed. Therefore, the key of this training is leading the Qi to the joints. First, practice only a single joint such as the wrist or elbow. After you have become more proficient in using your mind to lead the Qi, gradually, increase the number of joints. The final goal is to make the entire body's joints breathe with you at the same time. Once you reach this level, you can remove any stagnant Qi accumulated anywhere in your body. This is the best method of self-recovery after massage. We will discuss the practice of self-recovery later.

Respiration (Regulating the Breathing)

Breathing is considered as the strategy in Qigong practice. Correct breathing cannot only enhance the power and make it controllable, but can also bring you a higher level of relaxation and concentration. Normally, there are two common ways of breathing used in massage.

Normal Abdominal Breathing (Zheng Fu Hu Xi, 正腹呼吸 **).** Normal Abdominal Breathing is also commonly known as "Buddhist Breathing" (Fo Jia Hu Xi, 佛家呼吸). When you inhale, the abdominal area expands, and when you exhale, it withdraws. You should practice until the entire process becomes smooth and the entire body remains relaxed.

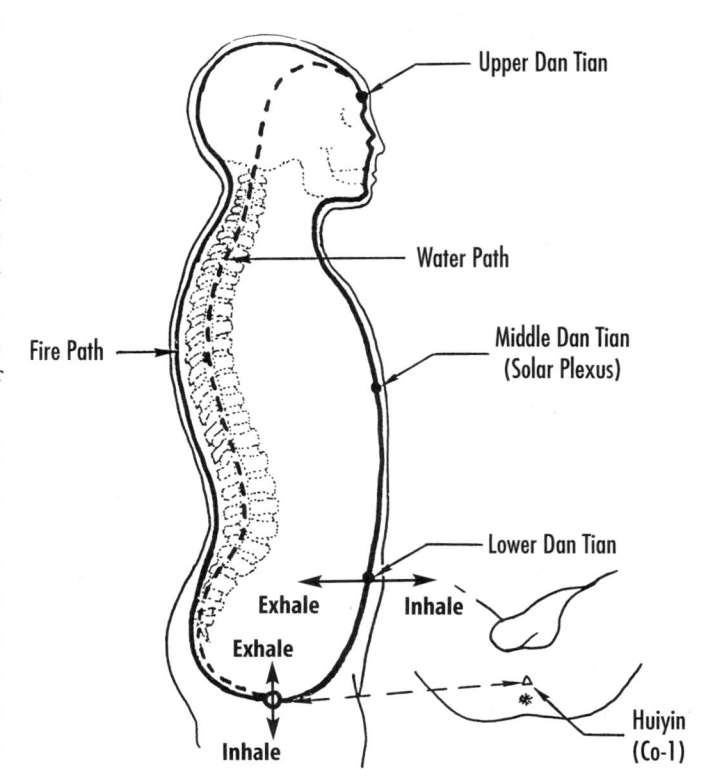

FIGURE 3-15. NORMAL ABDOMINAL BREATHING

Once you have reached this level, you should then coordinate your breathing with the movements of your Huiyin (Co-1) (會陰) (Perineum) and anus. When you inhale, relax the Huiyin and anus, and when you exhale hold them up (Figure 3-15). Remember, you are gently holding up the Huiyin and anus, not tightening them. When you hold them up, they can still remain relaxed. If you tighten them up, you will impede the Qi circulation. When you tense them, you also cause tension in the abdomen and stomach, which can generate other problems. At the beginning, naturally you will need to use your mind to control the muscles of the abdomen. However, with practice, you will realize that your mind does not have to be there to make it happen. That means you are regulating it without regulating. When you have reached this stage, you will feel a wonderful comfortable feeling in the area of the Huiyin and anus. Not only that, you will also feel that the Qi is led more strongly to the skin as though your entire body is breathing with you.

Normal Abdominal Breathing
Neutral (inhalation and exhalation equal length)
- Yin - Inhalation (Abdomen Expands, Huiyin Pushed Out Gently)
- Yang - Exhalation (Abdomen Withdraws, Huiyin Held Up Gently)

Body Yin (inhalation longer than exhalation)
- Inhalation (Abdomen Expands, Huiyin Pushed Out Gently)
- Exhalation (Abdomen Withdraws, Huiyin Relaxed)

Body Yang (exhalation longer than inhalation)
- Inhalation (Abdomen Expands, Huiyin Pushed Out Gently)
- Exhalation (Abdomen Withdraws, Huiyin Held Up Strongly)

Reverse Abdominal Breathing (Fan Fu Hu Xi, Ni Fu Hu Xi, 反腹呼吸・逆腹呼吸). Reverse Abdominal Breathing is also commonly called Daoist Breathing (Dao Jia Hu Xi, 道家呼吸). After you have mastered Normal Abdominal Breathing (Buddhist Breathing), you should then start this breathing. It is called Reverse Abdominal Breathing because the movement of the abdomen is the reverse of Normal Abdominal Breathing. In other words, the abdomen withdraws and Huiyin (Co-1) (會陰) (Perineum) is held up gently when you inhale, and the abdominen expands and Huiyin is gently pushed out when you exhale (Figure 3-16). Relatively speaking, Buddhist breathing is more relaxed compared with Daoist breathing, which is more aggressive. As a result, Daoist breathing can make the body more Yang (tensed and excited), while Buddhist breathing makes the body more Yin (calm and relaxed).

Many people today falsely believe that the reverse breathing technique is against the Dao, or nature's path. This is not true. If you observe your breathing carefully, you will realize that we use reverse breathing in two types of situations.

First, when we have an emotional disturbance, we often use reverse breathing. For example, when you are happy and laugh with the sound "Ha, Ha, Ha..." (哈) you are using reverse breathing. While you are making this sound, your stomach or abdominal area is expanding. When this happens, your exhalation is longer than your inhalation, your Guardian Qi (Wei Qi, 衛氣) expands, and you become hot and sweaty. This is the natural way of releasing the excess energy in your body caused from excitement or happiness.

Also, when you are sad and you cry, making a sound of "Hen" (哼) while inhaling, your abdominal area is withdrawn. When this happens, your inhalation is longer than your exhalation, your Guardian Qi shrinks, and you feel cold and chilly. This is the natural way of preventing energy loss from inside your body. When you are sad, your Shen (神) and your body's energy are low.

The second occasion in which we use reverse breathing is when we *intend* to energize our physical body, for example when pushing a car or lifting some heavy weight. In order to exert strenuous effort, you first must inhale deeply, and then exhale while pushing the object. If you pay attention, you will again see that you are using reverse breathing.

From the above discussion, we can generally conclude that when we are disturbed emotionally, or when we have a *focused intention* in our mind, for example to energize our physical body, we use reverse breathing naturally.

After you have practiced for a while, you may discover that you can now lead the Qi to the skin more efficiently when you exhale than with the Buddhist method. Not only that, you may also discover that you are able to lead the Qi to the bone marrow. To help you understand this more clearly, let us take a comparison of the Normal Abdominal Breathing with the Reverse Abdominal Breathing and see how the Qi can be led in these two different breathing strategies.

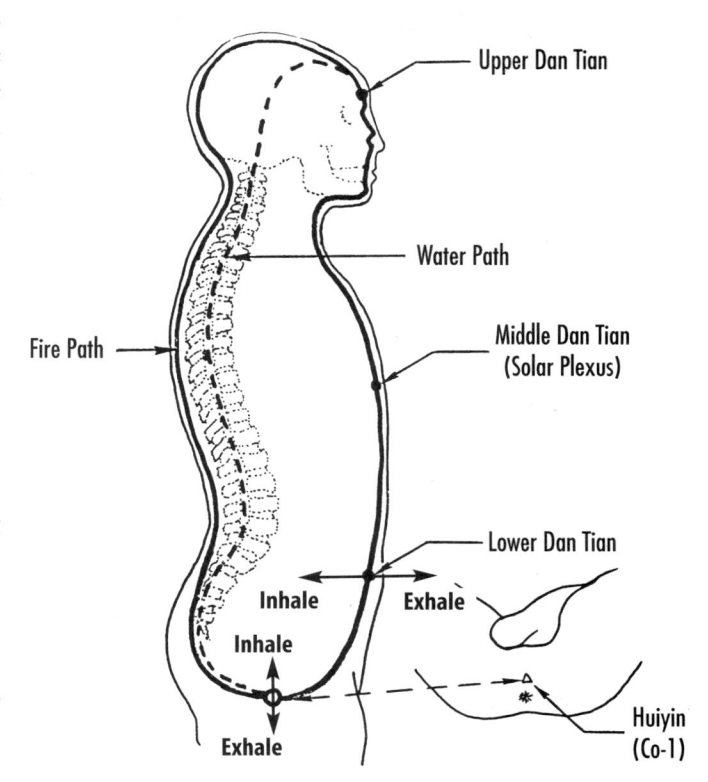

FIGURE 3-16. REVERSE ABDOMINAL BREATHING

In Normal Abdominal Breathing, the majority of Qi circulates in the primary Qi channels (Jing, 經) which connect the internal organs to the extremities. Some Qi also spreads out through the secondary Qi channels (Luo, 絡) and reaches the skin and bone marrow (Figure 3-17). Since the majority of Qi is not led away from the primary Qi channels, the physical body is not energized and therefore the body remains relaxed. Therefore, Normal Abdominal Breathing is able to bring a beginning practitioner to a state of deep relaxation. Normal Abdominal Breathing (Kan, 坎) is able to make the body Yin, while Reverse Abdominal Breathing (Li, 離) will cause the body to be Yang.

However, in Reverse Abdominal Breathing, the majority of Qi has been led sideways through the secondary Qi channels to the skin and also to the bone marrow, with the minority of Qi circulating in the primary Qi channels (Figure 3-18). As mentioned earlier, normally these Qi circulating behaviors are influenced by the emotional mind or intentional mind. Generally, patterns of Qi circulation related to the mind can be dis-

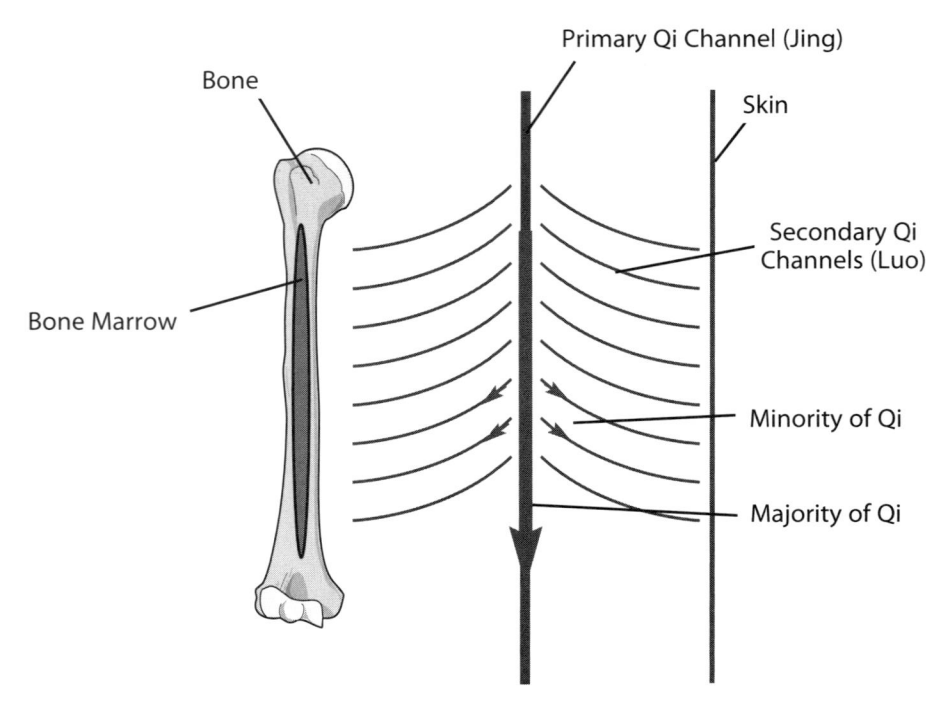

FIGURE 3-17. IN NORMAL ABDOMINAL BREATHING, A MAJORITY OF THE QI CIRCULATES IN THE PRIMARY QI CHANNELS

tinguished according to the breathing and emotional behavior. When you are excited and generate a sound of "Ha" (哈), exhalation is longer than inhalation. The Qi is led outward strongly to the skin surface from the primary Qi channels, the muscles are energized and you sweat. The Guardian Qi (Wei Qi, 衛氣) is strengthened and this will result in your body's becoming more Yang.

However, if you are scared or sad while making the "Hen" (哼) sound, your inhalation will be longer than your exhalation. The Qi is led inward to the marrow from the primary Qi channels and the Guardian Qi is weakened. You will feel cold. Naturally, this will result in the body's being more Yin.

From this brief discussion, you can see that skin breathing (or body breathing) (Ti Xi, Fu Xi, 體息 · 膚息) can be done much more effectively and efficiently through Reverse Abdominal Breathing. Naturally, the marrow breathing (Sui Xi, 髓息) can be reached more aggressively through Reverse Abdominal Breathing as well. Next, let us summarize some important concepts of Reverse Abdominal Breathing. If you wish to know about Qigong breathing, please refer to the book: *Qigong Meditation—Embryonic Breathing*, by YMAA.

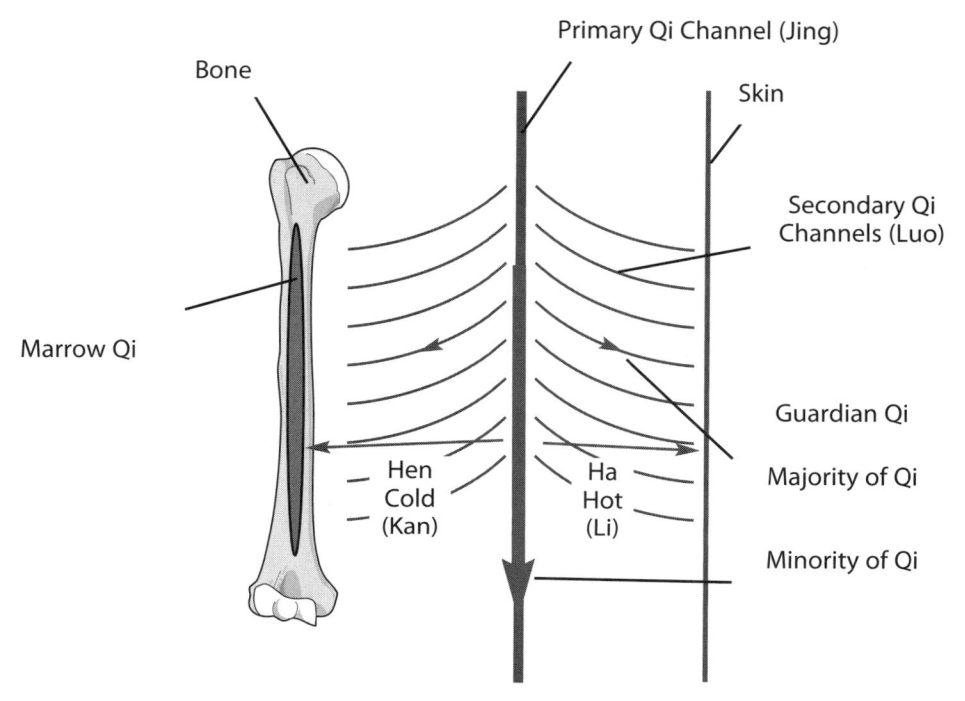

FIGURE 3-18. IN REVERSE ABDOMINAL BREATHING, A MAJORITY OF THE QI IS LED TO THE SKIN SURFACE AND BONE MARROW

Reverse Abdominal Breathing
(Emotionally Disturbed or the Mind has Intention of Yin or Yang)

Neutral (inhalation and exhalation equal length)
    Yin - Inhalation (Abdomen Withdraws, Huiyin Held Up Gently)
    Yang - Exhalation (Abdomen Expands, Huiyin Pushed Out Gently)

Body Yin (inhalation longer than exhalation)
    - Inhalation Longer (Abdomen Withdraws, Huiyin Held Up Firmly)
    - Exhalation (Abdomen Expands, Huiyin Relaxed)

Body Yang (exhalation longer than inhalation)
    - Inhalation (Abdomen Withdraws, Huiyin Held Up Gently)
    - Exhalation (Abdomen Expands, Huiyin Pushed Out Firmly)

Concentration (Regulating the Mind). The main purpose of training a concentrated mind is to build up a clear connection or communication between your mind and your physical/Qi bodies and also your mind with the patient's physical/Qi bodies. The success of the entire communication relies on the level of sensitivity in your feeling. Feeling is a language which makes these communications possible. Without this feeling, your massage will be shallow and ineffective. From this, you can see that the mind and the feeling cannot be separated. If your mind has separated from your feeling, then the communication will be interrupted. In this subsection, I will introduce a few Qigong massage concentration trainings which are commonly used to train a professional masseur in China.

There are two major goals in this training. The first one is to build up a clear communication between your mind and your patient's body. The area which you want to concentrate in your patient's body must be precise and the depth in which your power should reach must be accurate. This is specially important and crucial in Tui Na and Dian Xue massages.

The second goal is, through your concentrated mind, to direct and to enhance the Qi circulation in your body more efficiently. When this happens, your nerves will be more sensitive and your feeling will be more profound. This is crucial not only for treatment but also for your own safety and speedy recovery.

The first step for training how to focus your mind at the target is to build up a connection between your 'third eye' and the target. You should understand that it is through the third eye area, with the assistance of the eyes, that predators are able to focus on their prey. Through the third eye, you are able to concentrate better. In massage, since you cannot see the places under the skin where that you wish your massage to reach, you must rely on the feeling and the third eye's concentration to locate the position and to direct the power. The most common practice is placing many layers of clothes on a table (Figure 3-19) or on one of your palms (Figure 3-20). Place a few tiny beans between the layers (Figure 3-21). Place your finger or the base of your palm to press the clothes and find the beans. Then massage the bean and see if you are able to break it. If you are able to break it easily, then increase the thickness or layers of clothes and repeat the same training. Naturally, the thicker the clothes are, the more difficult it is to feel the bean. This training technique can also be used for any other area that you use for massage such as the finger knuckles, back of your palm, your forearm, or the side of the palm. There is another common way to train concentration that is used in Chinese martial arts society. This is watching the flame of a candle and paying attention to any slight movement of the flame (Figure 3-22). It is important to connect your mind with the movement of the flame. If your mind is not aware of the flame's action, even though your eyes are staring at the flame, the training is in vain.

To reach the second goal, the first step is to use your mind to lead the Qi to your joints such as fingers, wrists, and elbows. The reason for leading to these three joints is because they are used most often in massage manipulation. If you are able to lead abundant Qi to them, the feeling will be stronger and you can manipulate the Qi's circulation and manifest it into massage power.

In practice, first keep your mind at the Real Lower Lower Dan Tian and when you exhale, use your mind to lead the Qi to the joints. When you inhale again, lead it back to

Chapter 3: Qigong Practices for Massage

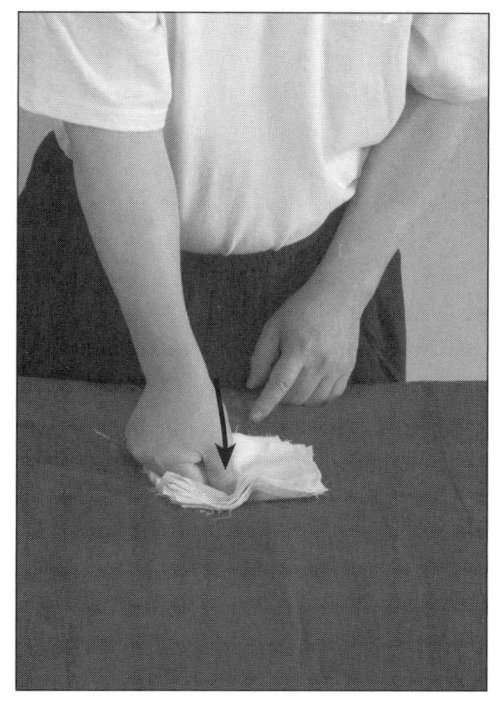

FIGURE 3-19

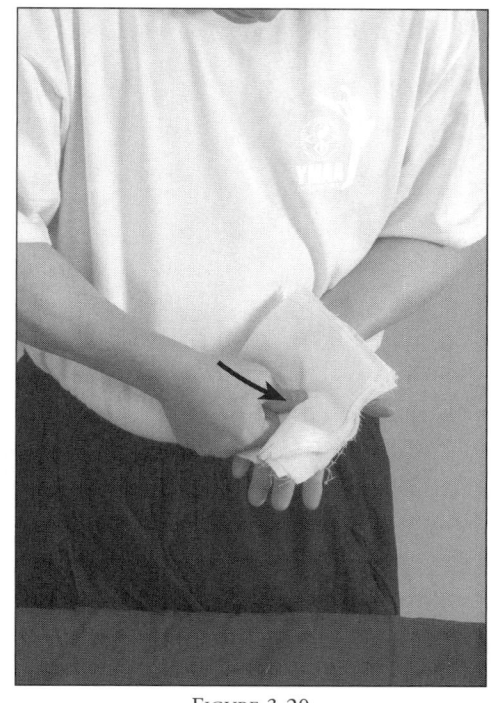

FIGURE 3-20

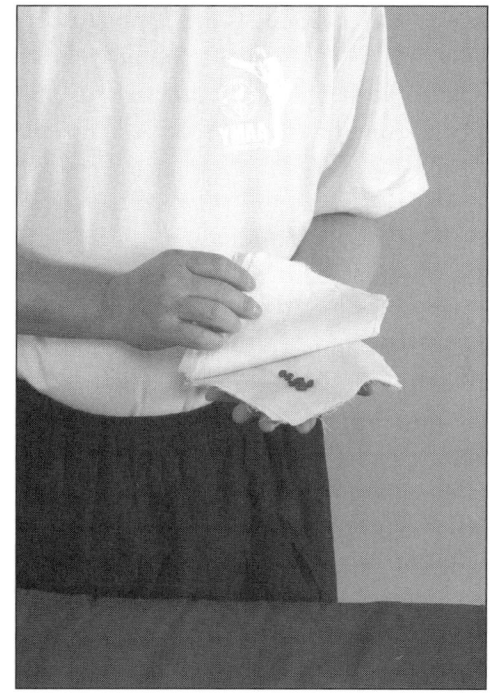

FIGURE 3-21

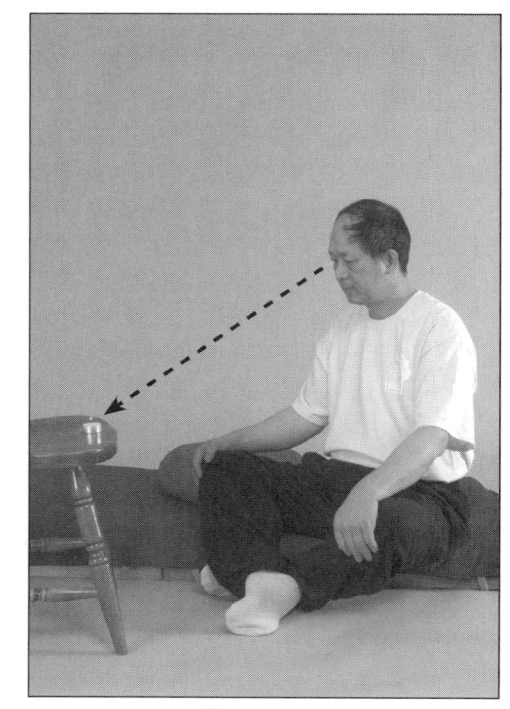

FIGURE 3-22

137

Qigong Massage

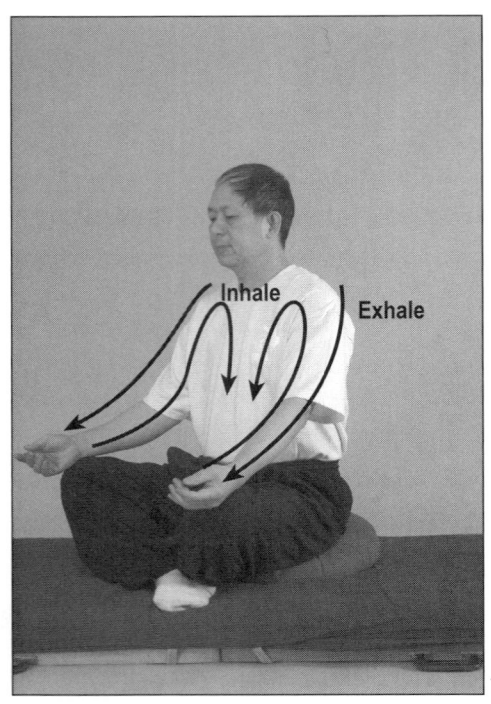

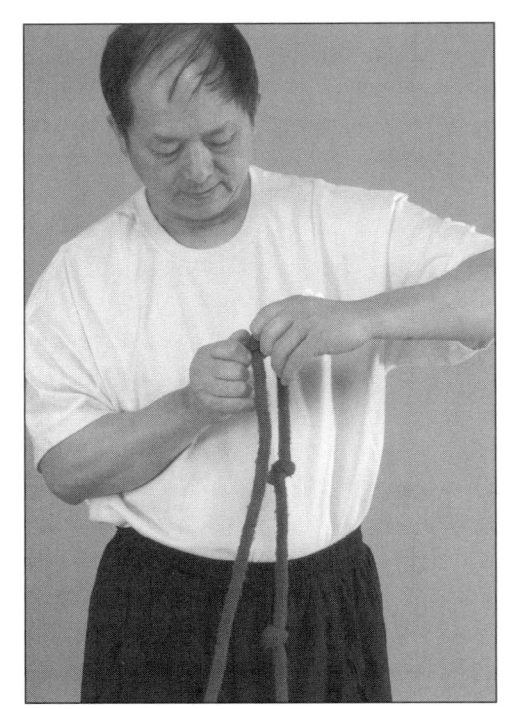

FIGURE 3-23

FIGURE 3-24

the Real Lower Dan Tian (Figure 3-23). If you know the technique of reverse abdominal breathing (Fan Fu Hu Xi, Ni Fu Hu Xi, 反腹呼吸・逆腹呼吸), you should use it. Whenever, your mind is involved, reverse abdominal breathing is more effective and efficient in leading the Qi. If you wish to know more about breathing, please refer to the book: *Qigong Meditation—Embryonic Breathing,* by YMAA.

The final stage of this Qigong concentration training is to combine the above two trainings. By using your mind and coordination of reversed abdominal breathing, you lead the Qi and power to the bean underneath the clothes and break it. Naturally, the more you practice, the better skill you will have.

Still, if you use Tui Na and Dian Xue massage for healing, you will need a greater level of sensitivity and power in your fingers. The best way of training this is to untie a tight knot made in a thick rope (Figure 3-24). Tie up as many knots as possible in different ways, then close your eyes to untie them one by one. After you practice for a few months, you will feel an increase in your fingers' strength and sensitivity.

Recovery (Regulating the Body and Regulating the Qi). It is very important that after you have treated many patients, you know how to recover your Qi and physical condition into a normal and balanced state again. The key to this is learning to relax your physical and Qi bodies. In order to reach this goal, you must first regulate your mind and allow it to return to its peaceful and calm state.

Next, if you know the technique of embryonic breathing (Tai Xi, 胎息), then you

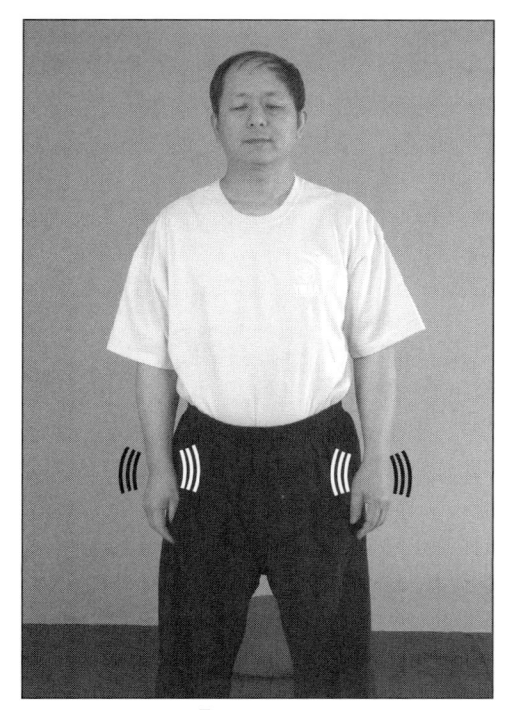

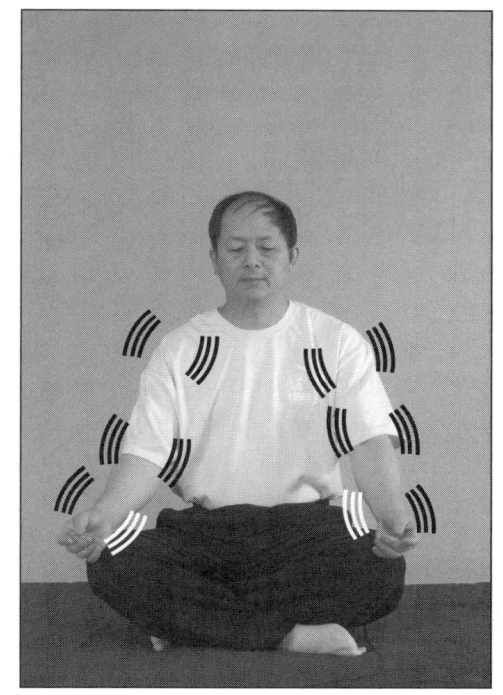

FIGURE 3-25

FIGURE 3-26

should practice this for a while. Through embryonic breathing, you will be able to lead the dispersed Qi back to its center, which helps you recover from your mental and physical fatigue quickly. Using this breathing for recovery is especially important for Tui Na and Dian Xue masseurs since they often have to use their Qi to manipulate the healing process. If you wish to know more about the theory and technique of embryonic breathing please refer to the book: *Qigong Meditation—Embryonic Breathing,* by YMAA.

However, if you don't know the technique of embryonic breathing, then you may simply use the normal abdominal breathing discussed earlier. This breathing will provide a good mental and physical condition for relaxation, thus allowing the Qi to return to its normal state.

To quickly recover the joint areas which are used for massage, you should learn joint breathing techniques (Guan Jie Hu Xi, 關節呼吸). In practice, if you wish to practice wrist joints breathing, first inhale deeply and use your mind to lead the Qi from the surface of the wrist area to the center of the wrist joint and when you exhale, you lead the Qi outward from the center (Figure 3-25). If you practice this with the coordination of reverse abdominal breathing (Ni Fu Hu Xi, 逆腹呼吸), the Qi can be led more efficiently and effectively. The more you practice, the easier and the better the Qi will be led. Soon, you will feel your entire wrists are breathing with you.

In the joint breathing exercises, if you are breathing the shoulder, elbow, wrist, and finger joints, you may sit with your both arms draped comfortably on your thighs (Figure 3-26). Naturally, you may also lie down and allow your arms to comfortably lay

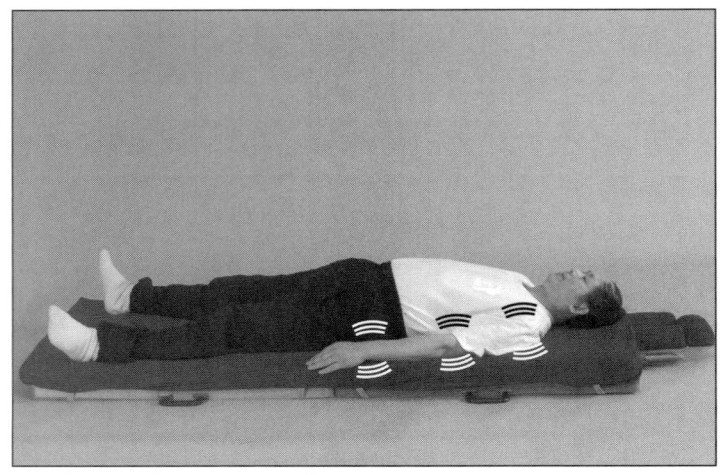

FIGURE 3-27

on the sides of your body (Figure 3-27). In this training, again, when you inhale, you lead the Qi at the center of three joints and when you exhale lead the Qi out the joints. After you have practiced for a few minutes, you will feel mild tingling or warmth at the joint areas. This breathing exercise is also commonly used by Qigong practitioners for joint self healing.

Attitudes (Regulating the Mind and Regulating the Spirit). The most difficult part of being a professional messeur is to maintain the same high spirit and nice attitude when you treat patients. Naturally, this spirit and attitude can be affected by your life style, mood, mental situation, and physical condition when massage is performed. For example, if you get to bed late, then your willingness and enthusiasm will not be the same as if you have obtained a nice rest the night before. If you have just had a argument with someone, then your mood and massaging spirit will also be affected. Not only that, if you have treated many patients and become fatigued, your energy will be low and your spirit will also be low. However, the most difficult part of massaging some patients is dealing with or handling the patient himself/herself. For example, do you like your patient? Does he/she have some weird Qi circulating around when you massage him/her? Does this patient appreciate your massage treatment? All of these concerns may influence your enthusiasm, willingness, and spirit in treating a patient.

To be a professional, you must know how to maintain your attitude. Not only that, you must also know how to recover yourself from Qi imbalance caused from massage. In addition, you must also know how to regain your normal status both mentally and physically.

Here, I have some suggestions to those who would like to become professional messeurs.

Be enthusiastic. If you are running a massage business, then enthusiasm will be the first key to your success. If you massage some friends, enthusiasm will also bring you the best joy in Qi's exchange. To build up an enthusiastic attitude, you should set up a goal when you massage someone each time. For example, when you massage the next ten people, you will train your sensitivity of their muscles and after that, you will train yourself to feel the next ten people's fasciae, ligaments, or bones. After you have gained so much experience in physical massage, then you will learn how to coordinate you breathing and mind so you are able to direct your feeling deeper and govern your Qi's circulation smoothly. Remember, there are unlimited levels or depths of massage. As long as you keep your mind humble and you ponder, you will soon see that every time you massage someone, it is a great opportunity for you to learn. It does not matter how deep you are, if you treat each massage case as an educational opportunity, then you will maintain your enthusiasm.

Be willing. To be willing to do something you do not want to do is a high level of spiritual cultivation. Whenever you encounter a patient whom you don't feel like massaging, you will lose your enthusiasm. In this case, you must learn how to conquer your emotional mind. You should treat it as a great opportunity to cultivate your spirit and temperament. Think, if you always do what you like, then your spirit will not grow. The main path of spiritual growth is initiated from encountering obstacles and bearing suffering or challenge both mentally and physically. Treating different patients will be a great challenge for you to conquer your emotional mind and allow your spirit to grow. Once you have this attitude, you will treat each case as a challenge to yourself. Once you have changed this thought, you will be willing and able accomplish the job joyfully.

Be meditative. When you massage someone, if you are able to bring your mind into a deeply meditative state, then your feeling will be deep and sensitive. Once you have this deep and clear feeling, your massage can be most effective. In addition, this will offer you a great opportunity to train your mind, feeling, and body. Different patients provide you different opportunities and cases for this meditation cultivation. For example, massaging an infant will be different from massaging an adult, massaging a lady will be different from a gentleman, massaging an over-weight person will be different from a under-weight person, and massaging a sick person will be different from massaging a healthy person. In addition, if you use massage for healing, then the feeling and the treatment will also be different from one case to another. The entire success of massage treatment depends on your feeling and this feeling can only be cultivated from a deep meditative mind.

Not only that, but as mentioned earlier, when you treat some patients, it is not uncommon to bring some Qi imbalance into your body. Therefore, you must have a good feeling or sensitivity of it, and know how to regain your balance. Meditation will not only help you to feel the imbalance, but can also help you recover. As mentioned before, the best way of regaining Qi balance is through the technique of embryonic breathing (Tai Xi, 胎息). If you wish to know more about this meditation technique, please refer to the book: *Qigong Meditation—Embryonic Breathing,* by YMAA.

References

1. Before birth, you have no Qi of your own, but rather you use your mother's Qi. When you are born, you start creating Qi from the Original Essence (Yuan Jing) which you received from your parents. This Qi is called Pre-Birth Qi, as well as Original Qi. It is also called Pre-Heaven Qi (Xian Tian Qi) because it comes from the Original Jing which you received before you saw the heavens (which here means the sky), i.e. before your birth.
2. 形不正，則氣不順。氣不順，則意不寧。意不寧，則氣散亂。
3. 李清庵詩云：〝調息要調無息息。〞
4. 廣成子曰：一呼則地氣上升，一吸則天氣下降，人之反覆呼吸於蒂，則我之真氣自然相接。
5. 唱道真言曰：一呼一吸通乎氣機，一動一靜同乎造化。
6. 黃庭經曰：呼吸元氣以求仙。
7. 伍真人曰：用後天之呼吸，尋真人呼吸處。
8. 靈源大道歌曰：元和內運即成真，呼吸外求終未了。
9. 大道教人先止念，念頭不住亦徒然。
10. 意不在氣，在氣則滯。
11. 孔子曰：先靜爾后有定，定爾后能安，安爾后能慮，慮爾后能得。

CHAPTER 4
Massage Techniques 按摩技術

4-1. Introduction 介紹

Before going into the specific practices of each category of massage, we would like to first introduce the most common techniques. Using the correct techniques will help you to treat problems effectively, while using the wrong techniques will often make matters worse. It is difficult to make general statements about what techniques you should use to treat particular problems, since what works well on one person may not work as well on another. Furthermore, even with the same technique, you may use a different amount of power with each person. One person may be extremely sensitive in a particular area, while another person may not feel anything but your strongest power. Experience is your greatest teacher. The more people you massage, the easier it will be for you to determine what needs to be done.

In this chapter, we will introduce many techniques. Over the years, many other techniques have been developed. However, because space is limited, and because some of the techniques have very specific uses, we will not be able to list them all. This chapter is meant to serve as a reference, and to give you guidelines for how to approach massage.

In the next section we will introduce the parts of the body that you will use in giving a massage, and in section 4-3 we will discuss the techniques.

4-2. The Tools of Massage 按摩施技位

Everyone knows that various areas of the hands are used in massage. However, many other parts of the body can also be used, such as the elbows, the forearms, and the heels. In this section, we will summarize the body areas that are commonly used for massage.

Finger Tips (指端). A fingertip covers a very small area, so its power can usually penetrate deep. Because of this, the fingertips are usually used to treat injuries deep inside the body, or to stimulate circulation in the primary Qi channels.

In Tui Na (推拿) massage, you usually rub with one or more fingertips when the injured area is small or deep, such as at particular points in the wrist, back of hand, or in the palm between the bases of the fingers (Figure 4-1). You would also use one or more fingertips to press inward on the skin and push along the Qi channels (Figure 4-2). The tips of the thumb, index finger, and sometimes the middle finger are used.

In Dian Xue (點穴) massage, the fingertip is also commonly used for pressing, usu-

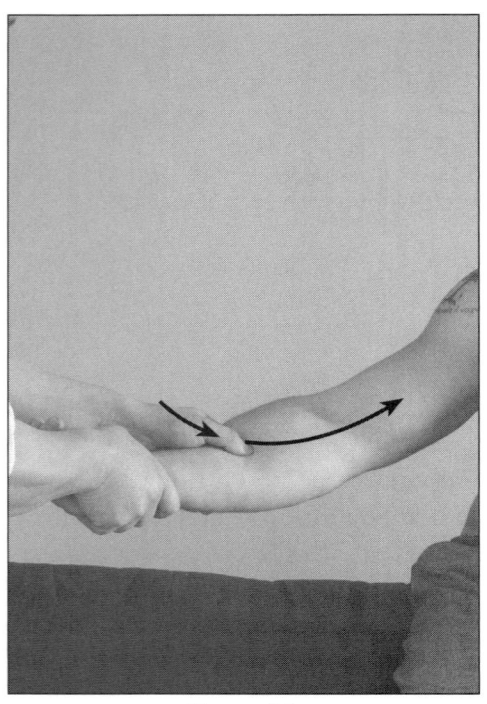

FIGURE 4-1 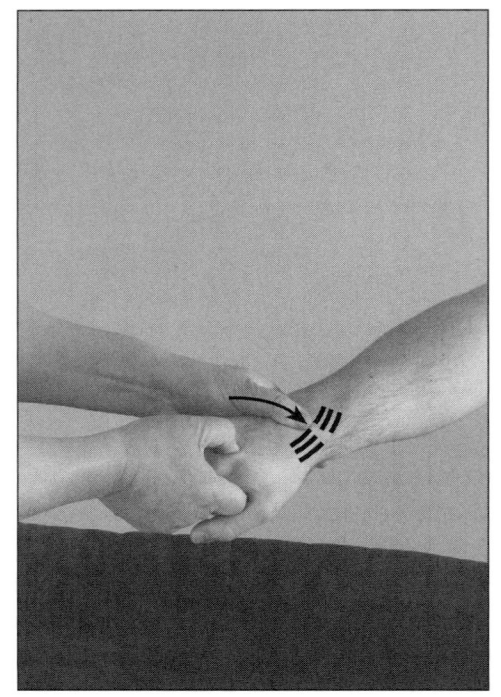   FIGURE 4-2

ally together with vibrating or shaking. To do this, you place your fingertip on the appropriate cavity, and then concentrate your mind so that your power reaches the Qi primary channel to either stimulate or soothe the Qi. Dian Xue usually uses the tip of the thumb (Figure 4-3) or the index finger (Figure 4-4). Sometimes the tip of the middle finger is also used (Figure 4-5). Since the Qi primary channel in the middle finger is connected to the pericardium, which is related to the heart, the Qi is usually strongest there.

In addition, since the fingertips are also Qi gates, they are often used in Qi massage to trace the Qi channels to adjust the circulation. This is usually done with the 'sword secret' (Jian Jue, 劍訣) hand form (Figure 4-6). Sometimes only the middle finger is used (Figure 4-7). When fingertips are used for Qi massage, they either touch the skin very lightly, or not at all.

In relaxation or general massage, the fingertips are commonly used to tap and stimulate the skin (Figure 4-8), which relaxes the patient and brings stagnant Qi to the surface.

The Last Section of the Fingers (最後指節). The last section of the fingers is the part most commonly used for rubbing and pressing. It covers a larger area than the fingertip does, and so a massage with it is gentler and softer than with the fingertip.

In Tui Na (推拿) massage, it is the most effective way of spreading out bruises and Qi stagnation so that waste material and stagnant Qi and/or blood can be removed. This is done by rubbing with a circular or straight motion. Usually, the last section of the

Chapter 4: Massage Techniques

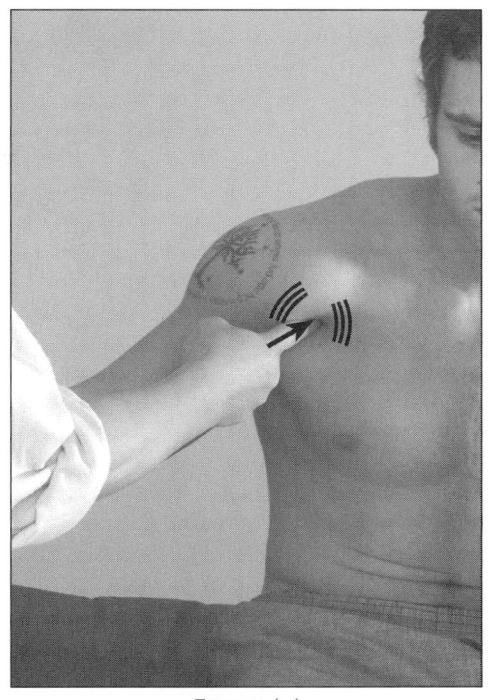

FIGURE 4-3

FIGURE 4-4

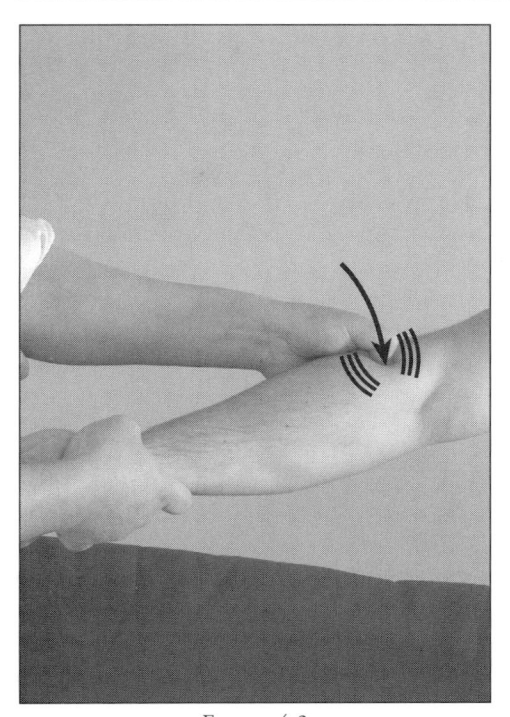

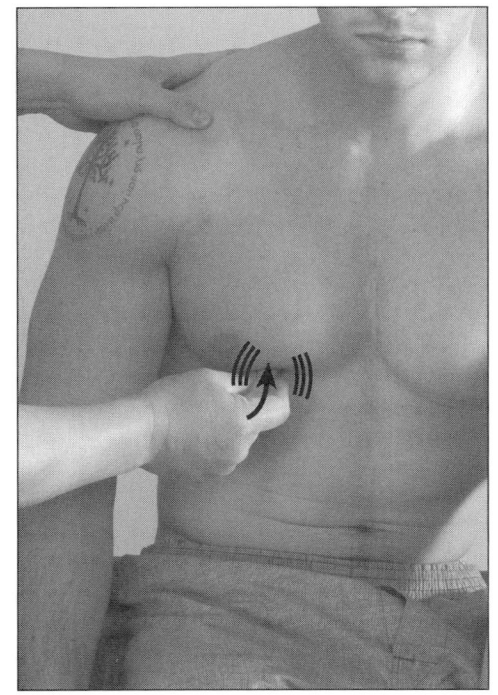

FIGURE 4-5

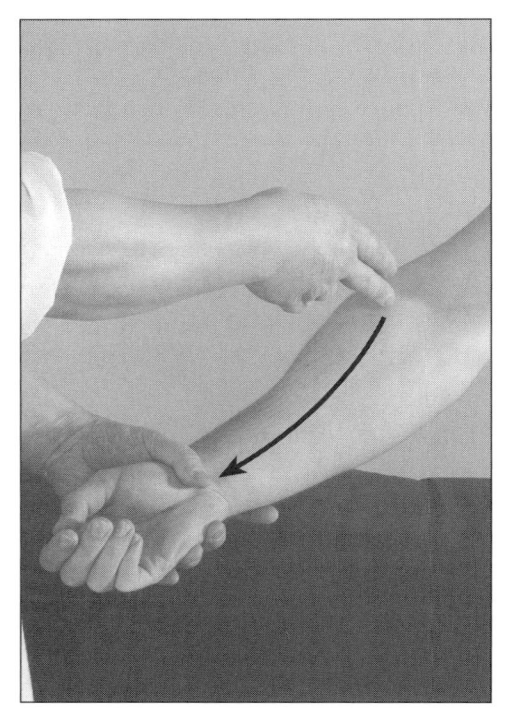

FIGURE 4-6

Qigong Massage

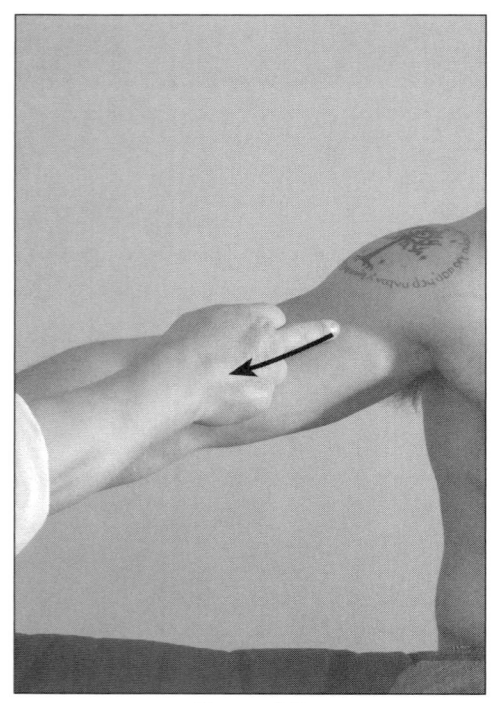

FIGURE 4-7

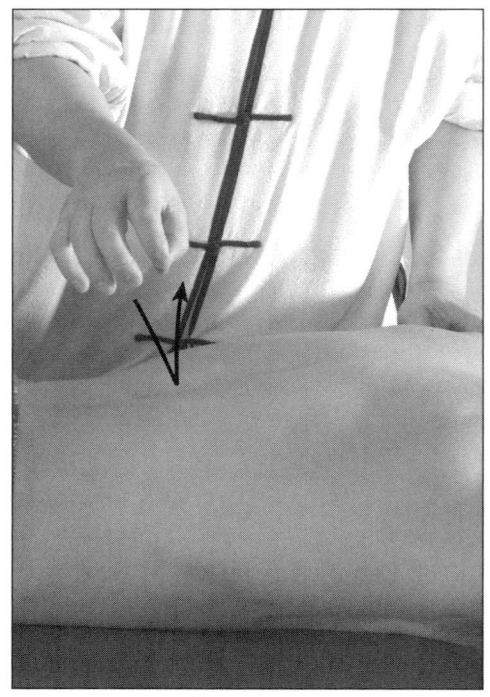

FIGURE 4-8

thumb is used (Figure 4-9). However, the last sections of the index and middle fingers are also commonly used together for this purpose (Figure 4-10). These areas are also used to press and push along the Qi channels to adjust the Qi.

In Dian Xue (點穴) massage, the last section of the fingers, especially of the thumb (Figure 4-11) and index finger (Figure 4-12), are commonly used for pressing cavities. This stimulates a larger area than a fingertip would, but it is the preferred method because it is not as painful for the patient. Since the patient stays more relaxed, recovery is quicker.

For relaxation or general massage, the last sections of the five fingers are used to adhere to the skin while using circular movements to relax an area (Figure 4-13). Sometimes, the last section of the thumb

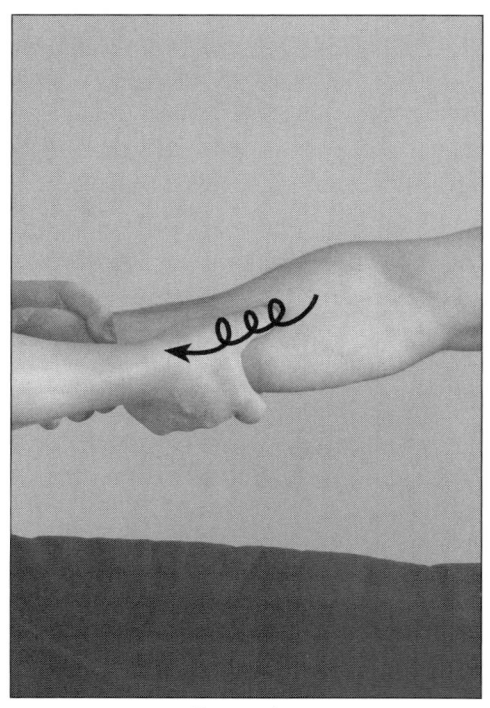

FIGURE 4-9

Chapter 4: Massage Techniques

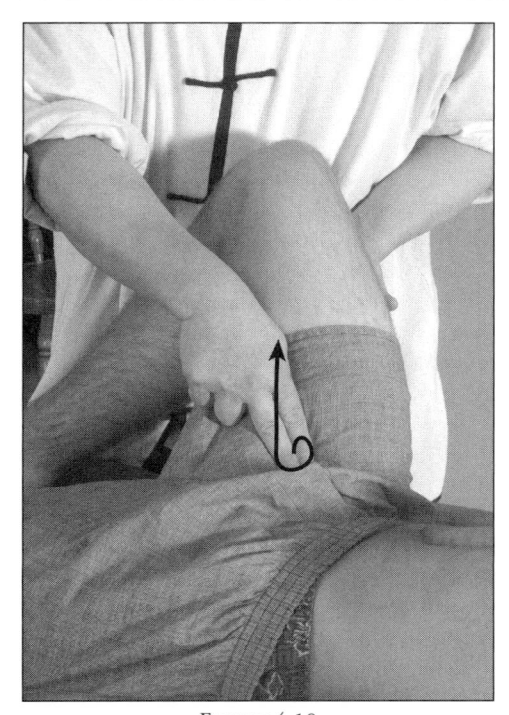

FIGURE 4-10

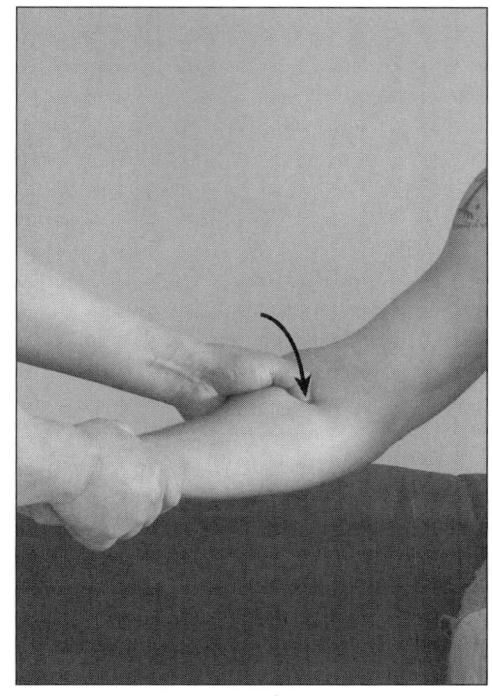

FIGURE 4-11

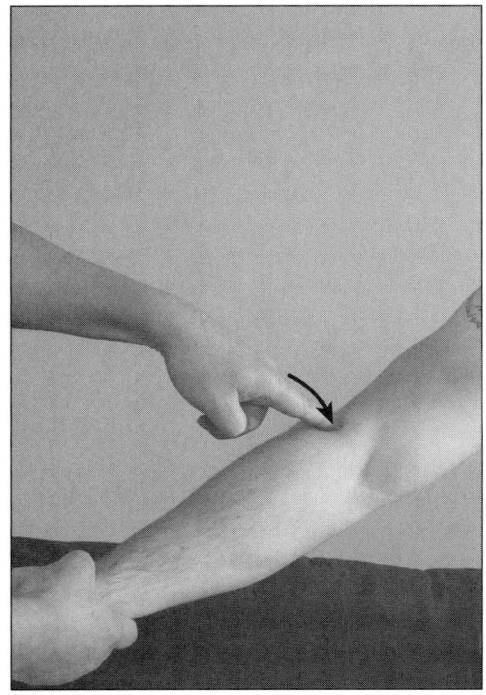

FIGURE 4-12

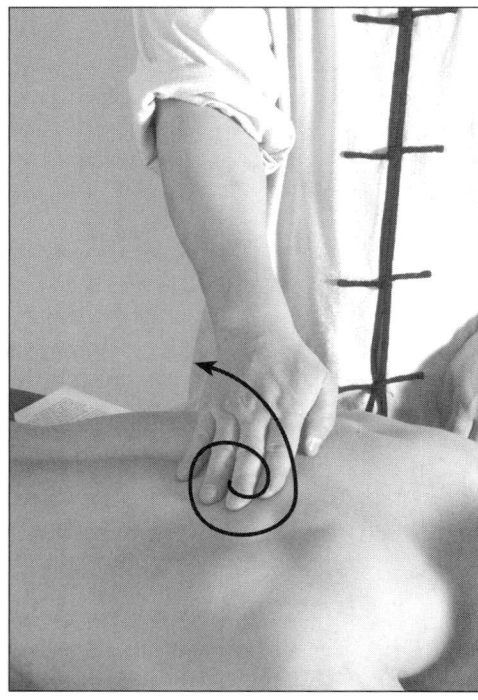

FIGURE 4-13

Qigong Massage

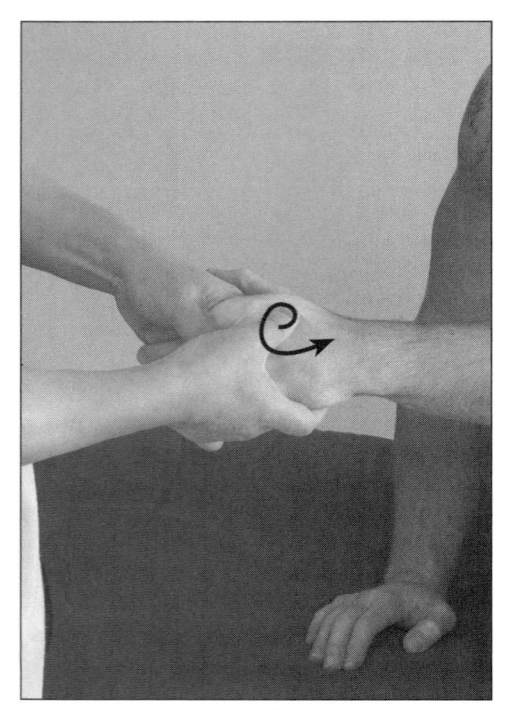

FIGURE 4-14

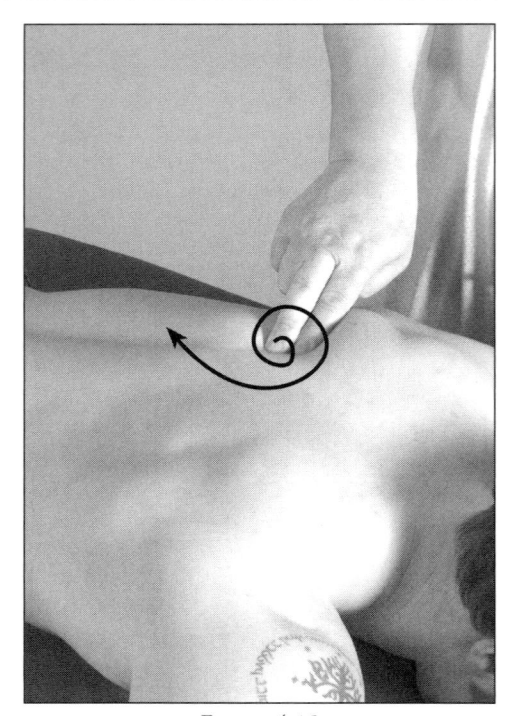

FIGURE 4-15

(Figure 4-14), or index and middle fingers (Figure 4-15), is used to rub a smaller area to disperse acid which has accumulated in the muscles and tendons.

The Last Two Sections of the Fingers (最後兩指節). The last two sections of the fingers are commonly used to grab muscles or tendons for Tui Na massage and relaxation massage. Usually, all five fingers are used at the same time. They are mainly used to massage the muscles on the limbs, such as on the arms (Figure 4-16), thighs (Figure 4-17), and calves (Figure 4-18). They are also often used to massage the big muscles, such as the muscles beside the armpit (Figure 4-19), and the muscles between the neck and shoulders (Figure 4-20).

This type of massage is usually used to spread out stagnant Qi and blood, as well as to stimulate areas to relax the patient.

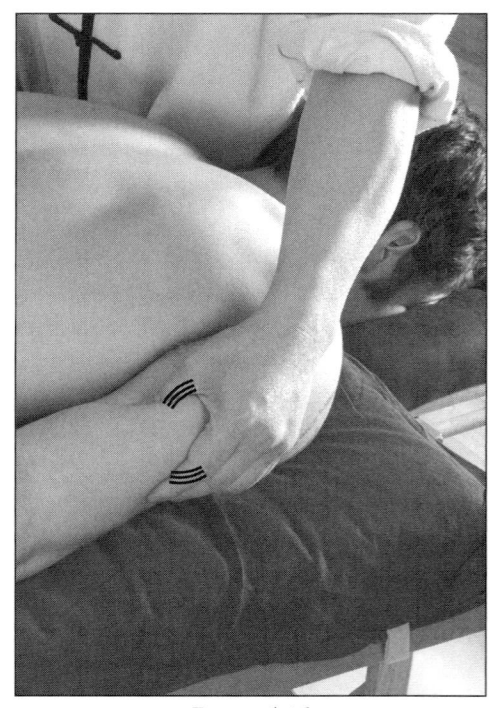

FIGURE 4-16

148

Chapter 4: Massage Techniques

FIGURE 4-17

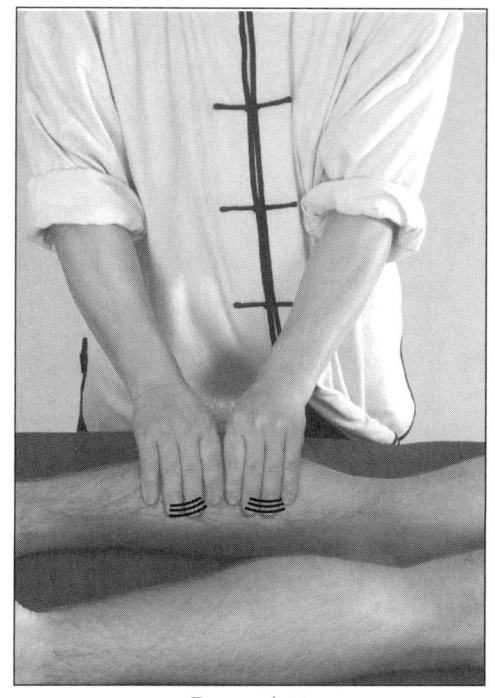

FIGURE 4-18

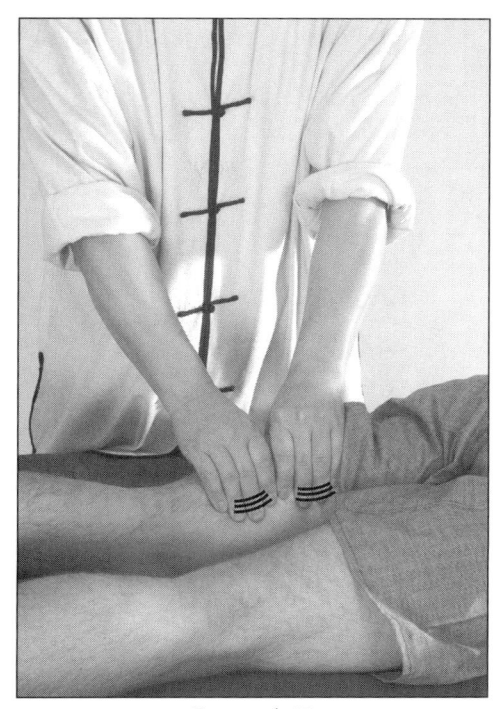

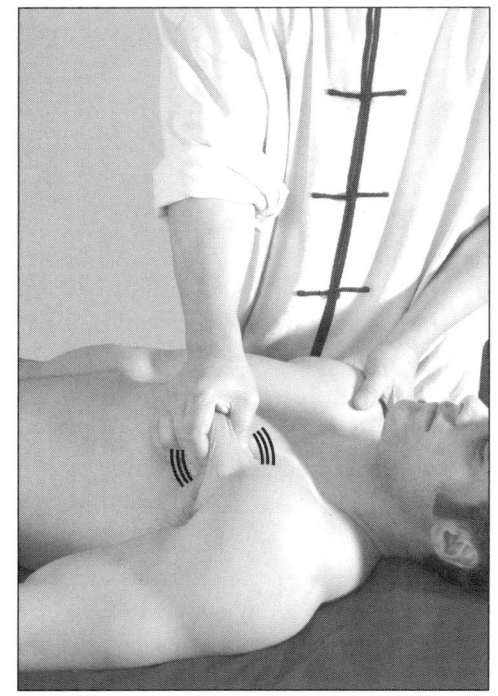

FIGURE 4-19

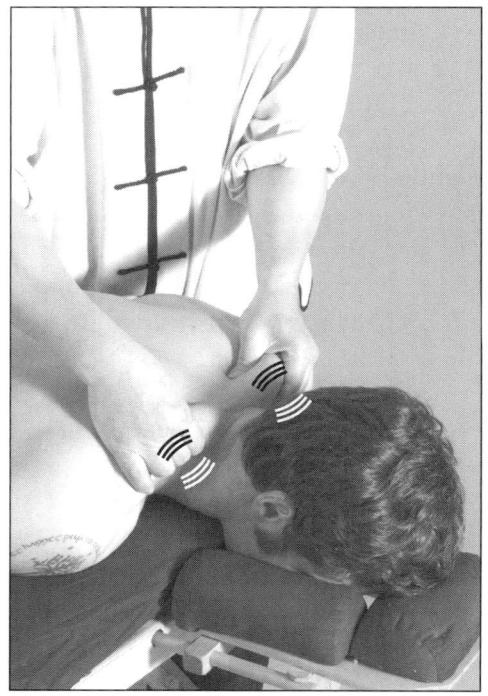

FIGURE 4-20

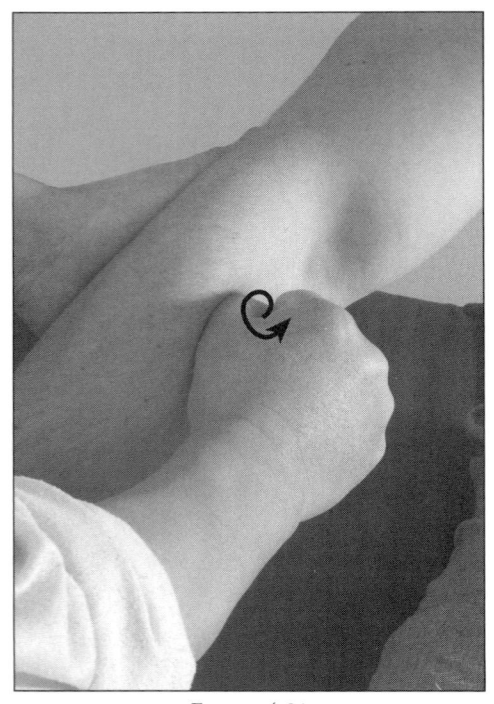

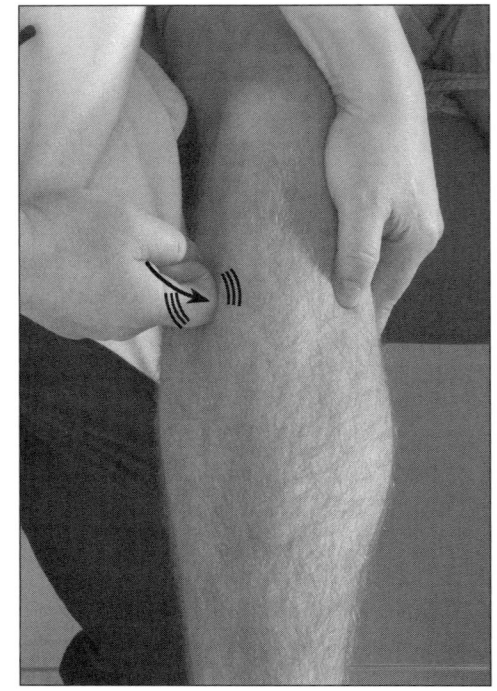

FIGURE 4-21   FIGURE 4-22

Knuckles (指關節). The knuckles are commonly used in Tui Na and Dian Xue massage, but only occasionally used in relaxation massage.

In Tui Na massage, the knuckle of the thumb (Figure 4-21) or the index finger (Figure 4-22) are normally used to press down and then push along the Qi channels to stimulate the Qi. Often, all of the knuckles except the thumb are used in a circular motion to massage areas where Qi and blood have become stagnate (Figure 4-23).

In Dian Xue massage, normally the knuckles of the thumb (Figure 4-24) or the index finger (Figure 4-25) are used to press inward through the cavities to stimulate the Qi circulation in the primary Qi channels. Quite often a vibrating motion will be used along with the pressure.

Side of the Palm (掌緣). The side of the palm is commonly used for Tui Na and relaxation massage. In Tui Na, after deep stimulation with other techniques, such as fingertip massage, has brought stagnant Qi and blood to the surface, then the side of the palm can be used to spread out the Qi and blood even more. The side of the palm covers a large area, and so it is used on large muscles on the torso or on joints such as the hip, knee, shoulder, or neck. The same techniques are also used in relaxation massage to spread acid accumulated in the muscles. The side of the palms are usually used for circular rubbing (Figure 4-26) and straight line pushing massage (Figure 4-27).

Base of the Palm (掌根). Like the side of the palm, the base of the palm is used to cover a larger area in Tui Na and relaxation massage. The base of the palm is stronger

Chapter 4: Massage Techniques

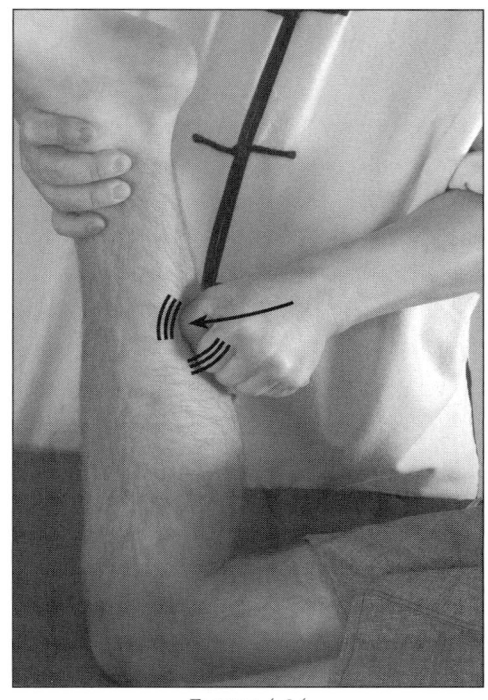

FIGURE 4-23

FIGURE 4-24

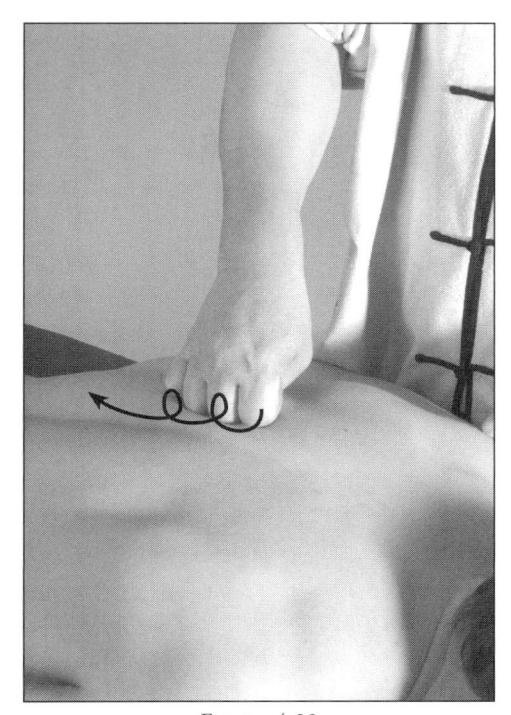

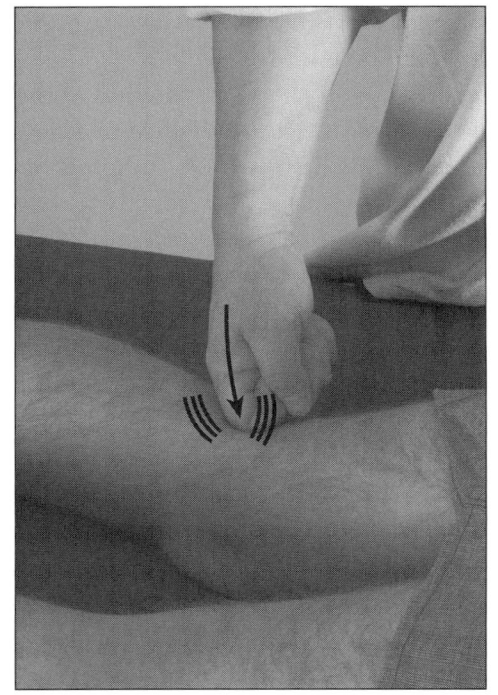

FIGURE 4-25

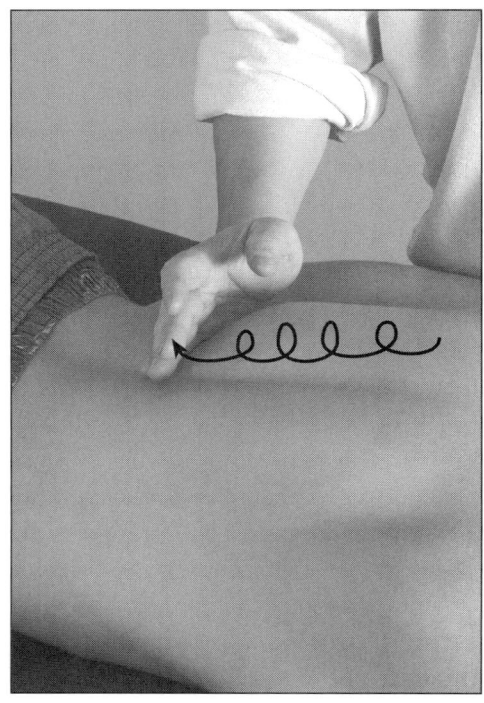

FIGURE 4-26

151

Qigong Massage

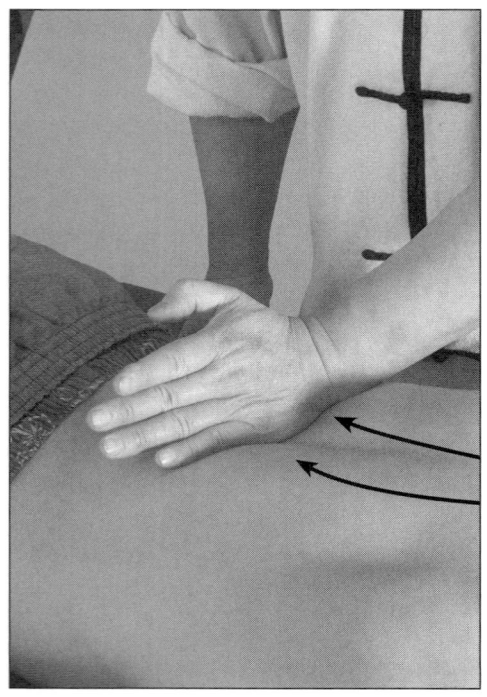

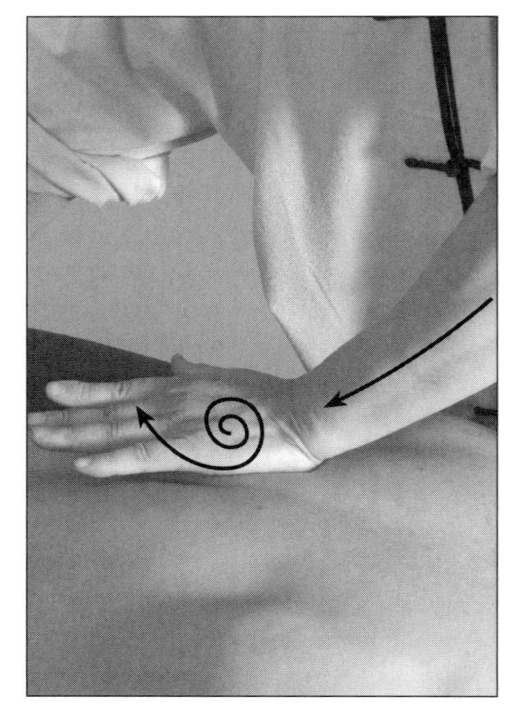

FIGURE 4-27

FIGURE 4-28

than the side because you can use your body as the root of the technique (Figure 4-28), whereas with the side of the palm you usually use your shoulder as the root.

The techniques for the base of the palm are the same as those for the side of the palm. However, there is one extra application for the base of the palm which is widely used, which is pressing without rubbing. This application is especially useful in loosening up the spine. It is done by pressing down on the joints between the vertebrae, one by one (Figure 4-29). This cannot be done easily with the side of the palm.

Center of the Palm (掌心). In the center of each palm is a cavity or Qi gate called Laogong (P-8) (勞宮) (Figure 4-30) which is used for dissipating extra heat in the heart. The Laogong cavity is on the Qi channel of the pericardium, which is the sack or membrane around the heart. Whenever there is too much 'fire' in the heart (i.e. when it is too Yang), the excess heat is conducted through the pericardium channel to the center of your palms. As long as you are healthy, the Qi in your heart is more positive than necessary, and the excess Qi is constantly being released through the Laogong cavities. This means that the Qi is stronger at the Laogong than elsewhere, and so this is the best cavity to use when you wish to lead a patient's Qi.

The center of the palm is commonly used for relaxation or general massage, as well as for Qi massage. In relaxation massage, the patient's Qi can be led while only lightly touching the skin (Figure 4-31) because the Qi released from your Laogong cavity can easily correspond with it. You only need to rub gently, and to let your hands flow

Chapter 4: Massage Techniques

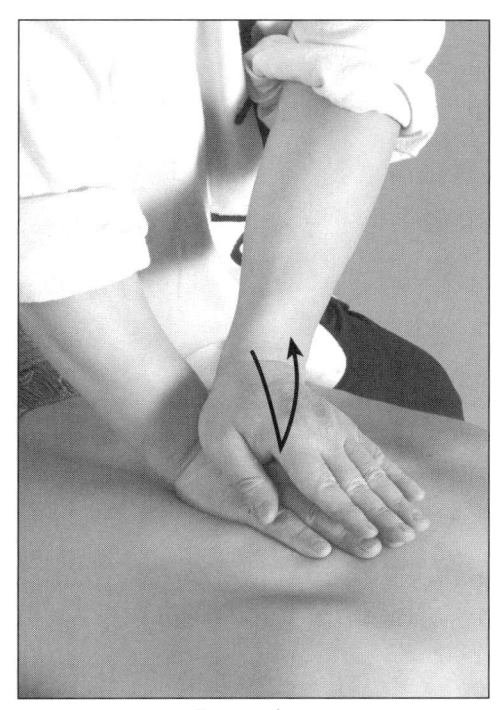

FIGURE 4-29

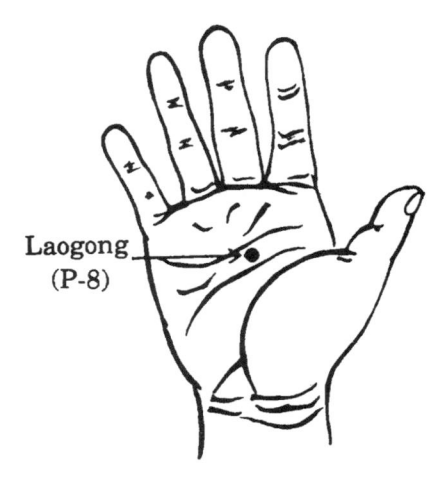

FIGURE 4-30. THE LAOGONG CAVITY.

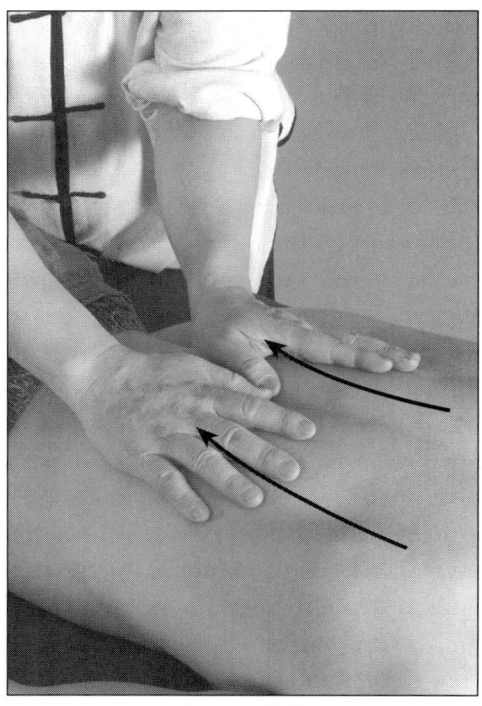

FIGURE 4-31

soothingly on their skin to relax them and open them up to your treatment. The hand is your main tool for regulating your patient's emotions, and therefore their Yi (意) and Qi. If you can skillfully use your hands to bring your patient into a relaxed state, you have already completed 50% of the treatment.

In Qi massage, you use the Qi released from your Laogong to correspond with the Qi in the patient's body (Figure 4-32). This allows you to restore smooth, healthy circulation, and to remove Qi stagnation from injuries or other causes.

Forearm and Elbow (前臂與肘關節). The forearm and elbow are not used very often in massage, however, there are times when they can be very useful. The forearm can be used in relaxation massage for large muscles when the hand is not strong

153

Qigong Massage

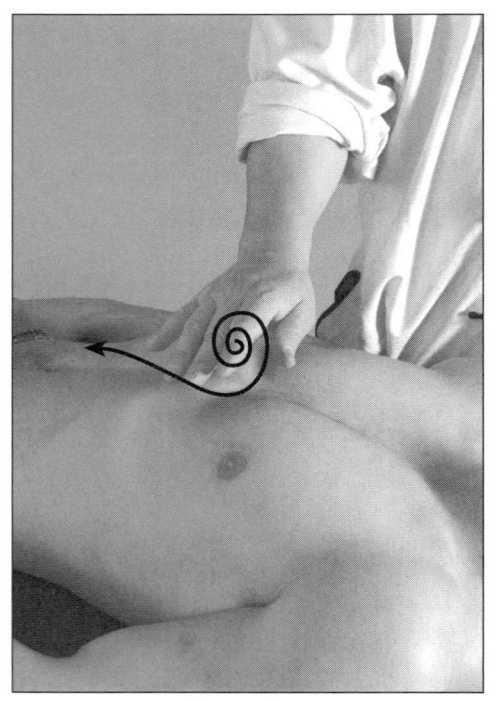

FIGURE 4-32

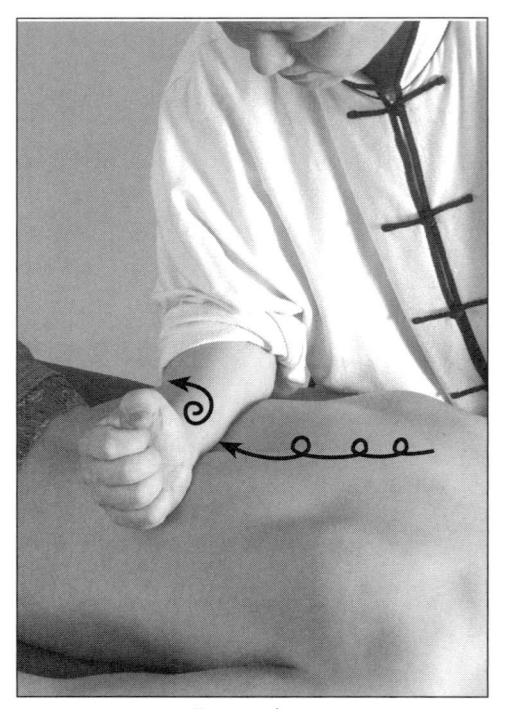

FIGURE 4-33

enough; for example, the trunk muscles on the back (Figure 4-33), or the thigh muscles (Figure 4-34). The forearm is sometimes used in Tui Na to spread out accumulated Qi and blood.

The elbow is sometimes used in Tui Na or Dian Xue massage because its power is stronger and more penetrating. It is used especially for cavities located in areas with big muscles, such as the hips and thighs (Figure 4-35).

Knee and Bottom of Foot (膝關節). The knee and the bottom of the feet are often used by women and by men with small builds in both Chinese and Japanese massage. They are used mainly for the back, hips, and thighs (Figures 4-36, 4-37, and 4-38) where the muscles are especially thick and strong, and the masseur therefore needs strong hands if the power is to penetrate.

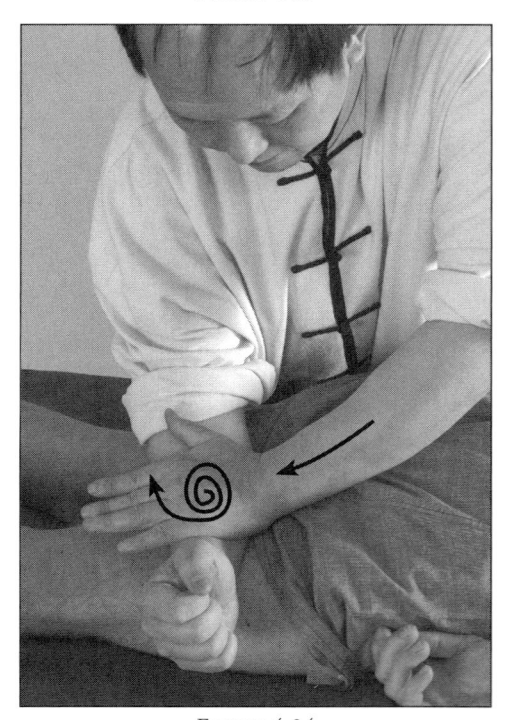

FIGURE 4-34

154

Chapter 4: Massage Techniques

FIGURE 4-35

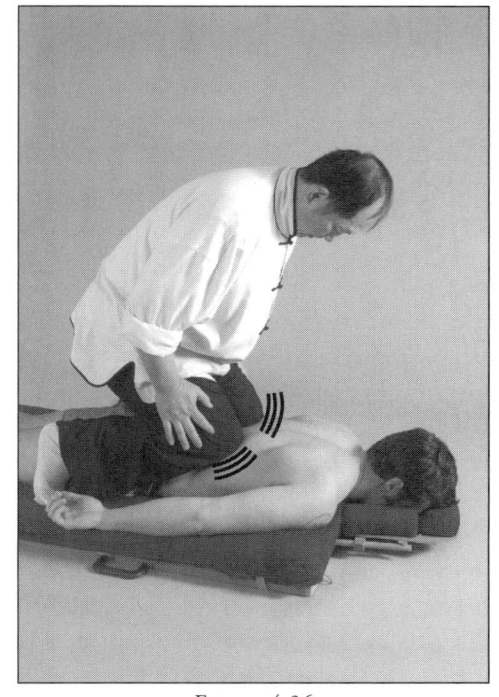

FIGURE 4-36

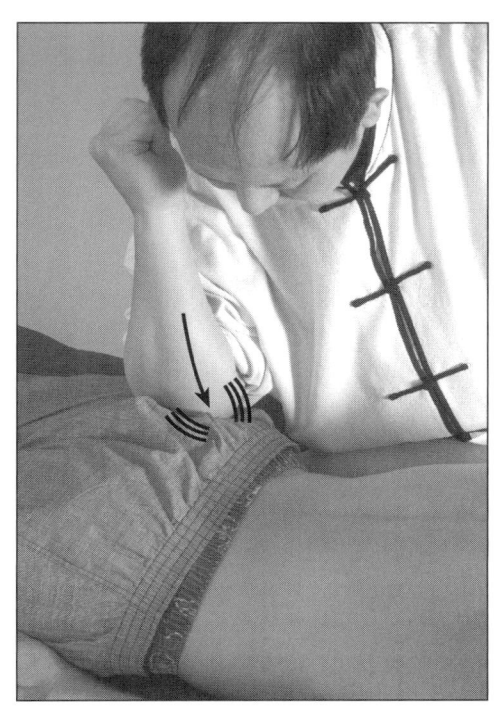

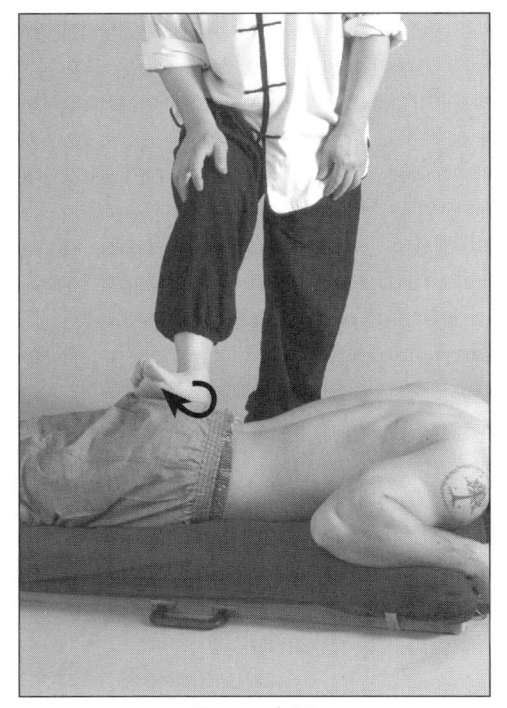

FIGURE 4-37

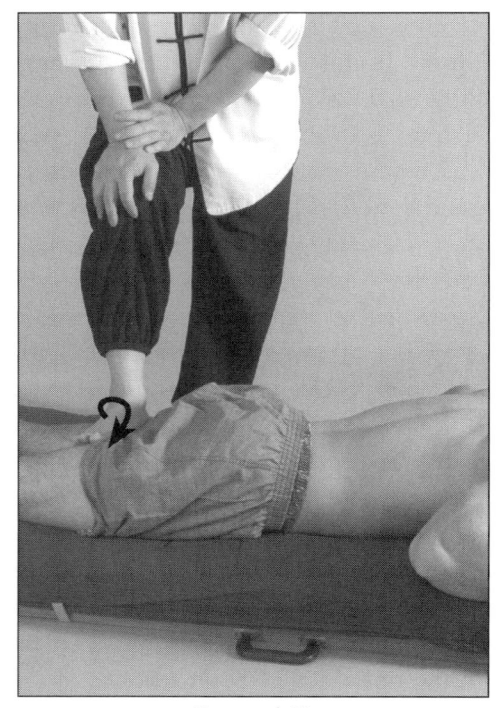

FIGURE 4-38

155

4-3. Massage Techniques and Training 按摩技術與訓練

In this section, we will introduce fifty basic massage techniques used in Chinese Qigong massage. Naturally, some of them are more effective for one category of massage than another. Once you have studied these techniques, you may discover others that are useful in some cases.

Rubbing (Rou or Mo) (揉、摩). The Chinese word Rou (揉) is made up of the two characters "hand" (才) and "soft"(柔). This implies that the Rubbing technique massages or rubs softly with the hand. It also implies that the hand doing the technique should be 'soft' or relaxed, with pressure coming from the whole body, guided by the relaxed and concentrated mind. There is no exact English word for this concept. "Mo" means almost the same thing, but implies a little larger movement, and includes some friction. Rou is generally a circular motion, while Mo is a straight, back and forth motion. In actual practice, there is almost no difference between the two.

Rubbing is the most common technique, and it can be used in general massage, Tui Na massage, and also Dian Xue massage. Naturally, although the theory and the basic movement are the same, the applications may be different in each category. For example, when Rubbing is used for an injury, it is used over a larger area because you want to get rid of local bruises and stagnant Qi. However, when Rubbing is used for healing illness, its power is focused on the primary channels or cavities to balance the Qi circulation. Also, the part of your hand you use for Rubbing will vary according to the application.

Rubbing is usually done with a circular motion. You may use the last section of your thumb (Figure 4-39), or the last section of one or more fingers (Figure 4-40), the last joint of the fingers (Figure 4-41), the side of the palm (Figure 4-42), base of the palm (Figure 4-43) or forearm (Figure 4-44).

When you use Rubbing, you do not actually rub the patient's skin, Instead, your hand contacts their skin and moves with it, so that you are actually rubbing under their skin. This lets you remove stagnant Qi and blood in the fascia between the skin and the muscles. Since your power is going beneath the skin, you can direct it to the muscles, the fascia between the muscles, or even to the fascia between the muscles and the bones.

Generally speaking, if you rub with your right hand in a clockwise direction (from your perspective), then you are releasing Qi to the patient. From the patient's perspective, your hand is moving counterclockwise, and the patient is absorbing the Qi (Figure 4-45). If you rub in a counterclockwise direction with your right hand, then you are absorbing Qi from the patient.

Rubbing is used to first relax the muscles or the injured area, and then to improve the Qi and blood circulation. Rubbing helps to remove stagnant Qi and blood and bring them to the skin. Finally, Rubbing spreads the Qi and blood even farther so that the body can remove it. Rubbing is very effective in removing the acid which accumulates in the muscles when you exercise.

Tui Na massage is frequently used for joint injuries. Rubbing is used first to bring

Chapter 4: Massage Techniques

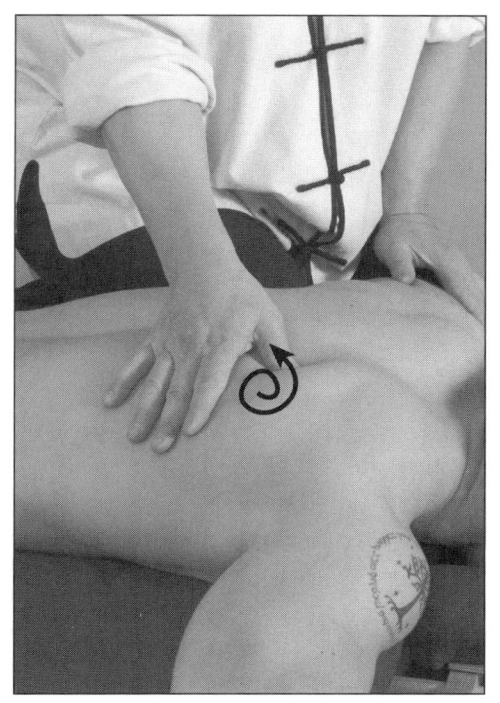

FIGURE 4-39

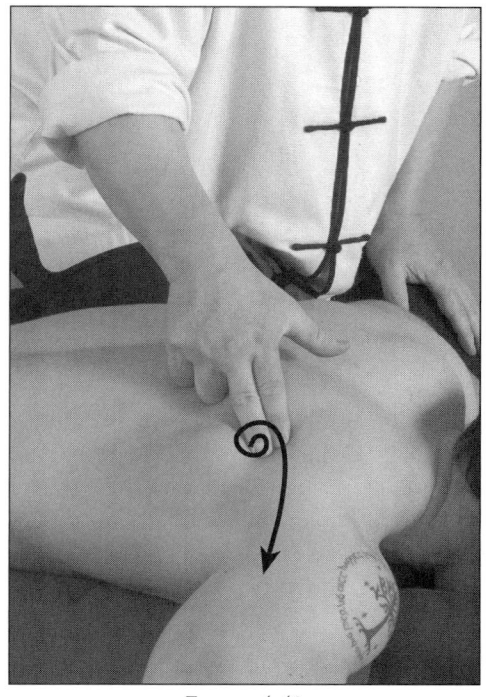

FIGURE 4-40

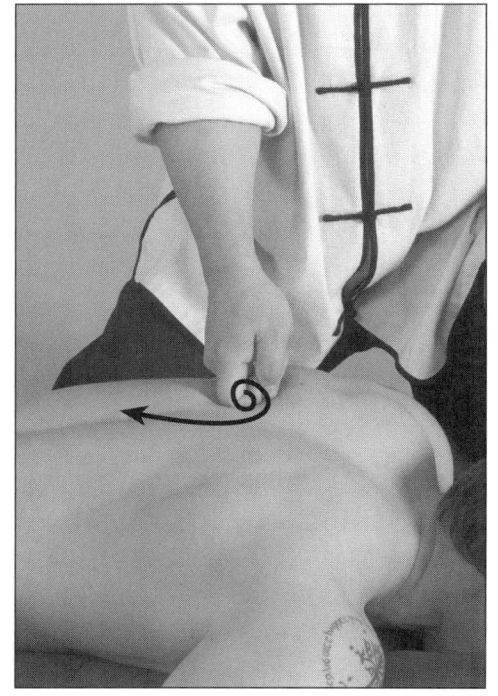

FIGURE 4-41

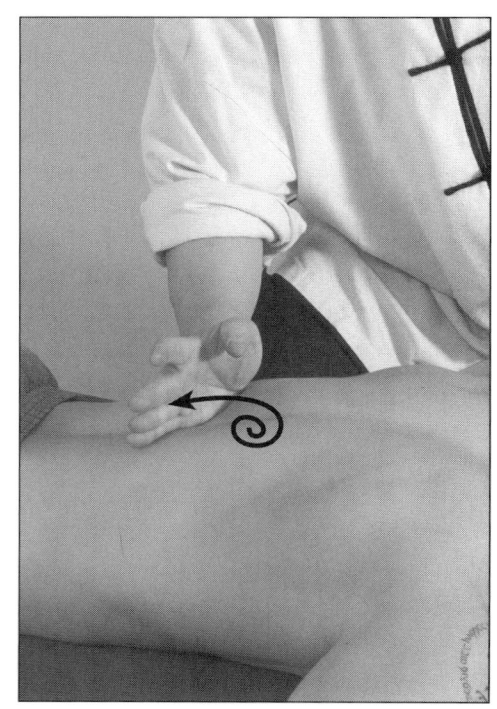

FIGURE 4-42

157

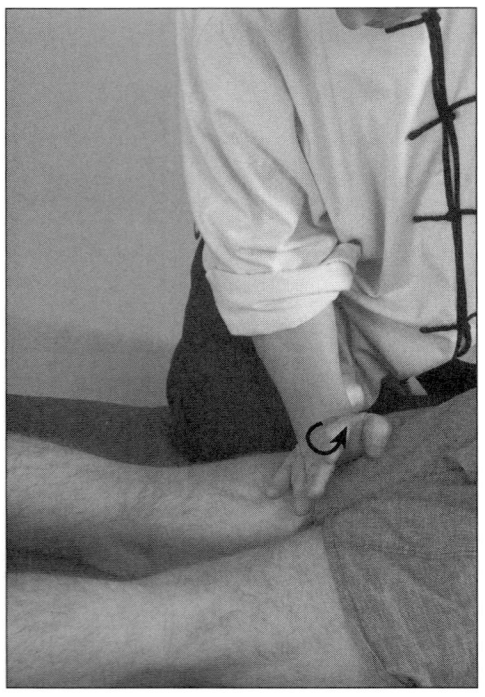

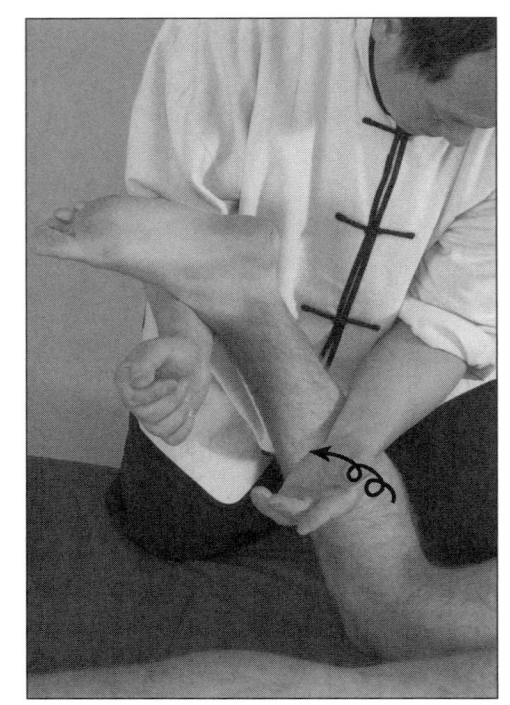

FIGURE 4-43

FIGURE 4-44

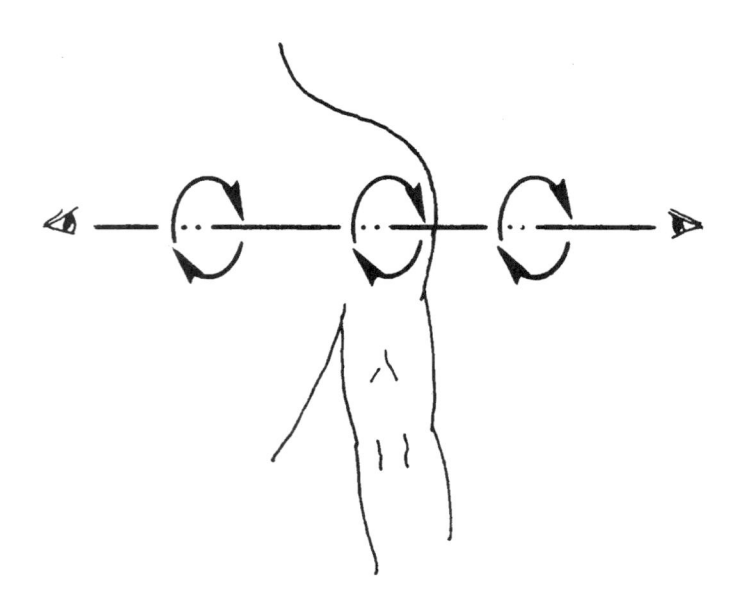

FIGURE 4-45. DIFFERENT VIEWPOINTS FOR THE DIRECTION OF MASSAGE.

Chapter 4: Massage Techniques

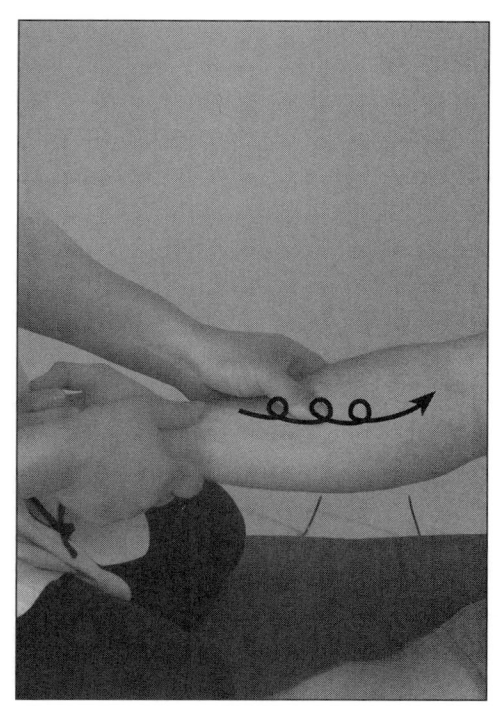

FIGURE 4-46

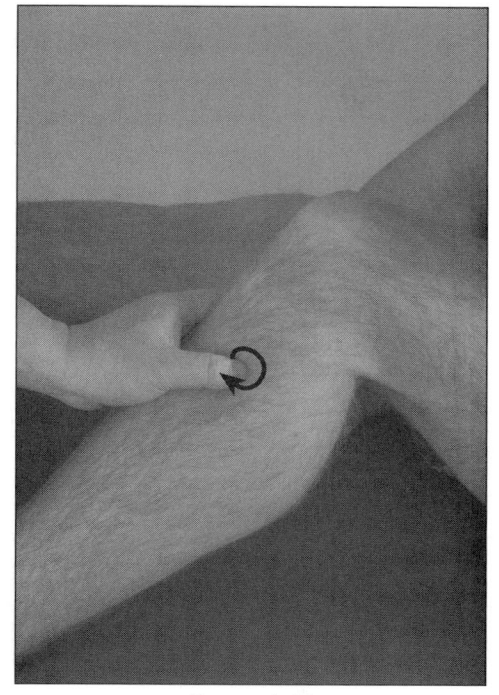

FIGURE 4-47

the Qi and bruise to the surface, and then circular and straight Rubbing (Figure 4-46) are used to push the stagnant Qi and blood away from the joint so that the body can take care of the residue.

In Dian Xue massage, the circular motion is very small. Normally, the first section of the finger is used to press down heavily on a cavity, then a small, circular rubbing motion is used to lead power into the cavity (Figure 4-47).

Pressing (An) (按). Pressing straight inward is called An (按). Pressing is often used together with other techniques. For example, in the Rubbing technique, Pressing is required to adjust the depth of the massage. Pressing can be applied through the fingertips (Figure 4-48), the last section of

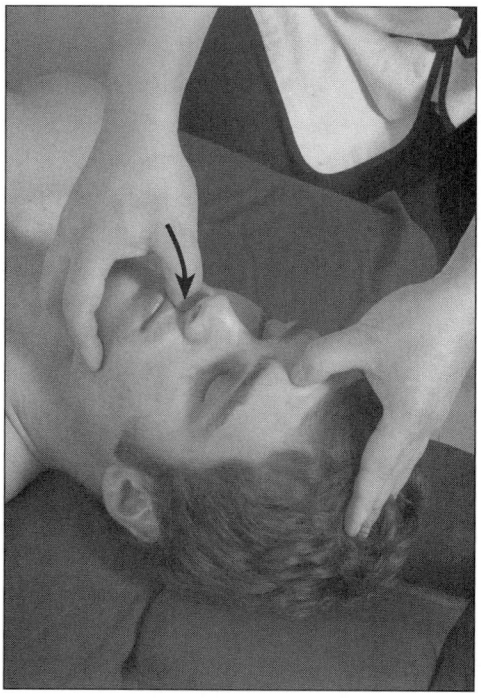

FIGURE 4-48

159

Qigong Massage

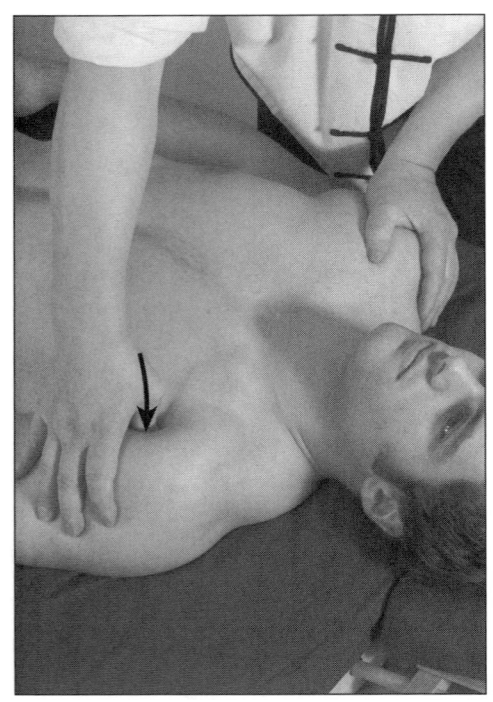

FIGURE 4-49

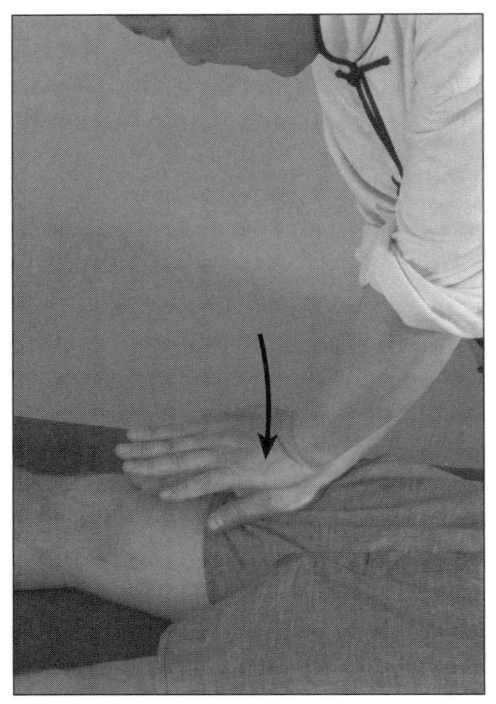

FIGURE 4-50

the fingers (Figure 4-49), the base of the palm (Figure 4-50), the forearm (Figure 4-51), or the elbow (Figure 4-52). Dian Xue massage normally uses Pressing with the fingertips and the last section of the fingers (especially the thumb and/or the index fingers) (Figure 4-53). In Tui Na or general massage, the base of the palm or the forearm are commonly used to press the spine, the trunk muscles, or even the kidneys.

In Dian Xue massage, you apply pressure with this technique and then release it. Doing this repeatedly stimulates the area or cavity and affects the Qi circulation there.

Pushing (Tui) (推). Pushing combines Pressing with straight movements. It is normally used right after circular Rubbing. Pushing can be done with the last section of the fingers (especially the thumb) (Figure 4-54), the side of the palm (Figure 4-55), the

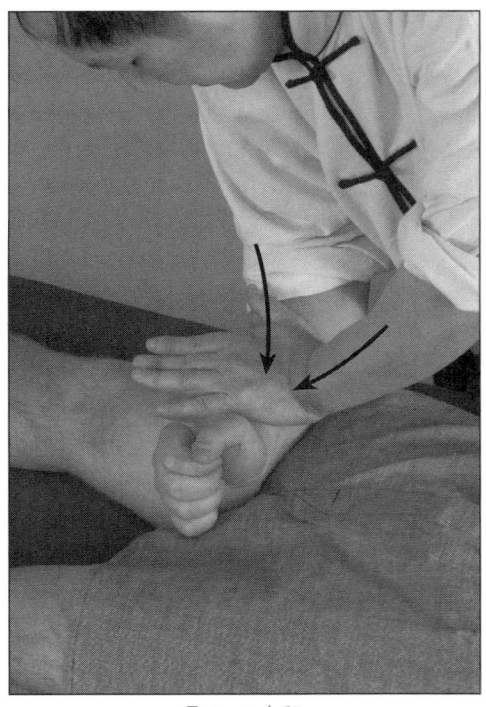

FIGURE 4-51

Chapter 4: Massage Techniques

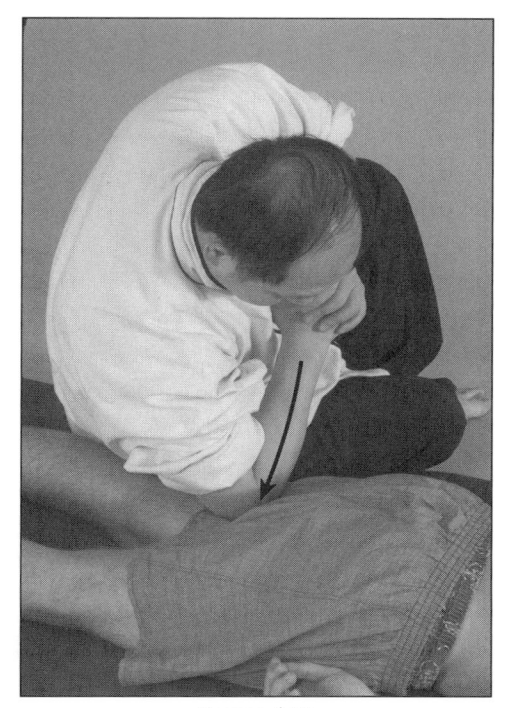

Figure 4-52

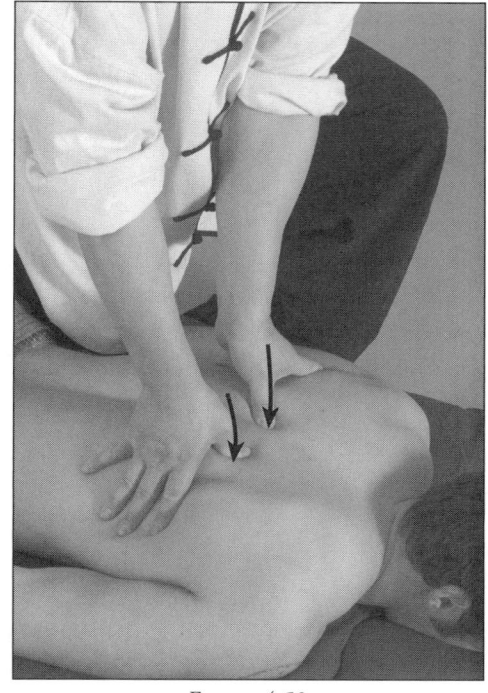

Figure 4-53

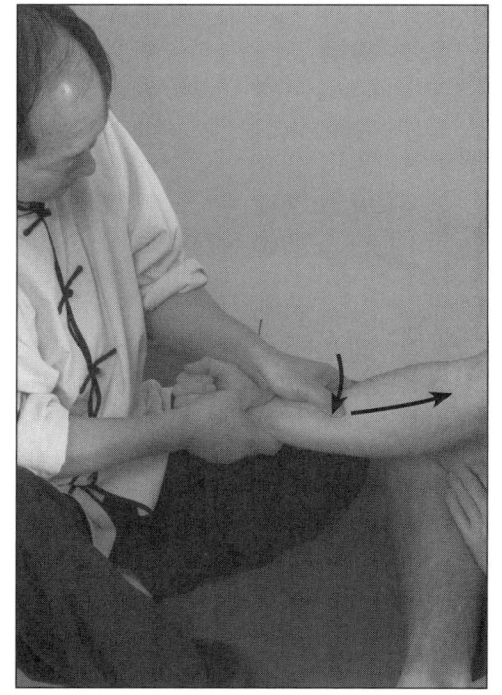

Figure 4-54

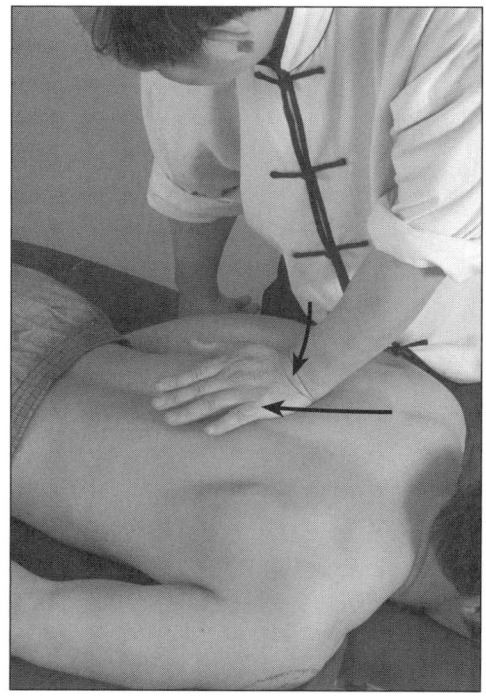

Figure 4-55

Qigong Massage

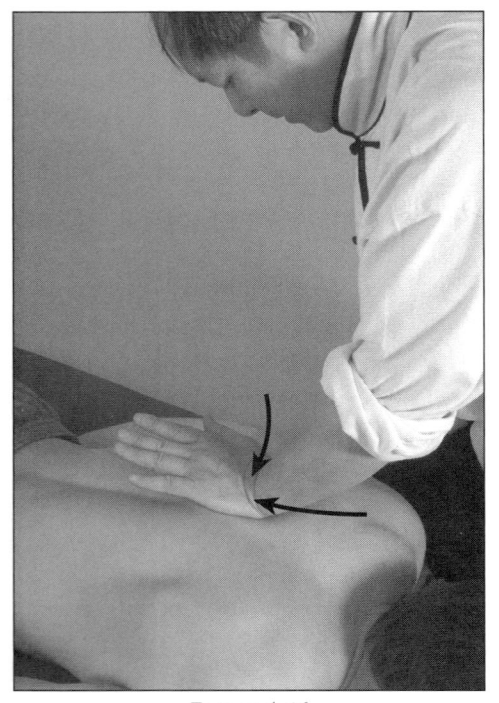

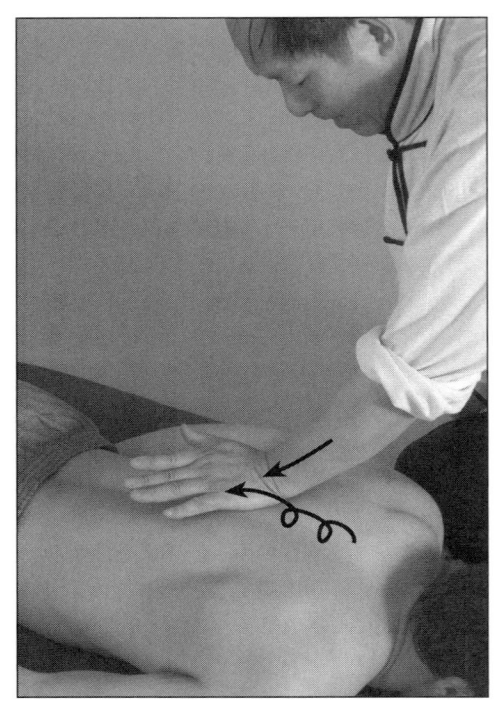

FIGURE 4-56

FIGURE 4-57

base of the palm (Figure 4-56), or the forearm. Pushing can also be combined with other techniques such as Rubbing (Rou, 揉) (Figure 4-57) or Vibrating (Zhen Zhan, 震顫).

Pushing is commonly used in both general and Tui Na massage. In general massage, Pushing is used to push and spread the acid accumulated in the muscles. In Tui Na massage, a straight pushing motion is used to spread bruises and Qi out away from the area of stagnation. The more the bruises and stagnant Qi are spread out, the easier it will be for the body's natural blood and Qi circulation to assist the healing. In general, you do not want the stagnation to be focused in a tiny area, because this is more difficult for the body's healing processes to handle.

Grabbing (Na) (拿). You can use Grabbing with one or both hands. Grabbing is used to stabilize a limb for pushing, to correct dislocated joints, or to connect broken bones (Figure 4-58). Grabbing is also used on the limbs for cavity press. The thumb presses on the cavity while the other four fingers provide support for the thumb (Figure 4-59). Another technique is to grab a muscle and rub or shake it. This is used particularly on the muscles beside the armpit, the arm muscles, the thigh muscles, and the calf muscles (Figure 4-60).

Caressing (Mo) (摸). Lightly touching the patient's skin can relax the patient and give them a very pleasant feeling. Simply move your hands lightly along the massage pathways. For a more delicate, sensitive feeling, use just your fingertips (Figure 4-61). Follow the simple rules, and massage from the top to the bottom, and from the center to the sides of the limbs. This will help the patient to lead the Qi from the top of the

Chapter 4: Massage Techniques

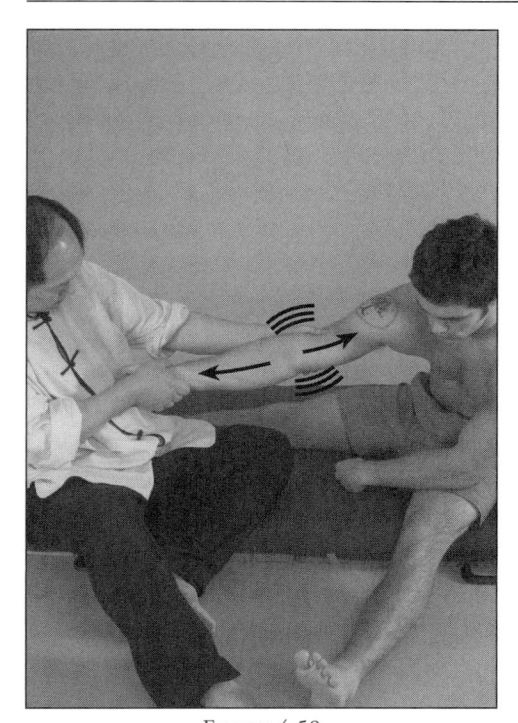

FIGURE 4-58

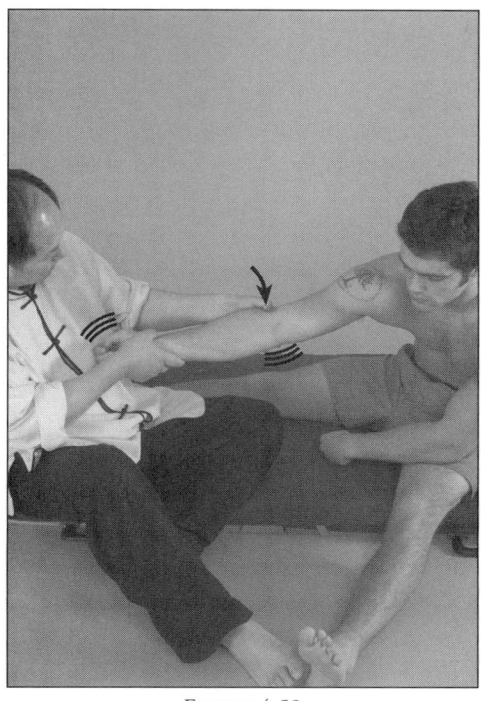

FIGURE 4-59

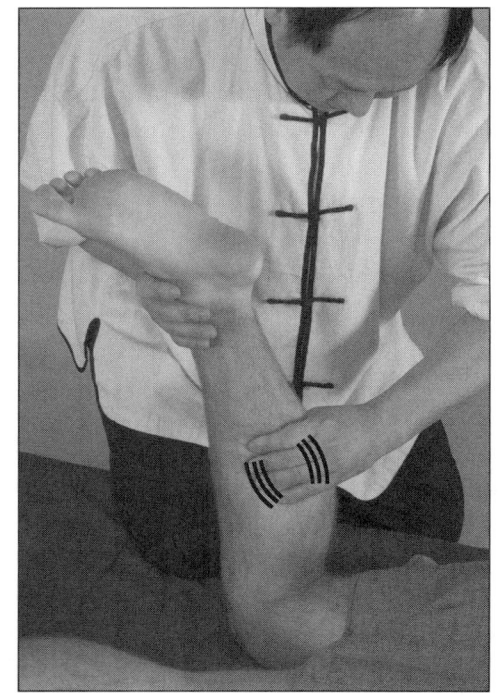

FIGURE 4-60

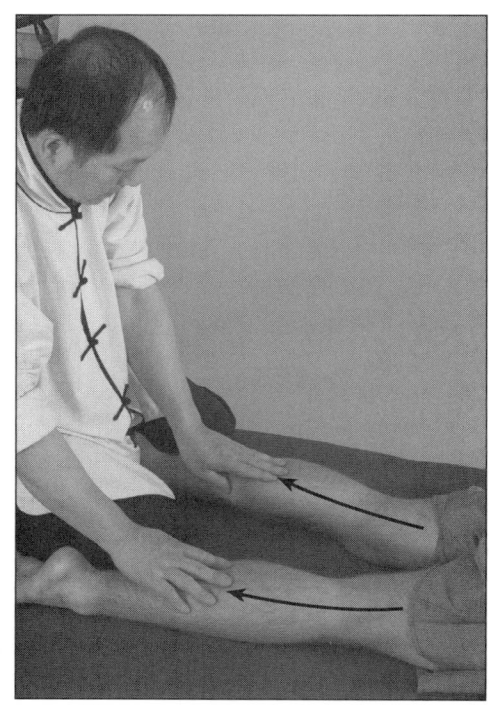

FIGURE 4-61

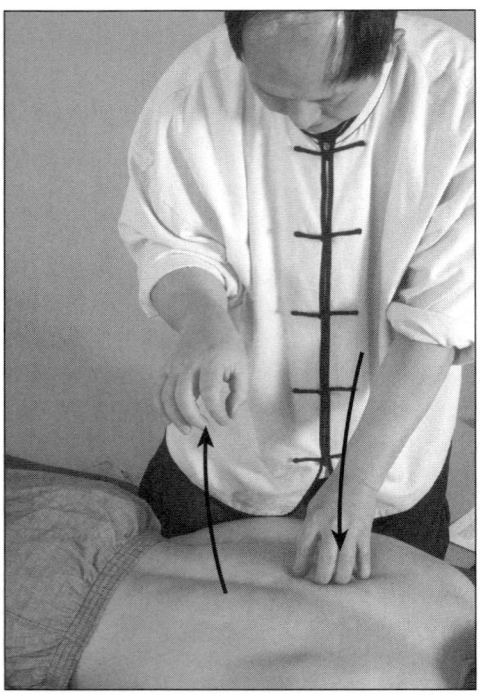

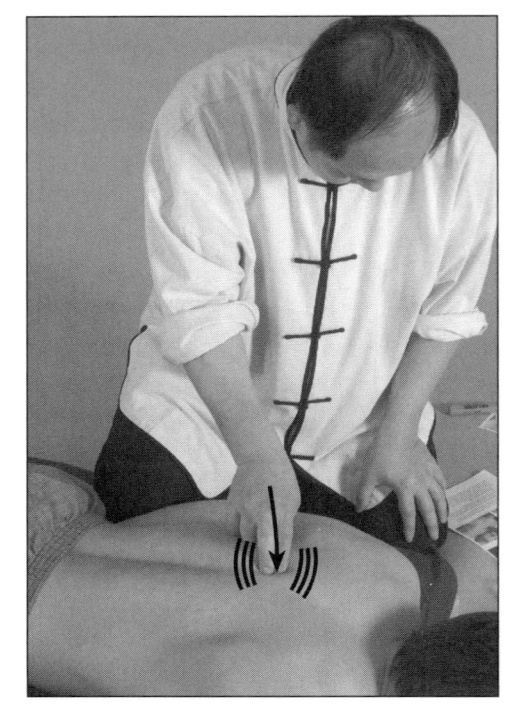

FIGURE 4-62

FIGURE 4-63

head to the feet and finally to the ground, and it can also help to spread stagnant Qi in the body out to the limbs and finally get rid of it.

Point Striking or Knocking (Dian Da, Qiao) (點打、敲). Point Striking is tapping or striking specific areas or cavities with the fingertips (Figure 4-62). This stimulates the skin or cavity, and raises stagnant Qi or blood to the surface.

Vibrating (Zhen Zhan) (震顫). Vibrating is a quick, shaking motion. Normally, this shaking motion is done together with another technique. For example, in Dian Xue massage you will frequently press a cavity with a finger and then shake or vibrate the finger to quickly raise the energy level in the cavity (Figure 4-63). In general and Tui Na massage, you may grab a muscle or tendon and shake it to stimulate it (Figure 4-64). You may also press with the base of your palm on big muscles such as the trunk and thigh muscles, and then shake them to loosen them up (Figure 4-65).

Vibrating is also commonly done with an up and down motion to stimulate the skin and muscles and increase Qi and blood circulation (Figure 4-66). Qigong masters will often use this technique to lead the Qi into the patient's body for nourishment.

Holding (Duan) (端). Holding is usually used to keep part of the body in a certain position, because different positions will cause the patient's body to respond in different ways. For example, when you are working in the armpit you will want to hold the patient's arm up. Although the muscles in the armpit will be slightly tensed, it will still be much easier for you to reach deeper into the body (Figure 4-67). In Tui Na massage,

Chapter 4: Massage Techniques

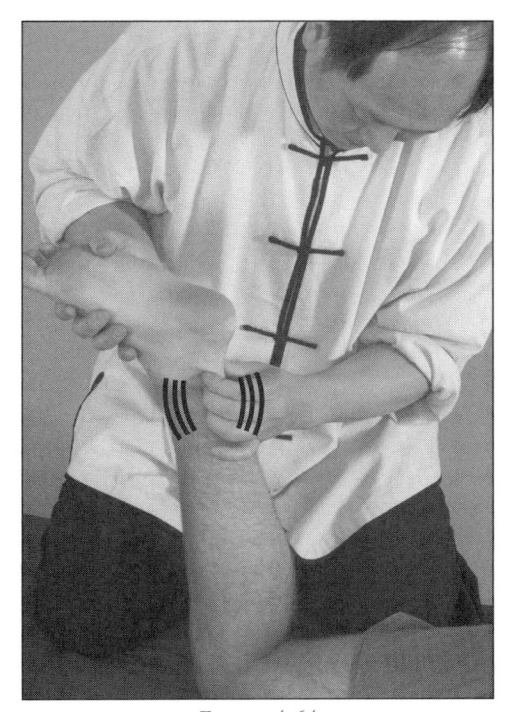

FIGURE 4-64

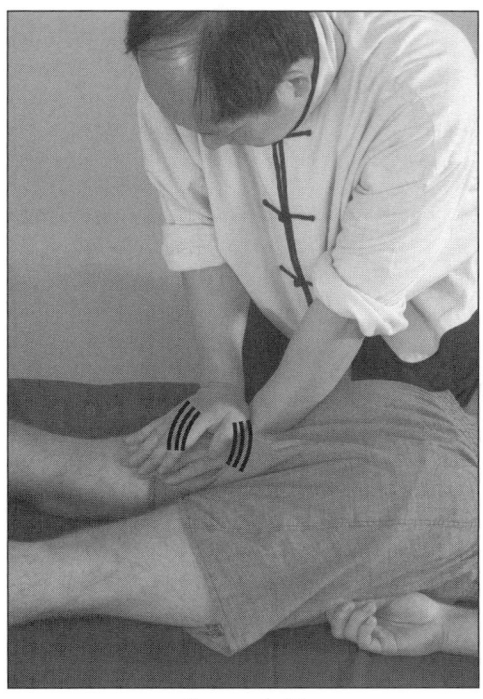

FIGURE 4-65

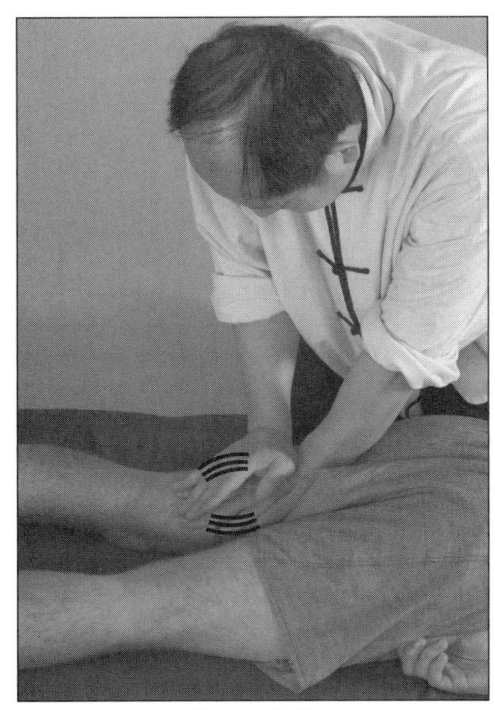

FIGURE 4-66

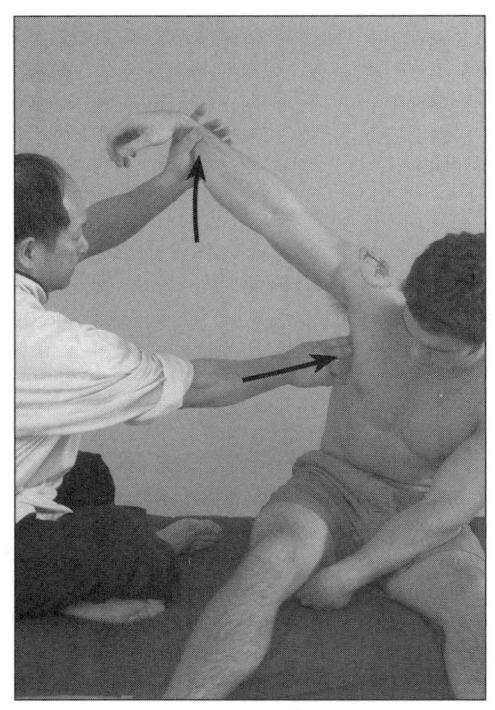

FIGURE 4-67

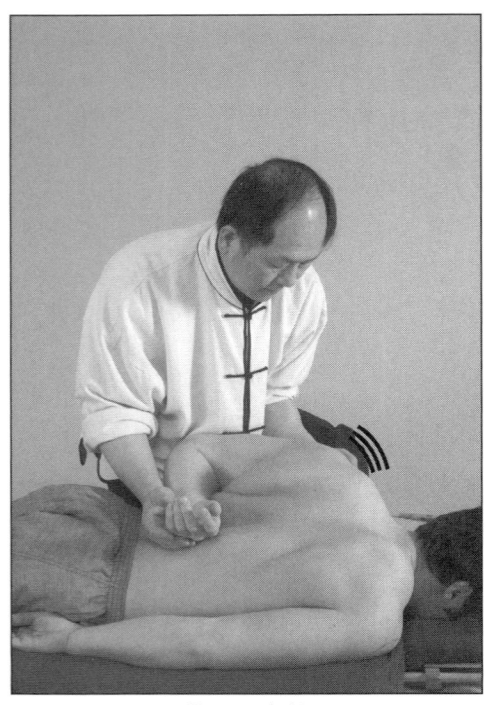

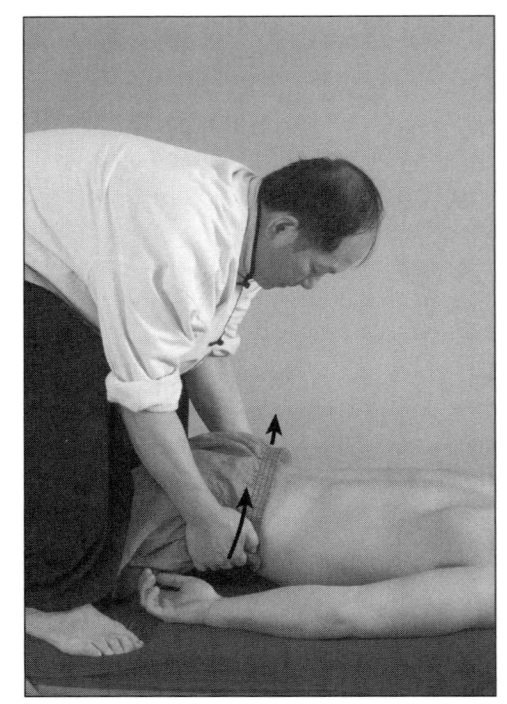

FIGURE 4-68

FIGURE 4-69

Holding is used to stabilize the body when you set or relocate bones. While holding part of the body, you may move it in certain ways to loosen it up. For example, in general massage you may lift the shoulder and move it to loosen up the shoulder blade and shoulder (Figure 4-68).

Raising or Lifting (Ti) (提). Raising or Lifting is moving part of the body upward. For example, when a patient is lying face downward, you may lift up and lower their waist area to loosen up the muscles there (Figure 4-69). You may also lift up a patient's head to loosen up the neck muscles and spine (Figure 4-70), or raise their arms or legs to loosen up the joints in general massage.

In Qi massage, a Qigong master will place his palms on a cavity and push down gently and firmly, and then, in coordination with his breathing, quickly lift up his palms (Figure 4-71). This sudden change on the surface of the skin will affect the Qi in the patient's body.

Pulling (La) (拉). Pulling is generally applied on the limbs. In general massage, the arms and legs are pulled to straighten out the muscles and tendons (Figure 4-72). In Tui Na massage, Pulling is generally used to set broken bones.

Kneading (Nie) (捏). Kneading is using the thumb and one or more fingers to grab a portion of the patient's body and then either squeeze or rub it. Kneading is different from Grabbing (Na, 拿), which is used for larger areas. Kneading is commonly used on the muscles in the back of the neck, the muscles between the neck and the shoulders,

Chapter 4: Massage Techniques

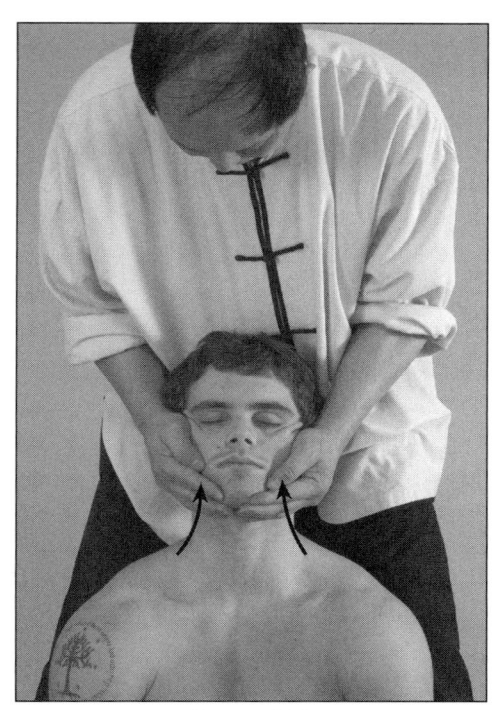

FIGURE 4-70

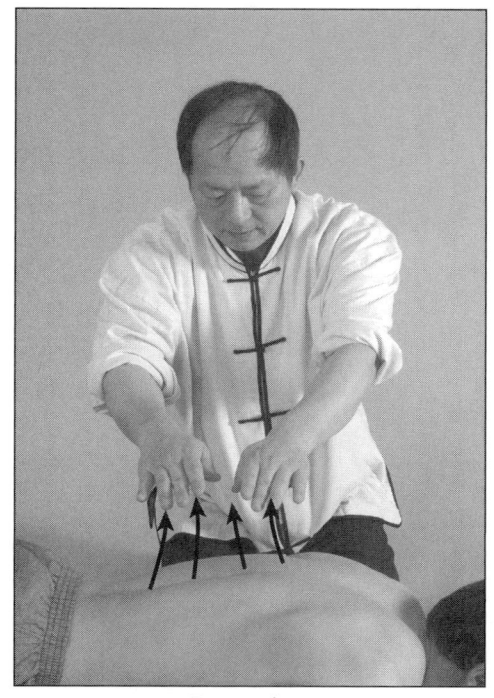

FIGURE 4-71

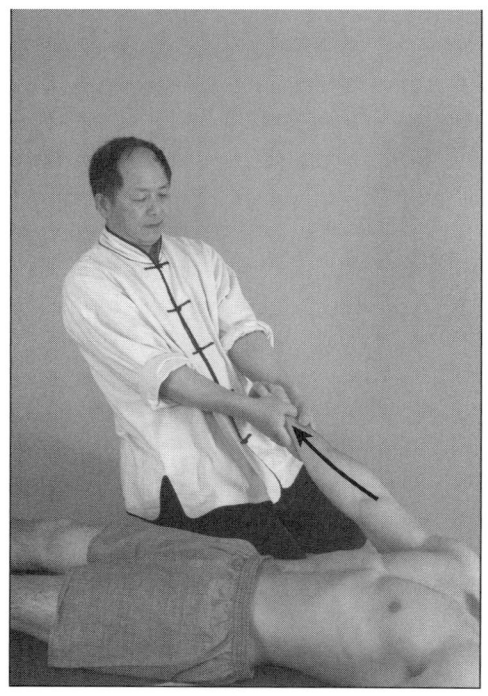

FIGURE 4-72

167

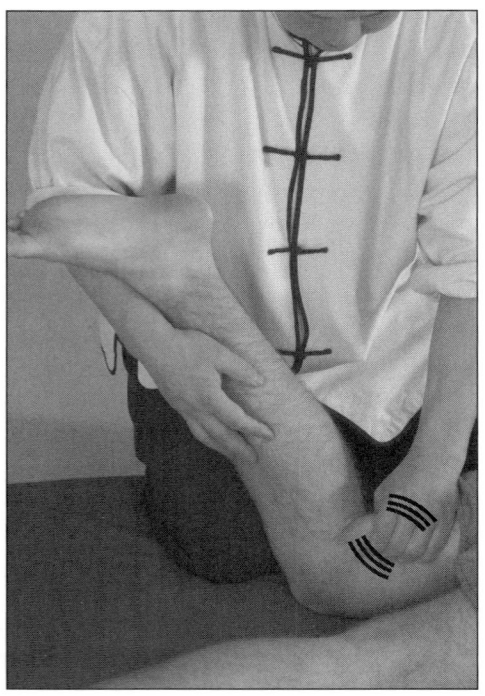

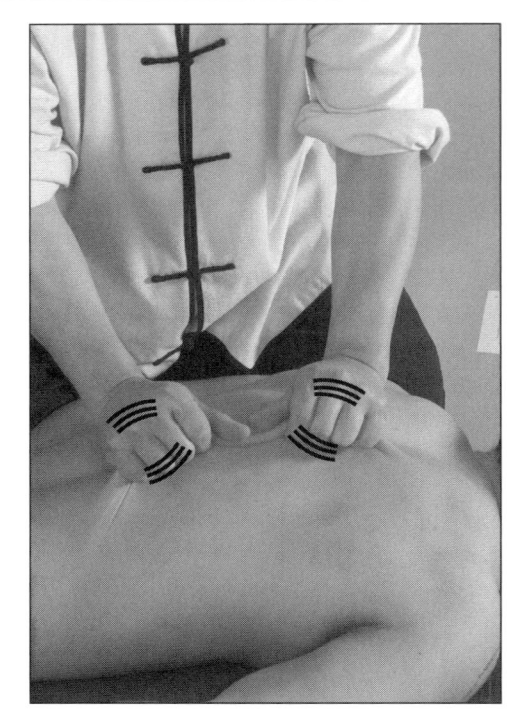

FIGURE 4-73

FIGURE 4-74

the muscles beside the armpit, and on the arms and legs. Very often tendons, such as the ones in the ankles or the back of the knees, are also kneaded in Tui Na massage (Figure 4-73), Sometimes the skin, especially on the back, is kneaded to stimulate the Qi there (Figure 4-74).

Supporting (Ding) (頂). Ding means to support, and it is different from Holding (Duan, 端) or Raising (Ti, 提). Supporting is using part of your body to support part of the patient's body so that you can massage it more easily. For example, you may place the patient's arm on your shoulder and massage the upper arm (Figure 4-75). You may also use your leg to support the patient's leg in order to loosen up the thigh muscles (Figure 4-76).

Shaking (Yao) (搖). Yao means to shake, but it is different from the Vibrating (Zhen Zhan, 震顫) discussed above. The motion of Vibrating is fast and the scale is much smaller, while Shaking is slower and the motion is larger. You may grab a muscle and shake it, such as the muscles between the neck and the shoulder (Figure 4-77), or the muscle on the back of the thigh (Figure 4-78), You may even simply use the

Chapter 4: Massage Techniques

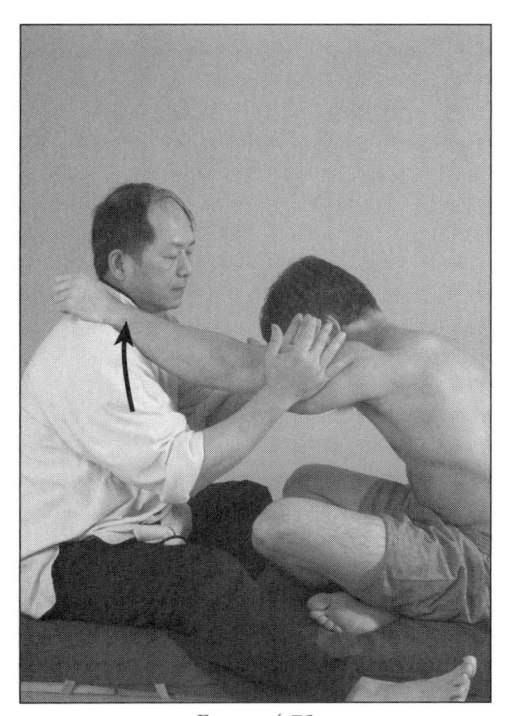

FIGURE 4-75

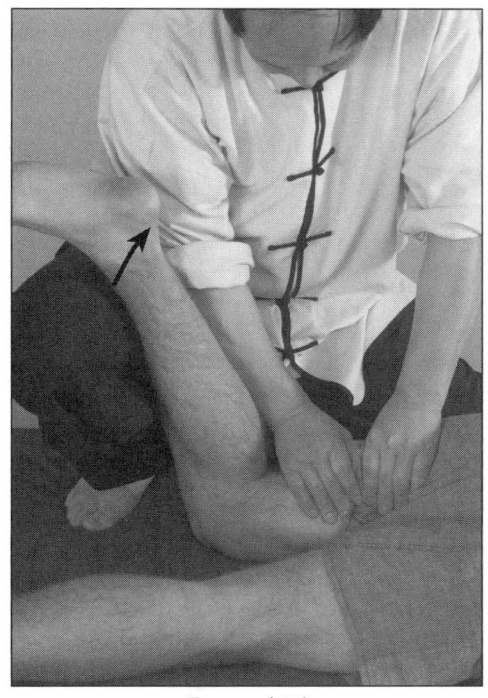

FIGURE 4-76

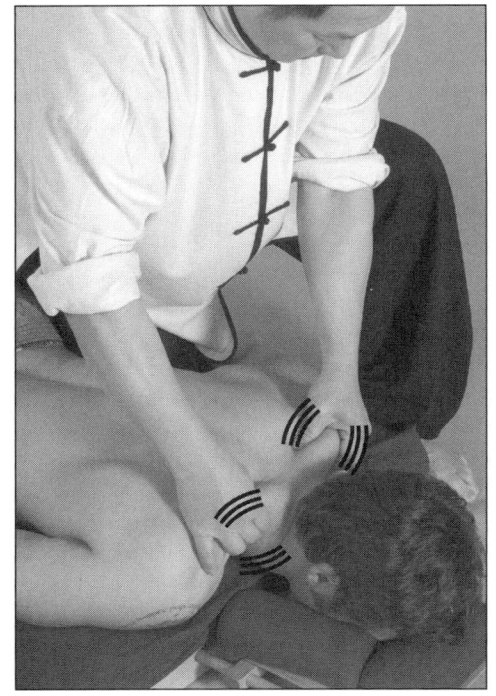

FIGURE 4-77

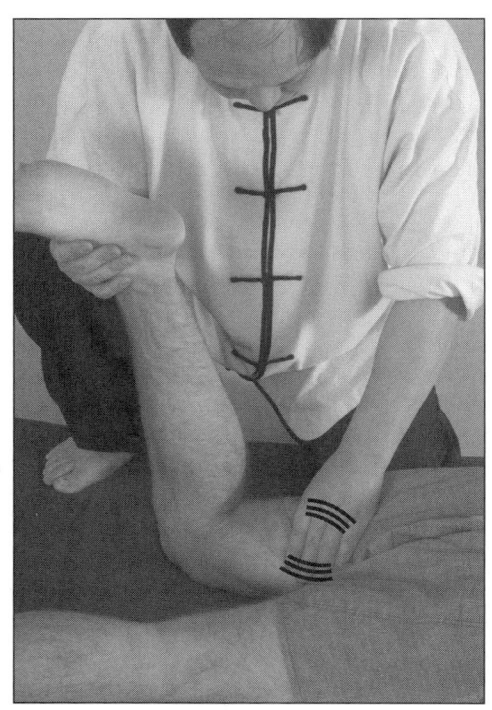

FIGURE 4-78

Qigong Massage

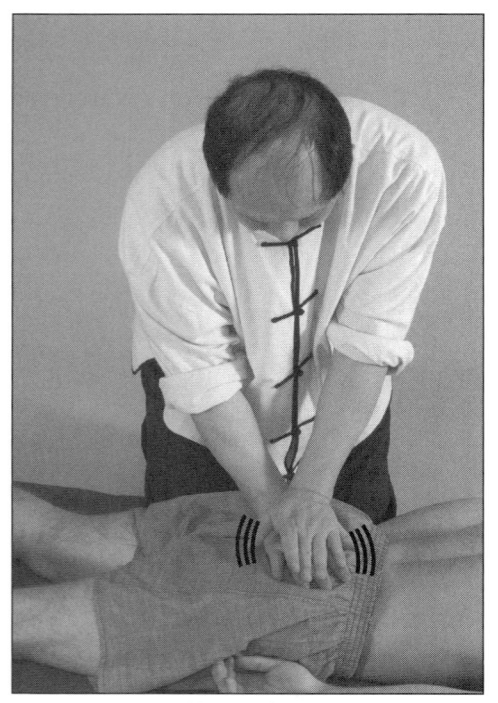

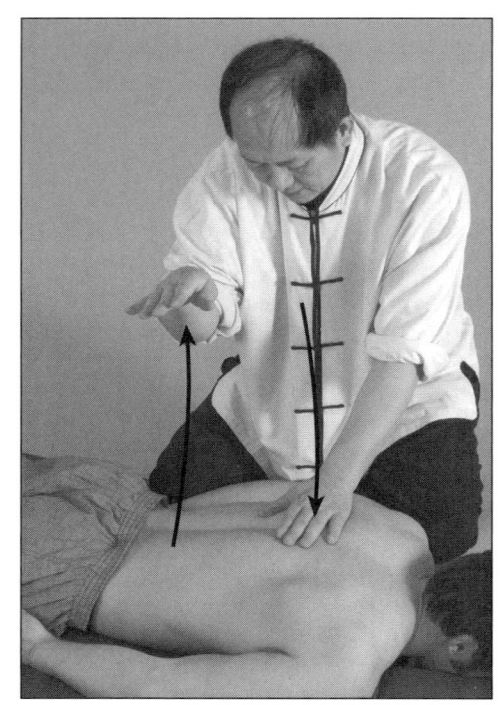

FIGURE 4-79

FIGURE 4-80

thumb or the base of the hand to press down and then shake a muscle to stimulate it (Figure 4-79).

Slapping (Pai) (拍). Slapping is done with either the front or the back of the fingers (Figure 4-80), After slapping to stimulate the Qi in the skin, you may use smooth, gentle pushes to push the stagnant Qi away.

Flicking (Tan) (彈). In Flicking, the thumb holds back the second or the middle finger and then releases it to snap against the skin (Figure 4-81). This stimulates the skin cells and improves Qi circulation in the skin.

Swinging (Shuai) (摔). Swinging is generally used for the limbs. For example, you may gently grab the shoulder or the upper arm and then swing the forearm and the wrist (Figure 4-82). You may also grab the calf and swing the ankle (Figure 4-83). Swinging loosens up a joint so that you can massage it more easily.

Filing (Cuo) (搓). Filing is rubbing the skin with the side of the palm or the forearm (Figure 4-84). Filing is different from Pushing (Tui, 推) in that you are rubbing the skin to stimulate it and generate heat. Filing opens the pores and releases the Qi accumulated under the skin.

Chapter 4: Massage Techniques

FIGURE 4-81

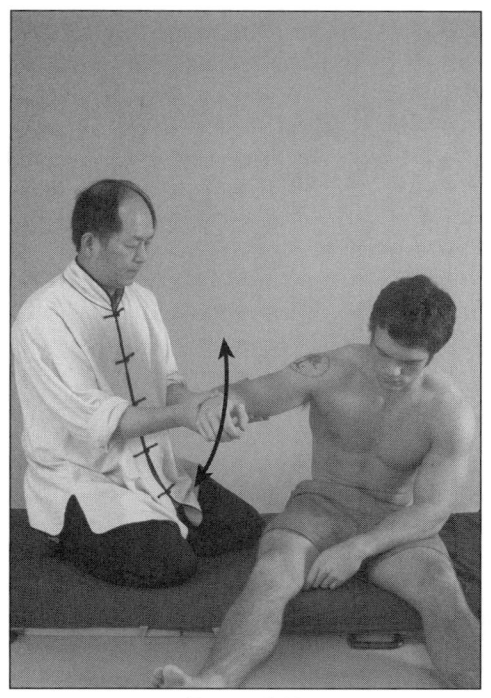

FIGURE 4-82

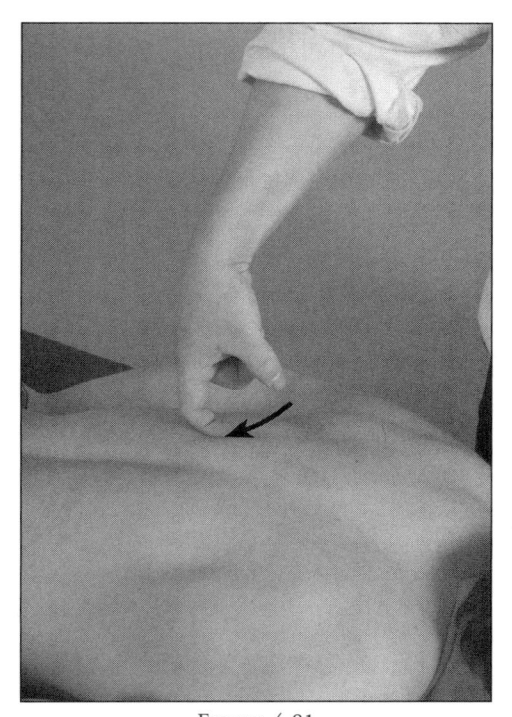

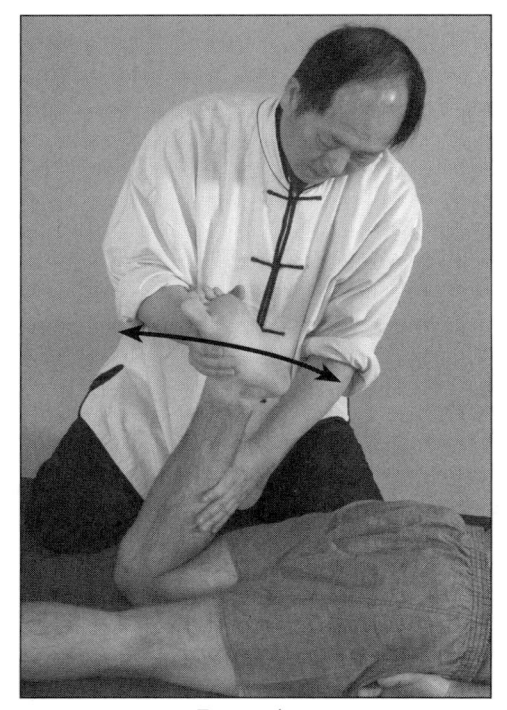

FIGURE 4-83

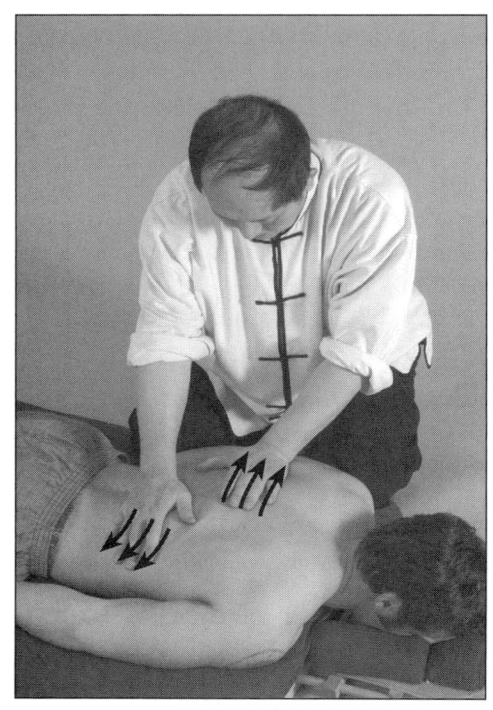

FIGURE 4-84

171

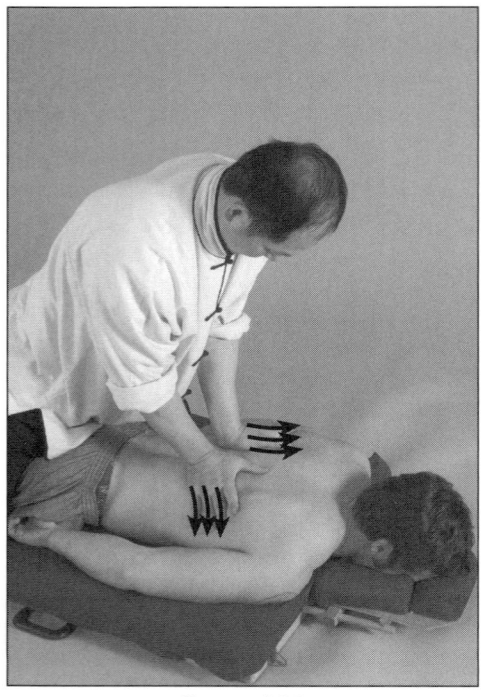

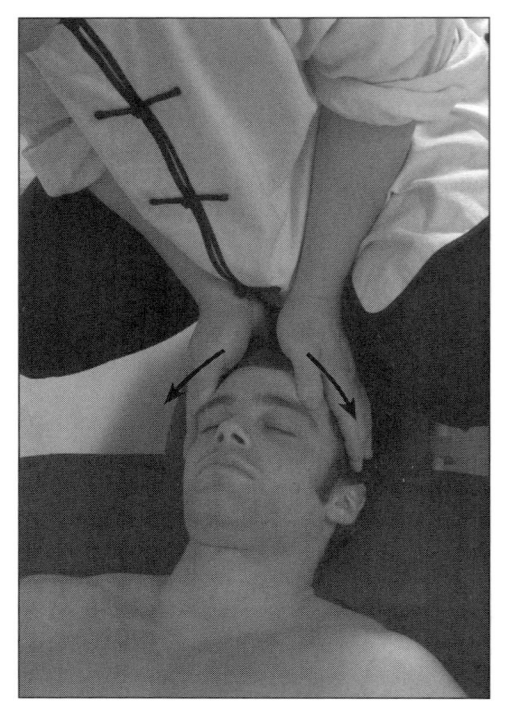

FIGURE 4-85

FIGURE 4-86

Dividing (Fen) (分). Dividing is using two forces in opposite directions on a part of the body. For example, you may place both palms on the patient's back and push away from the spine and then let up (Figure 4-85). This stretches the muscles, and when you let up the pressure, the muscles are stimulated. Another example is when you use both thumbs to push the accumulated Qi and blood to the sides of the forehead and spread them out (Figure 4-86).

Dividing can also be used to stretch the arms and legs. Stretching and then releasing the muscles will stimulate them and help to remove stagnant Qi and blood.

Combining (He) (合). Combining is using two forces to squeeze or bring together parts of the body. For example, you may use both hands to push the muscles or the skin on the sides of the back toward the center (Figure 4-87).

Folding (Die) (迭). Folding is generally used to loosen the joints of the spine or the chest. For example, you may use both hands to fold the entire body and then release it to loosen it up (Figure 4-88). You may also press both shoulders forward to fold in the chest area, and then release the pressure. This will loosen up the chest (Figure 4-89).

Rolling (Gun) (滚). Rolling is done with the back of the hand near the knuckles. Hold your hand slightly rounded, and keep it relaxed as you roll it back and forth on the area you are treating (Figure 4-90). If you need to apply more power, you may place

Chapter 4: Massage Techniques

FIGURE 4-87

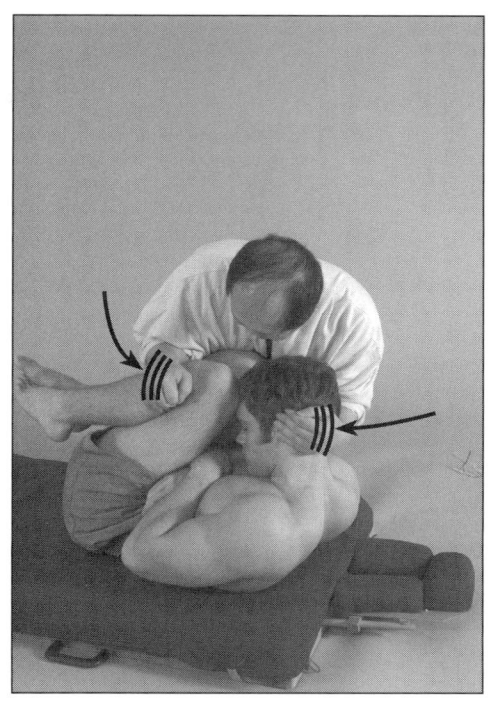

FIGURE 4-88

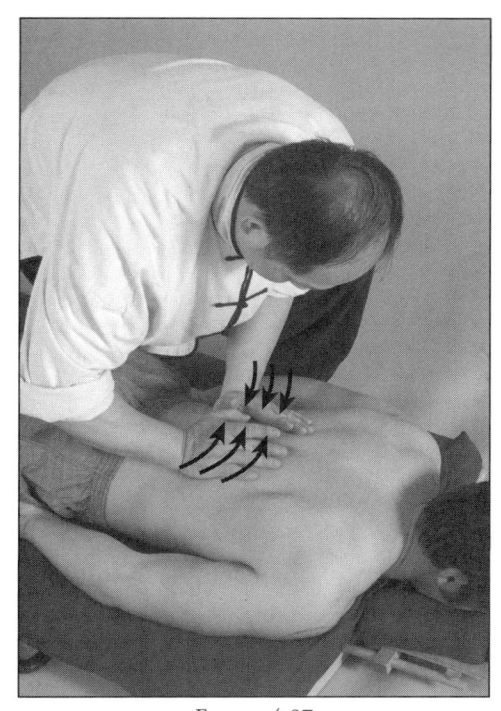

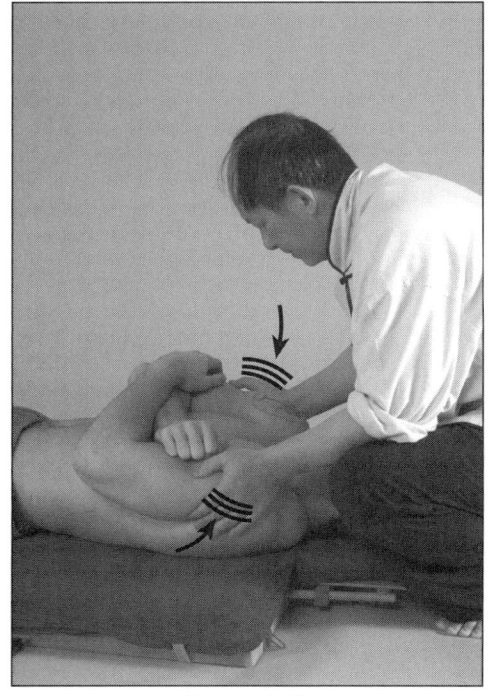

FIGURE 4-89

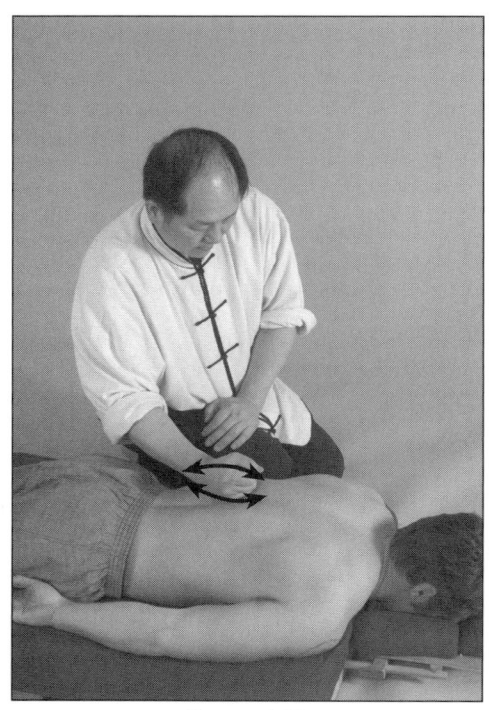

FIGURE 4-90

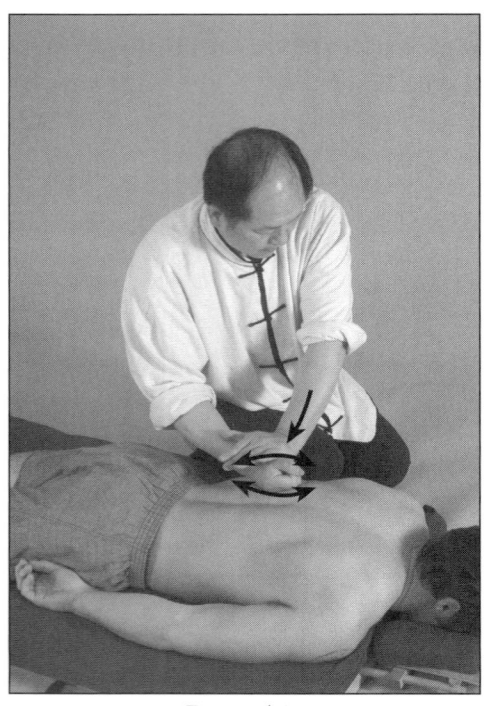

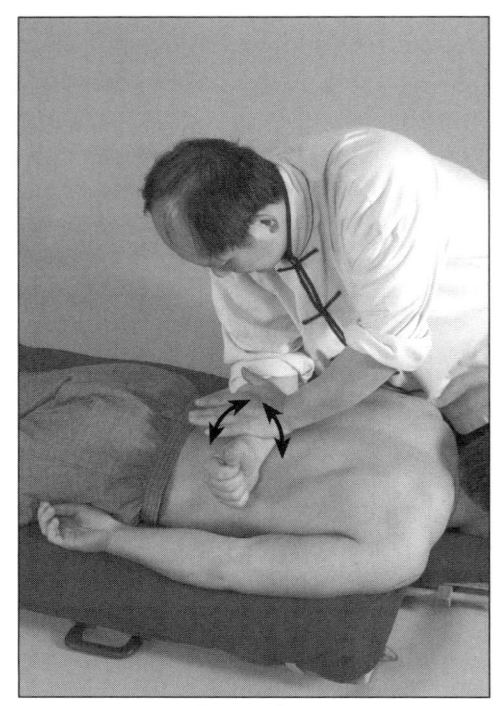

FIGURE 4-91

FIGURE 4-92

your other hand on the one you are rolling with and use the power of both arms (Figure 4-91). For rolling on larger areas, such as the back or the thigh, you may use a forearm (Figure 4-92). Rolling massage increases Qi and blood circulation, gets rid of the lactic acid which has accumulated in the muscles, and also restores feeling in numb areas.

Waving (Dou) (抖). Waving is different from Shaking (Yao, 搖) or Vibrating (Zhen Zhan, 震顫) in that it is a slower, larger motion. To do it, you simply grab one of the patient's limbs and shake it in a large, slow motion (Figure 4-93). Waving loosens the joints, stretches the muscles and tendons, and also increases the Qi and blood circulation.

Chopping (Pi) (劈). Chopping is a strike with the side of the palm (Figure 4-94). It is used when you need increased penetrating power to stimulate the deeper muscles. Chopping is commonly used on the back trunk muscles, the thigh muscles, or sometimes the calf muscles.

Carrying On the Back (Bei) (背). Carrying on the Back is a technique which is used for treating spine problems. As the name indicates, you carry the patient on your back facing either away from you (Figure 4-95) or toward you (Figure 4-96), and swing or shake them gently. This technique stretches the patient's spine and trunk muscles, and releases any tightness in the spine.

Chapter 4: Massage Techniques

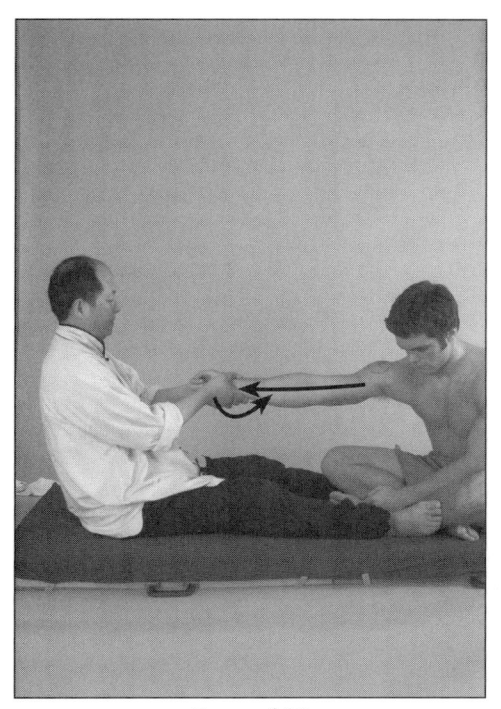

FIGURE 4-93

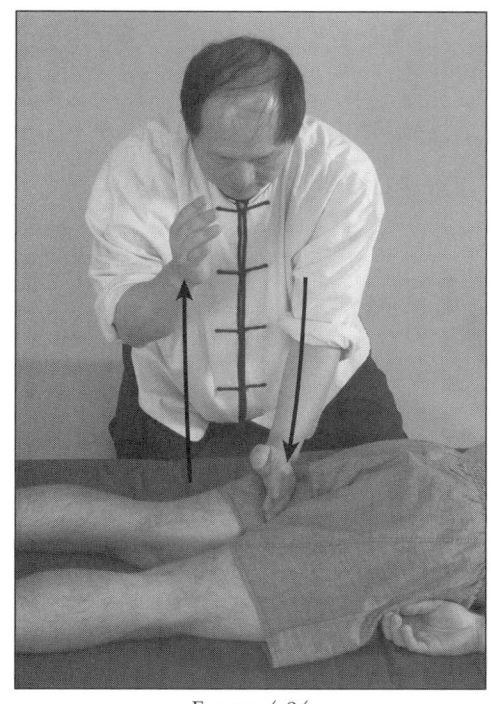

FIGURE 4-94

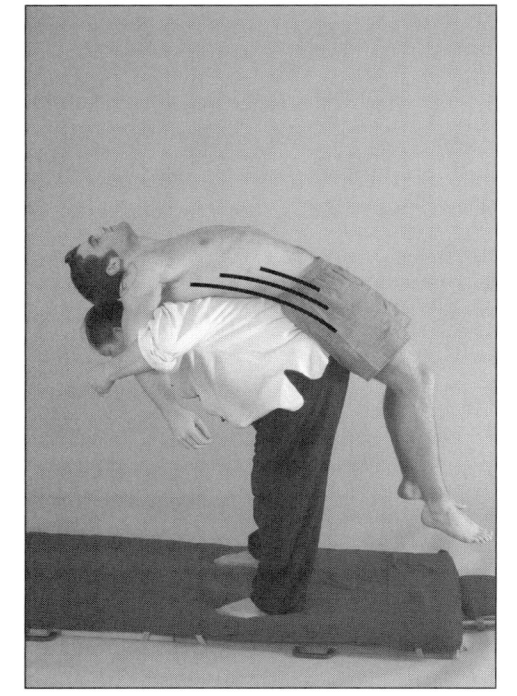

FIGURE 4-95

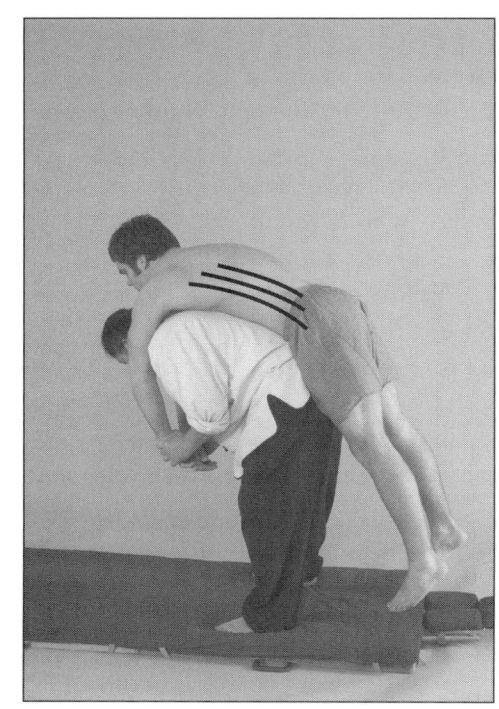

FIGURE 4-96

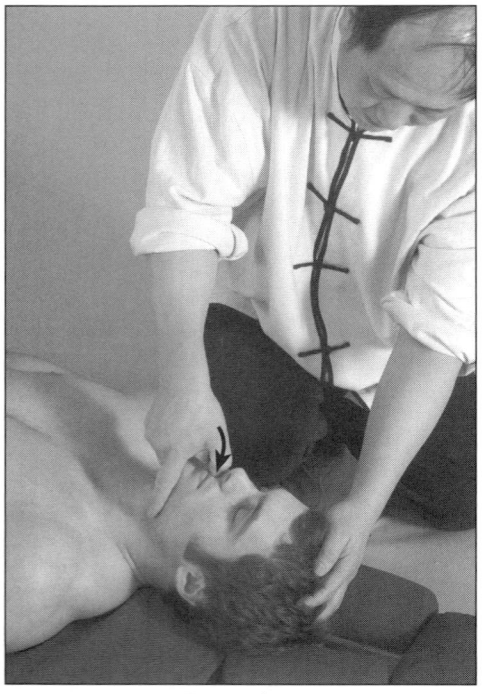

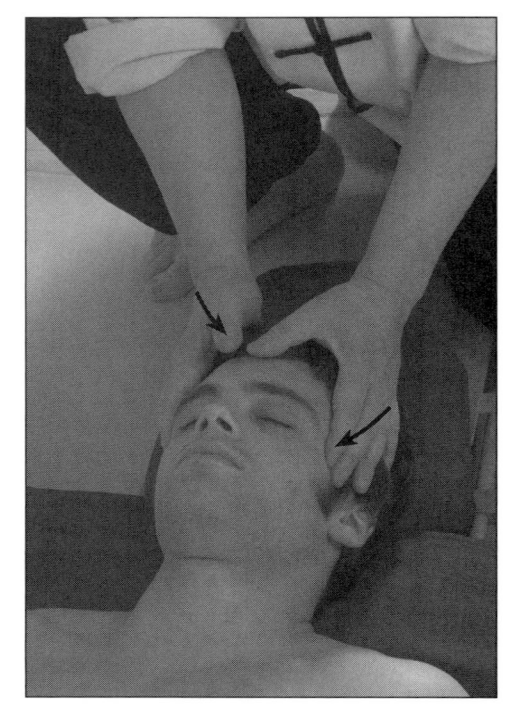

FIGURE 4-97   FIGURE 4-98

Piercing (Qia) (掐). Piercing uses a fingernail (often the thumbnail) to press cavities and stimulate the Qi circulation (Figure 4-97). Of course, the fingernail should not break the skin. Piercing is sometimes used by physicians who do not have acupuncture needles. Piercing is commonly used in both Tui Na and Dian Xue massage. Pressing in with a fingernail can quickly stimulate a cavity, so Piercing is commonly used to revive people who have fainted, or to quickly make the body more Yang, for example when a patient has a cold.

Pointing (Dian) (點). Pointing uses a finger (usually the thumb, or the index or middle finger or two fingers (usually the index and middle fingers) to press heavily on a cavity Figure 4-98). Pointing is different from Pressing (An, 按), which discussed previously. The area covered with Pressing can be large or small however, Pointing covers a much smaller area, and its power is more penetrating. Sometimes the elbow is used when you need more power to penetrate to a cavity which is covered by a thick layer of muscle, such as in the thigh (Figure 4-99). The Pointing technique is sometimes used when acupuncture needles are not available. Pointing is mainly used for Tui Na and Dian Xue massage.

Transporting (Yun) (運). Transporting uses the fingers to rub repeatedly in a straight line or circle until the skin is warm (Figure 4-100). This technique is usually applied on small children. However, it is sometimes used for adults in massaging the chest, abdomen, and face. When you are doing the Transporting technique, your fin-

Chapter 4: Massage Techniques

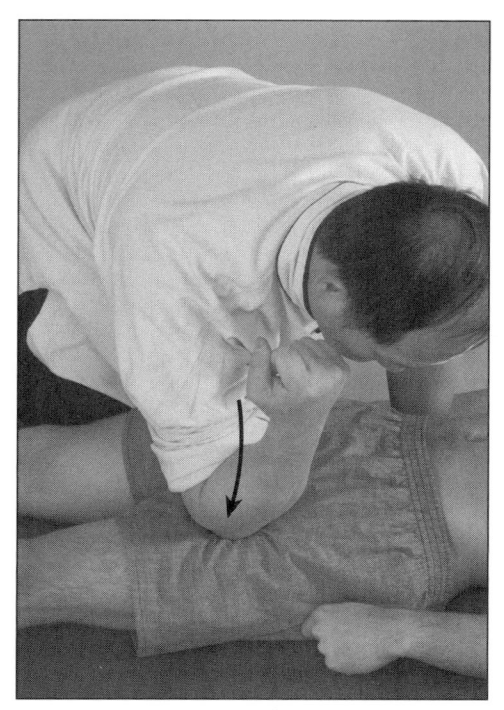

FIGURE 4-99

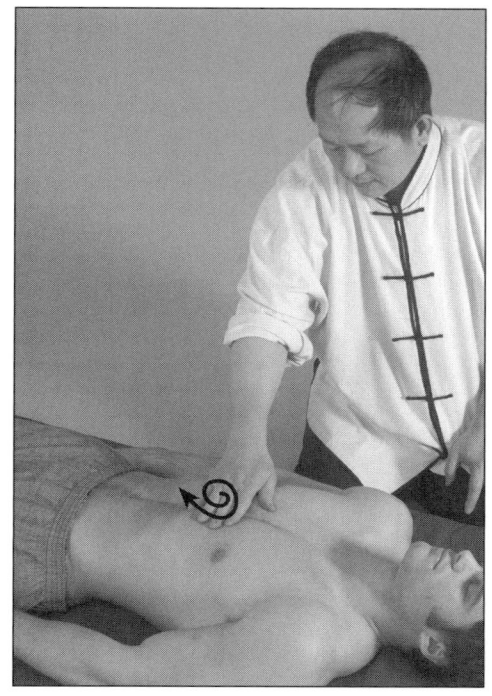

FIGURE 4-100

gers should lightly touch the skin as they rub with a fairly fast motion.

Quick Pull (Che) (扯). The Quick Pull technique is commonly used to loosen up joints in the arms and legs. To do this technique, hold a finger, a wrist, or ankle and move it around to loosen it up, and then give it a quick pull (Figure 4-101). This technique is different from the Pulling (La, 拉) technique described earlier. While Pulling uses a steady, firm power, Quick Pull uses a quick jerk. Quick Pull is commonly used on people who are strong but have very tense joints.

Extending (Shen) (伸). Extending is used to straighten a bent limb. Pain usually causes muscles and tendons to contract, which keeps the arm or leg in a bent position. Extending is needed to straighten the limb. To use Extending, hold the limb on

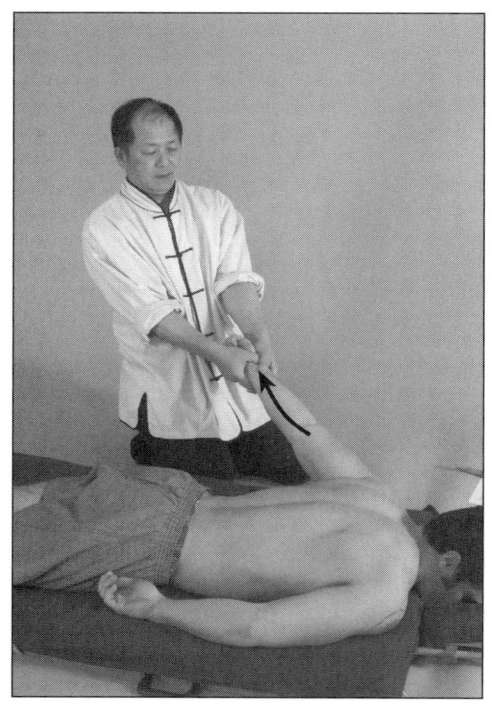

FIGURE 4-101

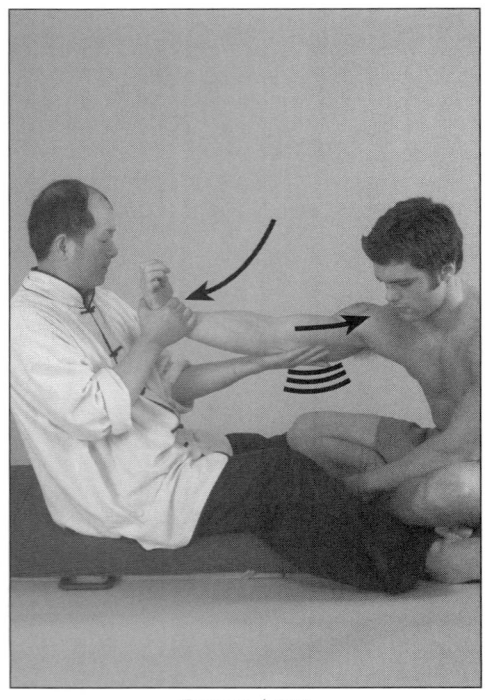

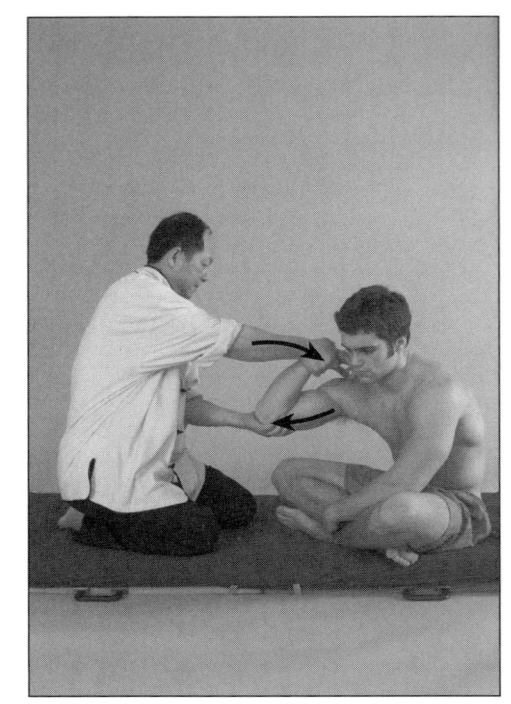

FIGURE 4-102

FIGURE 4-103

both sides of the constricted joint and pull in both directions with a firm and steady power (Figure 4-102). Do not use violent power, because that will only cause more tension.

Bending (Qu) (曲). Bending is the reverse of Extending (Shen, 伸). When a patient's arm or leg is straight and cannot be bent because of stiffness or numbness, you want to bend it to loosen up the joints. Hold the limb on both sides of the joint and bend it with steady, firm power (Figure 4-103). Normally, Bending and Extending are repeated until the joint is completely loose.

Striking (Da) (打). Striking uses the fists to strike an area (Figure 4-104). You need to carefully gauge the power, since too much force will cause bruises or other injuries, while too little force will not be effective. You want to stimulate the nervous system and Qi without causing any damage. Striking is used to quickly stimulate an area in the same way that, when your leg has fallen asleep, you punch it to restore feeling.

Shifting, Slipping (Nuo) (挪). To do Shifting, grab a piece of skin with one or both hands, and either shake it or let it slip out of your hand (Figure 4-105). Shifting is used to stimulate the skin, but be careful when you grab not to damage the skin. Shifting is commonly used on the back.

Chapter 4: Massage Techniques

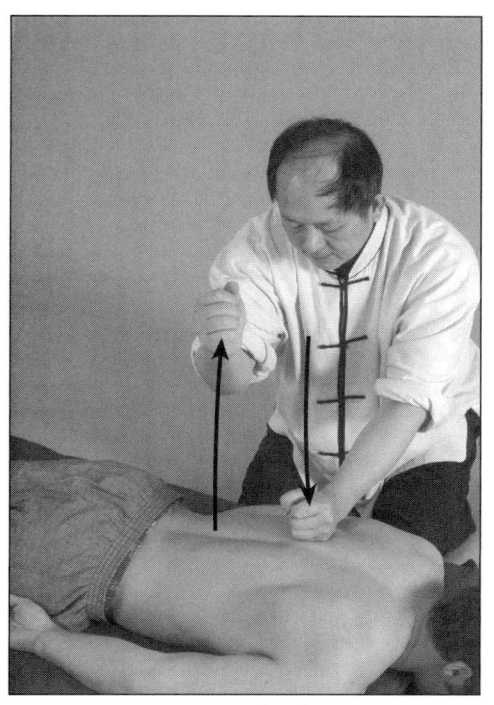

FIGURE 4-104

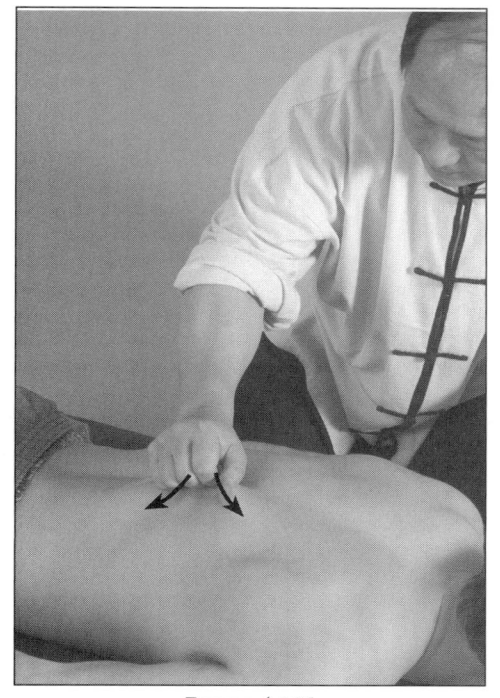

FIGURE 4-105

Reining (Le) (勒). Reining is commonly used to stretch the muscles or tendons on the joints of the fingers or toes. To do Reining, hold the patient's wrist or ankle with one hand, and hold the finger or toe you are treating with the thumb and index finger of your other hand. Pull the finger, and then let it quickly slip out of your grip (Figure 4-106). Reining is slightly different from Pulling (La, 拉), in which you hold the patient's limb steadily, without letting it slide out of your grip.

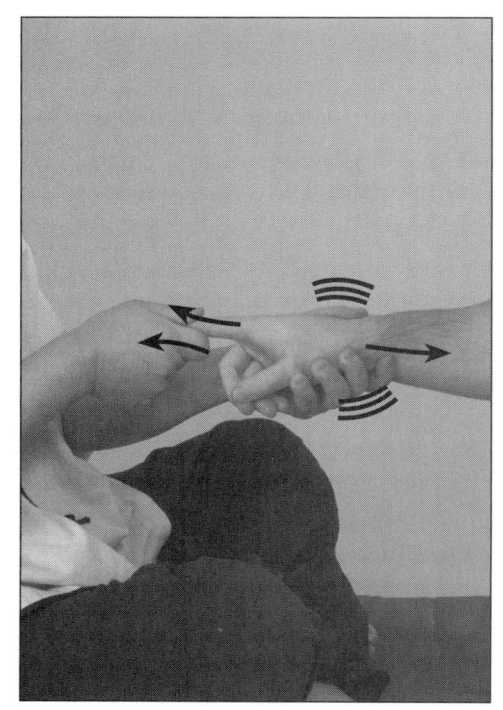

FIGURE 4-106

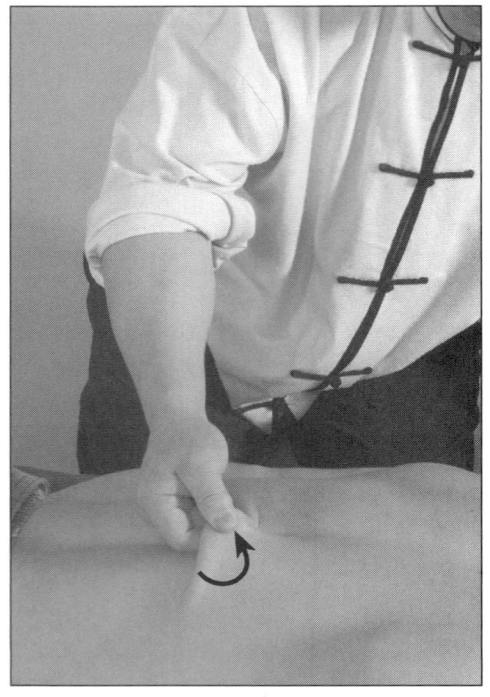

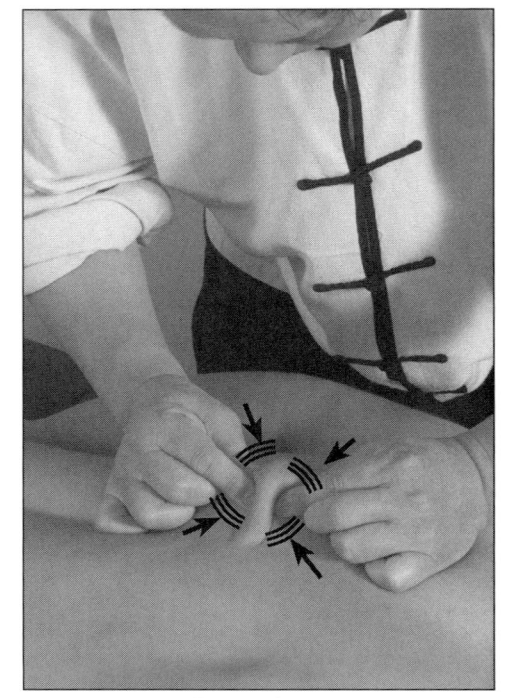

FIGURE 4-107

FIGURE 4-108

Uprooting (Ba) (拔). In Uprooting, you grab a piece of skin, muscle, or tendon and pull it away from the body (Figure 4-107). Uprooting is commonly used to stimulate the skin or the muscles located under the armpit, between the neck and the shoulder, elbows, or the hips.

Squeezing (Ji) (擠). Squeezing is commonly done with the fingers or palms. The fingers are used on smaller areas of skin, such as on the forehead or the smaller joints such as the spinal joints in the neck (Figure 4-108). The palms are used to squeeze the big muscles in the arms and legs (Figure 4-109).

Twisting (Ban) (板). Twisting is commonly used for the neck. Hold the back of the head and the chin, and give a quick twist to the side with both hands (Figure 4-110). Twisting is used to loosen the neck joints and also stretch the neck muscles and tendons.

Threshing (Dao) (搗). Threshing is commonly used to stimulate a cavity or a small, specific area with a continuous up and down or sideways movement. Threshing uses the index finger, supported by the thumb and middle finger (Figure 4-111), or a joint of the index finger (Figure 4-112). Press in on the cavity or area and move up and down or sideways with a steady speed until the area is sufficiently stimulated.

Chapter 4: Massage Techniques

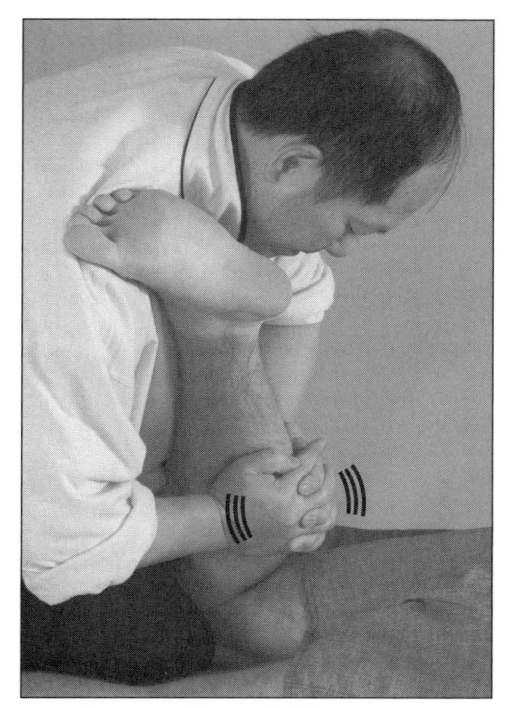

FIGURE 4-109

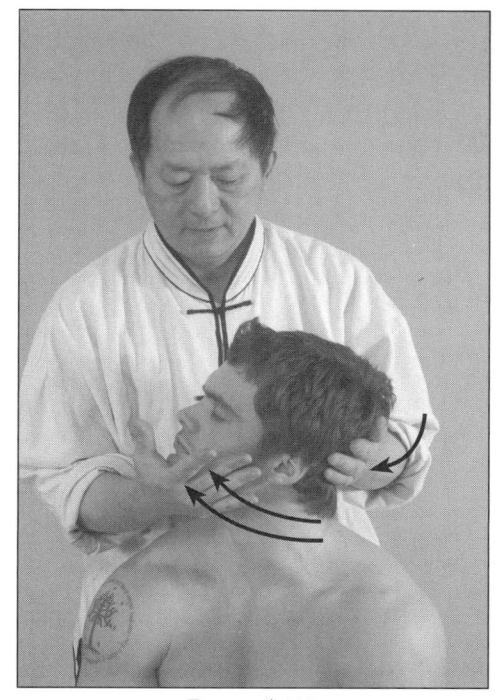

FIGURE 4-110

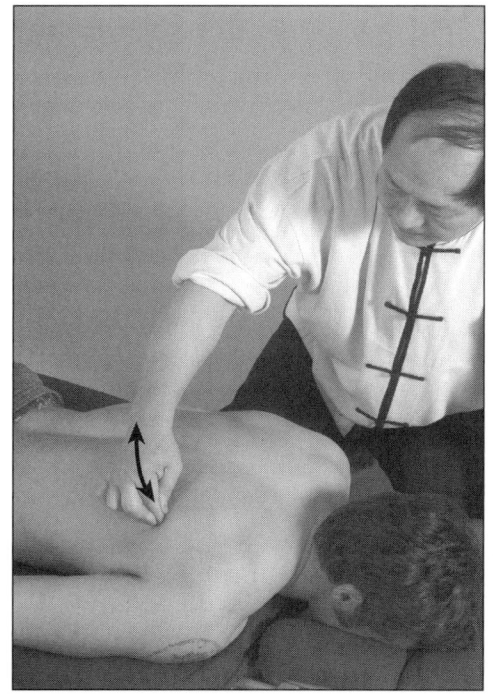

FIGURE 4-111

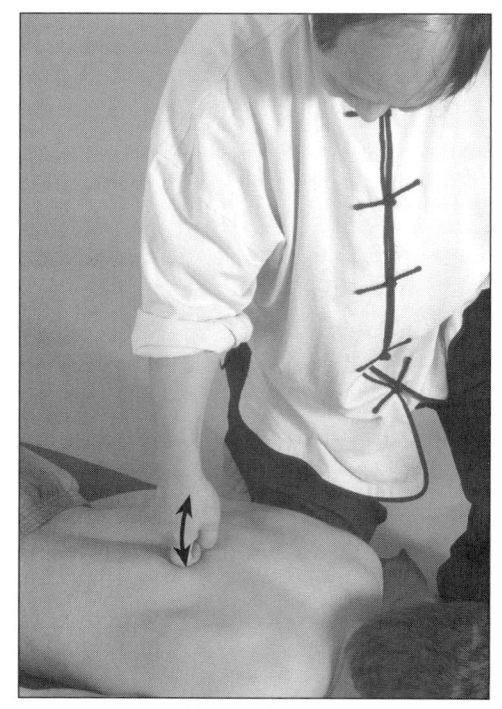

FIGURE 4-112

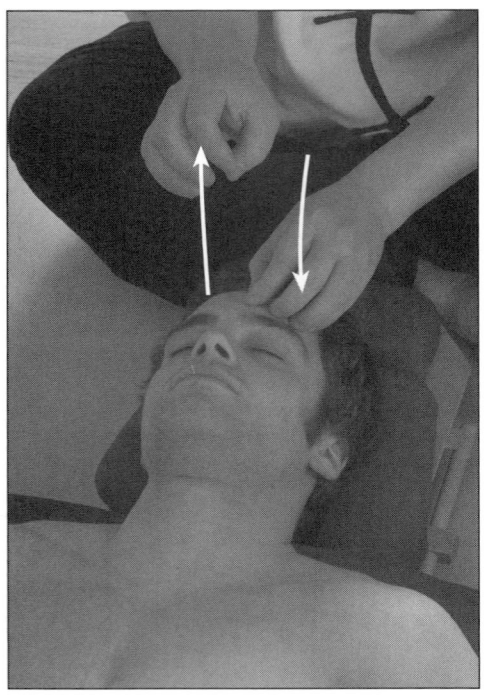

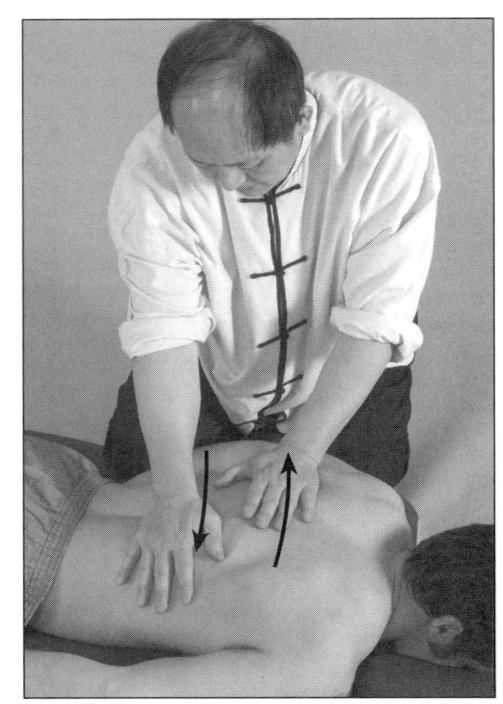

FIGURE 4-113

FIGURE 4-114

Pecking (Zhuo) (啄). Pecking uses the fingertips formed into a beak to stimulate the skin (Figure 4-113). Pecking is different from the Tapping (Dian Da, Qiao; 點打、敲) technique described earlier in that Pecking focuses on a smaller area, while Tapping covers a wider area.

Swaying (Huang) (晃). With the Swaying technique you place both hands on the patient's body and move the skin to and fro with a very slow motion (Figure 4-114). Swaying is used to relax the patient physically and mentally. Be sure not to rub the skin, just move it back and forth.

Rotating (Xuan) (旋). Rotating is commonly used for joints in the limbs. Hold the limb on both sides of the joint and twist (Figure 4-115) or rotate the joint (Figure 4-116). Twisting the limb will stretch the muscles, while rotating the joint will loosen the joint.

Combing (Shu) (梳). This technique uses the fingers or fingertips to comb along the ribs from the center of the body to the sides (Figure 4-117). Combing is one of the main techniques for leading Qi from the center of the body to the sides.

Scratching (Sao) (搔). Scratching, which is done just as the name indicates, is used on specific areas such as the head (Figure 4-118). This technique is used to stimulate an area, or to bring Qi to it. A light scratch will soothe, while a heavier scratch will stimulate.

Chapter 4: Massage Techniques

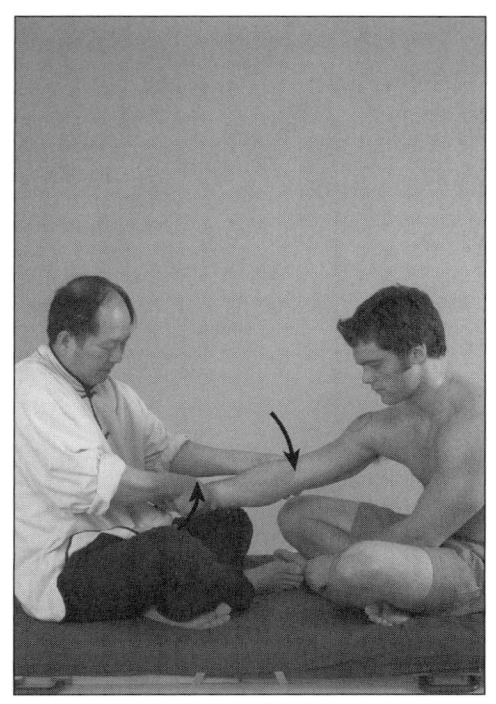

FIGURE 4-115

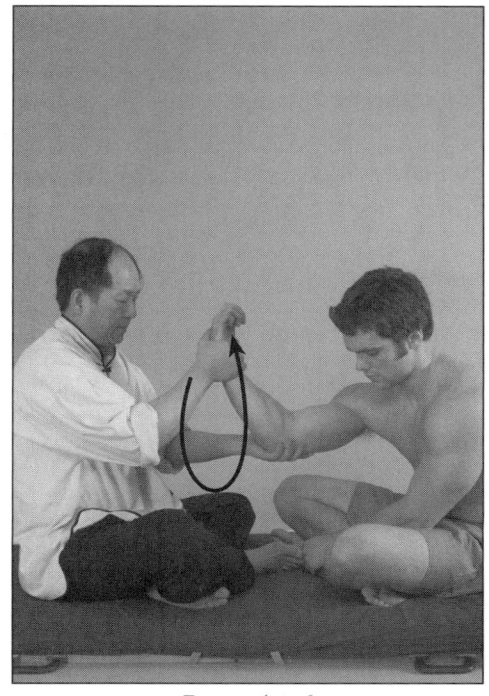

FIGURE 4-116

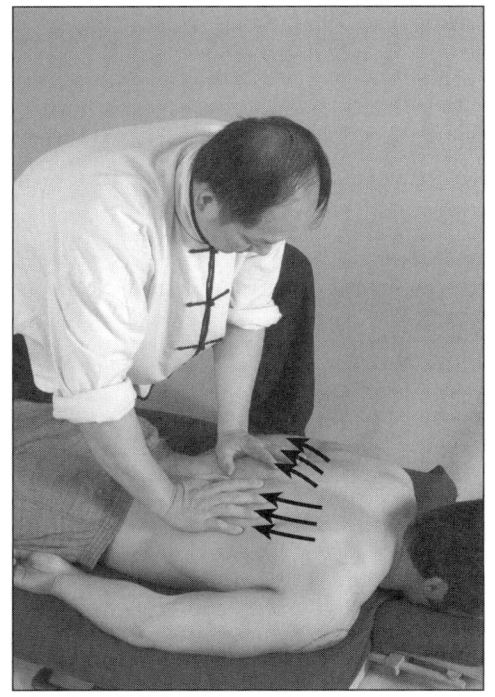

FIGURE 4-117

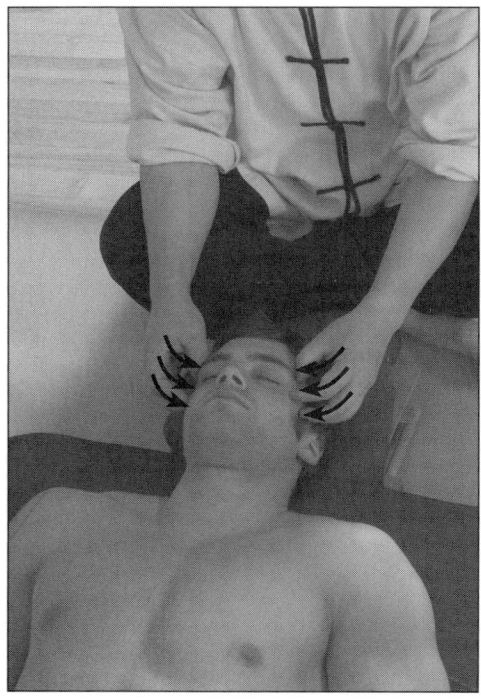

FIGURE 4-118

183

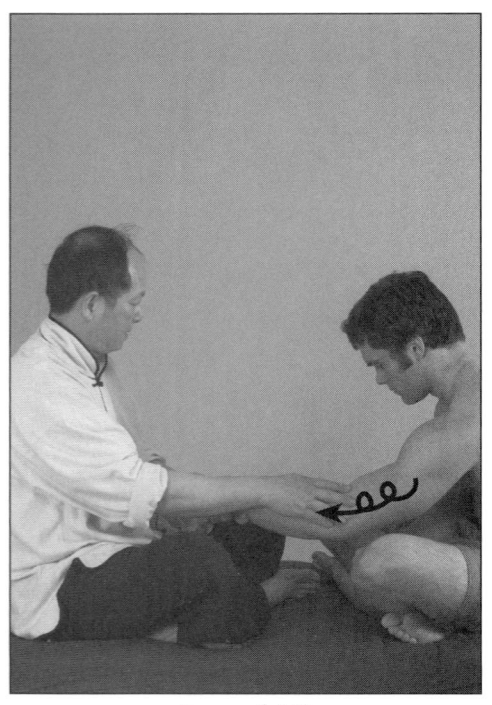

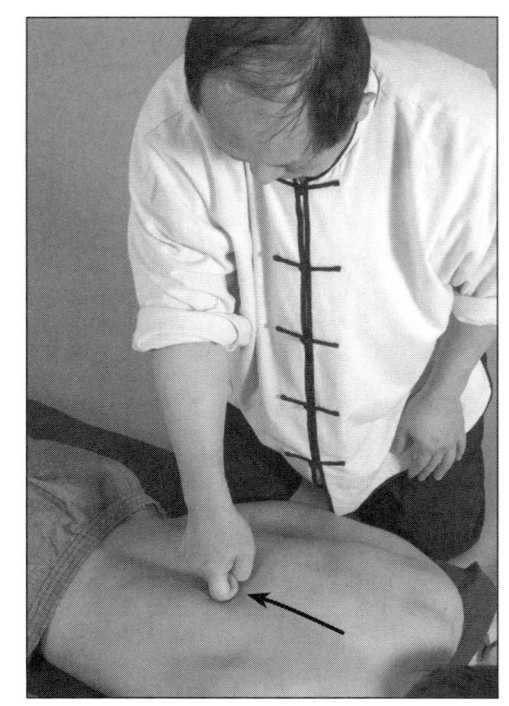

FIGURE 4-119

FIGURE 4-120

Reeling (Chan) (纏). Reeling uses the middle section of the fingers and palms to rub in a circular motion along a straight line (Figure 4-119). Reeling can be used on most of the body, such as the back, the chest, or the limbs.

Scraping (Gua) (刮). Scraping uses the fingernails or the knuckles to scrape the skin (Figure 4-120). This technique is commonly used in Tui Na along the Qi channels or on areas corresponding to specific internal organs to regulate the Qi there.

Jabbing (Lu) (戮). Jabbing uses a fingertip to press straight downward on a cavity to stimulate it (Figure 4-121). Usually the tip of the index or middle finger is used. Jabbing is a common technique in Dian Xue Massage. Jabbing is sometimes considered to be part of the Pointing (Dian, 點) technique; the main difference is that Jabbing is always used straight downward.

Pounding (Guan) (貫). Pounding is a technique for indirectly applying the force of a fist strike. Usually, one hand is placed on the area being treated, and it is struck with the other fist. This technique is usually used on the top of the head (Figure 4-122) or the bottom of the feet (Figure 4-123), and with only mild power.

Chapter 4: Massage Techniques

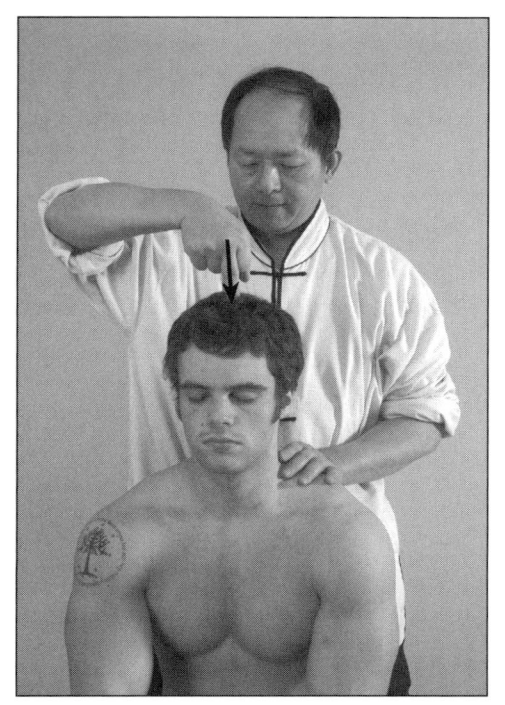

FIGURE 4-121

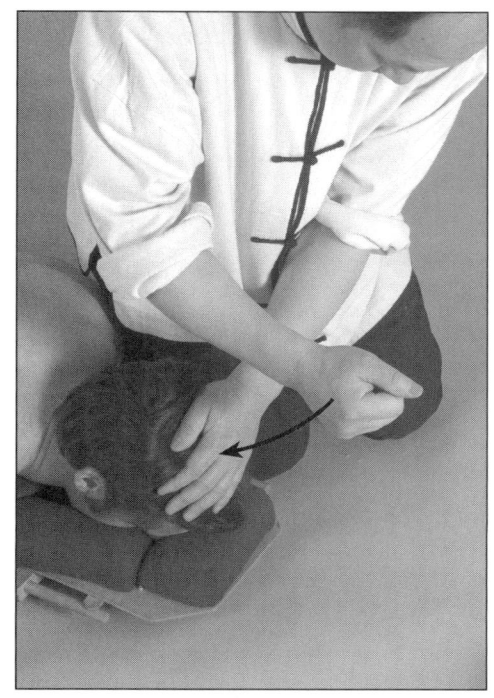

FIGURE 4-122

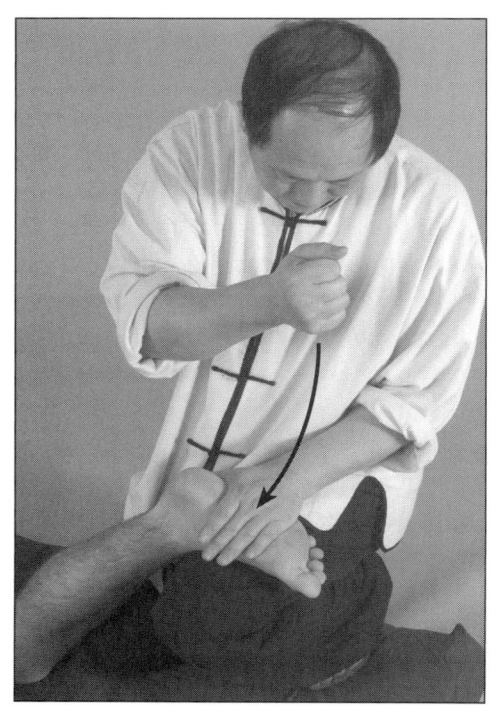

FIGURE 4-123

185

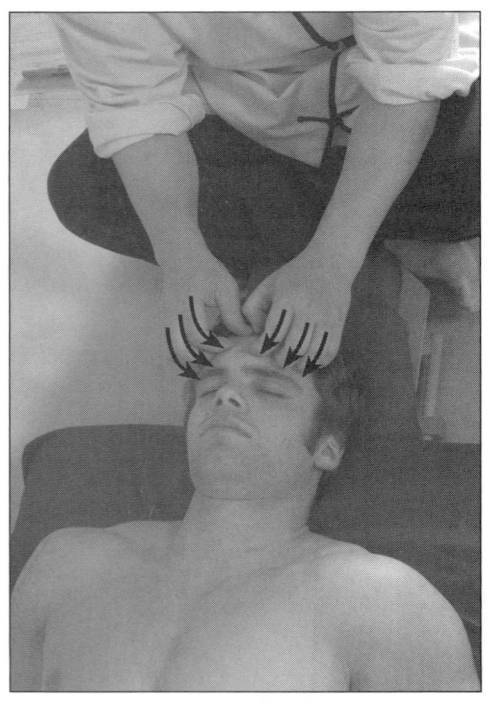

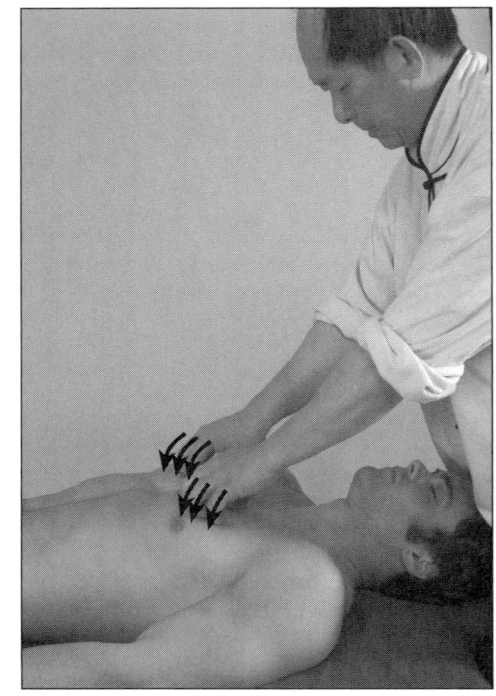

FIGURE 4-124

FIGURE 4-125

Cascading (Qie) (切). Cascading uses the fingernails to slowly stimulate many spots on an area of the body in a special order (Figures 4-124 and 4-125). Each finger stimulates a point in immediate succession, like a waterfall flowing through rocks. This strongly stimulates the skin, and leads Qi from under the skin to the surface.

Wiping (Ca) (擦). Wiping uses the fingers or palm to gently wipe or brush to and fro on the area being massaged (Figure 4-126). Wiping is an easy way to stimulate the skin cells. It is commonly used to strengthen deficient Guardian Qi (Wei Qi, 衛氣).

Dredging (Tao) (掏). Dredging uses the thumb or the last section of one or more fingers to press on a cavity and then drag outward (Figure 4-127). Dredging is commonly used in Tui Na and Dian Xue massage. When using Dredging, be careful not to break the skin.

Cupping (Kou) (叩). To use Cupping, cup your hand with all the fingers touching, and hit the area you are treating (Figure 4-128). Cupping can stimulate the skin efficiently without injuring it.

These are only some of the many techniques which have been used by masseurs around the world. This section is meant only to offer a guideline and some examples to help you understand the massage techniques. As long as you remember the purpose of massage and the theory behind it, you should be able to apply the different techniques skillfully.

Chapter 4: Massage Techniques

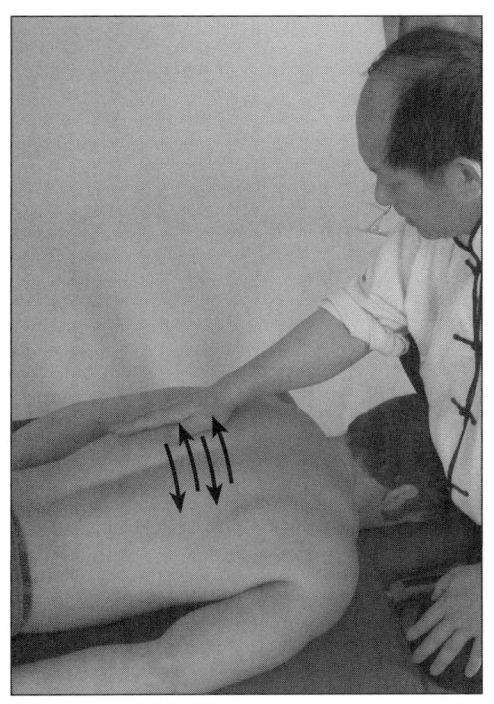

FIGURE 4-126

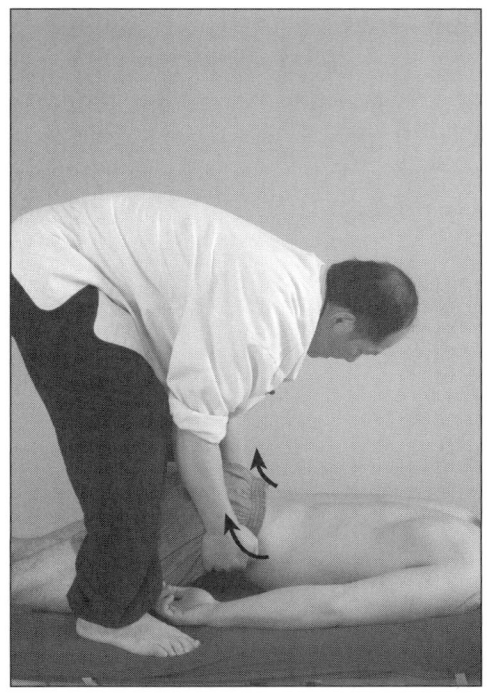

FIGURE 4-127

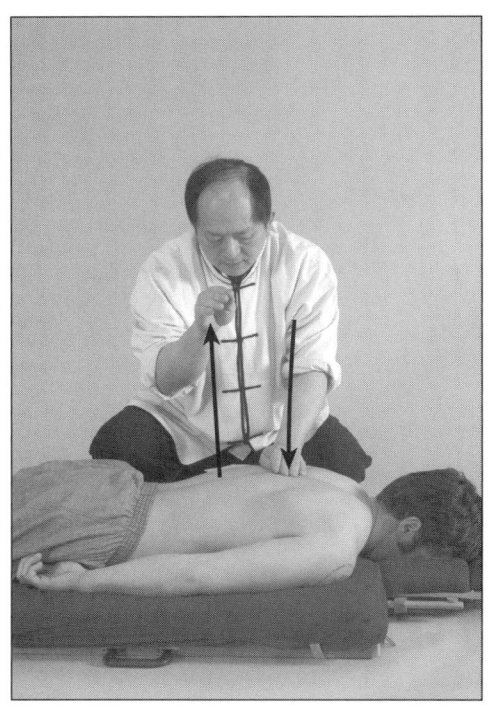

FIGURE 4-128

187

Reference

1. *The Body Electric* by Robert O. Becker, M.D. and Gary Selden, Quill, William Morrow, New York, 1985.

PART TWO
General Massage 普通按摩

CHAPTER 5

General Concepts 一般概念

5-1. Introduction 介紹

One of the more enjoyable experiences in life is to get a general massage to help you relax and recover from fatigue. Unlike Tui Na or Dian Xue massage, which are designed to heal, general massage can help you to relax mentally and spiritually, while physically it can help to disperse stagnant Qi and blood, speeding recovery from fatigue. This kind of massage is especially beneficial for older people, because it helps maintain the smooth circulation of Qi and blood consequently slowing down the aging process. Normally, the blood and Qi circulation gradually become sluggish as we get older.

The luxury of general massage is known in almost every culture, so there are many variations in theory and techniques. Even in China there are countless styles of general massage for relaxation. However, they all share the same basic theory. I believe that as long as you have mastered the theory and the techniques of one style, it will be easy for you to grasp the key to any other style. Remember, when you learn something. *Don't learn many things superficially. Instead, learn a few things deeply.* When you learn deeply, you will grasp the theory, which is the root. If your knowledge is wide and shallow, you have only learned about the branches.

In order to master general massage, you must learn and ponder the theory, study the techniques, and gain a lot of experience. The more you think and ponder, the more deeply you will understand. The more you practice, the greater your skill will be. The more experience you accumulate, the wider your knowledge will be. These three things are the keys to success. Keep on the path, and be humble, persevering, and patient. One day you will discover that the fruits of the seed you have planted are bigger and sweeter than any one else's.

Most people who learn massage start with general massage, because you do not need a deep understanding of the Qi circulation system or a high degree of skill. General massage teaches you the structure of the body and lets you feel the pattern of the Qi flow in the energy body. These understandings are crucial if you wish to learn Tui Na and Dian Xue massage.

General massage includes self-massage and massage with a partner. From the point of view of training, self-massage starts you on the path to mastering the skills of massage and building up a store of experience. It is therefore desirable to start with self-massage.

In our discussion, however, we will start with massage with a partner. It is important for the beginner to have a good understanding of the structure of the body as well as an overview of the complete massage procedure. However, this is difficult to learn in self-massage, since it is difficult to reach many parts of your own body, such as your back and hips.

In this chapter we will first review the purposes of general massage, then its theory, and finally its procedures and rules. In Chapter 6 we will discuss the techniques used in massaging the various parts of your partner's body. Before we introduce the techniques for each part of the body, we will review the structure of our physical and Qi bodies. We will focus especially on the networks of the nervous system and the Qi, blood, and lymph circulatory systems, as well as the gates or junctions. Finally, in Chapter 7 we will discuss self-massage. Since we have already discussed the basic theory and rules, we will not repeat them there. Self-massage will be divided into three sections: external self-massage, internal organ self-massage by hand, and finally, internal organ self-massage through movement.

5-2. Purposes of General Massage 普通按摩之目的

Before you practice general massage, you should first ponder several questions: 1. Why do you want to practice general massage, and what are your goals? 2. How do you intend to reach these goals? 3. What are the theories behind general massage? The first question shows you your motivation and also your target. Without knowing the answer to this question, your mind will be uncertain and confused. The second and third questions actually cannot be separated. Theory is the Yin side of practice, and it gives you the structured knowledge that lies behind the techniques. You need to have a profound understanding of the theory before you can choose the appropriate methods and techniques to reach your goals. These methods and techniques are the "how, which is the Yang (陽), the manifestation of Yin (陰).

In this and the following sections we will discuss the "why" and "what" of general massage. After explaining the theory, we will list a few general rules drawn from the theoretical analysis. After we have built this theoretical foundation, we will discuss the "how" in the following chapters.

Although we have already discussed the purposes of general massage in an earlier section, we would like to summarize them again here to develop the connection with the subjects that follow.

Releasing Mental Tension. Mental tension comes from thinking (i.e. from your mind). According to Chinese Qigong, the mind is the 'general' of your Qigong training, since it controls your entire being including both your Qi and physical bodies. Whenever your peace of mind is disturbed, the Qi circulation in your body will be immediately affected. For example, if your mind is disturbed by sadness, your Qi will be led inward to be stored in your bone marrow. When this happens you will feel cold, because the Qi in the muscles and skin is deficient (i.e. the Guardian Qi is condensed and weak). Conversely, if your mind is excited from happiness, there will be an excess of Qi in the muscles and skin, and you will feel hot (i.e. the Guardian Qi is expanding and strong). Whenever there is a deficiency of Qi (Yin) or an excess (Yang), the physical body will react accordingly, since its condition is decided by the Qi. Whenever the Qi supply to the physical body is abnormal (either Yin or Yang), the physical body will be tense, and this tension will cause the circulation of the Qi and blood to be sluggish.

Therefore, the first goal of general massage is to relieve mental tension. This restores normal Qi circulation, and insures that the cells of the physical body receive the proper amount of Qi nourishment. The greatest benefit of releasing mental tension is the relief from stress and depression, which brings the happiness back into your life.

Removing Stagnant Qi and Blood. Stagnant Qi and blood can have many causes such as mental stress and tension, improper life-style, fatigue, aging, and sickness.

Improper life-style includes the food you eat, the air you breathe, the time you get up and how long you sleep. In Chinese Qigong, food and air are the post-birth essences which can be converted into Qi. If you eat improper food and breathe unclean air, our body will produce poor quality Qi. Furthermore, some of the undesirable materials can remain in your body. For example, undigested fat can be stored in the body. We know that fat can cause sluggish circulation of Qi and blood. Our Qi circulation can also be affected by the time of day (i.e. by the sun's Qi). Therefore, working the night shift may disturb your Qi. Another example is that you usually need at least seven to eight hours of sleep to replenish the energy of our brain and body. If you do not get enough sleep, your Qi circulation can be affected and also the quality of your blood cells may be poor.

Another common cause of sluggish Qi and blood circulation is overwork and fatigue. Overwork causes your body to generate more waste (such as lactic acid) than the blood can remove. When the acid accumulates in the muscles, you feel tired, and your body becomes even more tense, which further affects the Qi circulation. One of the most effective methods of recovering from fatigue, other than rest, is general massage.

Aging is the next cause of stagnant Qi and blood circulation. As you get older, especially after thirty when the body stops producing growth hormones, your blood and muscle cells start to age. The blood cells are not as fresh and the Qi is not as abundant as when you were young. When this happens, the circulation of Qi and blood becomes sluggish. General massage will maintain and improve the circulation.

Finally, Qi and blood circulation can also be affected by illness. We will discuss this further in the sections on Tui Na and Dian Xue massage.

Maintaining a Healthy Nervous System. When the circulation of Qi and blood is smooth and healthy, it will provide proper nourishment to the entire body including the nervous system. Nerves connect the brain to the entire body, and enable the brain to govern it, and they also enable the body to respond to the brain. Without a good communication system, you will lose the war against sickness and aging. General massage helps the nervous system to function properly by insuring that it receives the proper amount of Qi nourishment.

Increasing Hormone Production and Strengthening the Immune System. The production of hormones and the condition of the lymphatic system are closely related to the immune system. Although we still do not understand exactly how the hormones work, we do know that they provide significant benefits. Only recently it was reported that the growth hormone can significantly extend the life span.

The endocrine and lymphatics systems are like factories. If we want to maintain or even increase production, we have to consider how to increase the energy supply to them. The lymphatic system is an important part of our body's defense against bacteria. I would like to point out again that the Qi circulatory system (the Yin system) is the root of all other circulatory systems.

For Enjoyment. The fact that it is so enjoyable is probably the main reason that most people are drawn to general massage. Not only does it help you to calm your mind and find peace, it can also bring you to a stage of deep relaxation and a feeling of complete comfort. In the beginning, it is difficult to bring your partner to this state. However, as your understanding of Qigong deepens, and as you gain experience, you will find that it happens more and more easily.

In conclusion, general massage has three areas of benefit: mental, Qi, and physical. The mental area is related to the mind, the Qi area to the inner energy which is the root of life, and the physical area is the body which manifests life. Although we discuss these three areas independently, they are closely related and cannot be separated. To maintain and improve your health, you need to be concerned with all three of them.

5-3. THEORY OF GENERAL MASSAGE 普通按摩之理論

We have explained in Part One that each category of massage has different purposes, and so each category has its own unique theory and somewhat different ways of reaching its goals. In general massage, to obtain the maximum result one needs to massage the mental body first, then the physical body, and finally the Qi body. No matter how hard you try to massage someone, or how strong your Qi is, if their mind is not calm and peaceful, you are wasting your time. However, when your partner can mentally coordinate with your massage, they will be able to relax deep inside and help you work. When the body is relaxed, the Qi can circulate more smoothly, and it can be led more easily. You have to massage your partner's mind before you massage the physical body. You can see that when you massage you are massaging three different bodies, yet you must treat them as one. They are mutually related and cannot be separated.

Massaging the Mental Body

When you are massaging someone, your first concern is how to gain their whole-hearted mental and physical cooperation. Since the main purpose of massage is to improve the Qi and blood circulation, if your partners mind remains tense, their physical body will also be tense and their Qi circulation stagnant. In addition, tense muscles may cause the pulse to speed up, and may even raise their blood pressure. Remember that *in a good massage, the person being massaged should be in a semi-hypnotic, relaxed and meditative state.* When this happens, the heart beat slows down and the mind is very peaceful. This does not mean that the person being massaged should be asleep. If you want to efficiently improve their Qi and blood circulation, you need their wholehearted cooperation. Remember, *it is the Yi which leads the Qi.* When your partner's Yi (意) (mind) is with your massage, they can regulate their Qi more efficiently, and your massage can be most effective. However, if your partner falls asleep, then the massage will not be as successful.

Furthermore, when you massage someone, you want your massage to reach well past their skin and muscles and deep into their body, as deep as the internal organs and bone marrow. However, when people give general massages they frequently cannot get their power to penetrate deeply enough. The cause of the problem is often with the person being massaged. They must be calm, they must be relaxed and balanced both mentally and physically, and most important of all, they must use their own meditative mind to regulate the Qi and blood circulation.

When you do have the cooperation of your massage partner, your Qi will unite with their Qi, your mind will unite with their mind, and both of you will enjoy the massage. As you can see, in general massage, your first task is to massage your partner's mind and spirit before you start on the physical massage.

Massaging the Physical Body

The main purpose of physical massage is to stimulate the cells of the body, enhancing Qi and blood circulation and removing Qi and blood stagnation. Massaging the physical body includes massage of the nerve endings (i.e. the skin), the sensory organs (ears, eyes, nose, and mouth), the fasciae and muscles, the joints including the spine, the internal organs, and the bone marrow.

Massaging the Nerve Endings. When you massage the nerve endings, you are actually also massaging the endings of the Qi channels in the skin. The nervous system communicates feelings and sensations to your brain, and your brain directs the Qi. Since the nervous system and the Qi system are so closely related, it is not surprising that massage techniques used on the skin can adjust both systems.

Massaging the nerve endings in the skin enables you to maintain or even improve the connection between them and the brain. Usually, when you touch the skin in the proper way, you can relax the entire part of the nervous system which is related to that area of the skin. This is why we can use touch to express our emotions so well and cause such varied sensations in our partners. So much love can be communicated through the sense of touch.

There are three ways to physically massage the skin. The first way is by using a gentle touch along the massage pathways (i.e. from the top to the bottom and from the center to the sides). This kind of massage can relax your partner and also lead them into a meditative state. Usually, this kind of skin massage is done at the very beginning of the massage.

The second way of massaging the skin is by slapping, grabbing and shaking, or even by whipping the body with the appropriate equipment. This type of massage causes some degree of pain, but it strongly stimulates the nerve endings and brings Qi and blood hidden deeply in or under the muscles to the surface of the skin allowing it to disperse. In Greece, this type of massage is done by gently hitting the skin with branches. This kind of skin massage is done near the end of the massage, when the Qi and blood accumulated deep within the body have already been loosened up. Slapping or gently whipping the skin will then lead the Qi and blood to the surface of the skin where it can be spread out.

The third way of massaging the skin is to rub it with the hands to generate heat, which leads the accumulated Qi and blood to the skin and spreads it out.

Massaging the Sensory Organs. In addition to massaging the skin, which is the sensory organ of touch, we must also massage the other sensory organs: the eyes, ears, nose, and mouth. In Chinese medicine, the areas near these organs are considered to be the endings of the Qi channels. As you get older, the Qi circulation to these organs gets weaker, and they don't function as well. The degeneration of vision and hearing are common occurrences in old age. Because of this, general massage places great emphasis on massaging the sensory organs.

Massaging around the sensory organs will gently stimulate the nervous system to lead Qi and blood to them. In fact, many people have had their vision and hearing improved through massage after years of deterioration.

Massaging the Muscles and Fasciae. Massaging the muscles and fasciae is probably the most important aspect of general massage for fatigue, although, of course, it can also greatly relax you even when you are not fatigued. When you are fatigued, an excessive amount of lactic acid has accumulated in the muscles. This causes muscle pain and the accumulation of Qi and blood.

When you massage the muscles, you are also massaging the fasciae between the skin and the muscles, and between the layers of muscle. The fat which is stored in the fascia hinders the Qi and blood circulation. General massage can remove much of this stored fat.

When you massage the muscles and fasciae, you stimulate them and increase the circulation of Qi and blood. This removes the lactic acid and spreads it out so that it can be removed from your system. Since most of the Qi channels are within the muscles, this will also restore smooth Qi circulation, which is one of the best ways of retarding the aging process.

Massaging the Spine. The spine consists of seven cervical vertebrae in the neck, twelve thoracic vertebrae in the back, five lumber vertebrae in the waist, as well as the sacrum and tailbone. Nerves branch out from the spinal cord to the limbs and the internal organs. Any problem with the spinal cord interferes with the brain's ability to sense and govern the body.

Inside the spinal column is a Qi vessel (the Thrusting Vessel; Chong Mai, 衝脈) which connects the brain to the Huiyin (Co-1) (會陰) cavity and communicates with the other two main vessels (the Conception and Governing Vessels; Ren Mai and Du Mai, 任脈、督脈). These three vessels are the most important ones in the body, and they are intimately related to your health and longevity. Whenever the Qi level in these three vessels is low, the whole body receives insufficient Qi nourishment, and consequently, the physical body (including the nervous system) cannot function normally.

In order to keep enough Qi coming into the central nervous system, the spine must be loose, and any accumulated Qi or blood must be removed. Since the trunk muscles around the spine have a very great influence on the condition of the spine, massaging the trunk muscles is a very important part of spine massage.

Massaging the Joints. This refers to the joints in the arms and legs. We know that in the area of the joints are gates which allow the exchange of Qi between the body and the environment. In addition, around the joints are areas where we can access the main nerves and arteries. And, of course, the joints allow us to move our limbs freely. Whenever there is any stagnation of Qi or blood in the joints, or any physical defect such as arthritis, we suffer pain and our mobility is limited. Injuries and aging affect the joints much more than the shafts of the bones. Therefore, general massage places great emphasis on keeping the joints healthy and functioning properly.

Massaging the Internal Organs. The internal organs can be massaged with the hands and also with movement. While another person can use the first method on you, you may use either one on yourself.

When you massage by hand, you place your hands on the skin above the organ, and use gentle rubbing movements in specific patterns to loosen the muscles around the organ. The gentle movements of your hands generate Qi under the skin. This Qi follows the movement of the hands, and therefore can be directed into the organ. Naturally, if the person being massaged uses their mind to relax the muscles and lead the Qi, the results will be significantly greater.

Massage by movement uses mainly the trunk muscles and the up and down movement of the diaphragm (from deep breathing) to massage the internal organs. Muscles in the torso wrap around the internal organs. When these muscles are tense, the Qi and blood circulation around the internal organs will be stagnant. Therefore, the first steps of self-massage of the internal organs with movement are learning how to loosen up the trunk muscles, and then using movements of the trunk muscles to massage the internal organs. You also need to learn how to breathe deeply to move the diaphragm smoothly, slowly, and gently while keeping it relaxed. This massages the organs under the diaphragm.

FIGURE 5-1

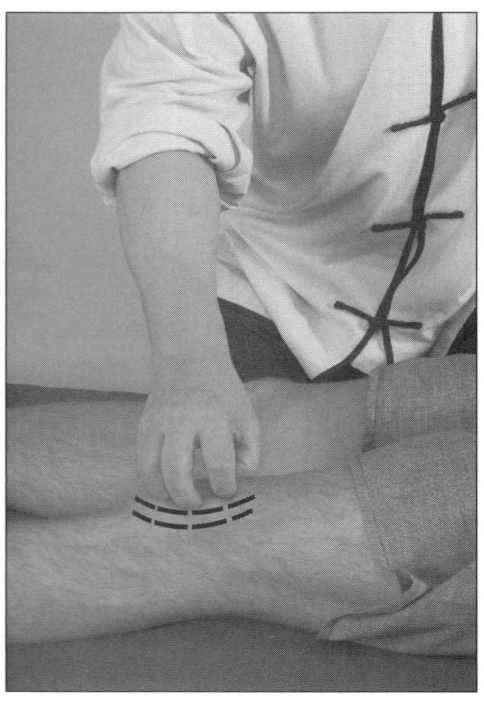

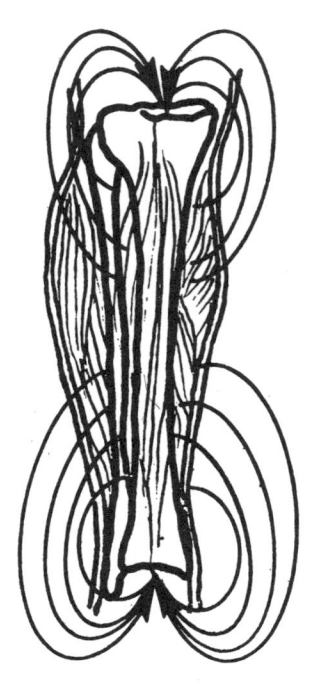

FIGURE 5-2. BONE BREATHING THROUGH MUSCLE STIMULATION.

In Qigong, it is desirable to learn how to control the muscles in the abdominal area so that you can move the abdomen in and out. This will enhance the effectiveness of the internal organ massage.

Massaging the Bone Marrow. Massaging the bone marrow is one of the most difficult parts of general massage. The main purpose of bone marrow massage is to lead Qi to the marrow to maintain the normal production of healthy blood cells. In Chinese Qigong, one of the most effective ways of leading Qi to the marrow is through correct breathing techniques and certain methods of meditation. These are discussed in the YMAA book, *Qigong—The Secret of Youth.*

Because the theory is difficult to understand, most practitioners of Qigong massage have ignored marrow massage. I would like to introduce several possible massage techniques which may stimulate the Qi circulation in the marrow.

The first technique is stimulating the bones in the area of the joints, where the bone is most exposed and closest to the skin. The shaft of the bone is protected by the muscles and difficult to reach. To stimulate the bone at the joint, press the bone with your fingernails and circle your fingers (Figure 5-1). Move the skin with your nails so that you do not scrape the skin. This will cause a slight amount of pain, and in some areas, such as the knees, it will cause an exciting, stimulating sensation deep within the body. You may also use your teeth to stimulate the bones at the joints or at places which do not have a thick layer of muscle over them, such as the shin. Go very carefully. Do not cause too much pain, and do not cause any bruising, because that would make the entire body more tense, and you will not be able to accomplish your goal.

In the areas which are protected by a thick layer of muscle, you can increase the exchange of Qi by stimulating the muscles so that Qi is led from the marrow to the skin (Figure 5-2). When this happens, the bone draws fresh Qi from around the joint. The easiest way to do this is to use a whip made of wire or a bar (Figure 5-3) to gently hit the muscles until they get warm.

Massaging the Qi Body

First, I would like to point out that massaging the Qi body is different from Qi massage, which we will discuss in the future volume. When you massage the Qi body,

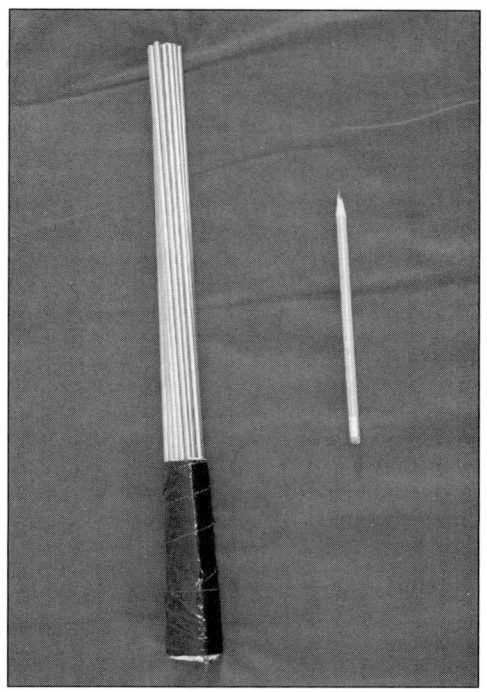

FIGURE 5-3. WIRE WHIP.

you use both physical techniques and Qi correspondence to regulate your partner's Qi. However, in Qi massage, you cause your Qi to correspond with your partner's Qi so that you can regulate and rebalance it. Massaging the Qi body smooths the Qi circulation for relaxation and health, while Qi massage is used to correct abnormal Qi circulation which was caused by illness or injury.

Before we discuss massaging the Qi body, I would like to remind you of a very important point we made in the first part of this book. According to both Chinese and Western medicine, every blood cell must have Qi or bioelectricity to stay alive. Furthermore, each blood cell functions like a battery, and stores and releases Qi as needed. Because of this, Qi and blood cannot be completely separated, and when you discuss either one of them, the other one is usually also involved to some degree.

In addition to the blood circulatory system, there are twelve primary channels which also circulate Qi in the body. Most of the course of each channel lies within the muscle, so when you tense your muscles you are limiting the Qi circulation to the organs (which are connected to these channels), and they may not receive the proper amount of Qi nourishment. This is why keeping your body relaxed is one of the main keys to health.

Next, we will discuss the theory of how to massage the Qi body.

Massaging the Qi Endings. Massaging the Qi endings cannot be separated from massaging the nerve endings. The reason for this is quite simple. Since Qi is necessary for keeping the nerve fibers alive, small Qi channels supply the nerves, and the endings of these tiny Qi channels are located near the endings of the nerves.

While the skin separates the insides of our bodies from the outside environment, the skin has thousands of pores, capillaries, nerve endings, and small Qi channels through which Qi and air pass in and out. According to Chinese medicine, all of the Qi channel endings in our skin are related to our internal organs. Stimulating the skin can maintain the exchange of air and Qi between our insides and the world outside, and can also stimulate our internal organs.

To massage the Qi endings in the skin, simply touch your partner lightly and move your hands along the massage paths (which are also the routes of the Qi channels and nerves). Move from the top to the bottom, and from the center to the sides. This allows several things to take place. If your Qi is in correspondence with your partner's, they will be able to use their own mind to lead their Qi in synchronization with your movements to smooth their own Qi. This skin-to-skin contact also allows the Qi to pass between you and your partner so that you can nourish each other. Mutual Qi nourishment is one of the methods which Chinese Qigong uses to balance irregular Qi conditions. For example, when you are sad, the Qi in your body is Yin and weak. If a friend holds your hands or hugs you, you immediately receive Qi nourishment from them. This allows you to smooth out your Qi, and helps them to relax. Touching is a natural, instinctive method of Qigong healing.

Massaging the Qi Gates. In general massage, you want to lead the excess Qi out of your partner's body to release the tension. In order to do this, you must know all of the Qi gates and junctions. This includes the gates between the body and the surrounding environment, and also the gates and junctions within the body. Stimulating the gates in sequence along the channels will lead the excess Qi to the limbs and finally release it from the body.

Massaging the Endocrine Glands. An important purpose of general massage is increasing the production of hormones and strengthening the immune system, The production of hormones can be increased in two places in men and in one place in women. In men, this can be done in the adrenal glands, which are on top of the kidneys, and in the testicles. In women, only the adrenal glands can be easily reached. Massaging the muscles around the kidneys and testicles will lead Qi to them and increase hormone production, and will also maintain smooth Qi circulation around them.

5-4. RULES OF GENERAL MASSAGE 普通按摩之原則

Now that you have a grasp of the theory, you probably already have an idea of what procedure you should follow. In this subsection. I would like to summarize the procedures of general massage, as well as the pathways you should follow, and also to discuss how much power you should use.

Procedures

When you massage, unless you are only massaging a portion of the body, you should follow the standard procedures which tell you where you should start, and where you should end. Following the correct procedures will make the massage more effective and more enjoyable.

Mental Massage. In order to achieve maximum effectiveness, and reach the deepest places in the body, your partner should be in a semi-hypnotic, meditative state. This lets them relax their body as much as possible, which allows the power of the massage to penetrate as deeply as possible. When their mind is calm, they are also able to regulate their own Qi and physical body. Therefore, before the physical massage, you should massage your partners mental body and help them to enter a deep meditative state.

Head and Neck. In physical massage, it is important to start from the head, because this is where a person's 'headquarters' is. Within the head is the brain, which controls the entire body through the nervous system. If the head is tense, the mind will also be tense, as well as the rest of the body.

The neck is the passageway of the Qi and blood. Whenever the neck is tense, the Qi and blood circulation will be stagnant, and the brain will not receive proper nourishment. The best way to remove the excess Qi and blood which has accumulated in the head, as well as to bring in plenty of nourishment, is to relax the neck and keep all of the Qi and blood vessels open.

Back. The next place to massage is the back. The spine is the central supply line of Qi, with the Governing Vessel (Du Mai, 督脈) running up the back of it. The Governing Vessel controls the six primary Yang Qi channels in the body. In addition, in the center of the spine is the Thrusting Vessel (Chong Mai, 衝脈), through which the Qi communicates between the lower part of the body and the brain. Furthermore, the spinal cord is a major part of the central nervous system, and all of the peripheral nervous system branches out from it. You can see that the spine is the connection between the brain and the entire body. Whenever there is any problem in the spine, there will be a malfunction in the related portion of the body. This is why loosening up the spine and improving the Qi circulation there is a crucial part of general massage.

After loosening up the spine, the next task is leading the accumulated Qi or blood away from the spine. This Qi and blood, which have accumulated deep inside the joints of the spine, are the main cause of problems with the nervous system. The Qi and blood must be brought up to the skin and spread out to the sides and downward.

Back of the Legs. Excess Qi is released out of the body at the ends of the limbs. The Qi which you have released from the back should be brought out to the limbs. You normally do the legs next, because the Qi channels in the legs are more open than those in the arms. In addition, it is easier to lead the Qi downward than to the sides. Therefore, the next step is to lead the Qi to the bottom of the feet.

Back of the Arms. After you have massaged the legs and feet, you massage the arms to smooth out the Qi flow and lead any excess Qi away from the body. Leading Qi to the arms is one of the most effective ways of releasing excess Qi in the head, simply because the arms are closer to the head than are the legs.

Chest and Abdomen. After you have completed the massage of the back, have your partner turn face upward.

Before you start massaging the chest and abdomen, you need to help your partner regain a meditative state, which was probably disturbed when they turned over. Spend a short time massaging their head to assist them in regaining a meditative state.

The chest and abdomen, which contain most of the internal organs, are the third most important area in general massage. Your goal in massaging this area is to loosen up and relax the muscles in the front of the body, and also to improve the Qi circulation in the internal organs. Your health is determined, in great part, by the condition of your internal organs. Bringing up the Qi and blood which have accumulated in and around the internal organs improves the Qi circulation and helps keep the organs healthy.

Front of the Legs. After you have loosened up the chest and abdomen and brought the accumulated Qi and blood up to the surface, lead the Qi and blood down the legs to the bottom of the feet. Follow the same theory that you used on the back of the legs.

Front of the Arms. Finally, massage the arms and lead the Qi from the head and the front of the body to the arms and get rid of it.

This suggested massage procedure for the entire body is drawn from the theoretical understanding of the Qi and the physical bodies. If you do not have time to massage the entire body, still follow the same sequence with the parts that you do massage. For example, when you massage the head to relieve a headache, also massage the back and arms in order to lead the Qi downward and sideways. If you fail to do this, the Qi and blood will remain in the head. Similarly, when you massage the back to relieve a backache, also massage the legs to lead the Qi further downward.

Pathways

One of the most important factors in successful Qigong massage is following the correct pathways. This is especially true in Tui Na, Dian Xue, and Qi massage. In this section we will discuss only the pathways used in general massage. Remember that the objectives of general massage are to get rid of excess Qi, smooth out the Qi circulation, and also relax the mental and physical bodies. These goals provide the rationale for the pathways.

Move From Top to Bottom. The first general rule in massaging pathways is to lead the Qi downward so as to release the Qi accumulated in the head and body (Figures 5-4 and 5-5). Therefore, when you massage, your hands move from the top of the body to the bottom. If you reverse the direction, you are nourishing the Qi and leading the Qi upward. This will prevent the release of Qi and result in the body becoming more Yang, which, in turn, will cause more tension in both the mental and physical bodies.

Move From the Center to the Sides. The next general rule in releasing the Qi accumulated in the body is to massage from the center of the body to the sides (Figures 5-4 and 5-5). Therefore, when you massage, your hands move from the center of the torso

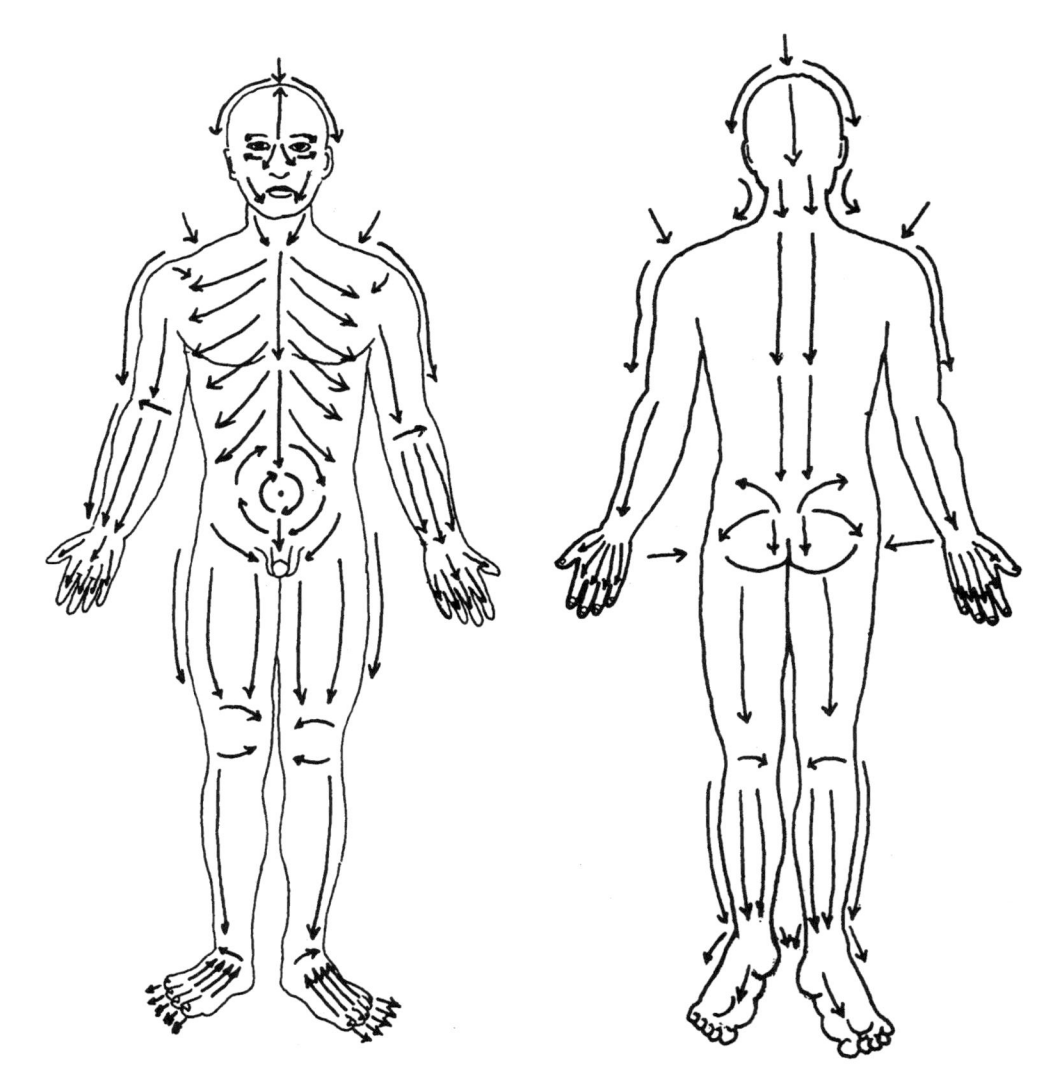

FIGURE 5-4. MASSAGE PATHWAYS ON THE FRONT OF THE BODY IN GENERAL MASSAGE.

FIGURE 5-5. MASSAGE PATHWAYS ON THE BACK OF THE BODY IN GENERAL MASSAGE.

out to the sides. If you reverse the direction, you are nourishing the body with Qi, and preventing the release of Qi. This will result in the body becoming more Yang, and will cause more tension in both the mental and physical bodies.

Move in Circles. There are many different rules for massaging in circles, and it can become very confusing. How you circle is usually more important in Tui Na (推拿), Dian Xue (點穴), and Qi massage, which are concerned with the condition of the Qi in the body. The direction of your circling determines whether you are drawing Qi in or out, and can have a great effect on whether healing takes place. The direction in which you circle is determined by the minds of the healer and the patient, and also by

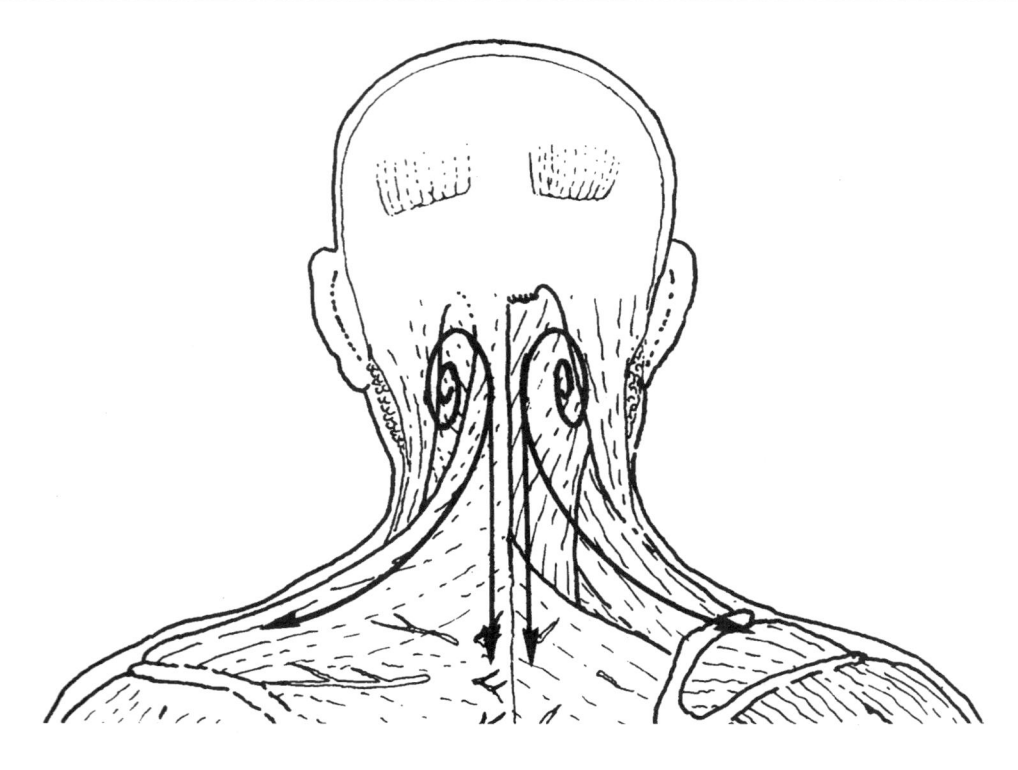

FIGURE 5-6. MASSAGE PATHWAYS ON THE BACK OF THE NECK.

the channel (whether it is a Yin or Yang channel), the cavities being used, and the time of day. You can see how it is much easier to learn general massage than the healing forms of massage.

In this subsection, we will discuss only the rules of general massage which focus on the release of mental and physical tension. If you ever become confused about which direction to circle, just take a little time to think about it, and then see the difference in how it feels to circle in either direction.

- **Leading the Qi and Blood Downward and to the Sides**

    In general massage, in order to release excess Qi and improve the Qi and blood circulation, lead the Qi and blood downward to the feet and also sideways to the arms. There are a few simple rules for this.

    Let us use two examples to explain these rules. First, when massaging the back of the neck, if you circle counterclockwise on the right-hand side and clockwise on the left-hand side, you are leading the Qi and blood downward (Figure 5-6). However, if you reverse the direction on both sides, then you are leading the Qi and blood upward, which may cause the head to become too Yang.

    When massaging the back, if you move in a counterclockwise circle while working

Chapter 5: General Concepts

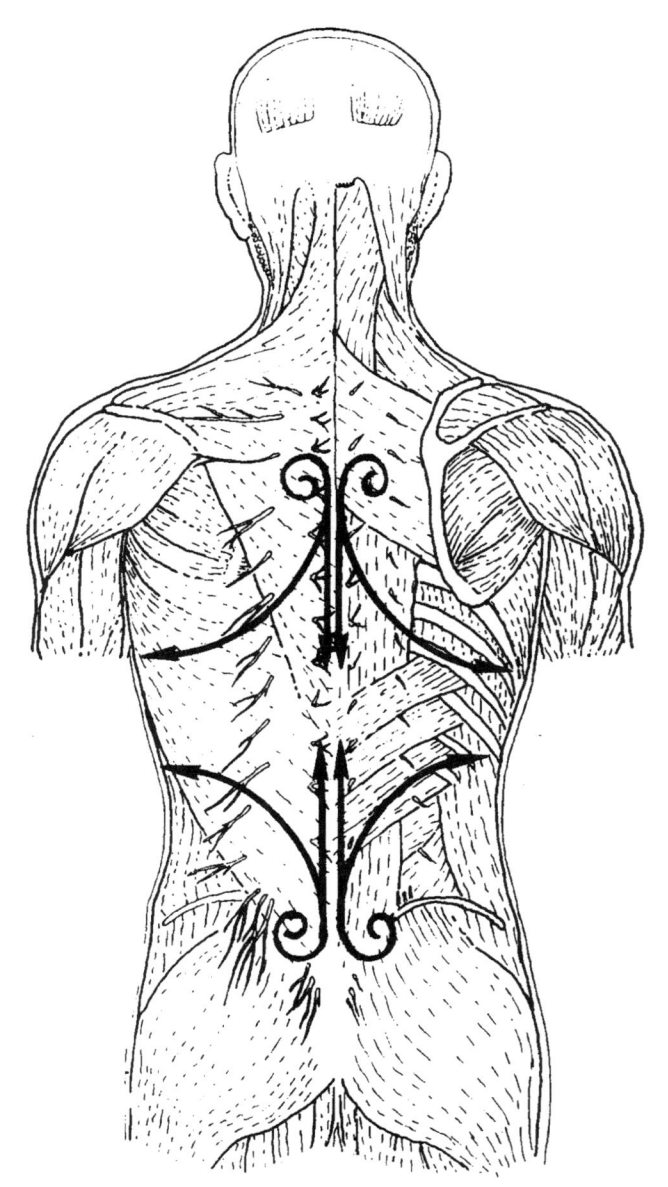

FIGURE 5-7. MASSAGE PATHWAYS ON THE BACK OF THE BODY.

on the right-hand side, and in a clockwise circle while working on the left-hand side, then you are leading the Qi downward and to the sides (Figure 5-7). However, if you reverse the directions, then you are leading the Qi upward and also to the sides. If you are trying to disperse excess Qi and release tension, then you would want to bring the Qi down and to the sides. However, sometimes you will want to lead Qi and blood from the back to the arms. In this case, you will circle in the other direction.

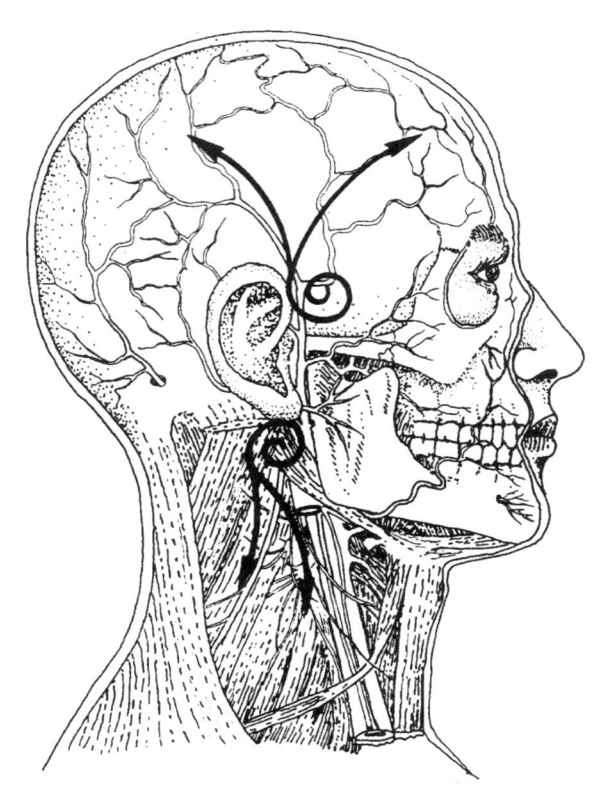

FIGURE 5-8. MASSAGE PATHWAYS NEAR THE EAR.

- **Massaging the Blood and Nerve Junctions**

    The blood and nerve junctions often become tense. For example, under each ear is a junction where arteries and nerves branch out and spread over the top of the head. If the top and sides of the neck are tense, the Qi and blood circulation will be affected. Massaging these junctions or knots will help the blood spread out smoothly and reduce the pressure on the junctions. Therefore, when you massage you may circle clockwise and then push upward, but you should also circle counterclockwise and then push downward (Figure 5-8). This will gently stretch the muscles around the junction and smooth out the blood and Qi circulation.

    The general rule is that when you use your right hand to massage, you circle clockwise to spread the Qi and blood upward or to the right (Figure 5-9), and counterclockwise to lead the blood and Qi downward or to the right. However, if you use your left hand to massage in a counterclockwise direction will spread the Qi and blood upward and to the left, while a clockwise direction it will lead the Qi and blood downward or to the left.

Power

The amount of power you use is probably the most critical factor in massage. General massage works on many places, including the skin, the fascia between the skin and muscles, the fascia between muscles, the fascia between muscles and bones, the muscles themselves, the tendons around the joints, the internal organs, and the bone marrow. Massage depth ranges from the surface of the body to deep inside it. How you reach these places depends not just on the techniques you use, but also on the power you apply.

The main rule in general massage is to relax your partner. If you use too much power and cause pain, your partner will tense up, and their mind will become upset. However, if you use too little power, the massage will not be effective.

There are a few general rules which will help you reach your goals. First, the power and the pattern of the massage should be consistent. This way your partner will know what to expect, and they will be able to relax more easily. Second, start massaging lightly, and gradually increase the power. Light power gently stimulates the nerves and soothes them, so that they will not so quickly send messages to the brain. Then you can use more power without disturbing your partner. Third, massage from shallow to deep. As you stimulate the outer layers of your partner's body, the reaction of the nerves will slow down, and their body can remain relaxed as you increase the power and reach a deeper layer.

Fourth, finish up from deep to shallow. Once your power can reach deep inside and remove the Qi and blood stagnation, you want to lead this accumulated Qi, blood, and acid to the surface of the skin and spread it out.

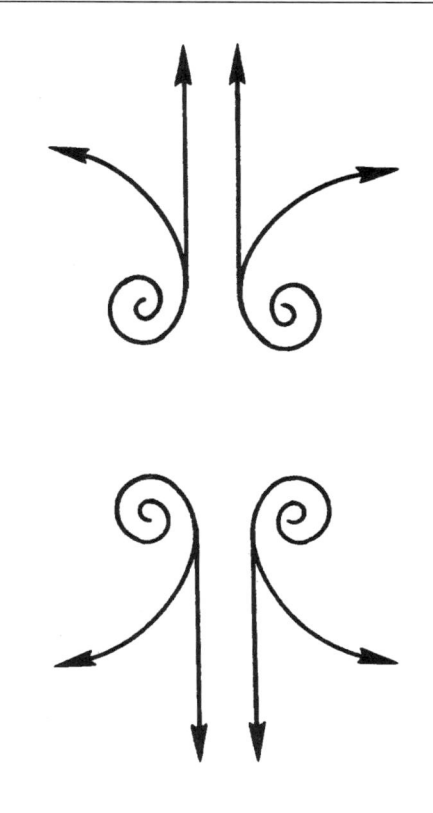

FIGURE 5-9. GENERAL MASSAGE PATHWAYS.

Qigong Massage

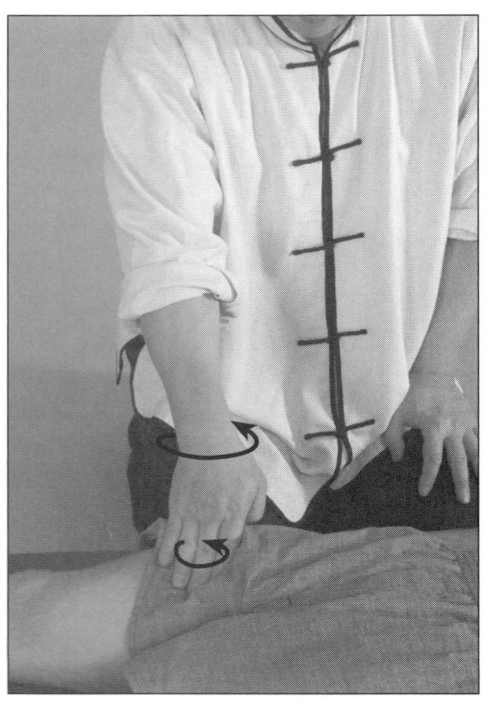

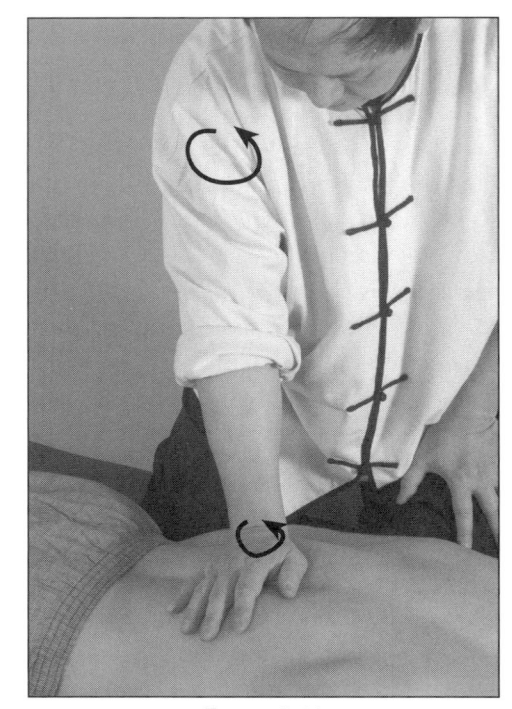

FIGURE 5-10

FIGURE 5-11

Finally, in order to keep the massage soft and enjoyable, your hands must be relaxed. The trick of doing this is, when you use your fingers to massage, generate the power and motion from your wrist (Figure 5-10), and when you use the palm or the base of the palm to massage, generate the power from your elbow and shoulder (Figure 5-11). If you try to generate power from the part of your body that your are massaging with, it will be tense, and you will not be able to apply the techniques gently. The best way to massage it to use your entire body to generate power, and not rely on muscular power. In addition to being the most effective way to massage, this is also very enjoyable for you, because you can feel your whole body moving harmoniously, and you won't tire out as quickly.

CHAPTER 6
General Massage 普通按摩

6-1. Introduction 介紹

In this and the next chapter we will introduce the "how" of general massage. As you practice massage, many questions will occur to you, such as: 1. What are the general problems which prevent us from reaching our goals? 2. How do we solve these problems? 3. Do we get the results that the theory leads us to expect? If you keep these questions in mind as you massage, you will be able to evaluate your progress and modify your approach as necessary. In Chapter 4, we introduced many massage techniques. You may try these techniques as you practice, or even create others.

We will first introduce the mental techniques of general massage. They are used to calm down your partner, and help them relax both mentally and physically. We will then discuss the physical aspect of general massage by dividing it into five sections: the head, the back, the back of the limbs, the chest and abdomen, and the front of the limbs. In the first part of this book we discussed the general environmental requirements for massage. It is important to create a relaxed, comfortable atmosphere for you and your massage partner; I urge you to study that section carefully.

In general massage with a partner, an entire body massage usually takes about two hours. While this is very enjoyable for your partner, it requires a masseur with a lot of patience and enthusiasm. Most of the time, only part of the whole routine is done, centering on what your partner needs. The head and back are the areas which most often need treatment. The next most common areas are the legs and arms, followed by the chest and upper abdomen. The lower abdominal area is rarely treated, simply because it is near the sexual organs, and most people would feel uncomfortable unless they had a close relationship with the masseur.

When you massage your partner's whole body, if they are not shy it is best if they disrobe. This will make for the best Qi communication. Usually a towel is used to cover the areas you are not working on so that the person does not catch a cold. Many people like to wear shorts when they are being massaged. This is somewhat inconvenient when you massage the lower abdomen and the hips. When you give a general massage on only a portion of the body, it is best to expose the area you will be working on. This will help you to exchange Qi with your partner, and will give you more sensitivity in your hands. However, it is not necessary that you do this, and if your partner is reluctant to expose

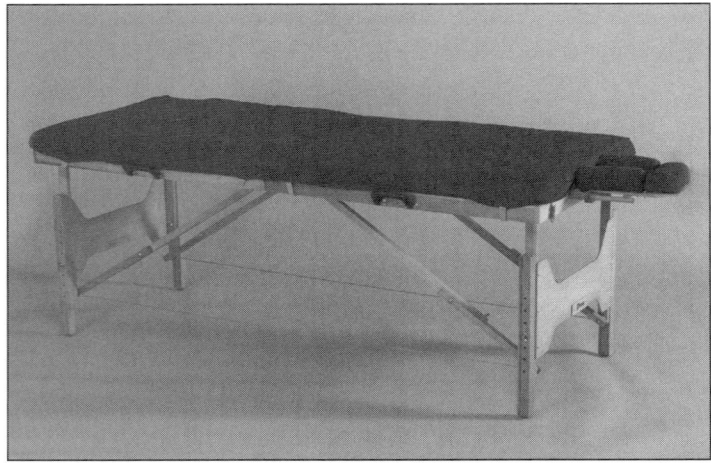

FIGURE 6-1

some part of his or her body, you needn't insist upon it.

Because general massage is not meant to treat injuries, herbal wines or ointments are not usually used. Some people use oil when they massage, such as baby oil or olive oil, on areas other than the head. While this can lubricate the skin and allow the hands to move more smoothly over it, it also seals the pores. This can interfere with the Qi communication between you and the person you are massaging. Because of this, many professional Chinese masseurs do not like to use any oil. Instead, they will often use a thin silk handkerchief to smooth the movement.

Before we introduce general massage, we would first like to discuss what the patient lies upon, be it the floor, a bed, or a specially designed wooden table. The first concern is the material beneath the patient. If you are massaging on the floor, you will need a material which provides good Qi insulation between the patient and the floor. It is best if it is made from natural materials such as cotton or wool. The thickness of the insulation is very important. If the insulation is too thin, the patient will continue to feel the Yin side of the ground and continue to lose Qi to the floor. If the material is made of synthetic material such as polyester, static charges will accumulate and make the patient feel uncomfortable. A futon is one of the most popular materials for massage, as well as for sleep and meditation.

If you use a bed for massage, it should not be too soft, which would be bad for spine massage. Padded, wooden massage tables of many different designs are available today, and are very popular (Figure 6-1).

The second concern is the neck area. When a person is lying face down on a flat surface, the head needs to be turned to the side. After a while, the neck muscles become tense and sore, and the patient is very uncomfortable. Because of this, many massage tables have an attachment which allows the patient to lie comfortably face down (Figure 6-2).

Chapter 6: General Massage

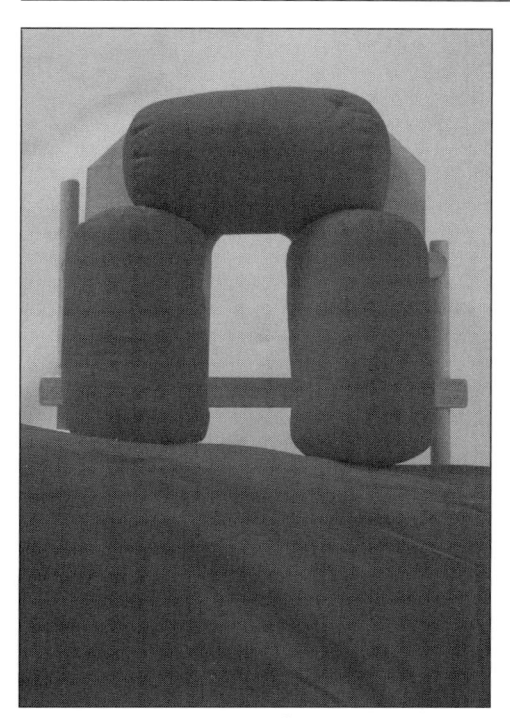

FIGURE 6-2

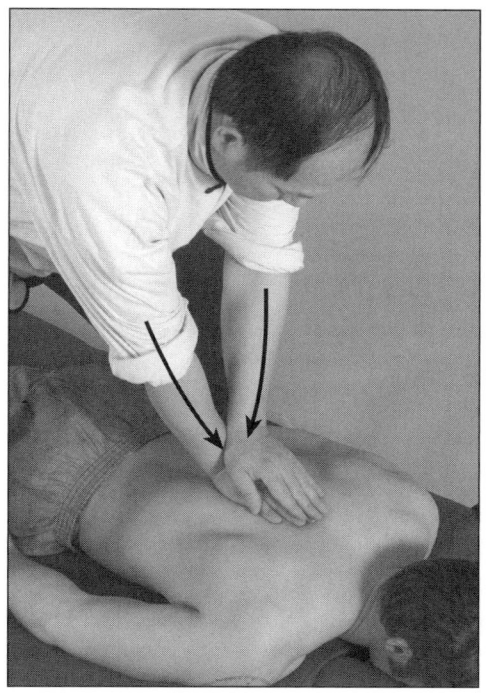

FIGURE 6-3

The third concern is the height of the massage table. If the table is too high, it will be difficult to massage the spine. You want to apply power easily and evenly, and it is especially important that the power of your press be even on both sides of the spinal joints. Therefore, you should be able to lower the table so that you may straddle the patient when you work on their back (Figure 6-3). However, when you massage other places such as the trunk muscles, the thighs, or the chest and abdomen, you would like the table to be about waist height so that you don't have to bend over all the time (Figure 6-4). The table needs to be the right height for you, so that you can use your whole body as you massage without expending too much effort. The best solution is a table with adjustable legs.

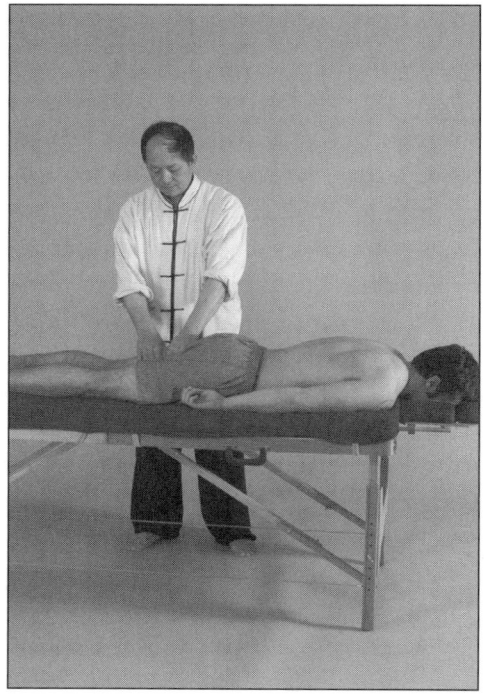

FIGURE 6-4

Qigong Massage

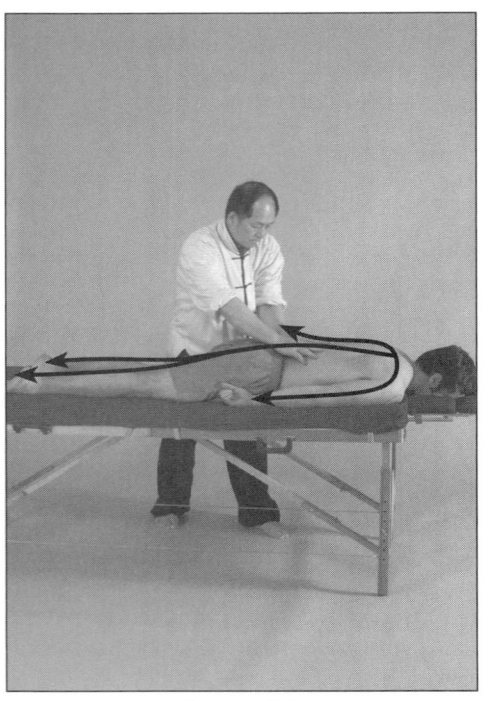

FIGURE 6-5

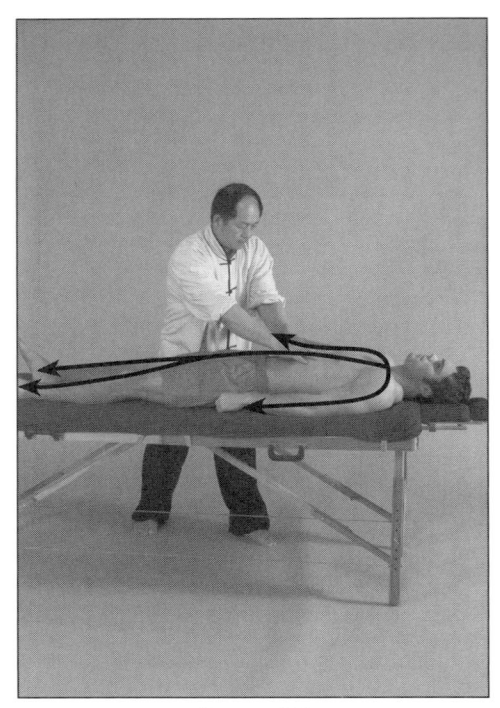

FIGURE 6-6

6-2. Massaging the Mental Body
心理按摩

As we explained earlier, the best results are obtained when the persons being massaged also uses their own mind to regulate their body and Qi. Therefore, the first step in massage is to massage the partner's mind and spirit. Once you have reached their spirit, you may lead it into a deep meditative and hypnotic state. This will let their thoughts be free and their mind relaxed. Their physical body will also be relaxed, allowing you to massage and regulate their Qi and blood effectively.

When you massage your partner's mind, there are a few things that you must do. First, make your partner feel relaxed and comfortable. This involves the ambiance of your surroundings as well as the relationship between you and your partner. Your

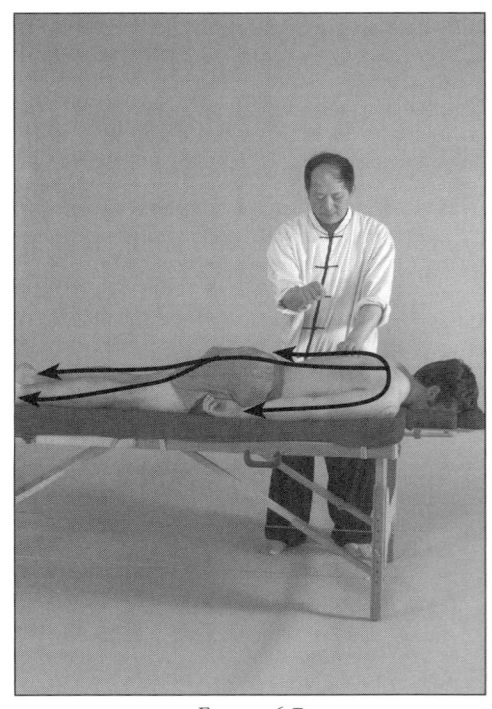

FIGURE 6-7

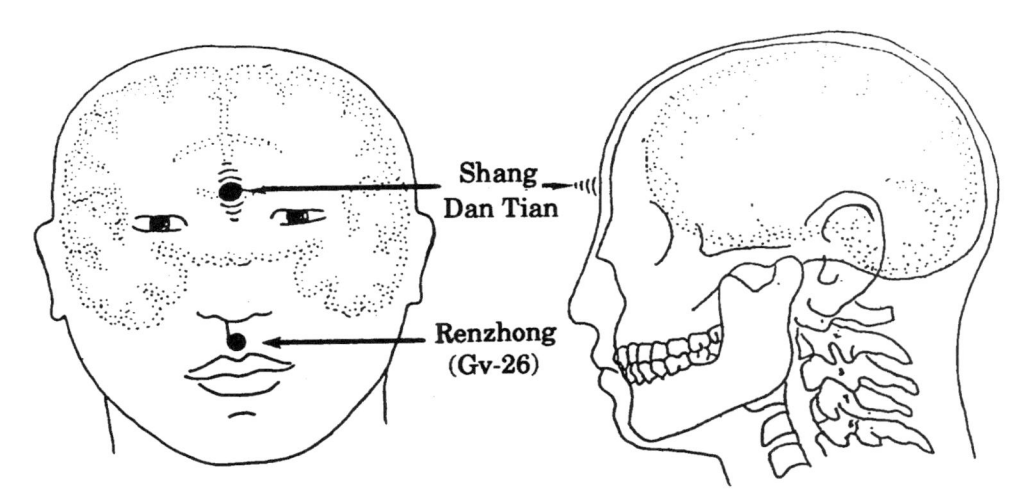

FIGURE 6-8. THE SHANG DAN TIAN (UPPER DAN TIAN) AND THE RENZHONG CAVITY.

partner needs to be able to relax totally so that they can pay attention to the condition of their body and enter a meditative state.

Next, you should draw your partner's mind away from all outside distractions and into total concentration on their body. Their attention should be totally on their Qi and your massage. There are two common ways to reach this goal. One is to ask your partner to lie face down, close their eyes, and try to relax as much as possible, and then lightly brush your hands over their body along the massage pathways, from the top of the body to the bottom, and from the center to the limbs (Figure 6-5). Repeat this several times. Then have your partner turn face upward and repeat the same process several times (Figure 6-6). Make sure that, before you actually lay your hands on them, you rub your hands together until they are warm. Few things are more startling than cold hands on your skin. Once you have brushed your partner down a few times, it will be very easy for you to bring their attention to your hands.

Some people use a different method. Instead of lightly brushing their hands over the person, they lightly slap or hit the body along the massage pathways mentioned earlier (Figure 6-7). However, according to my experience, this method is not as efficient as the previous one.

The last step of the mental massage is to massage your partner's spiritual center. The spiritual center is in the forehead, in a place called the Shang Dan Tian (上丹田) (Upper Elixir Field) by Chinese Qigong practitioners, and the 'third eye' by practitioners in the Western world. People in both Western and Asian cultures have recognized that this area can sense natural energy, and it is the center and headquarters of your spirit. With regard to physical structure, this spot is the gap between the two lobes of the brain

(Figure 6-8). It is believed in Chinese Qigong that the Qi in your brain is able to reach the outside world through this center, enabling you to sense and communicate with the natural energy. Some people who train this area are able to develop their intuition and their ability to sense things that other people cannot—almost as if they could see through an extra, special eye. Therefore, the Upper Dan Tian or third eye is considered to be the gate which allows you to reach the mental center and calm down the mind.

Another common approach when massaging the Upper Dan Tian is to also stimulate the Renzhong (Gv-26) (人中) cavity under the nose (Figure 6-8). Chinese physicians and Qigong practitioners know that stimulating the Renzhong cavity will raise the spirit of vitality and revive someone who has fainted. In massage, stimulating this cavity together with the Upper Dan Tian will help you to lead your partner's mind more easily to their center.

To massage your partner's spiritual center and Renzhong, help your partner to sit up, and let their head lean comfortably against your body. Then use your fingers or the center of your palm to massage the third eye or Upper Dan Tian slowly and gently, and at the same time press the Renzhong cavity firmly with the second or middle finger of the other hand (Figure 6-9). You may also do this when your partner is lying down (Figure 6-10).

While you are massaging their spiritual center, you should ask your partner to pay attention to your hands, relax their physical body as deeply as possible, and inhale and exhale deeply. This helps to bring them into a self-hypnotic state. People who have trained in meditation will be able to do this more easily. After massaging the Upper Dan Tian for a few minutes, you should be able to bring your partner into some level of meditation. Naturally, their cooperation is crucial in this.

Once you have led your partner into a meditative state, you can then start to massage their physical and Qi bodies. In the following sections, we will discuss the massage techniques for the head, back, back of the limbs, chest and abdomen, and the front of the limbs. In each section, we will first discuss the anatomical structure of the part being massaged, follow with massage theory, introduce the gates or junctions, and finally explain the massage techniques.

6-3. Massaging the Head 頭部按摩

We mentioned earlier that the head is the most important part of the body, and should be massaged first in general massage. This discussion will also include the neck, which is the passageway to the head for Qi and blood.

Anatomical Structure of the Head and Its Circulatory Systems

When we first look at the head, what we see is the hair or the skin. Under the surface is a layer of fat. Qi, oxygen, and nutrition are supplied to the hair and the skin by thousands of small capillaries and Qi branches. The skin also contains countless small nerves, which enable the brain to monitor the condition of the skin.

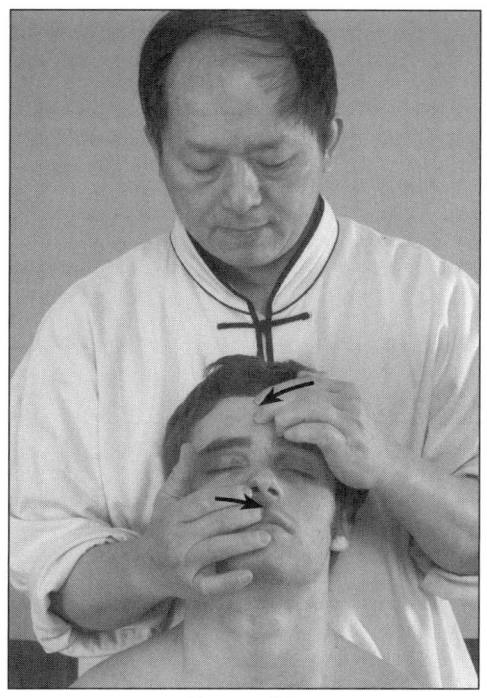

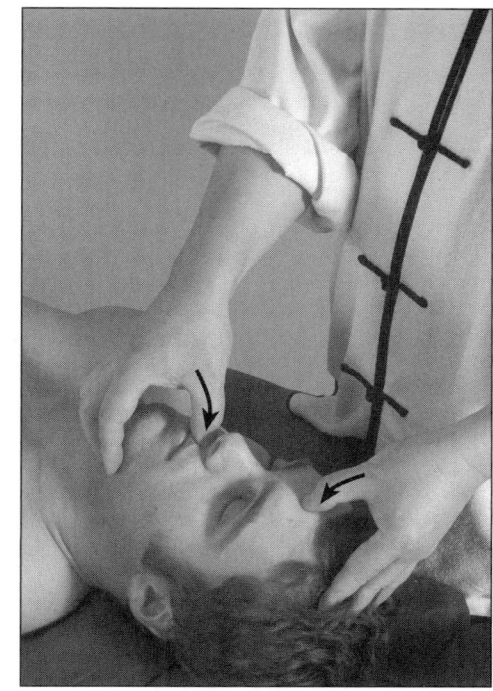

FIGURE 6-9

FIGURE 6-10

Next to the skin is the fascia. Fascia tissue can usually be found beneath the skin, between and around the muscles, between the muscles and bones, and between and around other structures such as internal organs. Under the fascia, we can see muscles, nerves, arteries, veins, lymphatics and glands. The muscles on the top of the head are usually very thin, but get thicker with different sets of muscles on the face area in order to control the movements of the eyes, nose, and mouth. Beneath the muscle is the skeleton, and again under the skeleton are many arteries, veins, and nerves which are connected to the brain.

When we look at the front of the head, under the neck muscles are large arteries, nerves, veins, lymphatics and glands, and behind them is the throat (Figure 6-11). On the side of the neck are many large sets of muscles, and underneath these muscles are big arteries, veins, and nerves (Figure 6-12). As you can see from the picture, all of the circulatory systems originate under the base of the neck, and extend to the brain and also to the top of the head.

When you look at the back of the head and neck, again you will see many arteries, veins, and nerves extending their networks from the neck to the top of the head (Figure 6-13). On the back of the neck, the spine is in the center with two large sets of muscles beside it. On each of the joints of the spine there are again arteries, veins, and nerves extending from the spinal cord to the surface of the muscles.

Remember that all of these circulatory systems are physical and therefore visible.

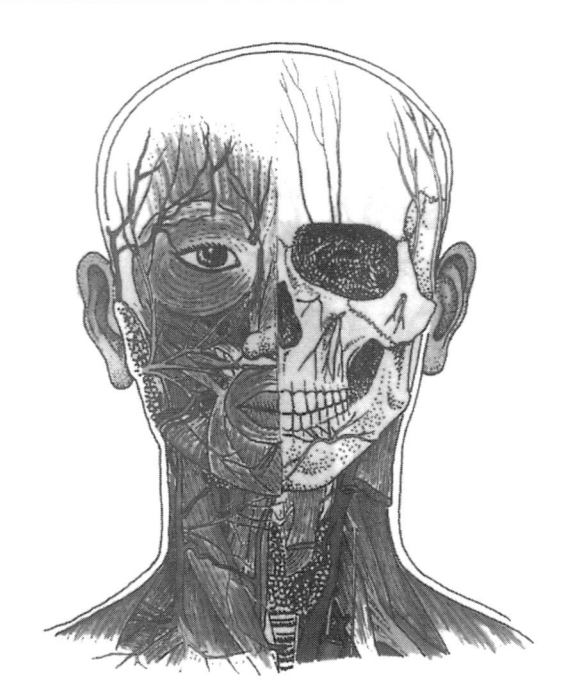

FIGURE 6-11. ANATOMICAL STRUCTURE OF THE HEAD (FRONT VIEW).

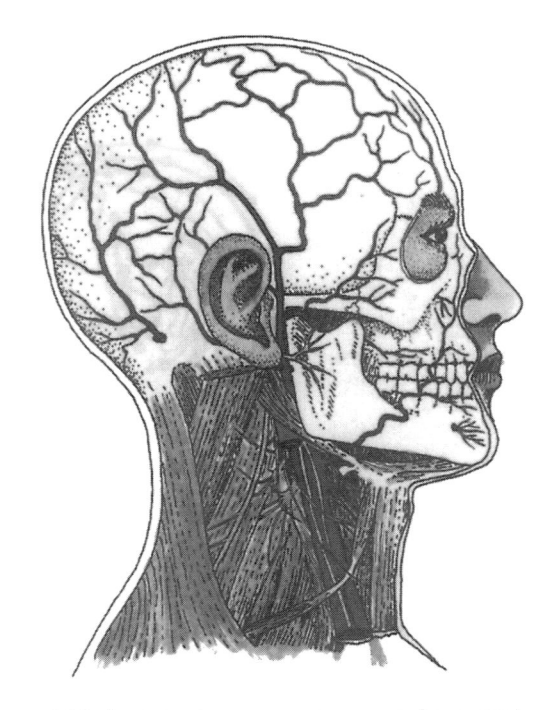

FIGURE 6-12. ANATOMICAL VIEW OF THE HEAD (SIDE VIEW).

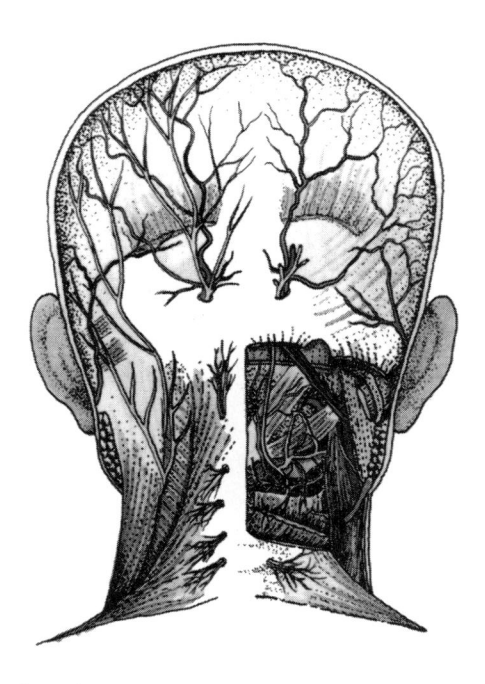

FIGURE 6-13. ANATOMICAL STRUCTURE OF THE HEAD (BACK VIEW).

However, in order to function, these physical systems need an invisible system to supply Qi or bioelectricity. Figures 6-14, 6-15, and 6-16 show the front, side, and back and top of the Qi circulatory system of the head.

Theory. The head is the center of your entire being, and it governs and influences your mental body, Qi body, and physical body. When you massage the head first and relax it, your partner's mind will become calm, and their entire body will stay relaxed.

A brain cell needs at least 10 times as much oxygen as any other cell. When you massage the head correctly you relax the muscles and soothe the nervous system. This lets the blood vessels expand and increases the flow of blood, thereby bringing the required oxygen.

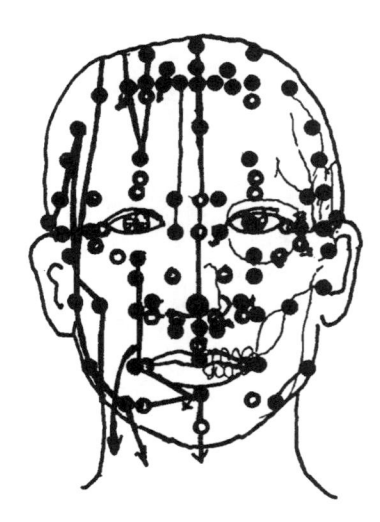

FIGURE 6-14. PRIMARY QI CHANNELS AND ACUPUNCTURE CAVITIES ON THE HEAD (FRONT VIEW).

Qigong Massage

In addition, when the muscles and the nerve network in the head are relaxed, the Qi channels will be wide open and the Qi will be able to circulate smoothly in the brain. Smooth Qi and blood circulation can prevent or even cure headaches. In addition, giving the brain cells enough Qi will slow down the natural process of degeneration. Chinese Qigong practitioners believe that the first requirement for a healthy body is to keep the brain cells healthy.

When your brain cells obtain enough oxygen and Qi, you will also be able to think more clearly. This, in turn, will increase the Qi nourishment to your spirit and raise your spirit of vitality, which is the key to longevity and health.

In massage, the head is divided into three sections: 1. the top, sides, and back of the head, 2. the face, and 3. the neck.

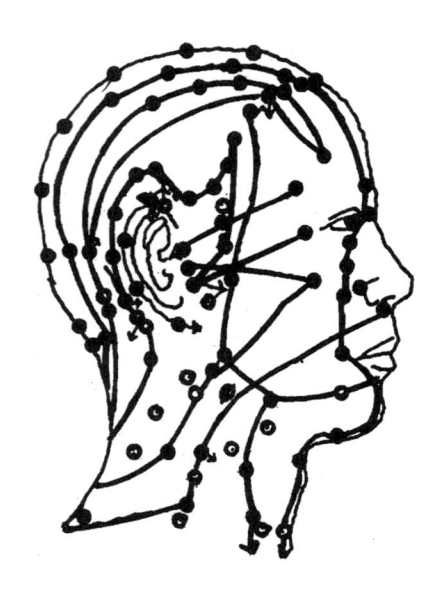

FIGURE 6-15. PRIMARY QI CHANNELS AND ACUPUNCTURE CAVITIES ON THE HEAD (SIDE VIEW).

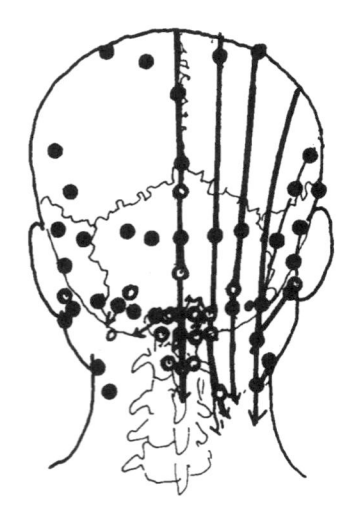

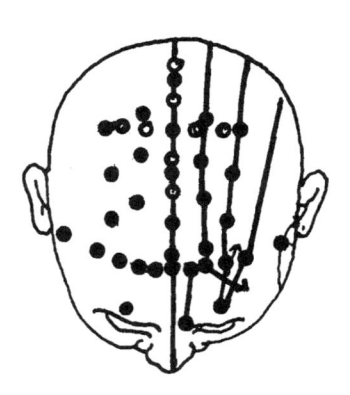

FIGURE 6-16. PRIMARY QI CHANNELS AND ACUPUNCTURE CAVITIES ON THE HEAD (BACK VIEW).

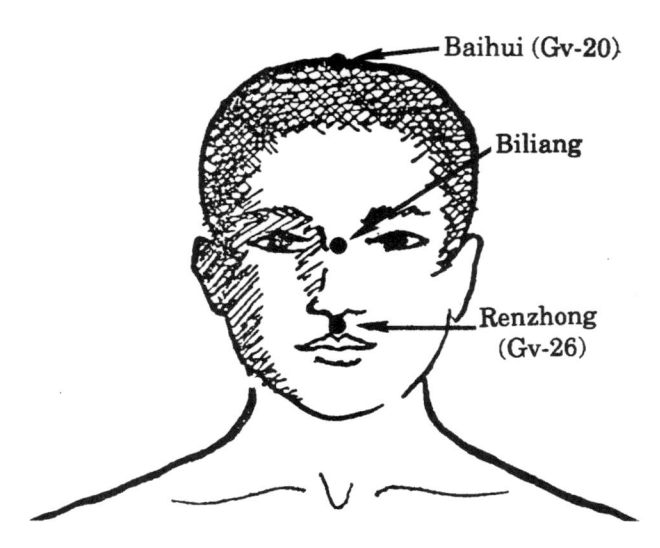

FIGURE 6-17. THE BAIHUI, BILIANG, AND RENZHONG CAVITIES.

The first section contains, as we have just seen, many nerves, blood vessels, and Qi channels hidden in the thin layer of muscle between the skin and the skull. If the nerves are tense for any reason, the muscles will tense up and hinder the smooth circulation of Qi and blood to the brain. This will result in a deficiency of Qi and blood on the top and the sides of the head, and the skin and hair will not receive the proper amount of Qi and nutrition. This deficiency is believed to be one of the main causes of gray hair and baldness.

Massaging the second section, the face, helps to keep the eyes and ears functioning well. These two senses tend to gradually fail as we get older. Massaging the face may also increase the Qi and blood circulation to the nose and mouth areas and keep them working normally.

Finally, the neck is the passageway or gate to the head for the Qi and blood. Anatomically, the neck consists of a center of bone, surrounded by many layers of muscle. Sandwiched between the layers of muscle are nerves, Qi channels, and blood vessels. The goal of massaging the neck is to relax the neck and open all of the channels and vessels.

In addition to the gate of the neck, there are many other small gates or pathways in the head. When you massage the head, you should focus on massaging and releasing the tension in these gates. They are the places where the Qi and blood can be blocked, causing problems such as headache (excess Qi and blood) or dizziness (deficient Qi and blood). Next, we will discuss the gates in the head.

Gates

Biliang (鼻樑). Biliang is not an acupuncture cavity, but it is an important gate in massage. The gate at the bridge of the nose is connected to your frontal sinuses, where your Upper Dan Tian is located (Figure 6-17). When you have a sinus problem, you get a stuffy nose. When this happens, you can lightly massage the bridge of the nose to relax

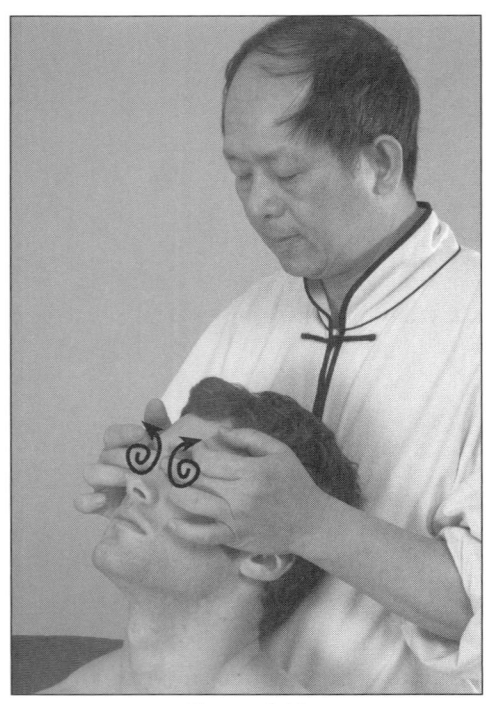

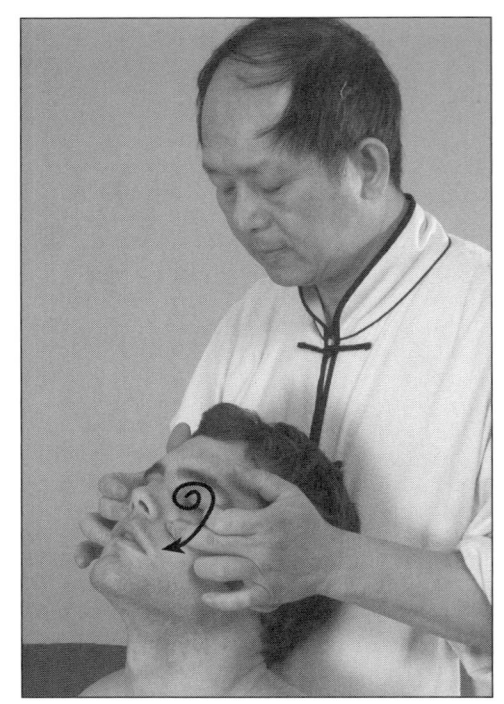

FIGURE 6-18

FIGURE 6-19

the muscles around the sinuses and nose, which will often relax the nerves there. When you have difficulty breathing, your Upper Dan Tian is disturbed and your mind will not be clear.

The bridge of the nose is right over the nasal cavity, through which air enters and leaves your body. When this area is tense, the membrane inside the nose will swell and interfere with the free flow of air. This is usually what happens when you have a cold.

The most common way to massage the bridge of the nose is to use both index fingers or middle fingers to lightly press the sides of the bridge of the nose and circle around. The circle should move in toward the center on the top of the nose, and out on the bottom, and then move up to the Upper Dan Tian (Figure 6-18). This leads the Qi upward to the forehead and then allows it to be spread upward or to the sides. Usually you circle a few times on the bridge of the nose and then lead the Qi up to the Upper Dan Tian.

Next, again use the middle finger to circle the bridge of the nose several times in the same direction mentioned, then lead the hands downward along the sides of the nose (Figure 6-19). Finally, spread the Qi to the sides of the face.

When you do this massage, your touch must be soft. Remember: *a soft touch helps relaxation, a harder press will tense up the muscles.* The motion should be smooth and continuous. This enables you to lead your partner's mind to follow your massage, and helps them to use their own Yi to lead their Qi.

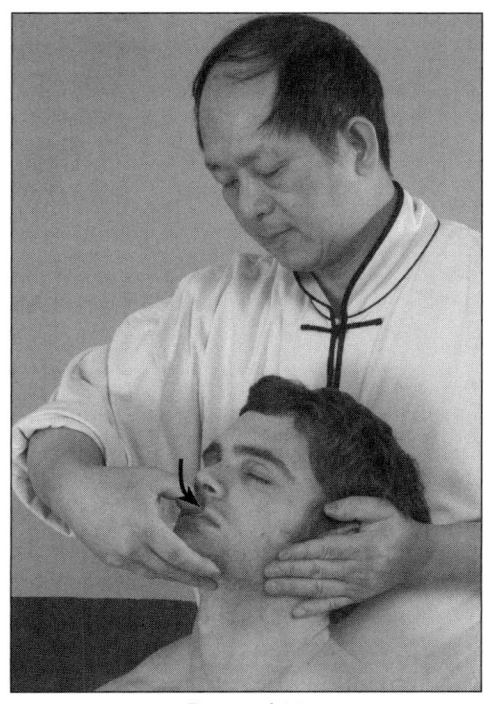

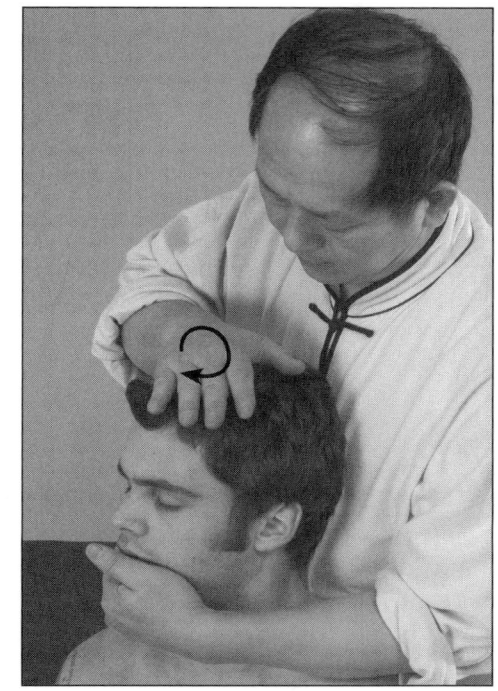

FIGURE 6-20   FIGURE 6-21

Renzhong (Gv-26) (人中). The Renzhong (Philtrum) cavity under the nose is well known to Chinese physicians and Qigong practitioners for its ability to stimulate awareness and wake people up (Figure 6-17). Stimulating this cavity will raise the Qi of the head and stop a sneeze, and it can raise the spirit and immediately revive a person out of a fainting spell. Massaging the Renzhong cavity will open blockage of the Qi channels in the head.

To massage the Renzhong, simply use the thumb or the tip of the middle finger to gently press inward firmly and vibrate (Figure 6-20).

Baihui (Gv-20) (百會). Baihui (Hundred Meetings) is the cavity or Qi gate on the top of the head which allows the brain to communicate with the Qi of nature (Figure 6-17). Qi can reach the brain easily through this gate to nourish the brain.

To massage this gate, simply place the center of your right palm on the crown of the head and gently circle your hand clockwise to nourish the brain (Figure 6-21). Reversing the direction and circling counterclockwise will release Qi from the brain and relieve a headache.

Qigong Massage

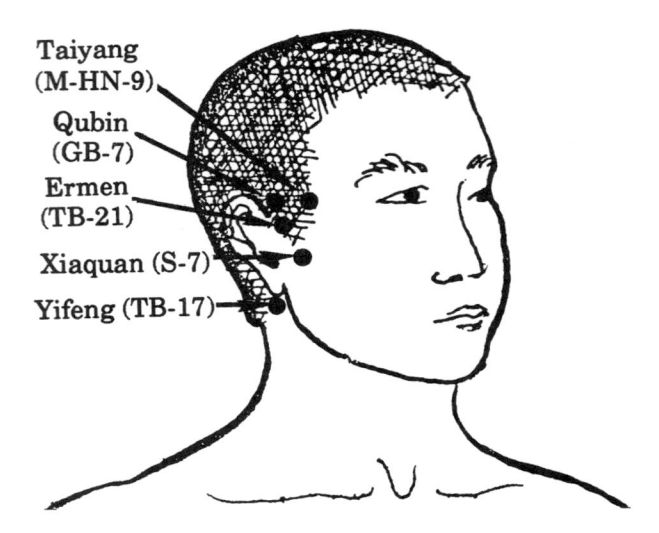

FIGURE 6-22. THE TAIYANG, QUBIN, ERMEN, XIAQUAN, AND YIFENG CAVITIES.

Taiyang (M-HN-9) (太陽). The Taiyang (Sun or Great Yang) cavities are also known as the temples (Figure 6-22). Whenever your brain gets fatigued from too much worry or thinking, the muscles in the temple area will tense up. This can disturb the supply of Qi and blood and cause a headache. It is therefore important to open this gate by lightly massaging the temple areas to loosen up the muscles, and let the blood circulate.

The index and middle fingers are usually used to massage the temples with a circular motion. When you massage the temples, you should circle down to the neck and then to your partner's front and up to the head and finally to the back with a gentle and soft power (Figure 6-23). After you have circled a few times, move the massage downward to the chin to dissipate the Qi and blood from the temples. You may repeat the process several times to release the pressure in the temple areas.

Yifeng (TB-17) (翳風). The two Yifeng (Shielding Wind) cavities are very important gates which are located under the ears. A major artery runs below each ear on its way to the brain (Figure 6-22). Whenever the muscles on the sides of the neck are tight, the arteries will be constricted and the brain will not receive enough oxygen. This will cause dizziness. Constriction here may also hinder the blood returning from the head to the heart and cause headache.

Massage with your thumbs or middle finger in a circular motion, up the front and down the back (Figure 5-24). This will spread the stagnant Qi backward to the neck muscles. After circling a few times, push downward to the bottom of the neck. Repeat the process several times until you feel the areas under the ears relax.

Ermen (TB-21) (耳門). Ermen (Ear's Door), which is located in front of the ear, is on the artery coming from the Yifeng cavity (Figure 6-22). In massage, the Yifeng (TB-17) (翳風), Ermen, and Qubin (GB-7) (曲鬢) cavities are frequently treated as one, since

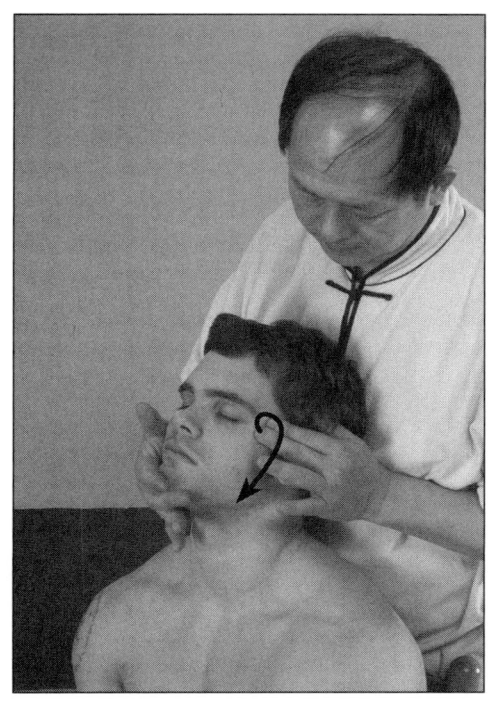

FIGURE 6-23

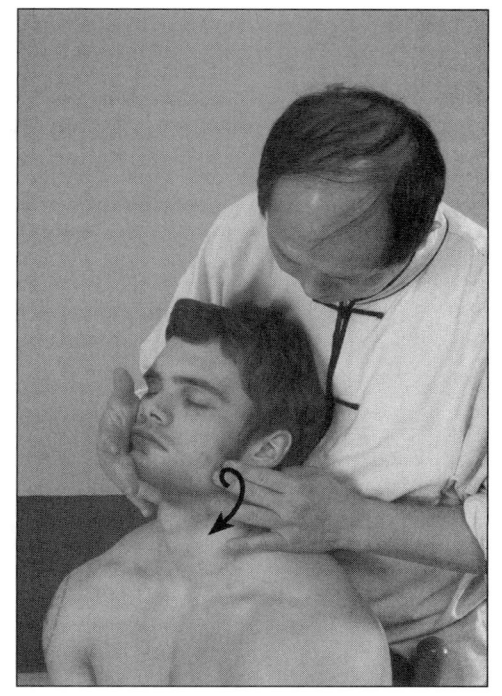

FIGURE 6-24

they are all in a line on the main artery.

While the Yifeng cavity is massaged downward, Ermen and Qubin are massaged upward to the top of the head. This helps in the blood distribution from the ears to the top of the head. To massage Ermen, simply use the middle finger or the second and middle fingers to gently rub the cavity with a circular motion a few times, and then gently push upward. Pass through Qubin and rub it a few times, and finish by pushing upward to lead the Qi and blood to the top of the head (Figure 6-25). When you circle, the direction should be downward to the neck, toward the back of the neck, upward, and finally forward. This will easily lead the accumulated Qi and blood upward to the top of the head.

Qubin (GB-7) (曲鬢). As mentioned above, Qubin (Crook of the Temple) is

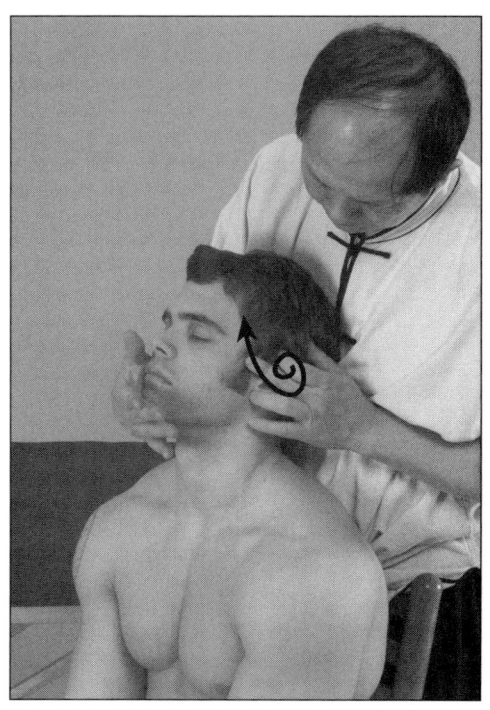

FIGURE 6-25

Qigong Massage

commonly treated together with Yifeng (TB-17) (翳風) and Ermen (TB-21) (耳門) (Figure 6-22). The Chinese believe that when a person is getting old and gray hairs are starting to appear on the sides of the head, it is because the blood and Qi are not circulating smoothly through these three cavities. See the above paragraph for the procedure for massaging this cavity.

Xiaguan (S-7) (下關). Xiaguan (Lower Hinge) is located on the joint of the jaw (Figure 6-22). Massaging Xiaguan can remove any Qi and blood stagnation in the jaw joint, and also maintain the normal functioning of the parotid gland. To massage Xiaguan, use the index and middle fingers to rub the cavity with a circular motion. Rub up and to the rear of the head, and down and forward (Figure 6-26). Circle a few times, and then gently push downward to the chin.

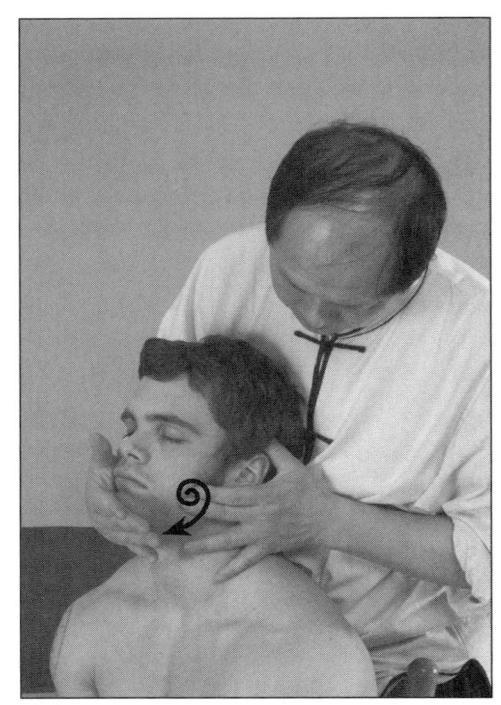

FIGURE 6-26

Tianzhu (B-10) (天柱). Tianzhu means "Heaven's Pillar," with 'heaven' referring to the head. Tianzhu is located on the back of the neck (Figure 6-27).

The neck is the gate through which Qi and blood move from the body to the head, and any tension there will interfere with this circulation. You have to massage the neck and loosen up the muscles before the head can be really relaxed.

There are two major sets of muscles in the back of the neck which support your

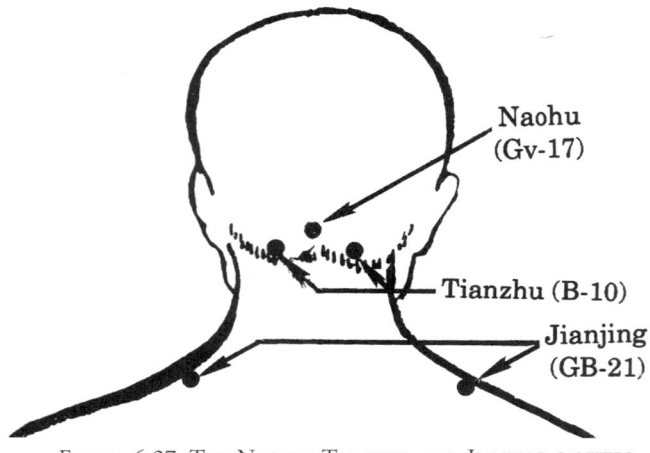

FIGURE 6-27. THE NAOHU, TIANZHU, AND JIANJING CAVITIES.

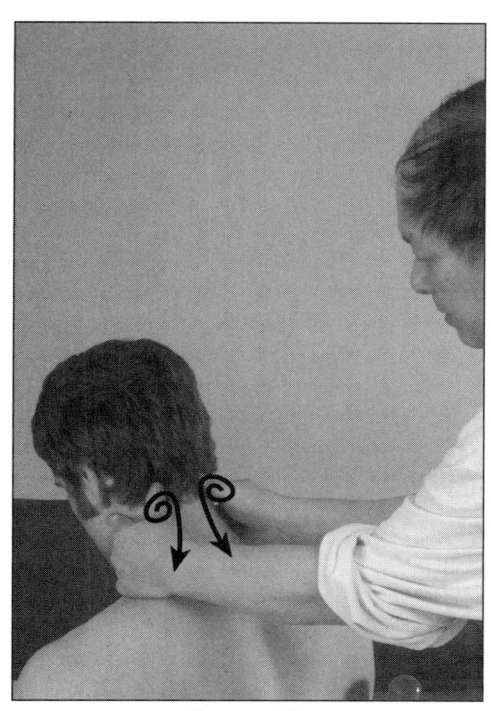

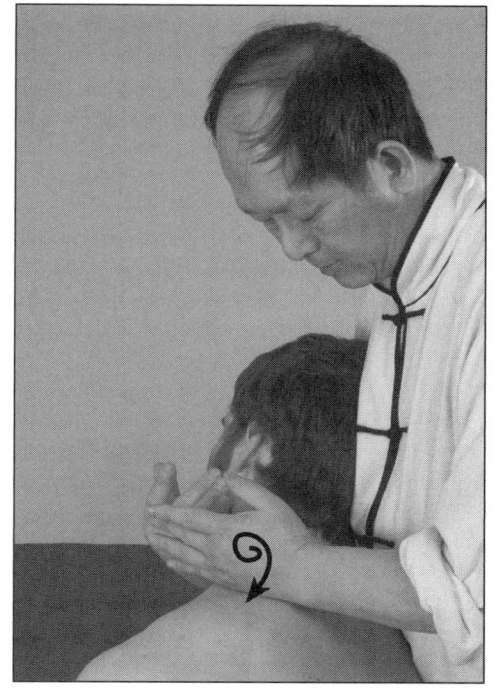

FIGURE 6-28

FIGURE 6-29

head. When you massage the neck, most of your attention should be on these two sets of muscles. Although there are some muscles on the side of the neck, they only turn the head, and you do not need to spend too much time with them. A light, brief massage here will be sufficient to help your partner to more fully relax. You can lightly touch the front of the neck and move your hand over it, but do not massage it, since there are no major muscles there.

When you massage the Tianzhu cavities, you will be able to loosen the muscles on the neck easily. Tianzhu is always massaged together with the cavity Naohu (Gv-17) (腦戶), which will be discussed next. When you massage the Tianzhu cavity, if your partner is sitting, you may use your thumbs to gently press the cavities and then circle a few times, and finally push gently downward to the back of the body. The direction of the circle should be downward at the center of the neck, then sideways, upward and then toward the center (Figure 6-28). Alternatively, you may use one of your hands to stabilize your partner's head while using the edge of the other hand to massage Tianzhu in the direction mentioned above (Figure 6-29).

You can usually achieve maximum relaxation of the neck by massaging it with your partner lying on their back. Since the neck muscles are not supporting the head, they are already relaxed. Sit or kneel above your partner's head and gently press upward on the cavities with your index and middle fingers. Move your fingers in a circular motion

Qigong Massage

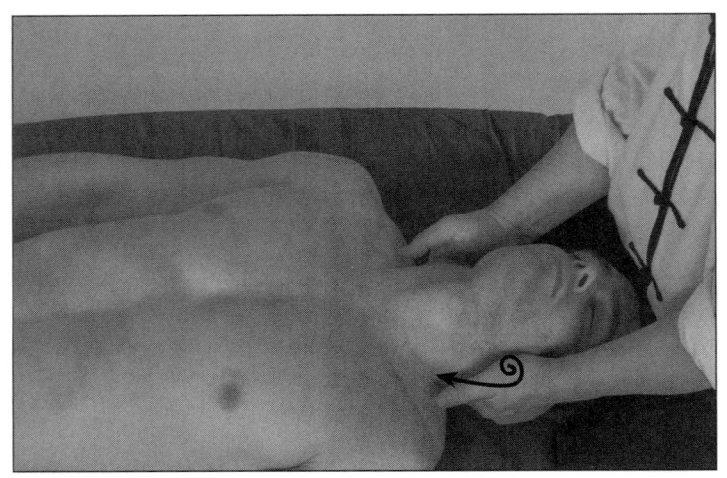

FIGURE 6-30

in the direction mentioned above and then lead the Qi sideward to the shoulders (Figure 6-30).

Naohu (Gv-17) (腦戶). Naohu means "Brain's Household." This cavity is located in the middle of the back of the neck, between the two main muscles and just under the skeleton (Figure 6-27). It is called Brain's Household because it is the entrance through which Qi enters the brain. Massaging this door and relaxing the muscles there is believed to improve Qi communication between the brain and the body.

To massage this cavity, simply use your right thumb (when your partner is sitting) or the right middle finger (when partner is lying down) to gently press the cavity with a circular rubbing motion (Figure 6-31). The clockwise direction is for nourishment, while counterclockwise is for releasing.

These ten gates should be done first when you massage the head. If the muscles around these gates remain tense, the Qi and blood circulation will be affected. When you massage these gates, do not cause any pain, since this will only make the muscles more tense. Simply massage them lightly in the appropriate direction before you start massaging the pathways. Remember to rub your hands together until they are warm before you touch your partner.

Massaging the Head

Next, we will introduce some of the common massage techniques and pathways on the head which are used in general massage. There are two common positions which can be used to massage the head: sitting, and lying face upward.

With your Partner Sitting

Your partner can sit cross-legged on the floor, with you kneeling behind; or in a chair, with you standing behind them. Your partner should be as comfortable as possi-

Chapter 6: General Massage

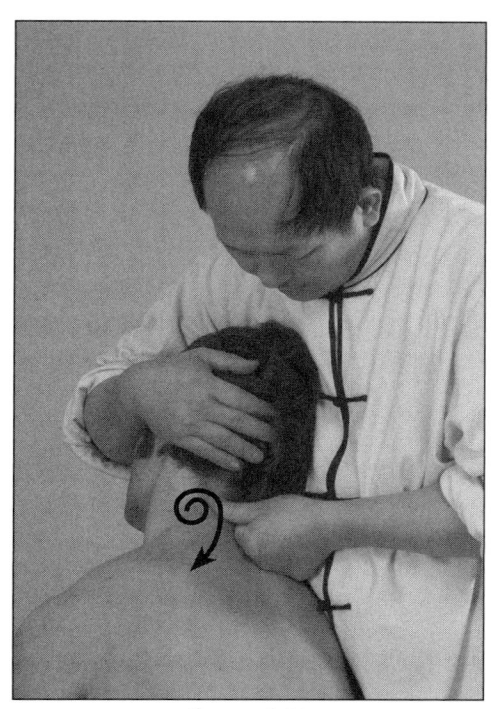

FIGURE 6-31

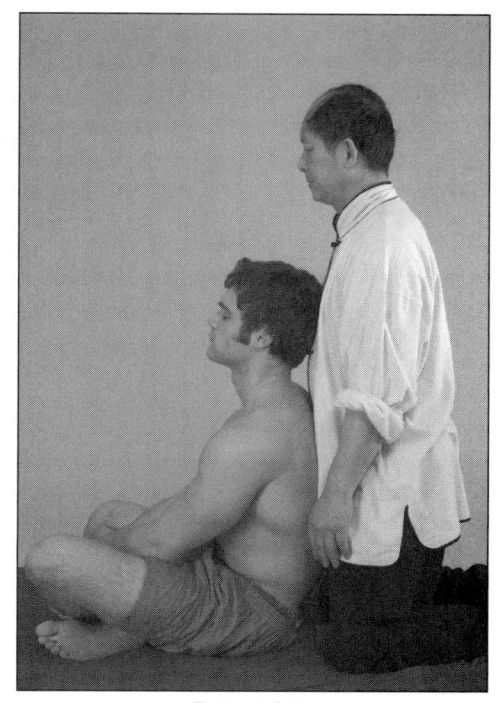

FIGURE 6-32

ble. If you let your partner lean their head against you, they will be able to relax their head and spine (Figure 6-32).

Step 1. Gently massage the bridge of the nose with your middle fingers in a circular motion about five times. Circle according to the rules discussed earlier. Then stroke the fingers upward to the center of the forehead. Finally, gently stroke your hands to the top of your partner's head, down the back of the neck, and out to the sides (Figure 6-33). Do this five to ten times. This path smoothes out the superficial circulation of the Qi and blood in the head. In order to lead the Qi out of the neck and head, after you complete each movement, grab the Jianjing (GB-21) (肩井) cavity (i.e. Shoulder Well) with the thumb and all of the fingers and massage the muscles

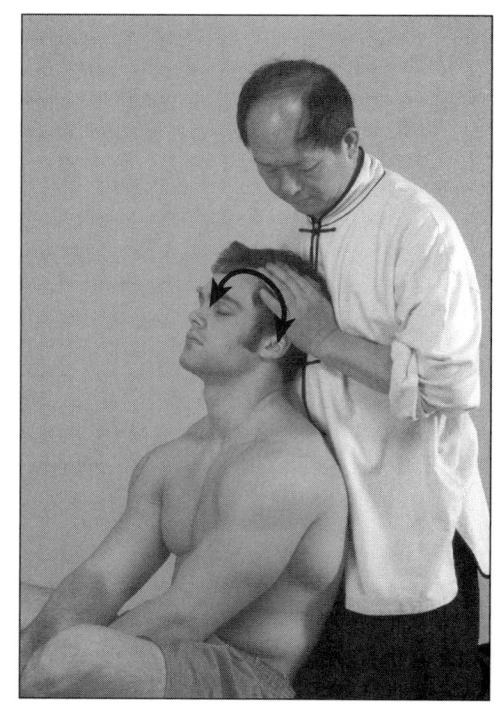

FIGURE 6-33

227

Qigong Massage

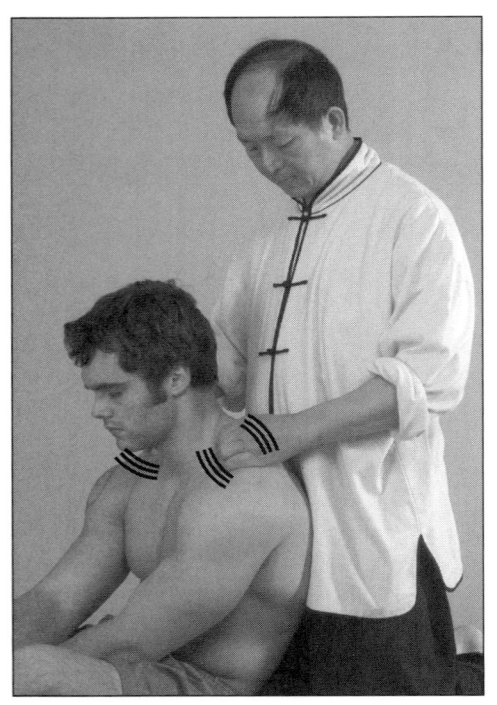

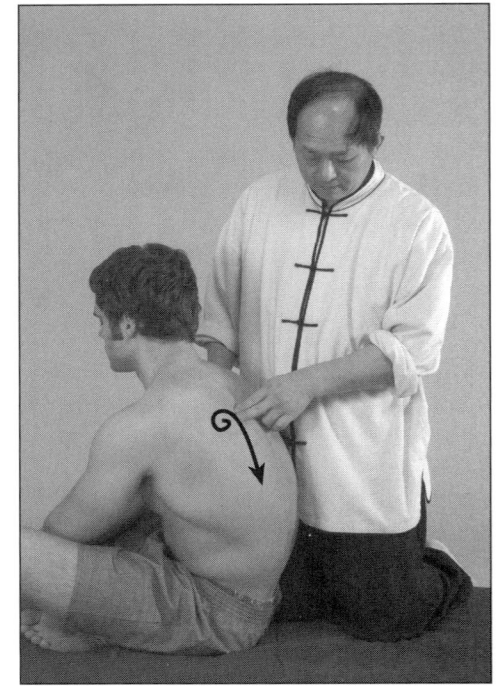

FIGURE 6-34

FIGURE 6-35

there (Figure 6-34). This will lead the Qi further out to the shoulders from the neck area. You may also massage the Gaohuang (B-38) (膏肓) cavity on the back and lead the Qi from the neck to the back (Figure 6-35). The Jianjing and Gaohuang cavities are important gates in back massage.

After you have completed this massage pathway, again circle the bridge of the nose with your middle fingers in the same direction and then gently press and brush downward along the sides of the nose. Repeat several times. Finally, use your fingers to spread from the nose area to the cheeks (Figure 6-36).

This massage will release tension in the sinus area, improve the Qi and blood circulation there, and spread the accumulated Qi and blood both upward and downward.

Step 2. Again circle your middle fingers on the bridge of your partner's nose about five times, and then move them up to the forehead. Brush with your middle and index fingers to the sides of the forehead, circle a few times on the temples (Taiyang, 太陽), brush down to the jaws and circle a few times, and finally brush down the front of the neck to the chest (Figure 6-37). Repeat the procedure five to ten times. This pathway can relax the temple and jaw areas and improve Qi and blood circulation in the face.

Step 3. Again start at the bridge of the nose. Circle your middle fingers five times, and then use your index and middle fingers to gently circle the eyes about five times. Finally, rub to the sides of the eyes and downward to the jaw (Figure 6-38). Repeat the procedure about five to ten times. Then rub your hands together until they are warm,

Chapter 6: General Massage

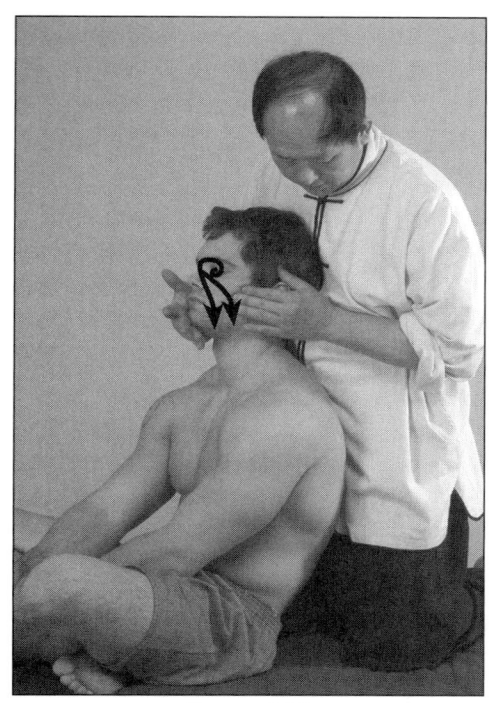

FIGURE 6-36

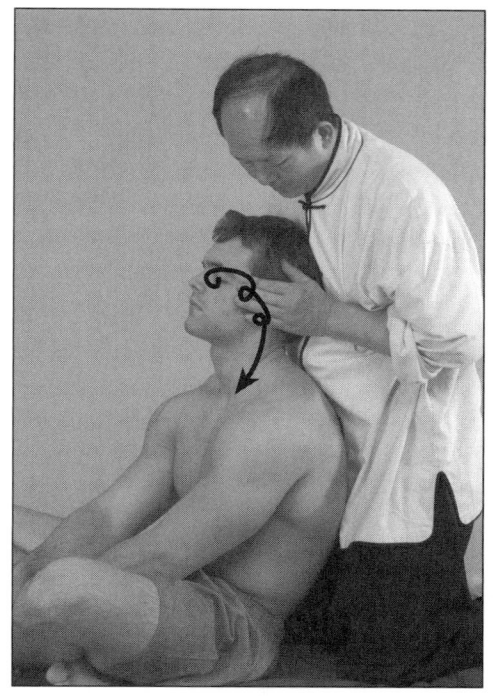

FIGURE 6-37

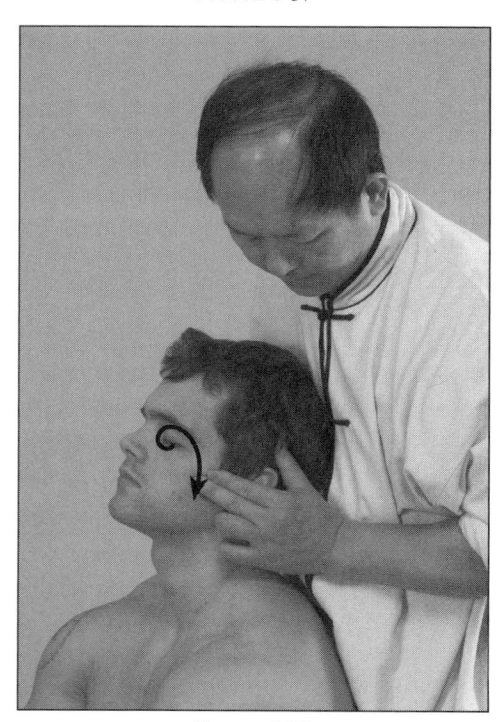

FIGURE 6-38

229

Qigong Massage

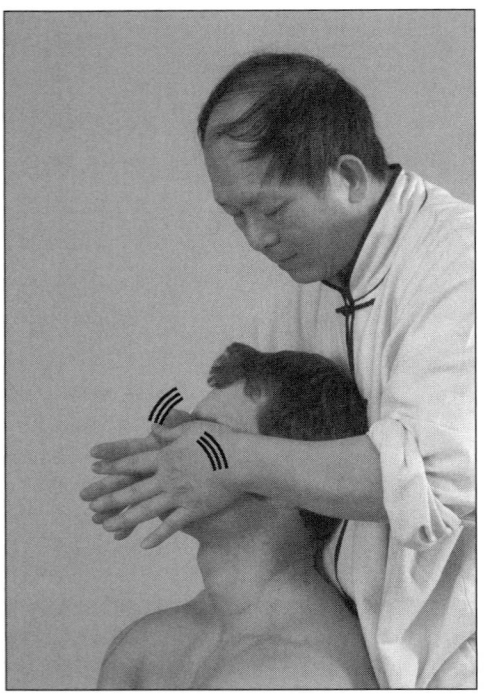

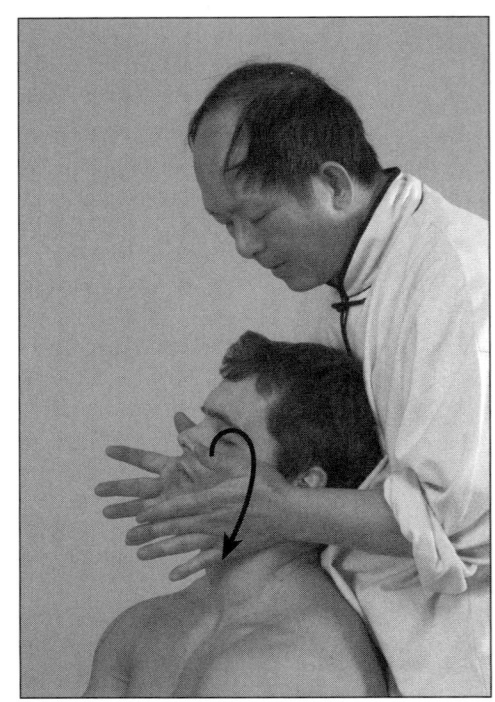

FIGURE 6-39

FIGURE 6-40

and gently place the base of your palms on your partner's eyes to nourish them with the Qi from your palms (Figure 6-39). Then stroke sideward with the base of the palms to the temples and downward to the cheeks (Figure 6-40). This is called 'ironing the eyes' (Tang Yan, 燙眼). This path improves the Qi and blood circulation around the eyes and slows the deterioration of the eyes.

Step 4. Gently press your index fingers in front of your partner's ears on the Ermen cavity, and rub lightly up and around the ears until your fingers reach the bottom of the ears, then stroke downward to the sides of the neck (Figure 6-41). Do this about five times. Next, press your hands on their ears, then circle the ears five times in one direction and then five times in the other direction (Figure 6-42). Next, press the ears and immediately release several times to pop the ears (Figure 6-43). Finally, massage the entire ear with your fingers (Figure 6-44). According to Chinese medicine, different portions of the ears correspond to different internal organs. Massaging the ears can stimulate and improve the functioning of the internal organs. This massaging path can also keep the ears functioning properly.

Chapter 6: General Massage

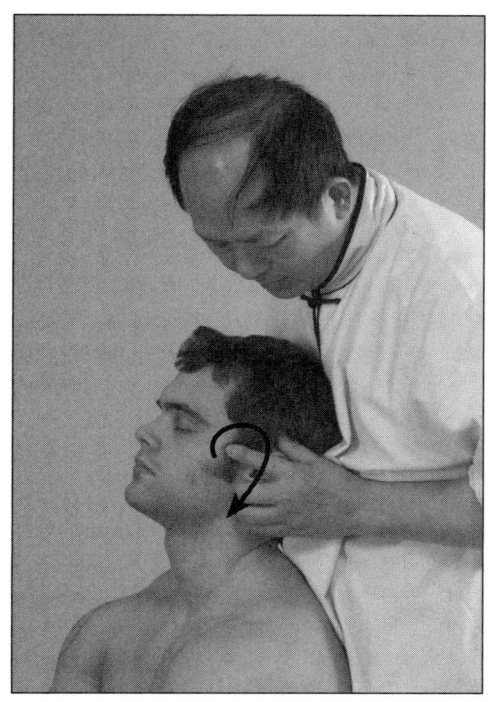

FIGURE 6-41

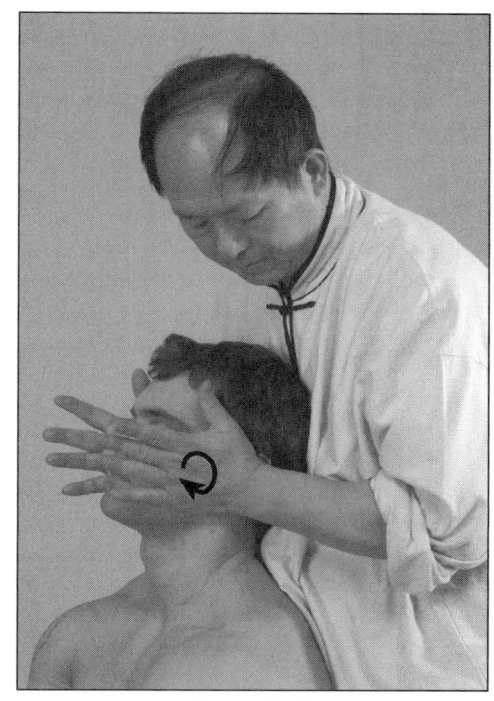

FIGURE 6-42

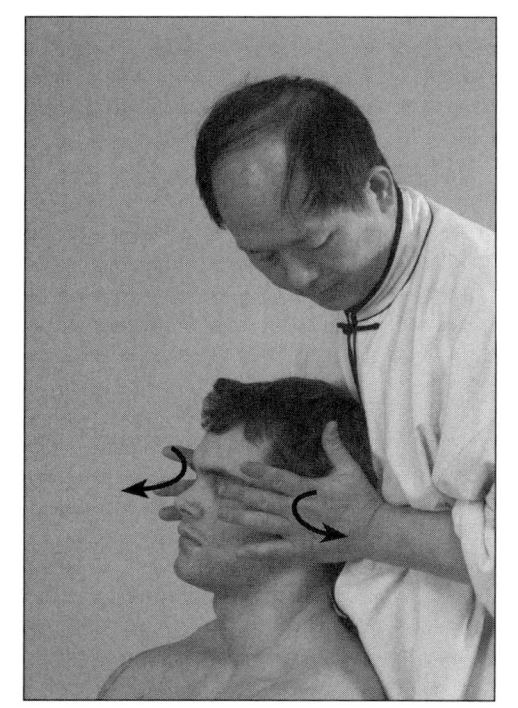

FIGURE 6-43

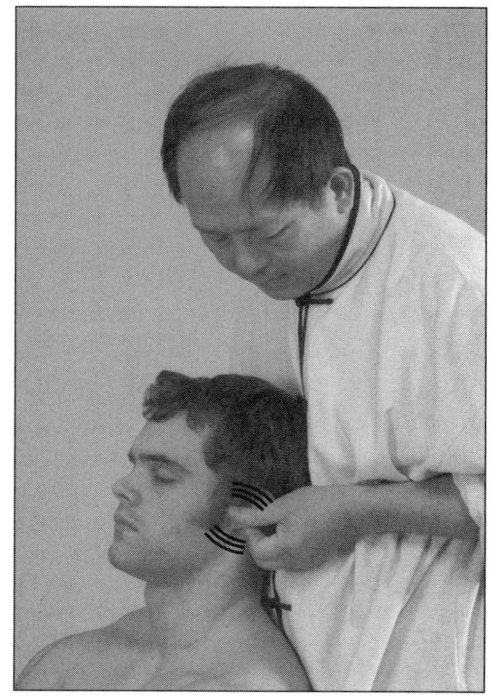

FIGURE 6-44

231

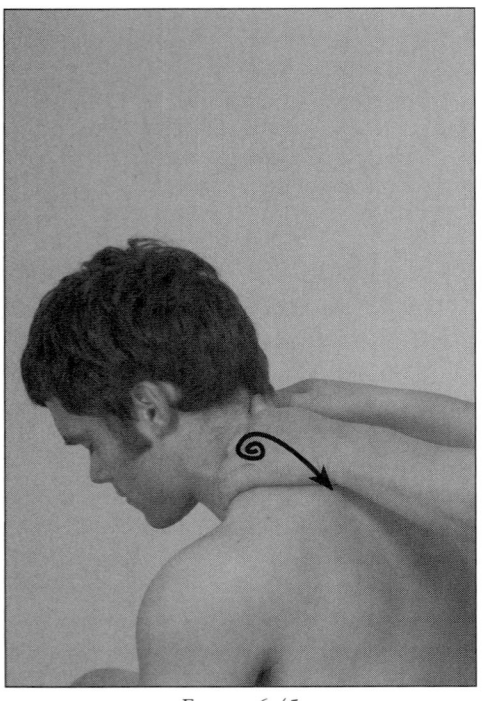

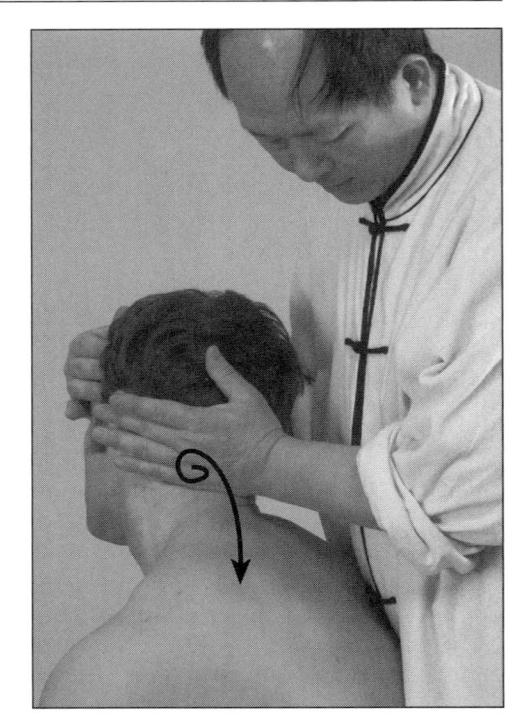

FIGURE 6-45

FIGURE 6-46

Step 5. Next, massage the muscles on the back of the neck, especially in the areas of the gates. When you massage the back of the neck, let your partner's head lean slightly backward to relax the muscles. Starting at the base of the skull, press and push with your thumbs down along the neck muscles on both sides of the spine (Figure 6-45). Alternatively, you may change your massage position and use one of your hands to support your partner's head by pressing gently forward on their forehead and using the edge of the other hand to gently rub downward on the back of the neck (Figure 6-46). Repeat ten times.

Then use the thumb and fingers of one hand to grab and rub the back of the neck ten times, paying particular attention to the Tianzhu and Naohu cavities. This loosens up the neck, and allows the Qi and blood to pass through the neck more smoothly. However, you also need to lead any excess Qi down and out of the head so that it doesn't stagnate there. Therefore, you should again grab and massage the shoulder muscles (Jianjing cavity) on both sides with your fingers (Figure 6-47). Naturally, you may again lead the Qi to the back by massaging the Gaohuang cavity on the back (Figure 6-48).

Chapter 6: General Massage

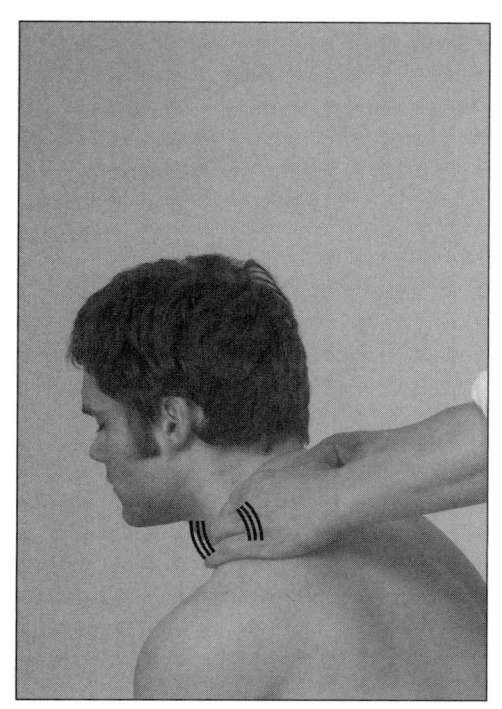

FIGURE 6-47

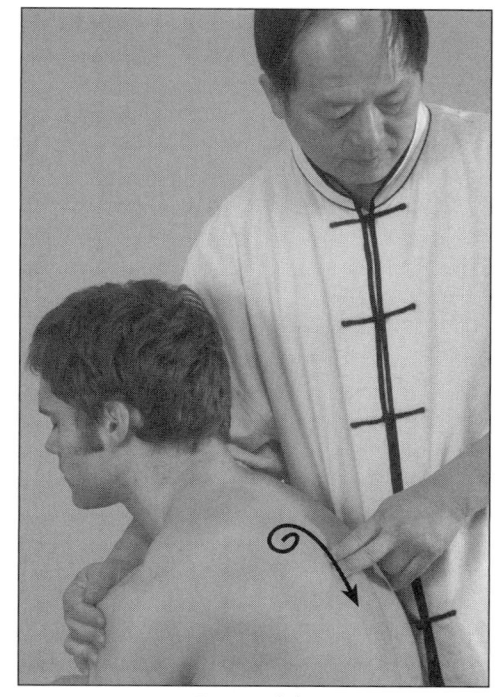

FIGURE 6-48

Step 1. This is the final pathway for massaging the head. After you have loosened up all of the gates and muscles on the head and neck, you now want to lead the Qi accumulated under the skin and in the muscles to the surface of the skin so that you can lead it downward to the neck and spread it out to the back of the body.

The first way to do this is to loosen up the fasciae between the skin and the skeleton. Simply place one or both palms on your partner's head. Gently press downward and move the skin in a circular motion (Figure 6-49). After circling a few times, stroke downward. Circle toward the center and downward to the back of the neck (Figure 6-50). You may also circle in the

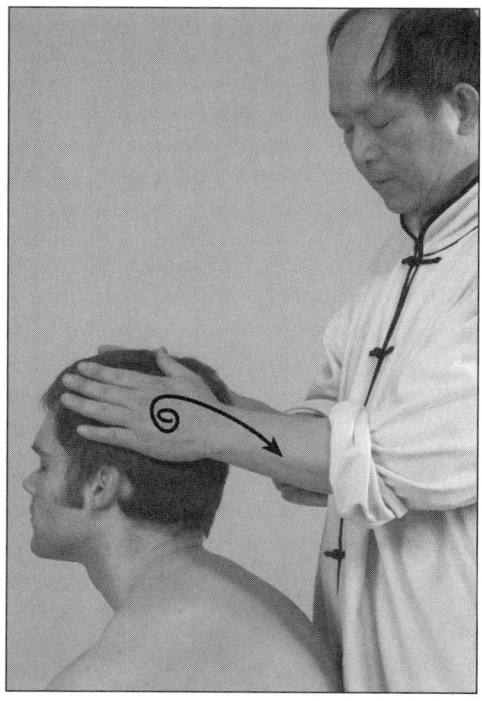

FIGURE 6-49

233

Qigong Massage

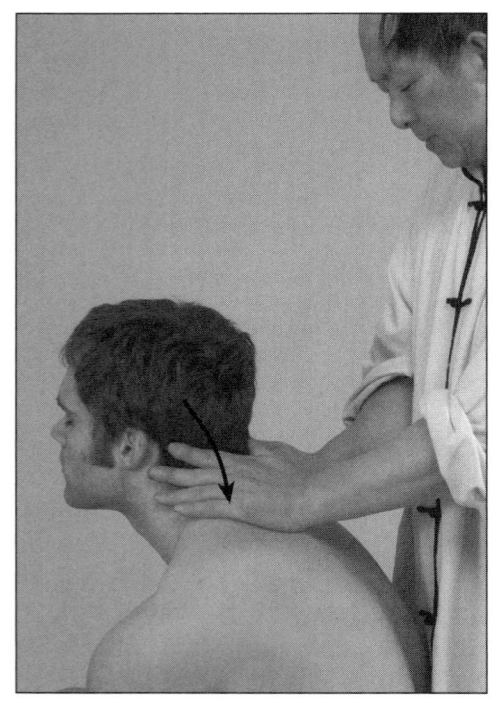

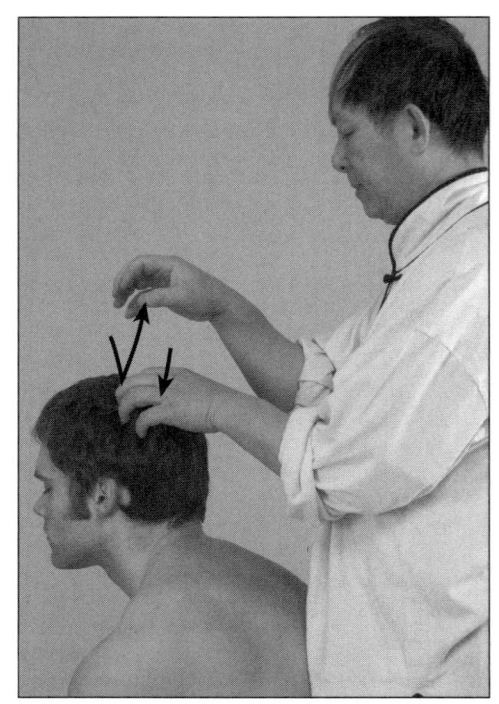

FIGURE 6-50   FIGURE 6-51

other direction to lead the Qi downward from the forehead to the face, however, experience shows that it is better to lead the Qi backward instead of forward.

Next, gently tap your fingertips over the entire head (Figure 6-51). This will lead the Qi to the surface of the skin. When you tap, you should always start at the center and move to the sides and back. After you finish tapping, again use your palms to brush the head from the top to the back of the neck and finally down to the shoulder and the back of the body.

With your Partner Lying Down

When you massage the neck, you may also have your partner lie on their back. This position has several advantages compared to the sitting position. First, the neck muscles can be very relaxed simply because they don't have to support the head. This allows you to penetrate more deeply into the neck. Second, lying down is more relaxed and more comfortable for the person being massaged, and therefore the massage can be more enjoyable.

When you massage someone who is lying down, you cannot always use the same techniques that you use when they are sitting, and sometimes you will use different parts of the hand to massage an area. However, whichever position you and your partner use, the goals and the theory of the massage remain the same.

When you massage, you should be sitting or kneeling comfortably above their head. If they are undressed, you should cover their body with a towel to keep them warm.

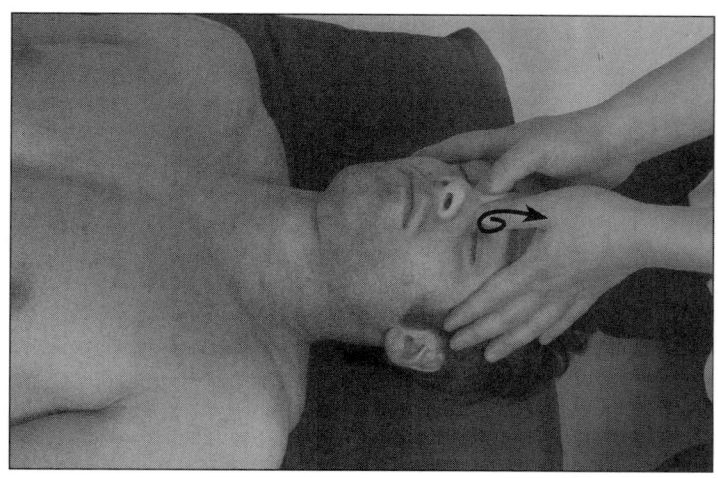

FIGURE 6-52

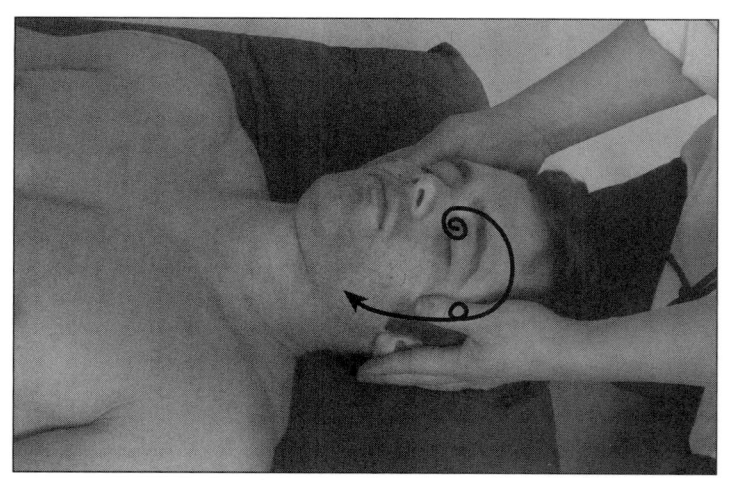

FIGURE 6-53

Step 1. Use your thumbs to gently massage the bridge of your partner's nose about five times with a circular motion (Figure 6-52). The direction of the circle should follow the rules discussed in the section on pathways in Chapter 5. Then stroke the thumbs upward to the center of the forehead. Finally, gently stroke your hands to the sides of your partner's head, circle a few times on the temples (Figure 6-53) and down the sides of their neck, and then out to the chest (Figure 6-54). Do this five to ten times.

Qigong Massage

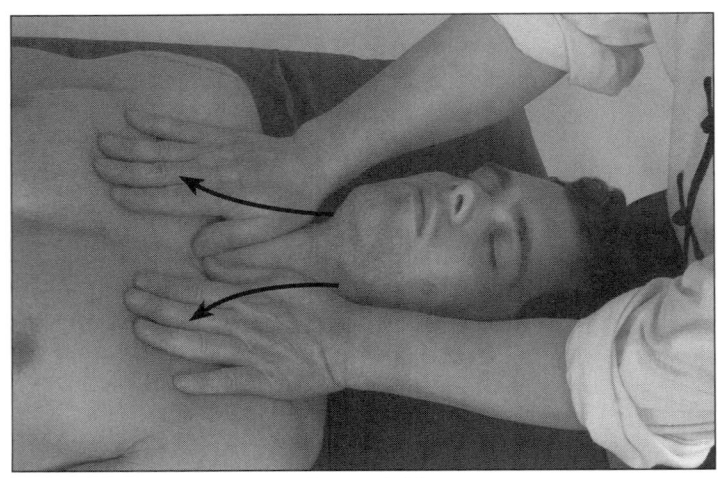

FIGURE 6-54

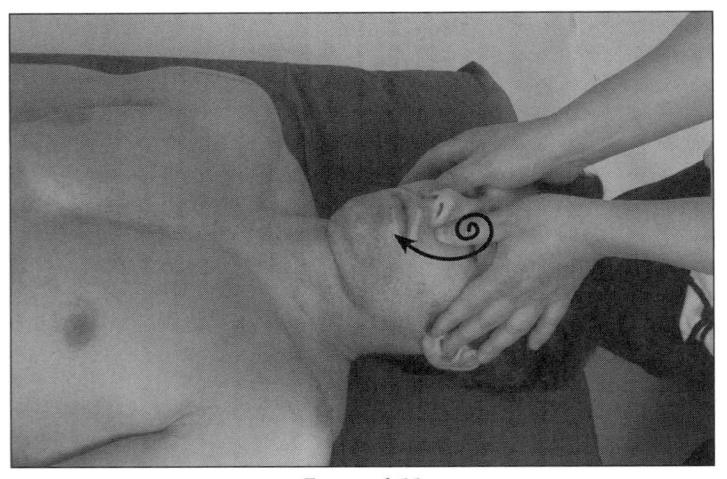

FIGURE 6-55

After you have completed this pathway, again use your thumbs or middle finger to circle the bridge of the nose in the same direction, and then gently press and brush downward along the sides of the nose. Finally, use your hands to spread from the nose area to the cheeks (Figure 6-55). Repeat several times.

This massage will release tension in the sinus area, improve Qi and blood circulation there, and disperse the accumulated Qi and blood both upward and downward.

Step 2. Again start at the bridge of the nose. Circle your thumbs five times, and then use your thumbs to gently circle the eyes about five times (Figure 6-56). Finally, rub to the sides of the eyes and downward to the jaw (Figure 6-57). Repeat the procedure five to ten times. Then rub your hands together until they are warm, and gently place the base of your thumbs on their eyes to nourish them with the Qi from your palms (Figure 6-58). Then stroke sideward with the base of the thumbs to the temples and downward to the cheeks

Chapter 6: General Massage

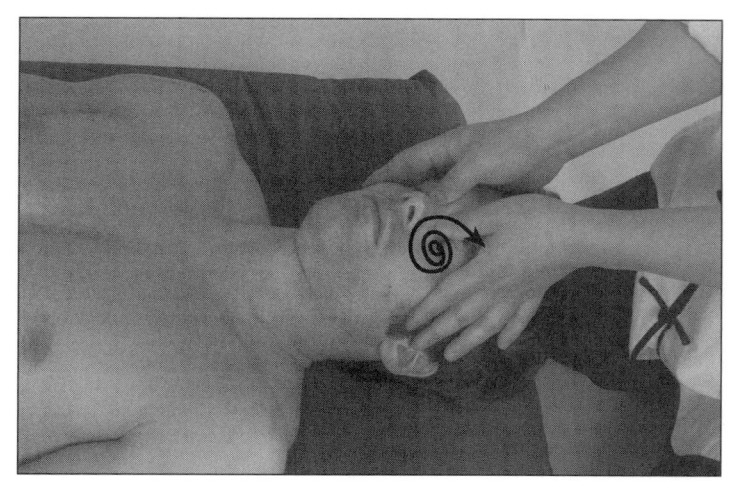

FIGURE 6-56

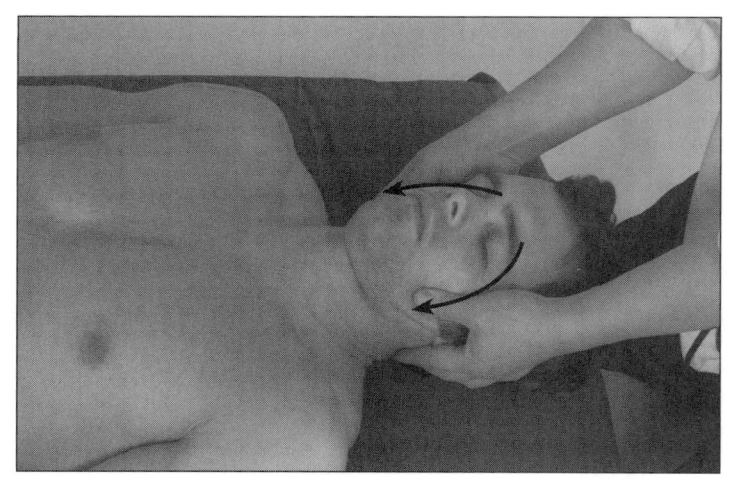

FIGURE 6-57

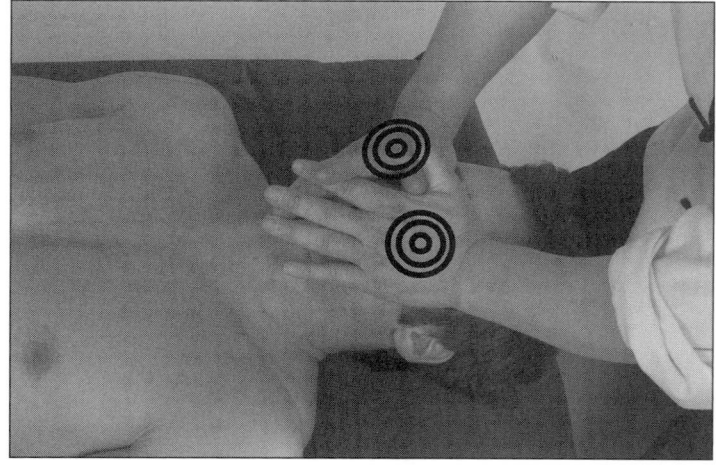

FIGURE 6-58

237

Qigong Massage

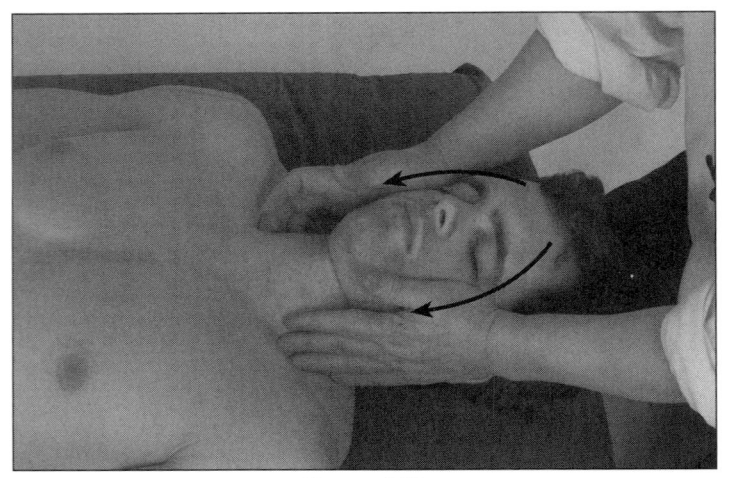

FIGURE 6-59

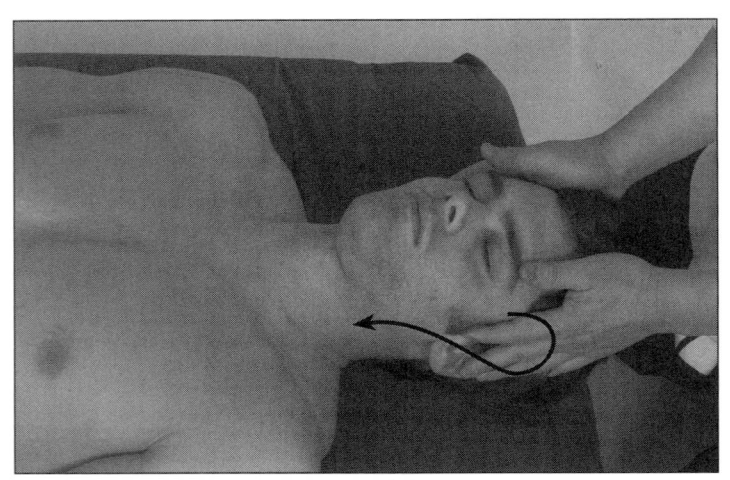

FIGURE 6-60

(Figure 6-59).

Step 3. Gently press your index fingers in front of your partner's ears on the Ermen cavity, and rub lightly up and around the ears until your fingers reach the bottoms of the ears, then stroke downward to the sides of the neck (Figure 6-60). Do this about five times. Next, press your hands on their ears, then circle the ears five times in one direction and then five times in the other direction (Figure 6-61). Then press on the ears and immediately release the pressure to pop the ears a few times (Figure 6-62). Finally, massage the entire ear with your fingers (Figure 6-63).

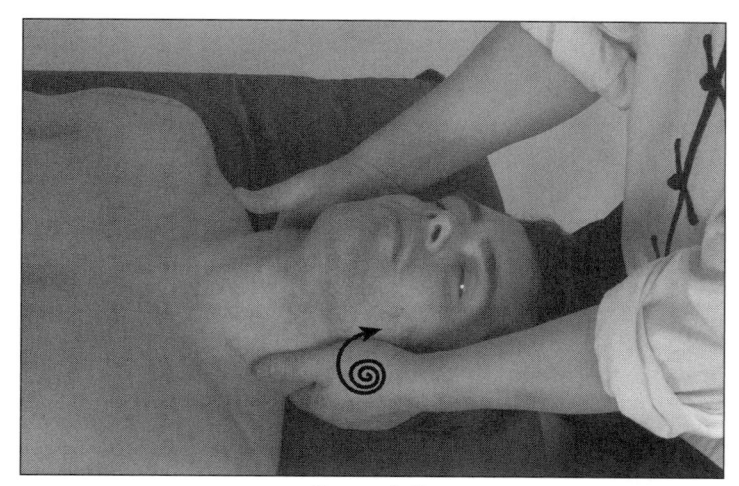

FIGURE 6-61

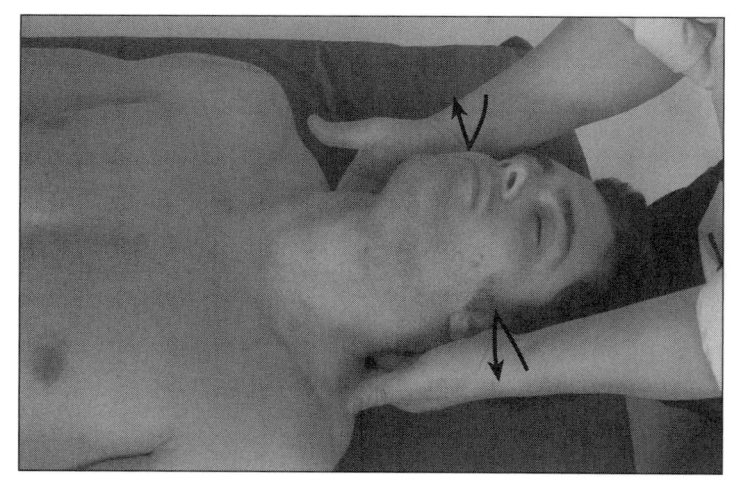

FIGURE 6-62

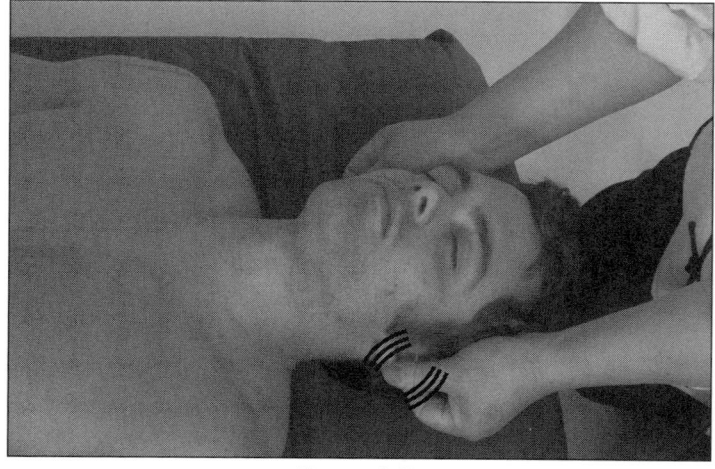

FIGURE 6-63

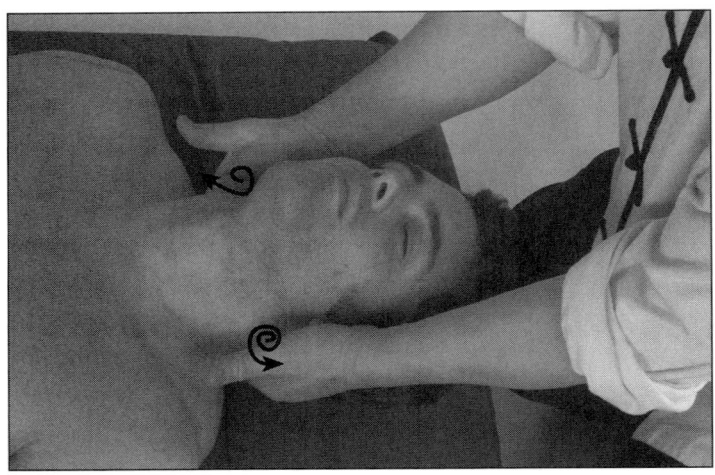

FIGURE 6-64

Step 4. Use your fingers to lift and rub the muscles on the back of the neck, especially on the gates (Figure 6-64). After you have loosened up the neck muscles, you also need to lead any excess Qi down out of the head so that it doesn't stagnate there. Therefore, grab and massage the shoulder muscles again (Jianjing cavity) on both sides (Figure 6-65). Finally, use your hands to stroke and brush from the neck to the shoulders (Figure 6-66).

Step 5. After you have loosened up all of the gates and muscles on the head and neck, you then want to loosen up the fasciae between the skin and the skeleton. Place one or both palms on your partner's head, press downward gently, and move the skin in a circular motion (Figure 6-67). After circling a few times, stroke to the sides and then downward. Finally, brush with your hands from the back of the neck to the shoulders and the chest.

Chapter 6: General Massage

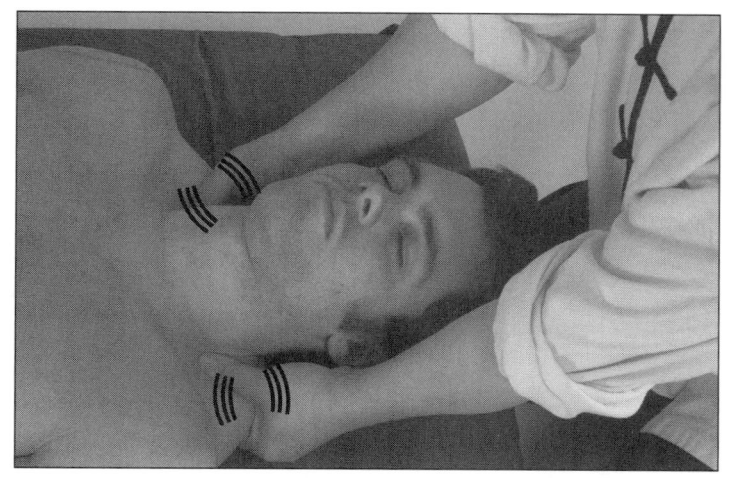

FIGURE 6-65

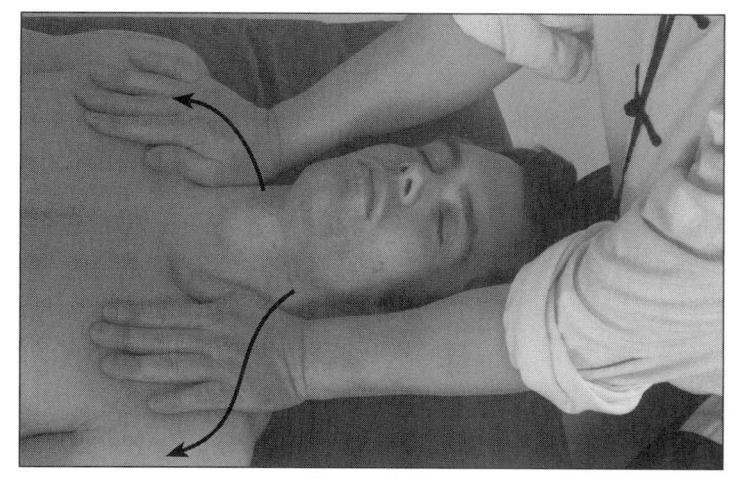

FIGURE 6-66

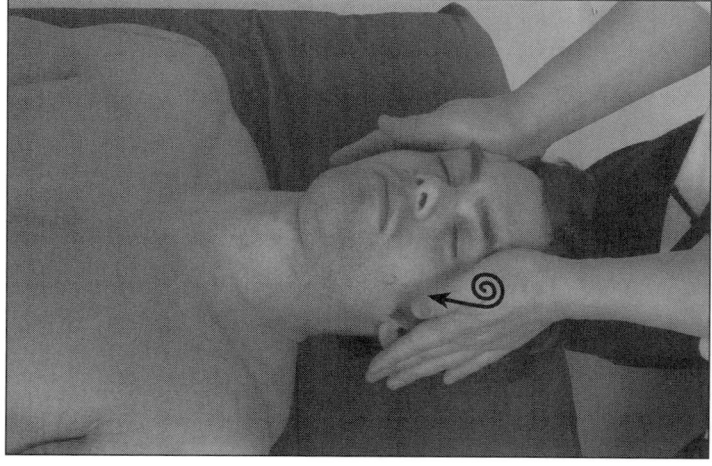

FIGURE 6-67

241

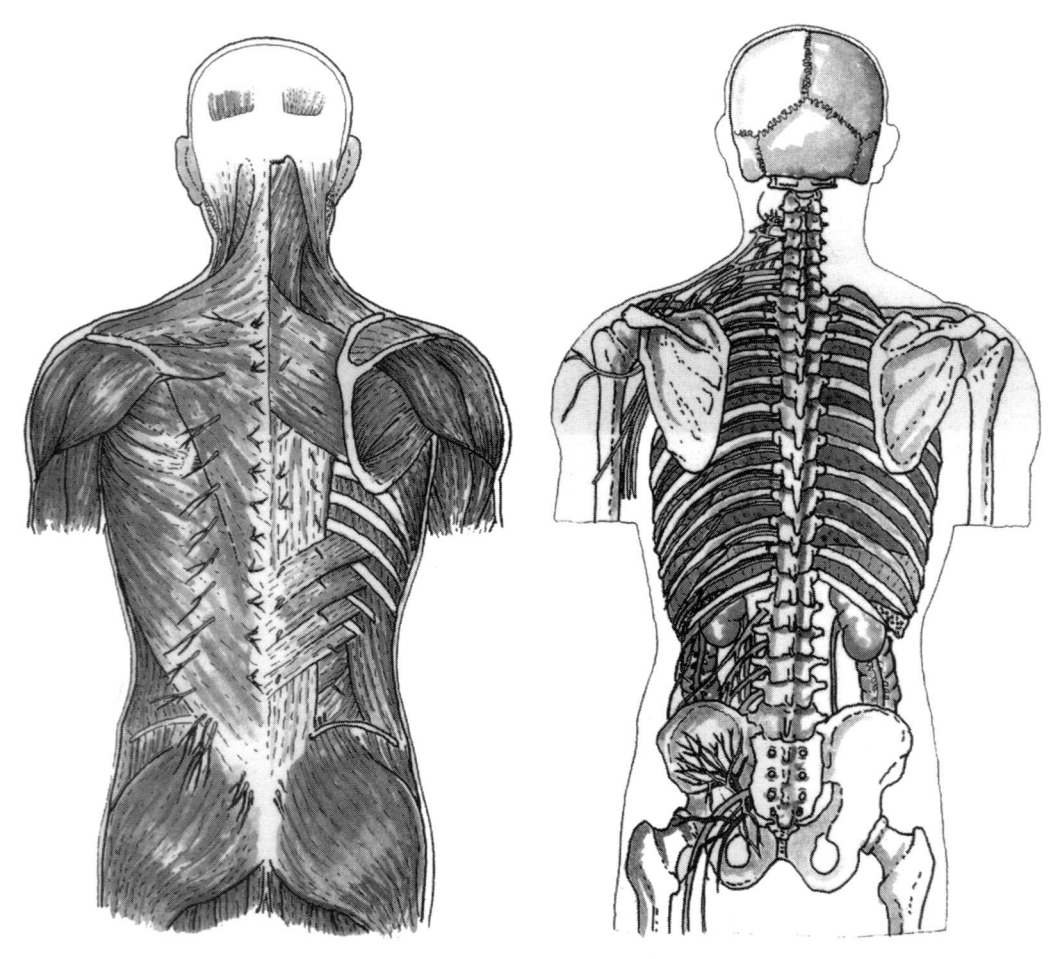

FIGURE 6-68. SUPERFICIAL ANATOMICAL STRUCTURE OF THE POSTERIOR ASPECT OF THE TRUNK.

FIGURE 6-69. DEEP ANATOMICAL STRUCTURE OF THE POSTERIOR ASPECT OF THE TRUNK.

6-4. Massaging the Back 背部按摩

The back, in this discussion, runs from the base of the neck down to the coccyx, and to the sides of the body from the armpit to the waist. Below the sides of the waist and the sacrum is considered to be part of the legs, and will be discussed in the next section.

Anatomical Structure of the Back and Its Circulatory Systems

Underneath the skin of the back are many sets of muscles and many nerves branching out from the center to the sides (Figure 6-68).

Beneath the muscles are the spine and ribs (Figure 6-69), with many nerves (PNS) branching out from the spine. The nerves from the neck vertebrae spread out to the arms, while the nerves from the lower portion of the spinal cord extend to the legs. The nerves from the middle section of the spine (the thoracic vertebrae) branch out and

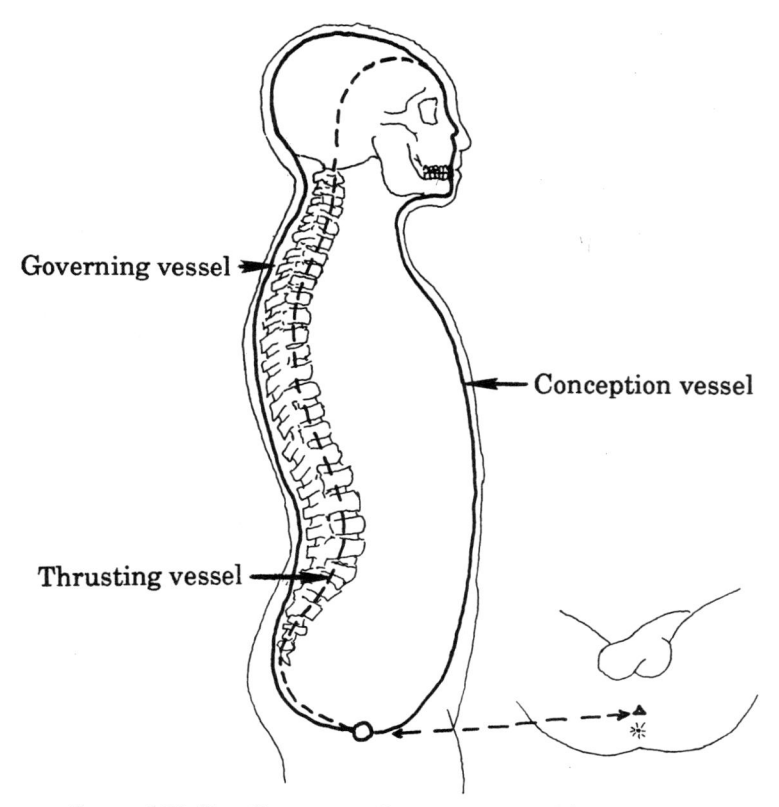

FIGURE 6-70. THE GOVERNING, CONCEPTION, AND THRUSTING VESSELS.

reach to the various internal organs.

Behind the ribs on the upper section of the back are the lungs. Behind the lowest ribs are the kidneys. Many nerves branch out to the hip area, and a big nerve passes through the pelvis to the back of the thighs.

Theory. The spine is the center of the nervous system, with nerves extending out to the brain, the limbs, and the internal organs (Figure 6-69). It is through this network that the brain controls the body.

From the point of view of Qi, the Governing Vessel (Du Mai, 督脈) runs along the back of the spine, and the Thrusting Vessel (Chong Mai, 衝脈) is inside the spinal cord (Figure 6-70). According to Chinese medicine and Qigong, the Governing Vessel is the Qi reservoir which supplies and regulates the Qi circulation in the six primary Yang channels, while the Thrusting Vessel is the reservoir which nourishes the Qi in the spinal cord and brain. The nervous system is constructed of physical cells which need to be nourished with Qi (bioelectricity) to function and stay alive. This tells us that Qi is ultimately responsible for the functioning of the nerves.

The spine is the center of our Qi distribution system, and also of our ability to sense our surroundings. If the muscles around the spine remain tense, the Qi circulation and

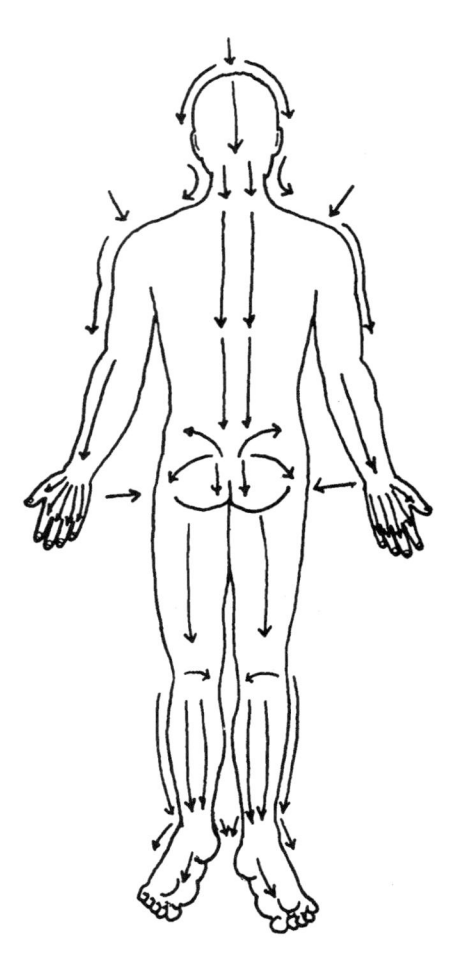

FIGURE 6-71. MASSAGE PATHWAYS ON THE BACK OF THE BODY IN GENERAL MASSAGE.

the functioning of the nerves can be affected in the whole body. Therefore, right after massaging the head, you should massage the spine and loosen up the muscles around it.

While your entire body is supported by the spine, the ability to move your body depends upon the four sets of large trunk muscles, two in the front of your body, and two in the back. Whenever these muscles are tense, your trunk will be tense, and the Qi circulation along and in the spine will be affected. Therefore, when you massage the back, you must pay particular attention to loosening up the two trunk muscles on the sides of the spine. This will also relax the kidneys beneath the muscles, and improve the Qi circulation in them.

Therefore, when you massage the back, you must first focus on the spinal area, and lead the Qi downward to the sacrum and spread it out to the hips and legs. You must also spread the Qi in the center of the back out to the sides (Figure 6-71). Next, you will focus on the trunk muscles in the back. The rule is to first lead the Qi from deep

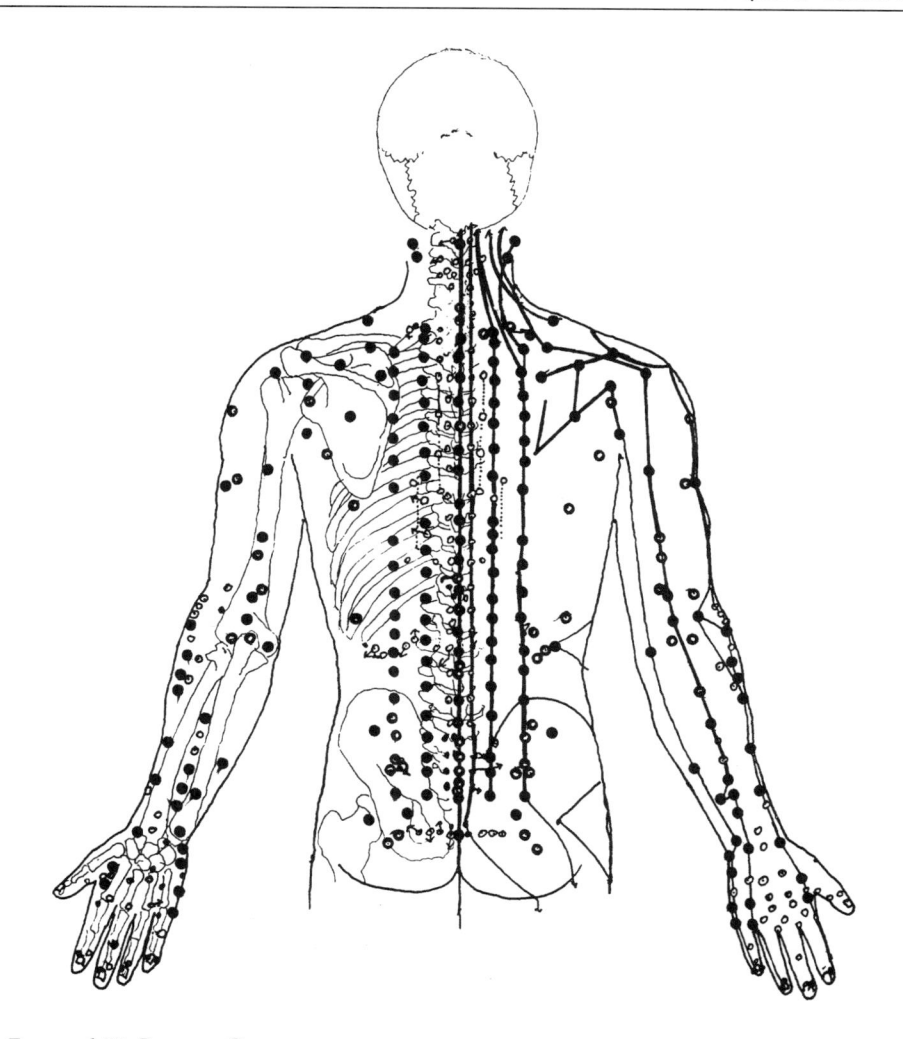

FIGURE 6-72. PRIMARY QI CHANNELS AND ACUPUNCTURE CAVITIES ON THE BACK OF THE BODY.

inside the body to the surface, and then spread it out from the top to the bottom and from the center to the sides.

Before we discuss the gates, let us first review the Qi channels in the back. As mentioned earlier, the Governing Vessel is in the center of the back along the outside of the spine, and the Thrusting Vessel is inside the spine. The Qi circulating in the Governing Vessel is used to nourish the Yang channels and the development of the physical body, while the Thrusting Vessel nourishes the marrow and the brain. In addition to the cavities on these two vessels, there are thirty-eight miscellaneous cavities (M-BW-1 to M-BW-38) on the sides of the vertebrae where the nerves branch out from the spinal cord (Figure 6-72). Stimulating these cavities properly can relax all the nerve junctions and also affect the Qi circulation in the Governing Vessel.

On each side of these cavities are two branches of the Urinary Bladder Channel of the foot (Zu Taiyang Pang Guang Jing, 足太陽膀胱經). This channel runs straight down from the top of the head to the bottom of the feet, splitting into two parallel branches in the back (Figure 6-72). On the inner branch are cavities which are closely related to the health of the internal organs. These cavities are: Feishu (B-13) (肺俞) (Lung Admittance), Xinshu (B-15) (心俞) (Heart Admittance), Ganshu (B-18) (肝俞) (Liver Admittance), Danshu (B-19) (Gall Bladder Admittance) (膽俞), Pishu (B-20) (脾俞) (Spleen Admittance), Weishu (B-21) (胃俞) (Stomach Admittance), Sanjiaoshu (三焦俞) (B-22) (Triple Burner Admittance), Shenshu (B-23) (腎俞) (Kidney Admittance), and Dachangshu (B-25) (大腸俞) (Large Intestine Admittance). Shu (俞) in Chinese means "allowance" or "admittance." Sometimes they are translated as "doors."

These cavities are related to many of the internal organs, and are the Qi entrances from the back. Actually, if you take a detailed look, you can also see that almost all of the cavities on these channels are entrances which allow the Qi to communicate with the front of the body. All of these cavities are located on the inner branch of the Urinary Bladder channel. In order to open all of these gates or doors, the spine and the trunk muscles must first be relaxed. Next, we will discuss a number of additional gates which are also important.

Gates on the Back

Jianjing (GB-21) (肩井). Jianjing means "Shoulder Well" and is the passageway between the neck and the arms. Stimulating the Jianjing cavity correctly will not only open up the Qi channels from the head to the arms, but also stimulate the skin and open all the pores. Stimulating this cavity causes a very pleasant, exciting feeling in the patient, and often gives them goose bumps all over the body. Jianjing is frequently used in acupuncture and Qigong to draw out the Qi which has accumulated in the head and thereby relieve headaches and other Qi over-concentrations in the head.

You can see that the massage of the head does not end with the neck. Once you have loosened up the neck muscles and the Qi and blood start to circulate smoothly, you need to lead the Qi which was there and has come up to the surface. Therefore you should continue on to the Jianjing cavity area (Figure 6-73), which will lead Qi from the neck to the shoulders and spread it out so that it can get back into circulation.

To open this gate, simply grasp the shoulder muscles with your thumb and fingers, and rub the muscles forward and backward, vibrating them gently (Figure 6-74). Do not use too much power when you do this, as it will be painful and cause the muscles to tense. This will seal the gates, rather than open them. After rubbing a few times the shoulder muscles should be loose and more relaxed. Then press the cavity with your index and middle fingers, and make a circular motion to stimulate the cavity more deeply (Figure 6-75). Finally, slide your hands or the edge of your hands along the

Chapter 6: General Massage

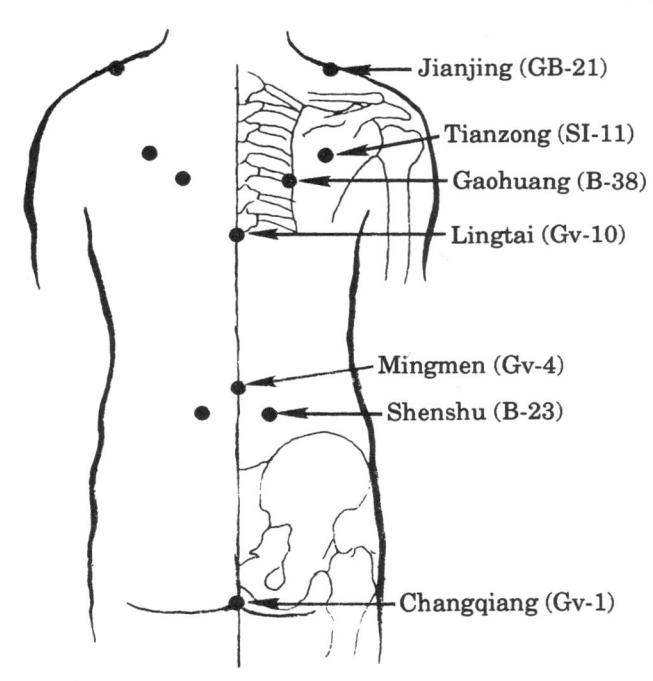

FIGURE 6-73. THE JIANJING, TIANZONG, GAOHUANG, LINGTAI, MINGMEN, SHENSHU, AND CHANGQUANG CAVITIES.

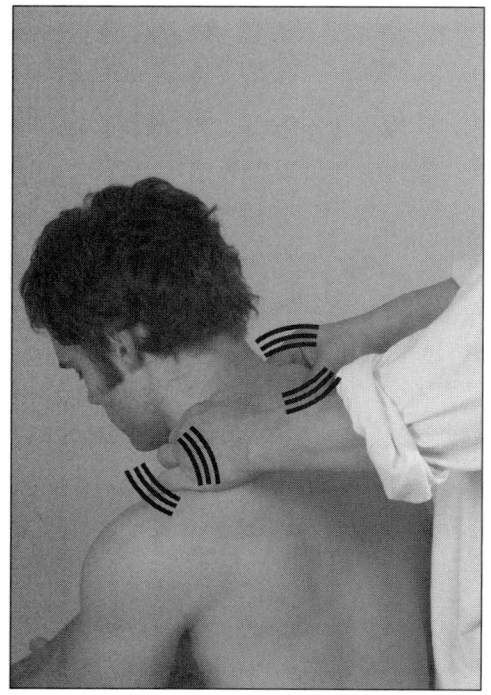

FIGURE 6-74

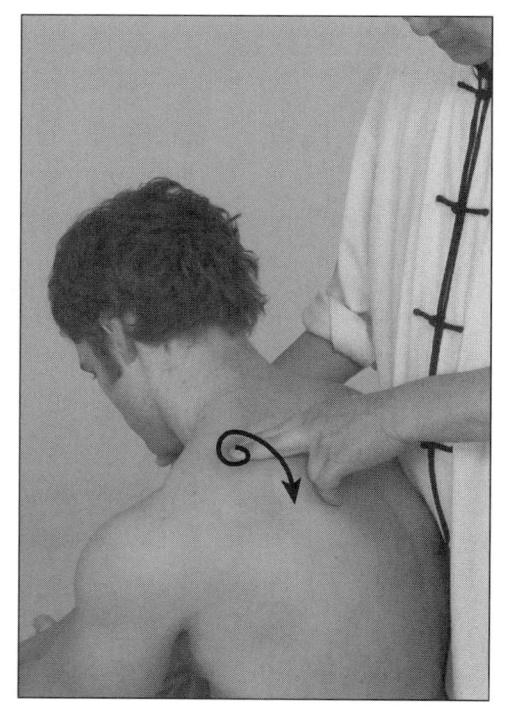

FIGURE 6-75

247

Qigong Massage

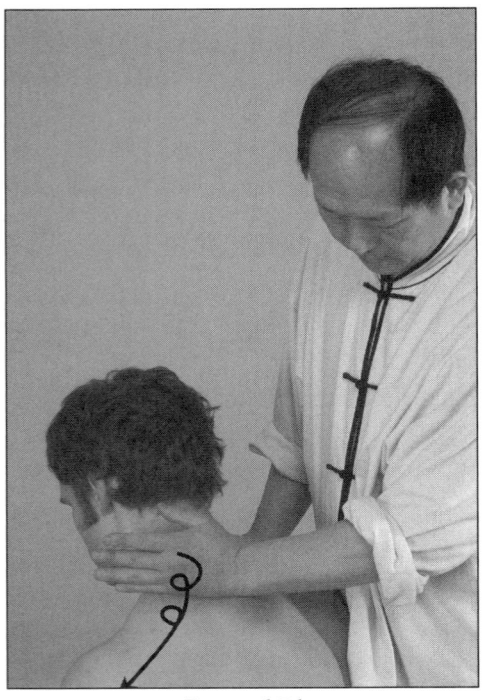

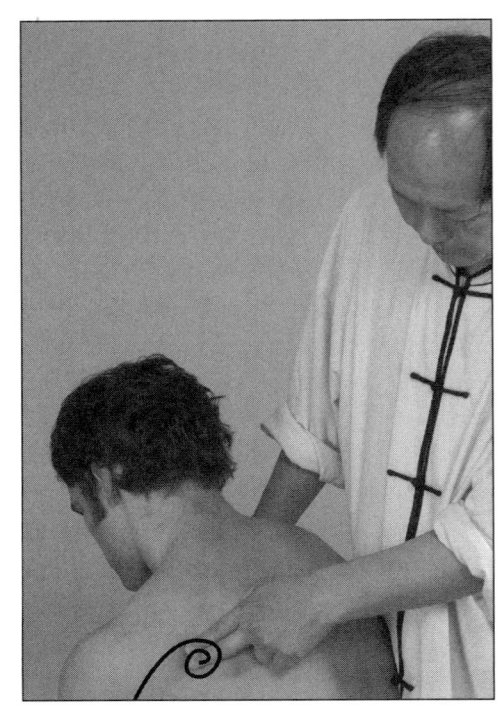

FIGURE 6-76

FIGURE 6-77

shoulder muscles and down to the shoulder joints (Figure 6-76).

Tianzong (SI-11) (天宗). The Tianzong (Heaven's Ancestor) cavity is located in the center of the shoulder blade and belongs to the small intestine channel (Figure 6-73). Tianzong is the Qi passageway between the arm and the back. In the martial arts, this cavity may be struck to paralyze the entire arm. A gentle massage, however, can open this passage and allow smooth Qi communication between the arm and the back.

To massage this cavity, use your index and middle fingers to press gently with a circular motion. If you use your right hand on the cavity located on the right, circling clockwise will lead Qi to the arms, while circling counterclockwise will lead Qi downward (Figure 6-77). You may also use the base of the palm to massage this gate.

Gaohuang (B-38) (膏肓). The Gaohuang (Vital's Hollow) cavity is located right beside the shoulder blade near the spine (Figure 6-73). In the martial arts, this cavity is struck to contract the lungs and seal the breath (Bi Qi, 閉氣). It is believed that when this cavity is seriously injured, the Qi circulation in the heart and certain other internal organs can be affected. In China, when a person is very sick and near death, it is said "Bin Ru Gaohuang" (病入膏肓), which means that "the sickness has reached the Gaohuang." The situation is then hopeless, because when the Qi is stagnant there, death is imminent.

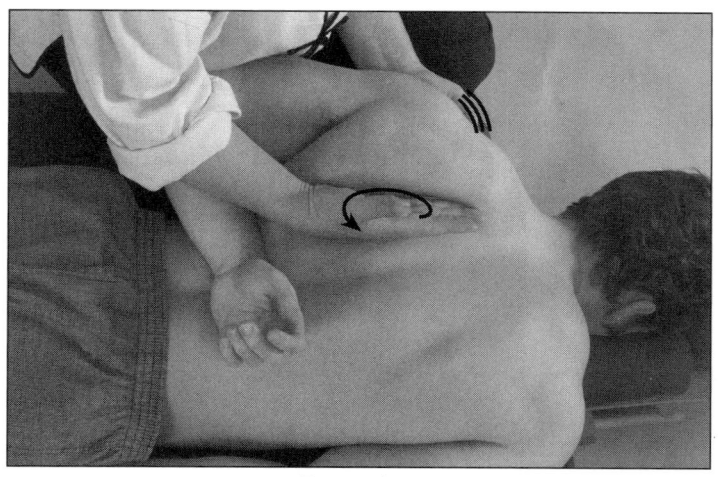

FIGURE 6-78

To massage the Gaohuang cavity, push the shoulder back slightly with one hand to loosen up the area, and then use the edge of the other hand to circle the cavity and push downward (Figure 6-78).

Lingtai (Gv-l0) (靈臺). The Lingtai cavity, or the "Spirit's Platform," is so called because it is opposite the heart (Figure 6-73). Stimulating this cavity correctly will relax the heart. However, very strong stimulation may cause a heart attack. Massaging this cavity can balance the Qi in the front and the back of the body.

When you massage Lingtai, you should not put pressure on the bones directly and cause pain. The best way to massage this cavity is to press gently with the base of the palm or side of your fist and circle. When you circle clockwise, you are nourishing the heart. However, there is usually too much Qi in the heart, so you would normally circle in a counterclockwise direction, and then lead the Qi downward to the lower back (Figure 6-79).

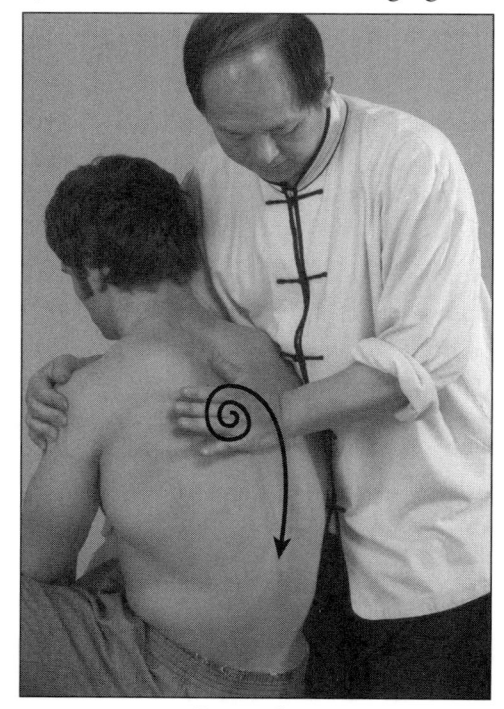

FIGURE 6-79

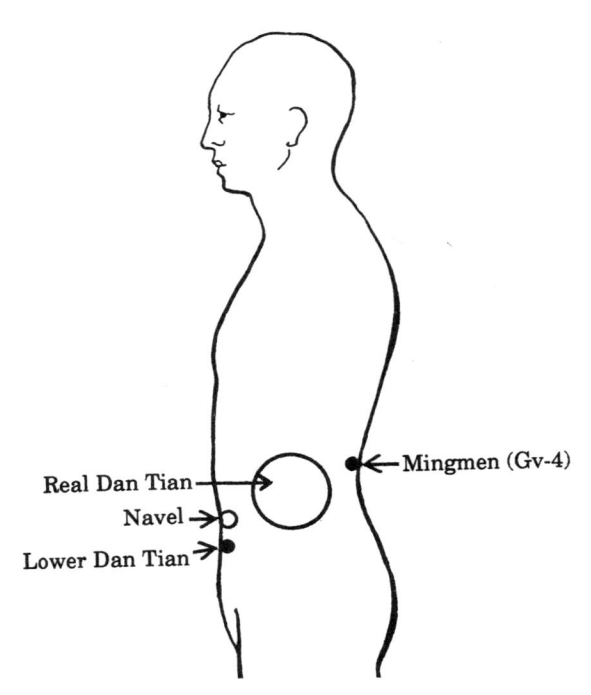

FIGURE 6-80. THE REAL DAN TIAN.

Mingmen (Gv-4) (命門). Mingmen means "Life's Door." It is called this because it is the gate through which you can reach the residence of the Qi: the Lower Dan Tian (Xia Dan Tian, 下丹田). In Qigong theory, the Lower Dan Tian in your lower abdomen is called Jia Dan Tian (假丹田), which means the "false Dan Tian," while the space between the false Dan Tian and the Mingmen is called Zhen Dan Tian (真丹田) or the "real Dan Tian" (Figure 6-80). While the false Dan Tian is the furnace which generates Qi, the real Dan Tian is the residence which stores the Qi which has been generated. According to Chinese medicine, Qi is the origin of life. The Mingmen is therefore the door to reach this Qi storage place.

On the sides of the Mingmen are the two Shenshu (B-23) (腎俞) (Kidney Admittance) cavities (Figure 6-73). Massaging these two doors can improve the Qi communication between the kidneys and the surrounding environment. When you massage Mingmen, you should also massage the Shenshu cavities.

When you massage Mingmen and Shenshu to open them, you may use the base of the palm or the side of the fist to circle them. Theoretically, you would like to nourish and increase the Qi in the Qi residence, and also nourish the Qi in your kidneys, since it is usually deficient there. Therefore, when you massage these gates, your right hand should circle clockwise while the left hand should circle counterclockwise (Figure 6-81).

Sacrum (Jian Gu) 薦骨. In Chinese Qigong, the sacrum is the junction where the Qi enters the spinal cord and reaches up to the brain. The sacrum is called Xian Gu

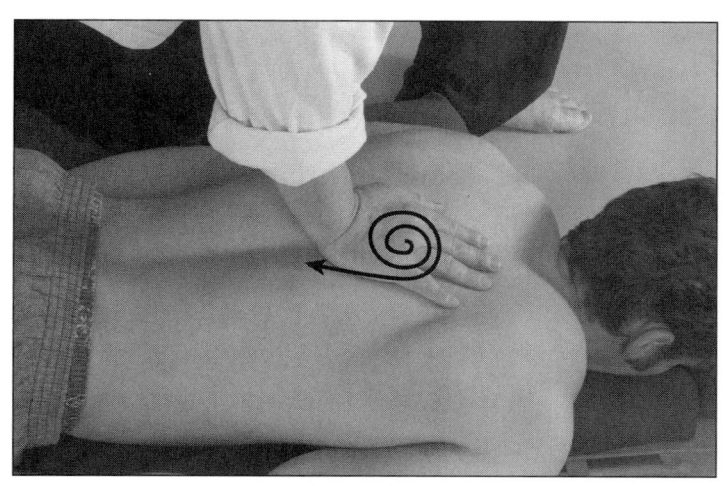

FIGURE 6-81

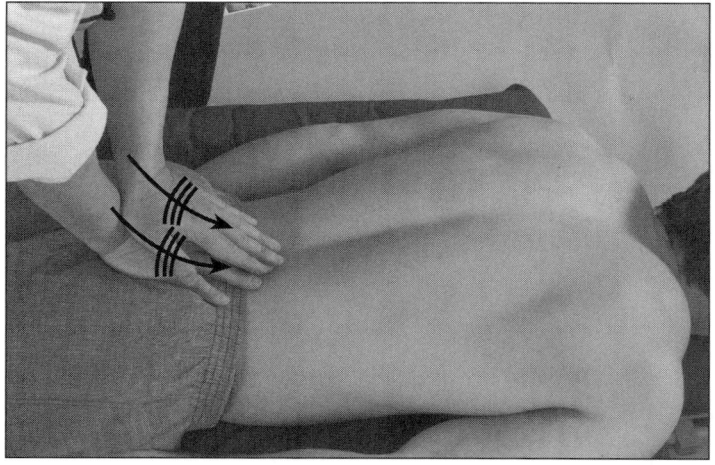

FIGURE 6-82

(仙骨), which means "immortal bone." This is because, in the advanced Qigong practices which lead the practitioner to Buddhahood or enlightenment and then immortality, the Qi must be led upward through the Thrusting Vessel (Chong Mai, 衝脈) in the spinal cord to reach the brain and nourish the spirit. To do this, you need to learn how to lead the Qi into the spinal cord through the sacrum.

Massaging the sacrum, in addition to sending a pleasant sensation to the brain, also sends Qi from the back to the bottom of the feet. This is because the sacrum connects the Qi from the legs with the Qi which goes all the way to the brain.

To massage the sacrum, use the base of your palm or the side of the fist to rub the area with a circular motion. Since this is the junction of the upward Qi and downward Qi, you should circle in both directions the same number of times (Figure 6-82).

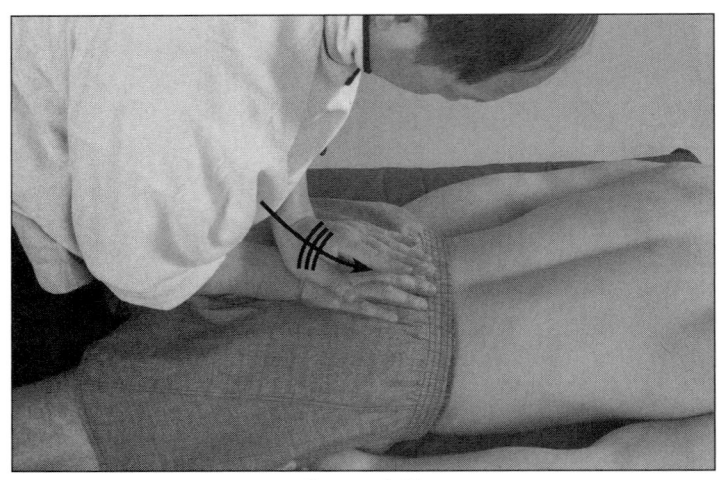

FIGURE 6-83

Changqiang (Gv-1) (長強). Changqiang (Long Strength) is also called Weilu (尾閭), which means "tailbone." The Changqiang cavity is the first cavity on the Yang Governing Vessel where the Qi circulation leaves the Yin Conception Vessel (Figure 6-73). It is believed in Chinese Qigong that, as you get older, this cavity seals up more and more, which interferes with normal Qi circulation in the Governing and Conception Vessels. When this happens, the Qi circulating in the twelve primary Qi channels will be affected and the Qi level in the twelve internal organs will not be regulated smoothly. It is believed that this is the cause of aging.

In the Chinese martial arts, Changqiang is one of the death cavities, and when it is struck it has a severe or even fatal effect.

When you massage the Changqiang cavity, first use the base of your palm to push inward and upward a few times (Figure 6-83). Next, use the base of the palm or the second and middle fingers to rub the cavity gently. If you use your right hand, massage clockwise and then push upward (Figure 6-84). This will follow the natural Qi circulation which is upward to the back from the Changqiang cavity. This can also lead the Qi to the sacrum and enter the spinal cord and bone marrow in the spine.

Before you massage the entire back, you may wish to first massage each of the above gates. You may also simply use the following techniques to massage the whole back, and pay extra attention to these gates.

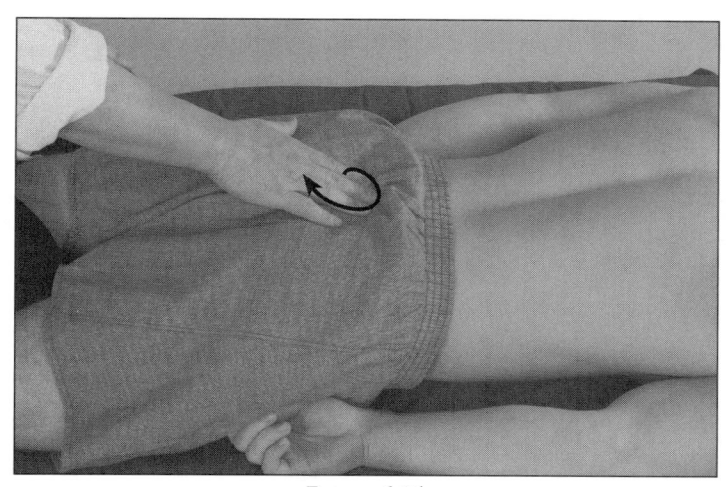

FIGURE 6-84

Massaging the Back

After you have completed the head and neck massage, you should let your partner lie face down. Ideally, you should have a massage table with a special extension for the head. If you do not, or if your partner is lying on the floor, you may place a soft pillow under their chest to keep the neck muscles relaxed, and to facilitate breathing (Figure 6-85).

Step 1. The first thing to do when you massage the back is to lead Qi from the neck to the arms and back. If you fail to do this, even though you have loosened up the head and neck the Qi will still be in the head, and it will eventually return to the problem sites. It is therefore important to remember to lead the Qi away from the head and neck.

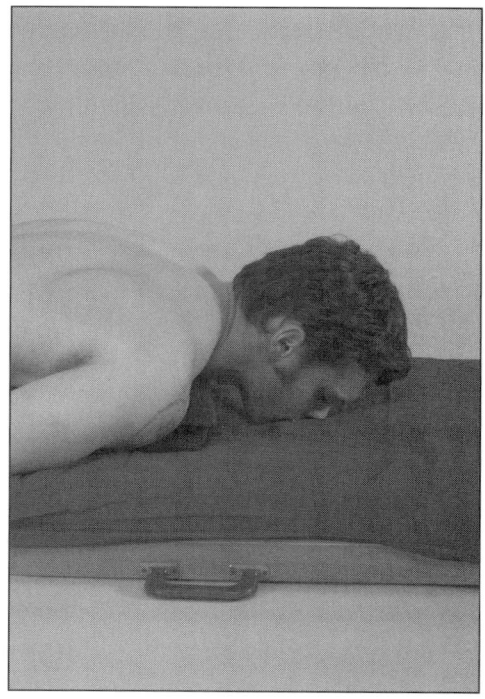

FIGURE 6-85

253

Qigong Massage

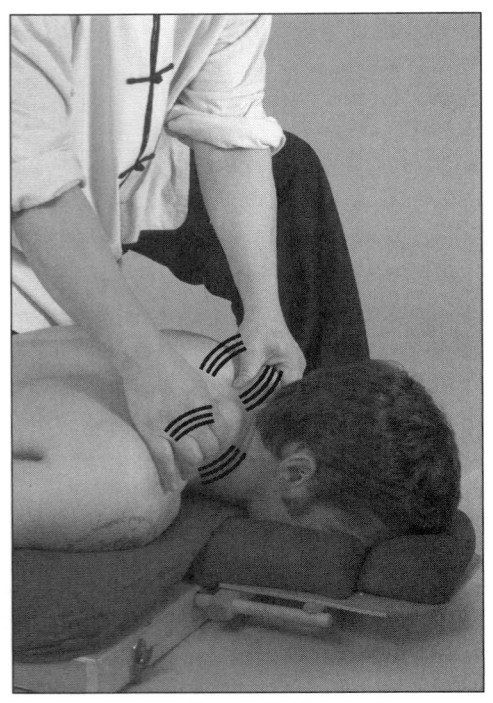

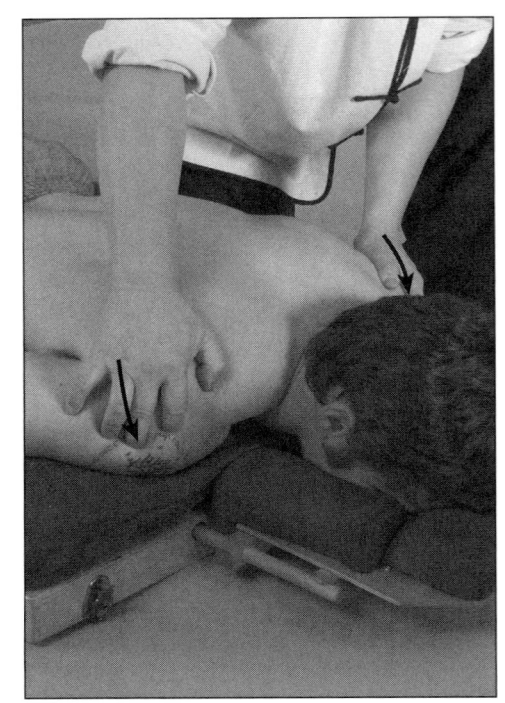

FIGURE 6-86

FIGURE 6-87

The first step is to grab and gently squeeze the Jianjing (GB-21) (肩井) cavities on the muscles between the neck and the shoulders (Figure 6-86). While you are grabbing, use your thumb to press the Jianjing cavity and rub around. Finally, use your second or middle finger to press the Jianliao (TB-14) (肩髎) cavity located on the top of the shoulder joint (Figure 6-87). This will lead the Qi to the top of the arms and spread it out there.

Next, lift your partner's shoulder up with one hand, and rub and massage the Tianzong (SI-11) (天宗) with the second and middle fingers (Figure 6-88). Continue to rub the Gaohuang (B-38) (膏肓) cavities with the edge of the other hand (Figure 6-89). This will lead Qi from the neck downward to the back.

Finally, use the base of your palms (Figure 6-90) to press the two back trunk muscles, moving down from the head to the lower back with a circular massaging motion. Massage both sides and repeat the same process about five times. This will loosen up the trunk muscles and release tension in the spine. Do not massage upward, because it would lead Qi back to the neck and cause problems.

Step 2. Once you have finished the circular pressing massage of the back trunk muscles, place one hand on top of the other and press down on each joint in the spine. Do not press on the neck. Be sure that you press on the joints, and not on the vertebrae. The purpose is to bend and loosen the joints a little (Figure 6-91). Press in coordination with your partner's breathing. Place your hands in position and ask your partner to

Chapter 6: General Massage

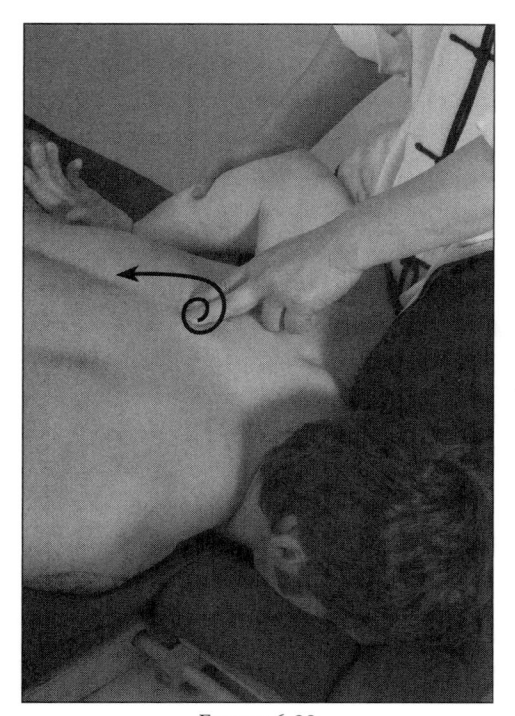

FIGURE 6-88

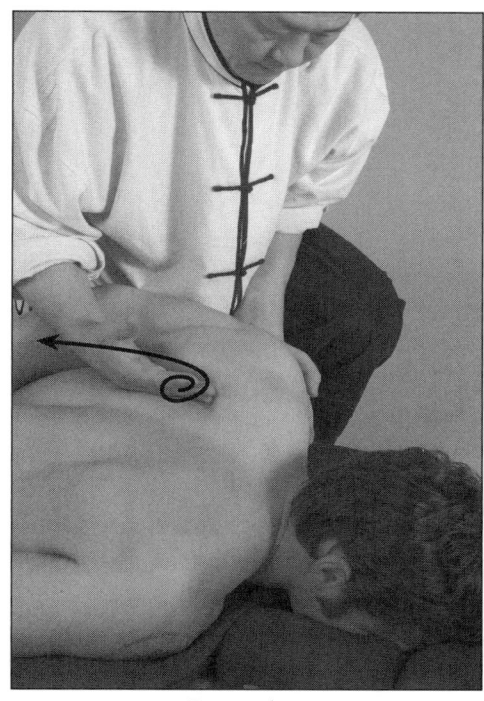

FIGURE 6-89

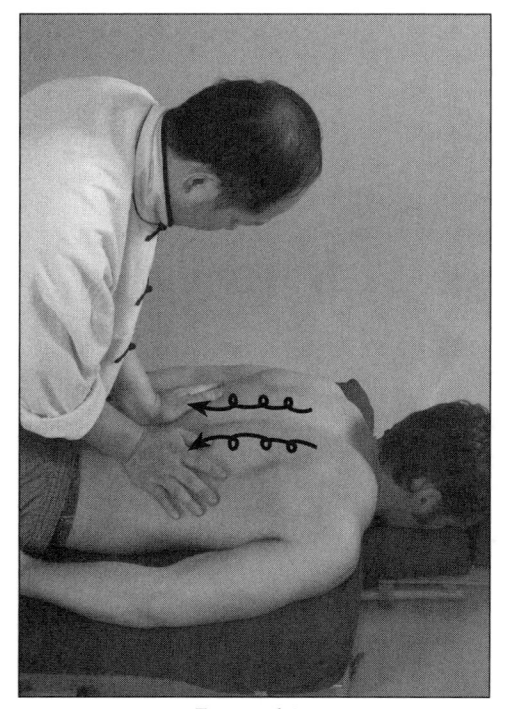

FIGURE 6-90

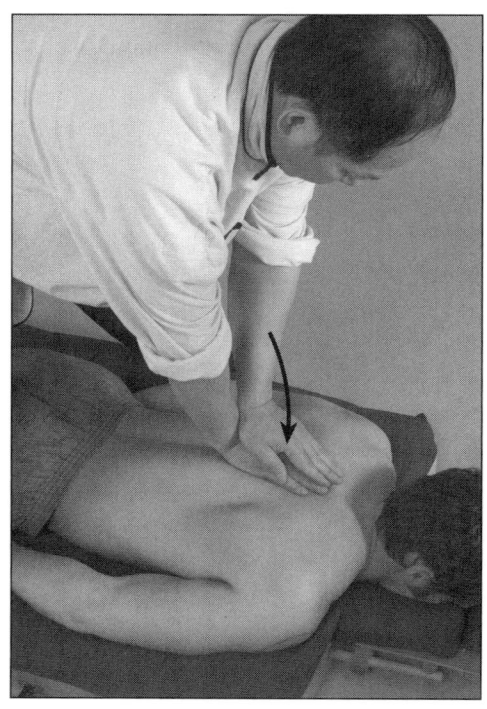

FIGURE 6-91

255

Qigong Massage

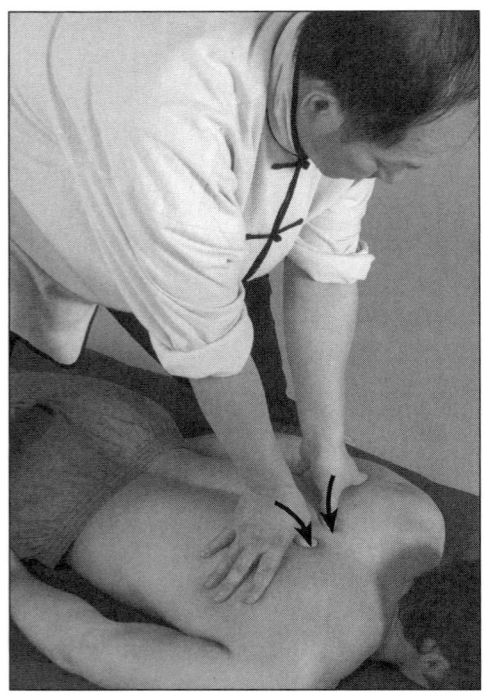

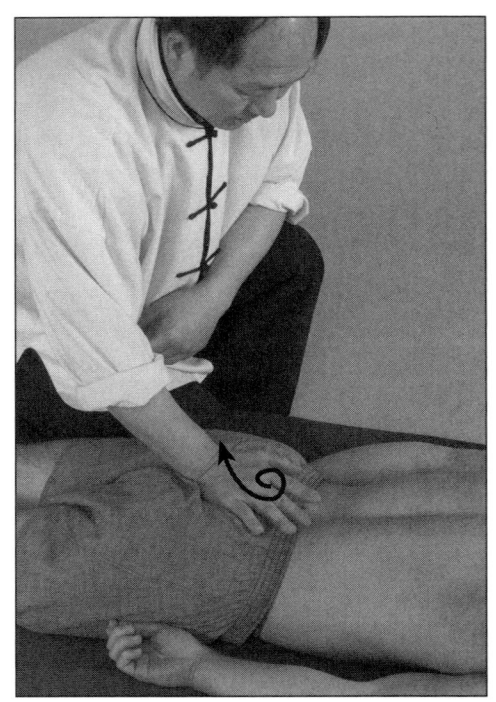

FIGURE 6-92

FIGURE 6-93

inhale deeply and then exhale. When your partner is exhaling, press down. How hard you press depends on your partner. Start with light power and observe your partner's reaction. If they hold their breath and tense up, then you are pressing too hard. Make sure that your posture is comfortable and your power is even and firm. You may repeat the entire procedure once.

Next, starting from the neck and moving down the length of the spine, press your thumbs into the gaps between the joints to stimulate the miscellaneous cavities just beside the center of the spine (Figure 6-92). When you reach the sacrum, massage it with the base of your palm (Figure 6-93).

After you have finished pressing on the sides of the spine, repeat the procedure, only now press about two inches away from the spine on the cavities on the inner branch of Urine Bladder channel (Figure 6-94). After pressing, again use the forearm, the palm, or the edge of the palm to rub the trunk muscles in small circles, pushing to the sides and also downward (Figure 6-95). This procedure leads stagnant Qi sideways and downward away from the spine. Repeat the process several times.

Chapter 6: General Massage

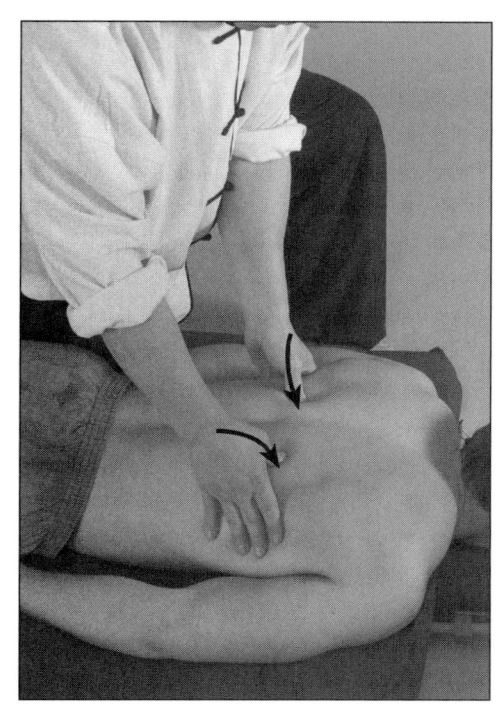

FIGURE 6-94

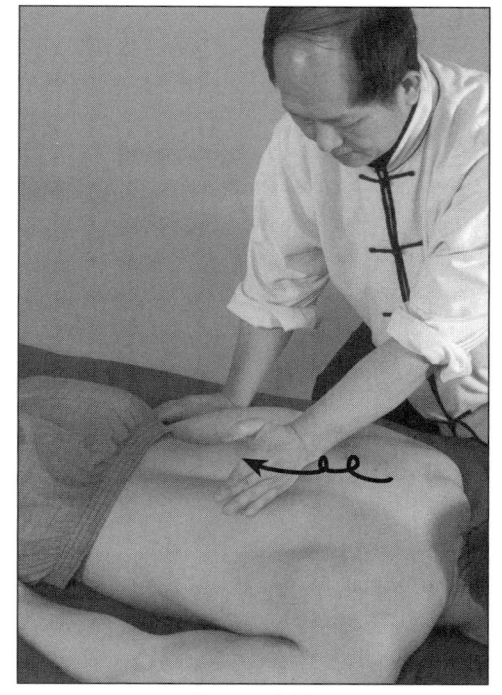

FIGURE 6-95

Step 3. Once you have loosened up the spine and the trunk muscles, you should now lead the Qi to the arms, the sides of the body, and downward to the legs.

To lead the Qi to the arms, first loosen up the area of the shoulder blades. To do this, place your partner's arm behind them, then lift up the shoulder with both hands and gently move it in a circle. Move the right shoulder clockwise (Figure 6-96) and the left shoulder counterclockwise to loosen the entire shoulder area.

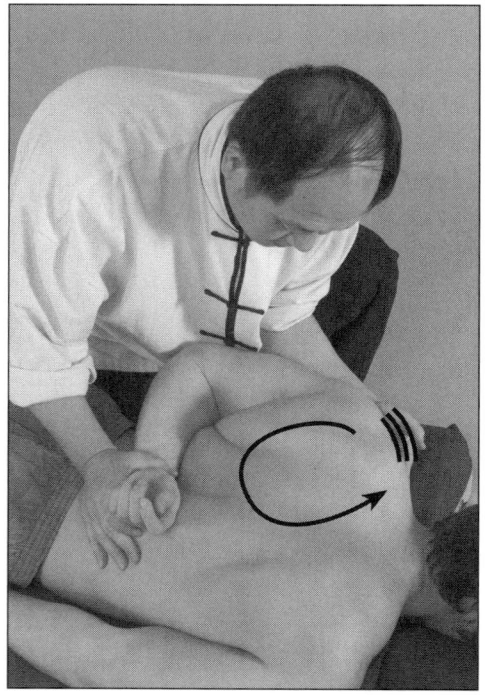

FIGURE 6-96

257

Qigong Massage

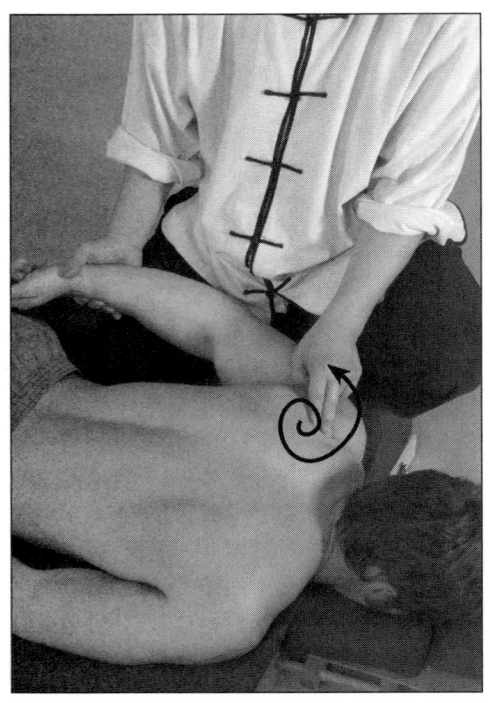

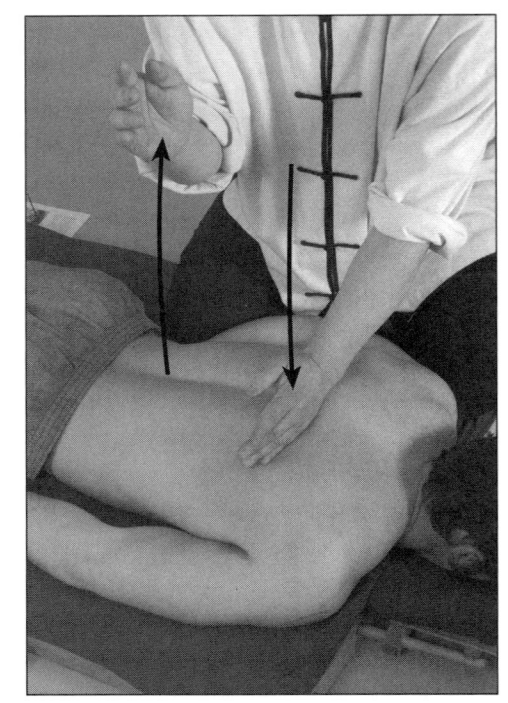

FIGURE 6-97

FIGURE 6-98

Next, press with your second and middle fingers on the Tianzong (SI-11) (天宗) cavity in the center of the shoulder blade and gently rub around. To lead Qi to the arms, circle clockwise with your right hand on the right shoulder blade (Figure 6-97), and counterclockwise with your left hand on the left shoulder blade.

After you have massaged the Tianzong cavity, use your hand to brush the skin from the spine over the Tianzong cavity and out to the arms. This will lead stagnant Qi from the back to the arms.

Step 4. You now want to spread the accumulated Qi to the sides of the back. To do this, first you may want to use the sides of your palms to hit the entire back gently from the top to the bottom and from the center to the sides (Figure 6-98). Alternatively, you may want to grab the skin on the back and shake it a little (Figure 6-99). This will bring up any Qi still hidden under the skin.

Next, brush with your hands from the top to the bottom and from the center to the sides (Figure 6-100). After brushing several times, grab the muscles under the armpits with both hands and rub and shake them (Figure 6-101). Next, use your hands to brush from the armpit areas downward to the sides of the waist.

Finally, follow the gaps in the ribs with your fingers, pushing from the center of the back to the sides (Figure 6-102). Repeat several times.

Chapter 6: General Massage

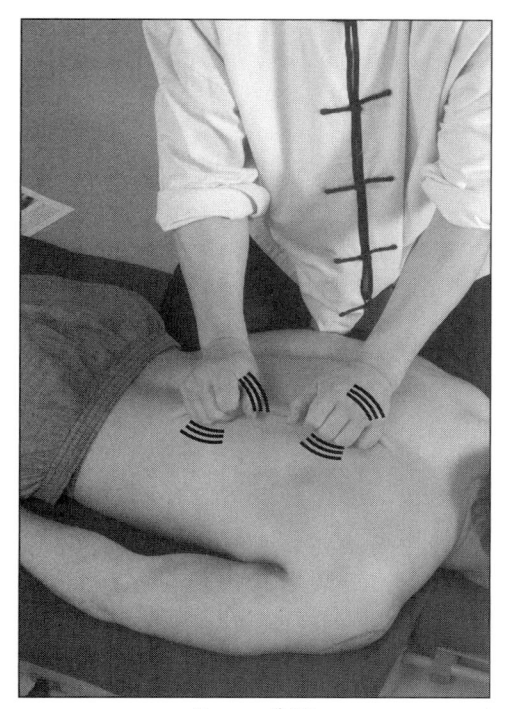

FIGURE 6-99

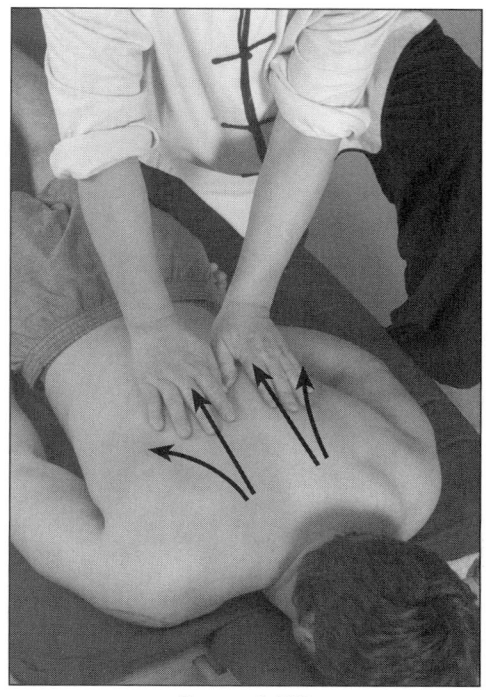

FIGURE 6-100

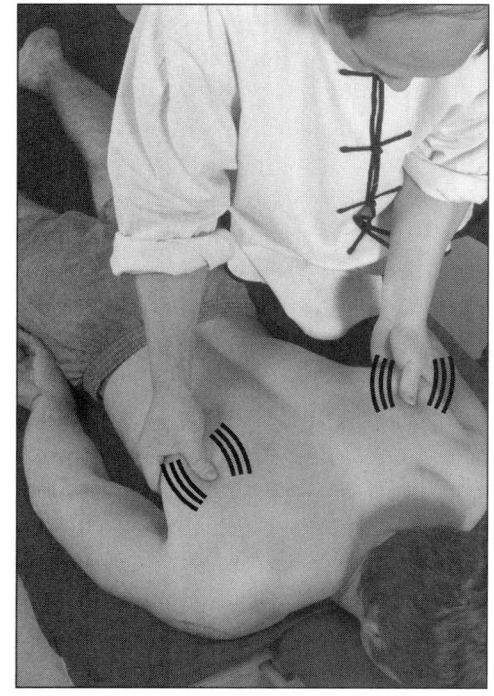

FIGURE 6-101

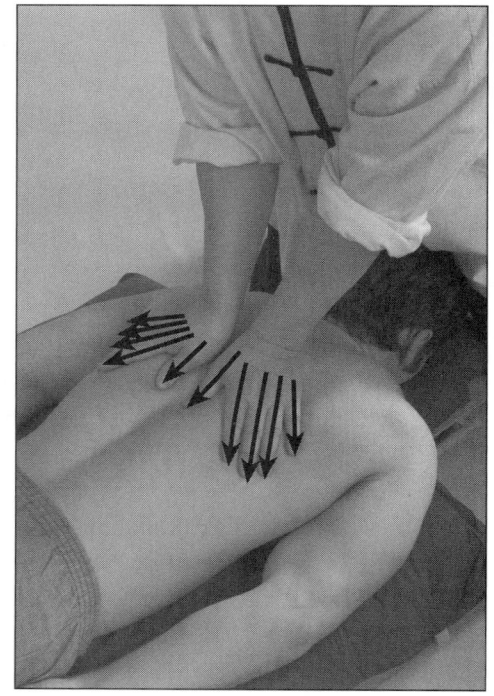

FIGURE 6-102

259

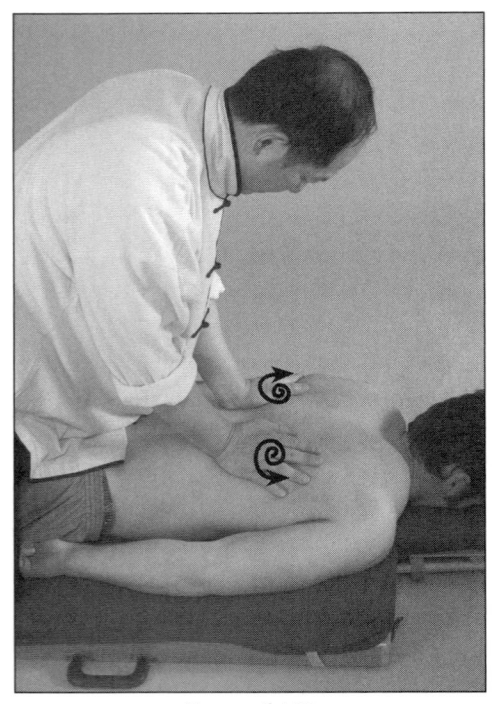

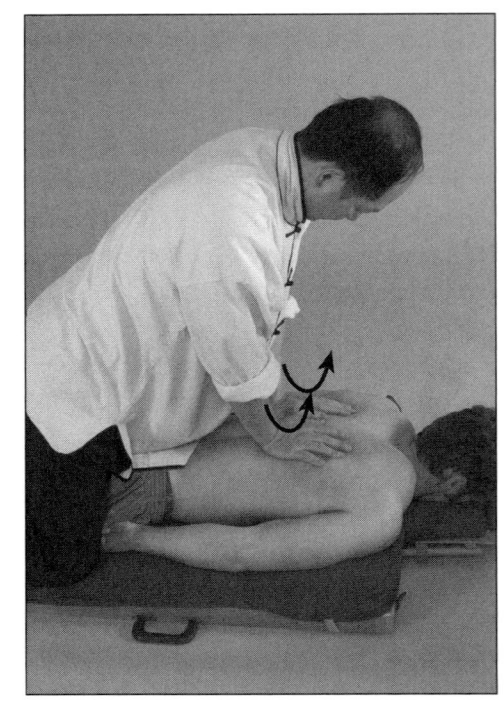

FIGURE 6-103

FIGURE 6-104

Step 5. Finally, you want to spread the Qi downward to the legs. To do this, you must first loosen the waist area. Start with the kidneys. Good Qi circulation in the kidneys is very important. When it is abnormal, the surrounding area will also be affected.

To massage the kidneys, use a circular motion. The right hand should move clockwise on the right kidney, while the left hand should move counterclockwise on the left kidney (Figure 6-103). These circular motions will nourish the kidneys, and they can also spread the accumulated Qi to the sides of the body. When you massage the kidneys, you may also press gently down on them with your palms, and then release the pressure (Figure 6-104). Do this about ten times and you will feel the tension in the kidneys release and the Qi circulation improve. Finally, use both palms to push from the kidneys to the sides of the body and also downward to the hips.

In order to loosen the waist area more, you may simply hold the sides of the waist with both hands and gently raise and lower it a few times (Figure 6-105).

Next, press and release with your palms on the joint between the sacrum and the first vertebra about ten times (Figure 6-106), and then push to the sides and to the hips to lead the Qi there (Figure 6-107). In the next section, we will introduce the gates in the hip area which lead Qi to the legs.

Chapter 6: General Massage

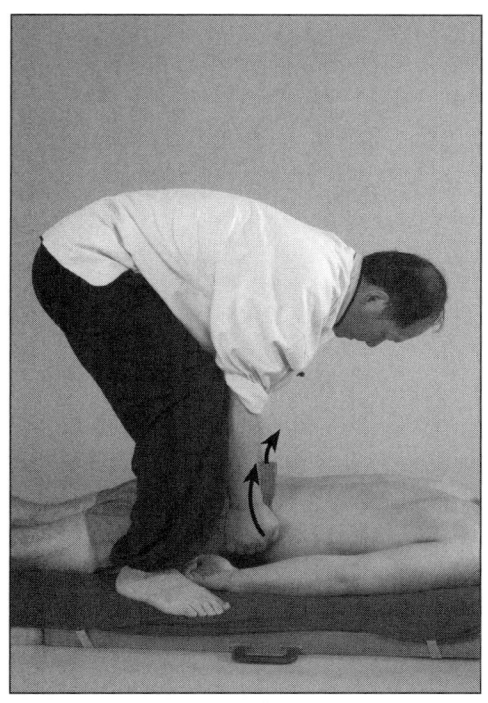

FIGURE 6-105

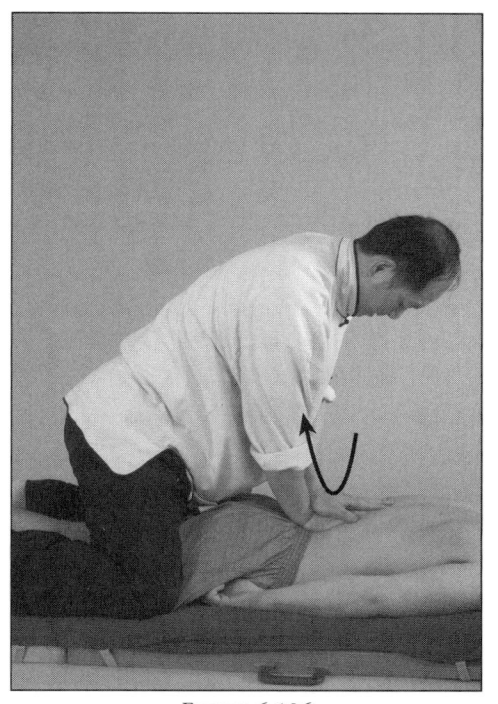

FIGURE 6-106

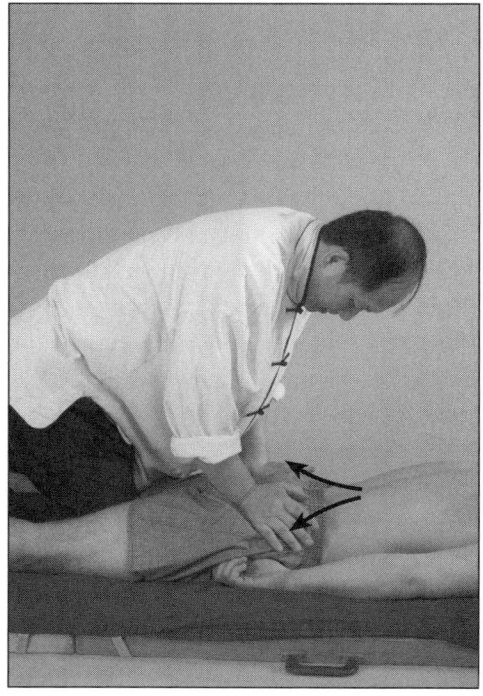

FIGURE 6-107

6-5. Massaging the Back of the Limbs 四肢背部之按摩

There are twelve Qi channels in the limbs, six in the arms and the other six in the legs. The other ends of these channels are connected to the twelve internal organs. There are three Yang channels and three Yin channels in the arms, and also in the legs. Generally, the Yang channels are on the external sides of the limbs, while the Yin channels run along the internal sides. The Qi in the Yang channels is relatively stronger than the Qi in the Yin channels. Consequently, the parts of the physical body which are nourished by the Yang channels are more developed, and more able to resist outside force. The internal parts of the limbs are relatively weaker, but, because they are under less strain, the Qi flow can be smoother, and Qi

261

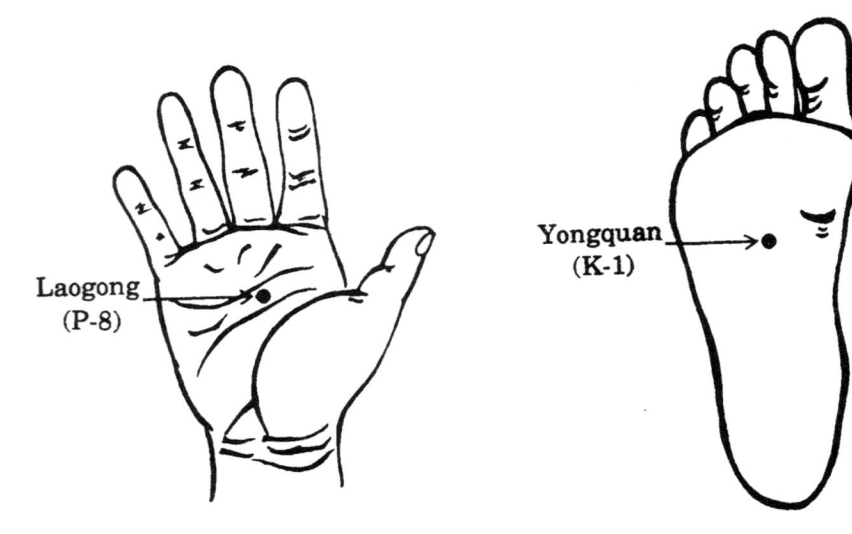

FIGURE 6-108. THE LAOGONG CAVITY.

FIGURE 6-109. THE YONGQUAN CAVITY.

disturbances on the Yin parts of the body can be sensed more easily by the brain.

For example, when you pinch or strike the external sides of the limbs you will feel less pain than you would on the internal sides. You are also more ticklish on the internal sides. Because of this, the Chinese martial arts emphasize using the external sides of the limbs for blocking, while they aim their attacks at the opponent's internal sides. This Yin and Yang theory can also apply to the torso. The front side is Yin and is more vital than the back side which is Yang. It is important to remember this when you massage, and to use less power on the internal sides of the limbs, or you may cause bruises.

You also need to be aware of the importance of massaging the limbs. The torso contains the internal organs, which absorb the essence of food and air and convert it through a biochemical reaction into Qi. This Qi is then supplied to the entire body. However, when there is an excess of Qi, or when the Qi loses its balance and affects the mutual cooperation among the organs, then the excess Qi is released through the limbs until balance is restored.

For example, your heart can be energized when you are excited. When this happens, the Qi in the heart is Yang (excessive), and the normal functioning of the heart may be impaired. The excess Qi is therefore led through the pericardium channel to the centers of your palms and released into the air. As this happens, you will feel warm and your palms will perspire. The pericardium is the membrane which encloses the heart, and is considered an organ in Chinese medicine. On the pericardium channel in the center of each palm is a cavity called Laogong (P-8) (勞宮) (Labor Palace). These cavities are the main gates for regulating the condition of the heart (Figure 6-108).

There are many important cavities on the legs. For example, the Yongquan (K-1) (湧泉) (Gushing Spring) cavities on the soles of the feet regulate the Qi in another important internal organ, the kidneys (Figure 6-109). In addition to the cavity gates, there are also thousands of pores, which are also considered gates.

In addition to acting as gates for releasing excess Qi from the organs, the limbs also play a role in Qi nourishment. Whenever you move or exercise, the food essence accumulated in your body as fat is converted into Qi and flows through the Qi channels to the internal organs. This is how Wai Dan Qigong (外丹氣功) (External Elixir Qigong) works.

In this section, we will discuss massaging the back of the limbs. Actually, we will discuss not just the back of the thighs and upper arms, but also both sides of the calves, feet, forearms, and hands. The reason for this is simply that, since the elbows and knees bend so easily, it is easy to massage the calves and forearms even when your partner is lying face down. We will start this discussion with the legs, and then cover the arms.

The front of the thighs and upper arms will be discussed after the front of the body has been dealt with. Once the chest and abdomen are massaged, the front of the body is relaxed and the Qi is flowing smoothly. The limbs should then be massaged to lead the Qi to the feet and hands.

Massaging the Back of the Thighs, Calves, and Feet

Anatomical Structure of the Leg and Its Circulatory Systems. Beneath the skin on the back of the leg are the muscles, some nerves which extend from the hip to the foot, and also some veins on the back and inner side of the calf. Under a layer of muscle is the main nerve coming down from the hip, and also several smaller branches extending upward to the hip area (Figure 6-110).

In addition, the main artery runs from in front of the hip joint and extends downward to the back of the thigh, where it runs parallel to the main nerve. There are also several smaller arteries branching out from the lower hip to the center of the hip. You can see in the last two illustrations how it is possible for you to reach the main nerve and blood vessel on the back of the knee.

Beneath the last layer of muscle are the main nerves and muscles in the legs (Figure 6-110). The area around the sacrum is very important in massage because it is the main gate for Qi channels, nerves, and blood vessels into the legs.

Just beneath the skin in the front of the leg, in addition to the muscles are many nerves and some veins extending downward from the hip joint. There are also some major nerves, veins and arteries near the joint. Beneath the muscles are the main nerve and artery systems running downward to the toes (Figure 6-111).

Finally, Figures 6-112 and 6-113 show the anatomical structure of the feet from the bottom and the top. You can see that most of the nerve and blood circulatory systems are hidden in the gaps between the bones.

Qigong Massage

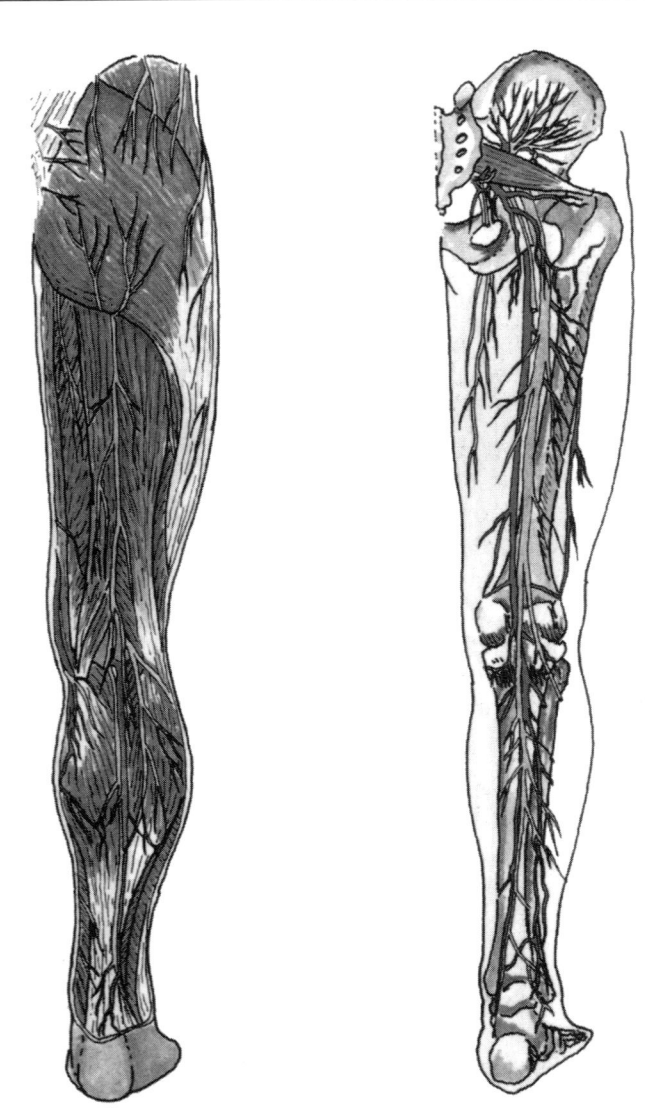

FIGURE 6-110. ANATOMICAL STRUCTURE OF THE POSTERIOR ASPECT OF THE LEG (BACK VIEW).

Theory. The nerves connected to the legs originate in the lower portion of the spine, which, in turn, is connected to the brain. To maintain and improve the functioning of this network of nerves which connects the brain and the legs, you start by loosening up the lower part of the spine. Once you have relieved tension in the lower part of the body, the Qi will be able to circulate smoothly between the brain and the legs. Always remember, *Qi is the root and life of the physical body.* Uneven Qi circulation will interfere with the functioning of the physical nervous system.

The hips are the gate for Qi and blood communication between the lower spine and the legs. Therefore, massaging the hips is the most important part of massaging the legs.

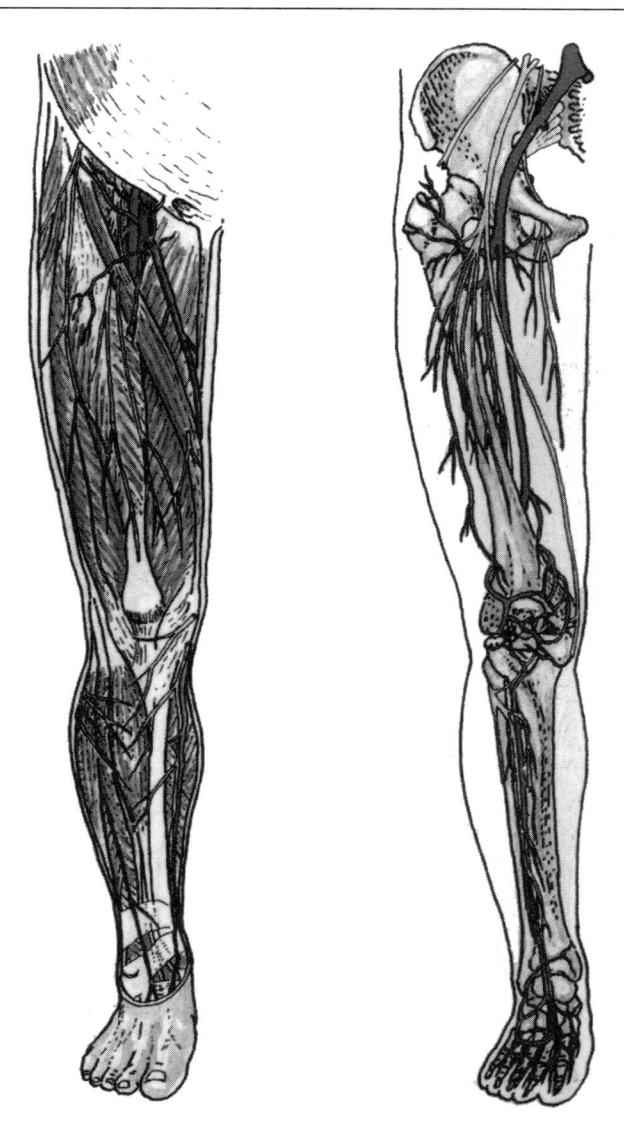

FIGURE 6-111. ANATOMICAL STRUCTURE OF THE ANTERIOR ASPECT OF THE LEG (FRONT VIEW).

The key to successful leg massage is relaxing the big muscles in the hips and opening and stimulating the Qi gates in the hips.

After massaging the hips and opening the gates there, you then move down to the thighs. The thigh muscles are big and thick, and you need very strong fingers to reach the muscles deep inside. Positioning your partner's legs correctly will make it easier. For example, when you massage the thigh and the calf, lift the foot up about twelve inches; with the leg bent, the muscles and tendons will be more relaxed, and it will be easier for you to penetrate.

You may find that it is difficult for you to generate enough power when using finger techniques. If this is the case, then using your feet may prove more effective. In the

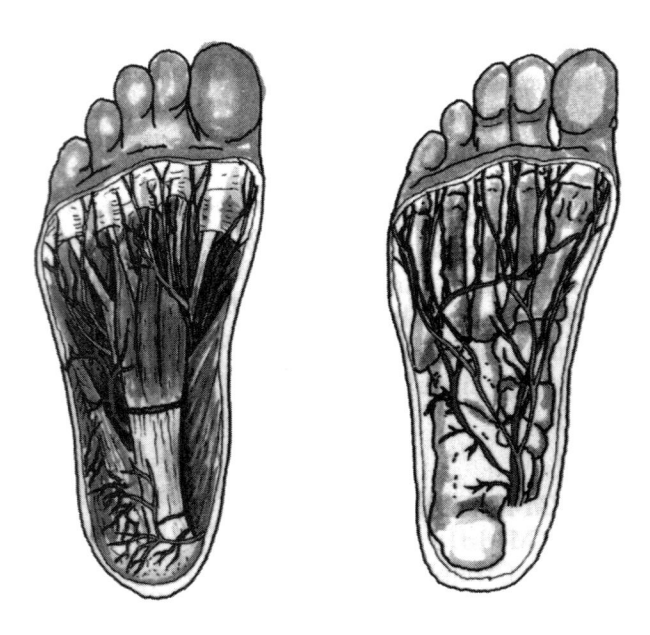

FIGURE 6-112. ANATOMICAL STRUCTURE OF THE POSTERIOR ASPECT OF THE FOOT (BOTTOM VIEW).

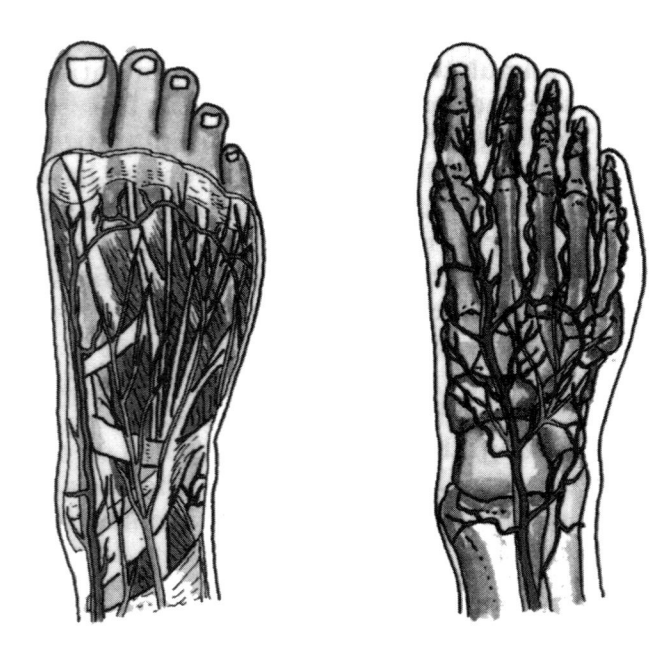

FIGURE 6-113. ANATOMICAL STRUCTURE OF THE ANTERIOR ASPECT OF THE FOOT (TOP VIEW).

Chapter 6: General Massage

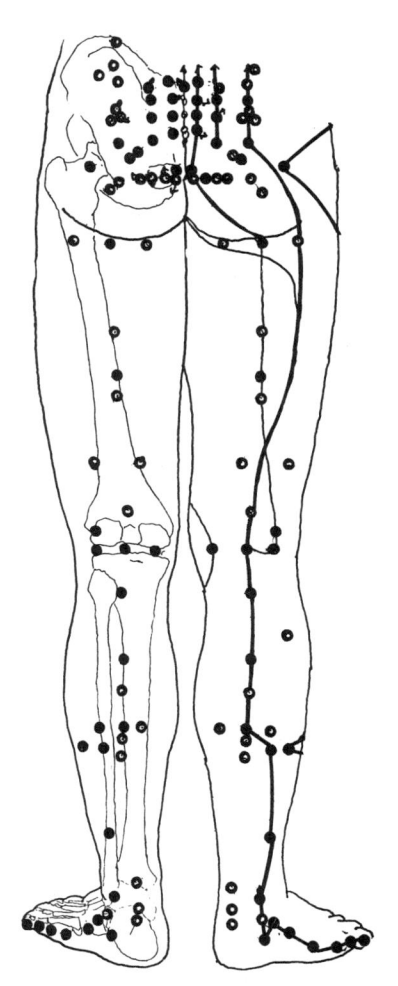

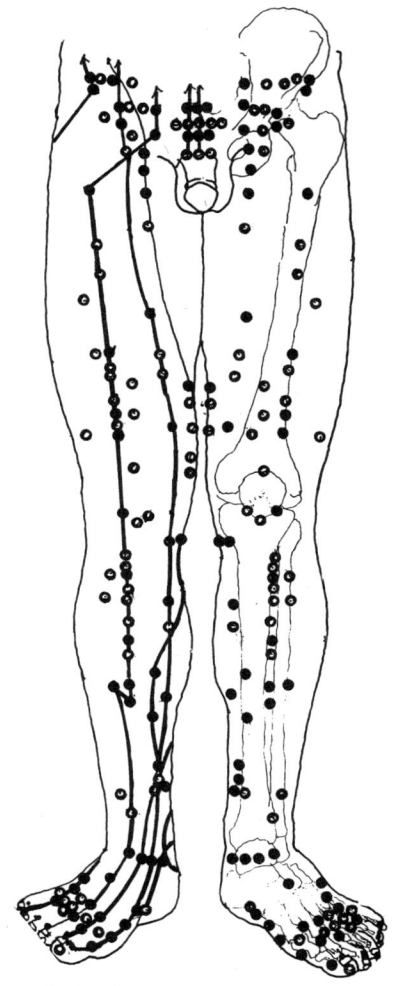

FIGURE 6-114. PRIMARY QI CHANNELS AND ACUPUNCTURE CAVITIES ON THE LEG (BACK VIEW).

FIGURE 6-115. PRIMARY QI CHANNELS AND ACUPUNCTURE CAVITIES ON THE LEG (FRONT VIEW).

first part of this book we discussed how many parts of the body could be used for giving a massage. Feel free to experiment with them, and discover which ones work best for you in various circumstances. As long as your partner stays relaxed and you can achieve your massage goals, they are good techniques. Do not feel that you must restrict yourself to the techniques we mention in this chapter.

After massaging the thighs, you then move on to the calves. First massage the tendons and open the Qi gates around the knees, which are the gates between the thighs and the calves. When you massage the calf muscles, the position of the foot should be the same as when you massaged the thigh. It should be easier to massage the calf, since the muscles there are not as thick as in the thigh, and the gate cavities are shallower.

Next massage the ankles, which are the junctions between the calves and the feet

Qigong Massage

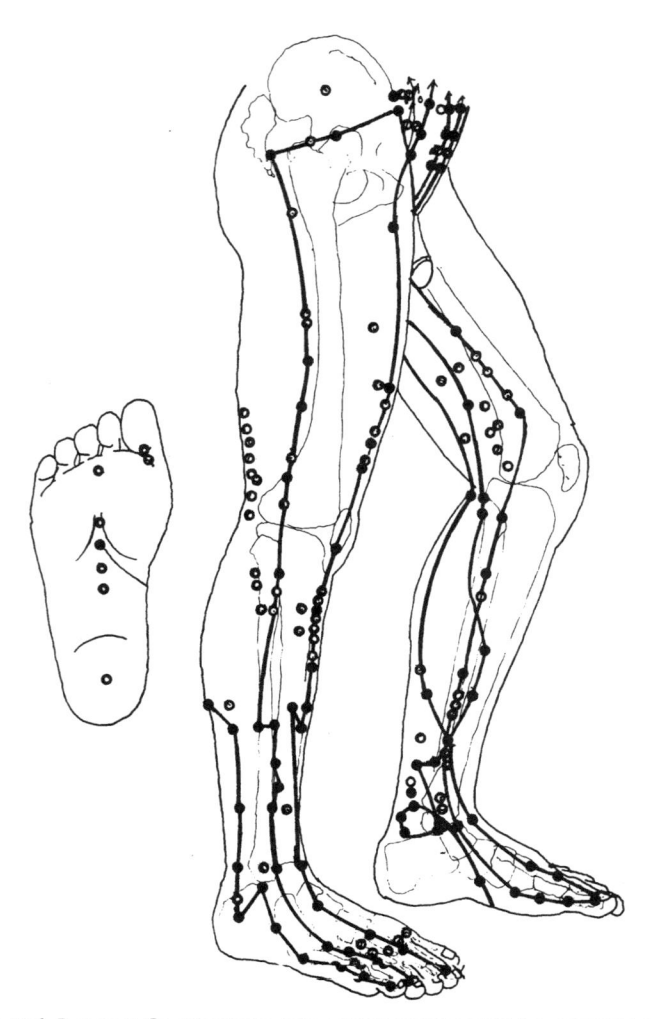

FIGURE 6-116. PRIMARY QI CHANNELS AND ACUPUNCTURE CAVITIES ON THE LEG (SIDE VIEW).

and finally massage the feet. The bottoms of the feet are more important than the tops because that is where the Yongquan cavity is located. Massaging the feet is very effective in calming people down, and can even put them to sleep.

Next, we will describe the gates on the legs, and follow this with a discussion of massage techniques. But first, please familiarize yourself with the Qi circulatory system in the legs, as shown in Figures 6-114 to 6-116.

Gates

Zhongkong (M-BW-26) (中空), **Zhibian (B-49)** (秩邊), **and Baihuanshu (B-30)** (白環俞). Zhongkong (Middle Space), Zhibian (Order's Edge), and Baihuanshu (White Circle's Hollow) are the gates which open up the Qi circulation from the lower back to the

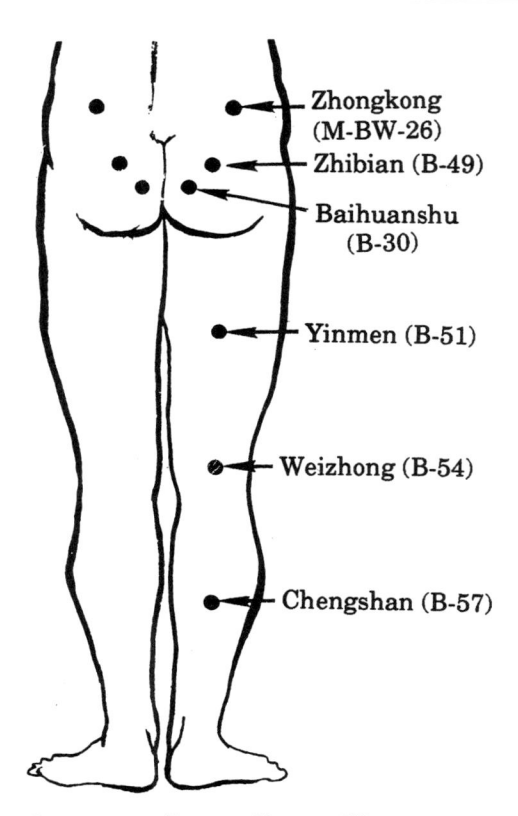

FIGURE 6-117. THE ZHONGKONG, BAIHUANSHU, ZHIBIAN, YINMEN, WEIZHONG, AND CHENGSHAN CAVITIES.

back of the thigh (Figure 6-117). Stimulating these three gates properly can generate a strong sensation which moves from the lower back to the feet. Frequently, stimulating any of these cavities will also cause the cavity on the back of the knee (Weizhong, B-54, 委中) or the Yongquan (K-1) (湧泉) cavity on the bottom of the foot to also be stimulated. This multiple stimulation leads the Qi straight down to the knee or to the bottom of the feet.

When you massage these cavities, you may simply use your thumb, the second and middle fingers, or even the base of the palm to press firmly on the cavity and then rub around (Figure 6-118). The direction of the circle is not as critical here as elsewhere, since you are either spreading the Qi to the side or leading it downward. When you massage these cavities, start with the top one and move downward to the bottom ones. It is important not to use too much power when you massage these cavities, since any pain will cause the hip muscles to tense and hinder the massage.

In order to build up the connection, the gates on the back of the legs will often be stimulated right after the ones on the hips. Additional gates on the back of the leg are Yinmen (B-51) (殷門), Weizhong (B-54) (委中), and Chengshan (B-57) (承山), which will be discussed later.

Qigong Massage

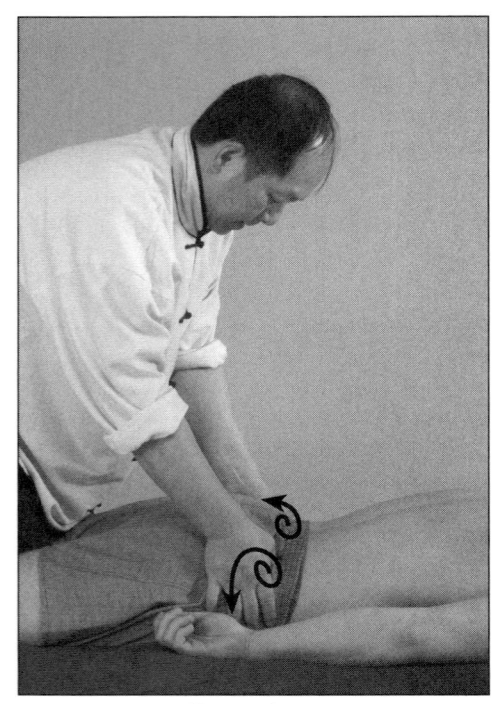

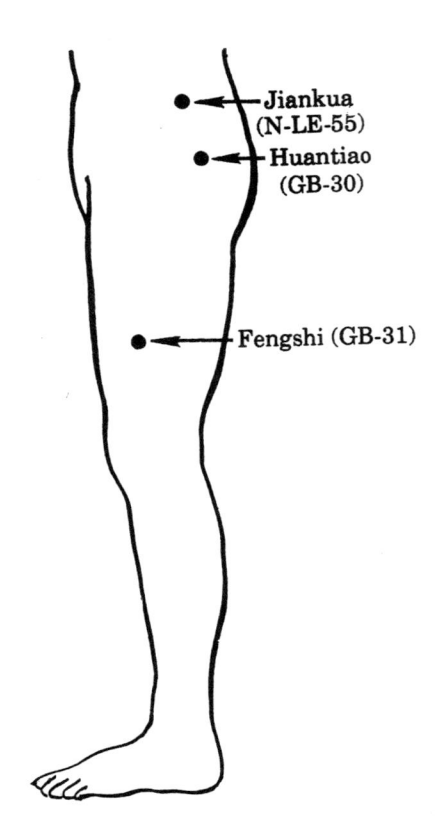

FIGURE 6-118

FIGURE 6-119. THE JIANKUA, HUANTIAO, AND FENGSHI CAVITIES.

Jiankua (N-LE-55) (健胯) **and Huantiao (GB-30)** (環跳). Jiankua (Strengthen Thigh) and Huantiao (Encircling Leap) are two important cavities located on the external sides of the thighs, and which are the gates which connect the waist to the sides of the legs (Figure 6-119).

You can use the same techniques on these two cavities that you used on the back of the hip: the thumb, the second and middle fingers, or the base of the palm (Figure 6-120). Press and rub in a circle. When you massage these cavities, start from the top one and move down to the bottom one. Again, do not use too much power, or you will cause tension.

In order to lead the Qi further downward, another cavity called Fengshi (GB-31) (風市) on the side of the thigh is also stimulated right after the above two cavities. We will discuss this cavity later.

Huiyin (Co-1) (會陰). The Huiyin (Meeting Yin) is located in the perineum midway between the genitals and the anus (Figure 6-121). In Chinese medicine and Qigong, the Huiyin is considered one of the most important cavities. It is the junction of many vessels, including the Conception (Ren Mai, 任脈), Governing (Du Mai, 督脈),

Chapter 6: General Massage

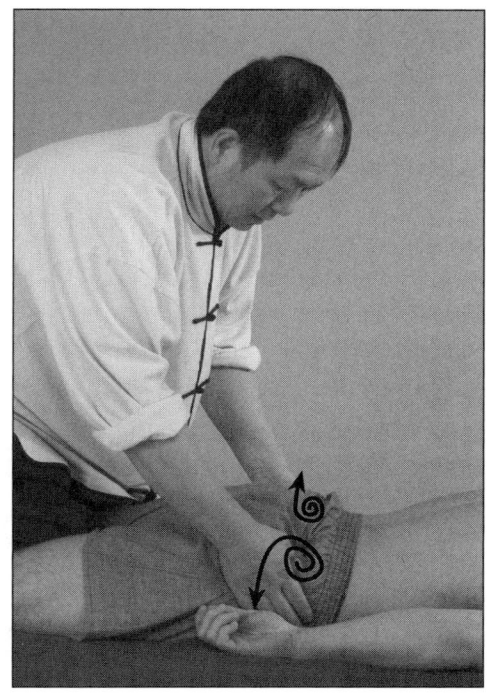

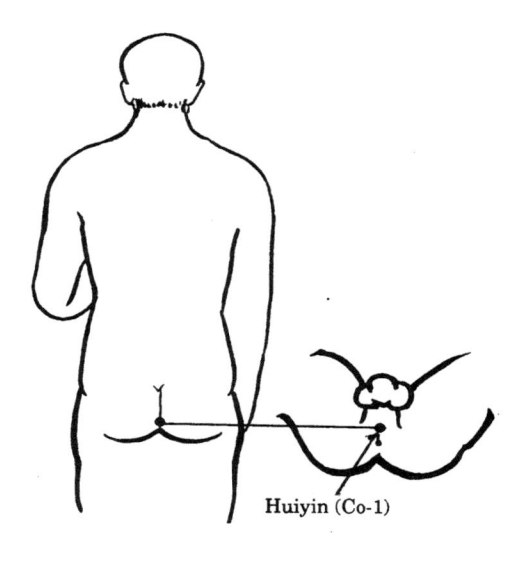

FIGURE 6-120

FIGURE 6-121. THE HUIYIN CAVITY (CO-1).

Thrusting (Chong Mai, 衝脈), Yin Heel Vessels (Yinqiao Mai, 陰蹻脈), and Yin Linking Vessel (Yinwei Mai, 陰維脈). Remember, according to Chinese medicine, vessels are like reservoirs which regulate the Qi circulating in the twelve channels.

Stimulating the Huiyin cavity will improve the exchange of Qi among the vessels. According to Marrow/Brain Washing Qigong, holding up this area or pressing it correctly will lead Qi from the lower body upward through the Thrusting Vessel to nourish the marrow in the spine and also the brain. Experience in massage has shown that through stimulating this cavity, the Qi converted from the Pre-essence (Yuan Jing, 元精) (hormone) which is produced by the testicles can be led downward to fill up the Qi in the Yin Heel Vessel. The Qi condition of this vessel is crucial for your leg strength. If you would like to know more about this subject, please refer to YMAA book, *Qigong—The Secret of Youth*.

When you massage this gate, spread your partner's legs a comfortable distance apart. Press gently on the Huiyin cavity with your middle finger and circle around. If you use your right hand, circling clockwise will lead Qi upward to the brain, and counterclockwise will lead Qi downward to the legs (Figure 6-122). Frequently, the Xuehai (Sp-10) (血海) cavity is massaged at the same time; this will be discussed later.

Yinmen (B-51) (殷門), **Weizhong (B-54)** (委中), **and Chengshan (B-57)** (承山). Yinmen (Door of Abundance) is located in the middle of the back of the thigh, Weizhong (Commission the Middle) is right behind the knee, and Chengshan (Support

Qigong Massage

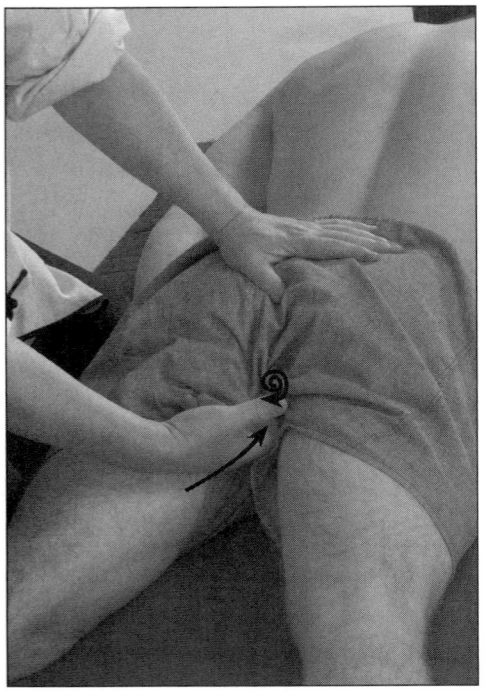

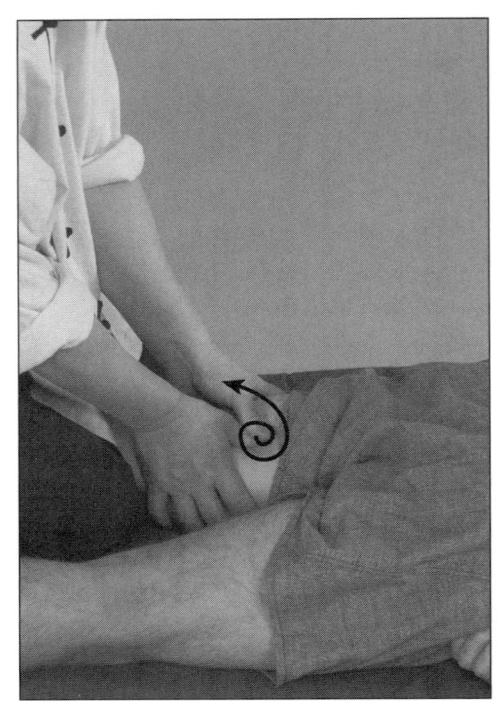

FIGURE 6-122

FIGURE 6-123

the Mountain) is on the back of the calf (Figure 6-117). All of these gates belong to the Urine Bladder Qi channel. If you massage these three cavities right after you have loosened up the hip, you will be able to lead the Qi very quickly to the feet.

Because of the thick layer of muscle over Yinmen, the best way to massage it is to use a thumb, with the other thumb on top of it for support (Figure 6-123), though some people use the elbow or the bottom of the feet.

When you massage Weizhong and Chengshan, you can simply use the thumb or the second and middle fingers to rub the cavity (Figure 6-124). Again, it is common practice when working on these cavities to massage the Yongquan (K-1) (湧泉) cavity at the same time to lead the Qi to the bottom of the feet.

Fengshi (GB-31) (風市). Fengshi (Wind's Market) is located in the center of the outside of the thigh (Figure 6-119). If you stimulate this cavity right after you have stimulated Jiankua (N-LE-55) (健胯) and Huantiao (GB-30) (環跳) on the side of the hip, you will be able to lead Qi from the waist downward to the legs very easily.

When you stimulate this cavity, you may use a thumb or the base of a palm to press in firmly and then vibrate (Figure 6-125). Frequently, the Jiexi cavity on the ankle will also be pressed to build up the connection. Jiexi (S-41) (解溪) will be discussed below.

Xuehai (Sp-10) (血海) **and Sanyinjiao (Sp-6)** (三陰交). Xuehai (Sea of Blood) is located on the inner side of the thigh near the knee. Sanyinjiao (Three Yin Junction) is located on the lower inner section of the calf (Figure 6-126). When these cavities

Chapter 6: General Massage

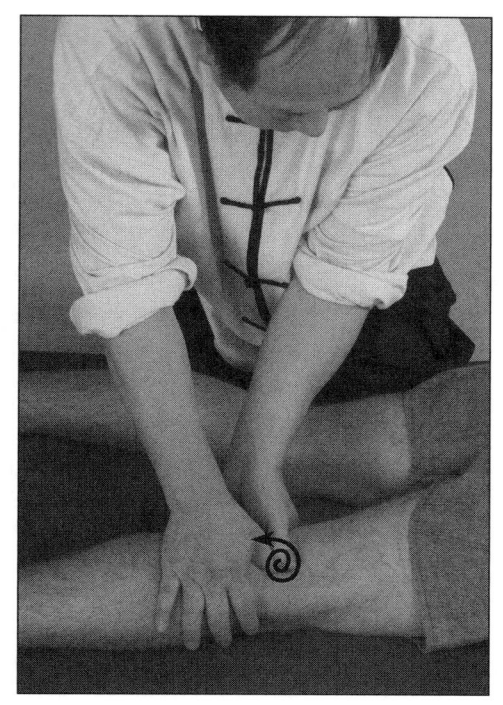

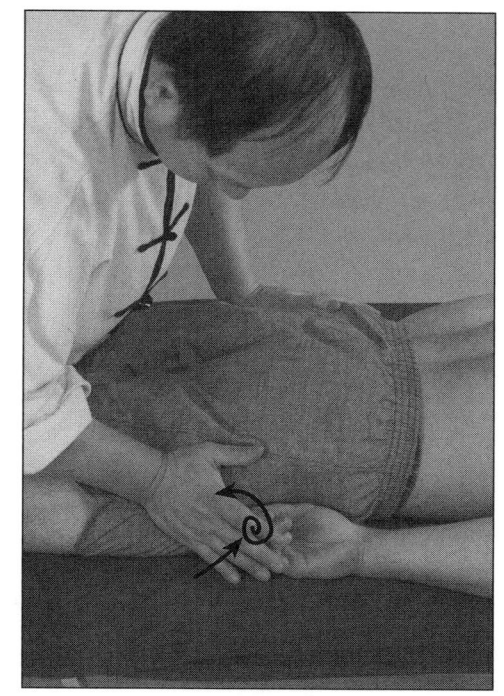

FIGURE 6-124

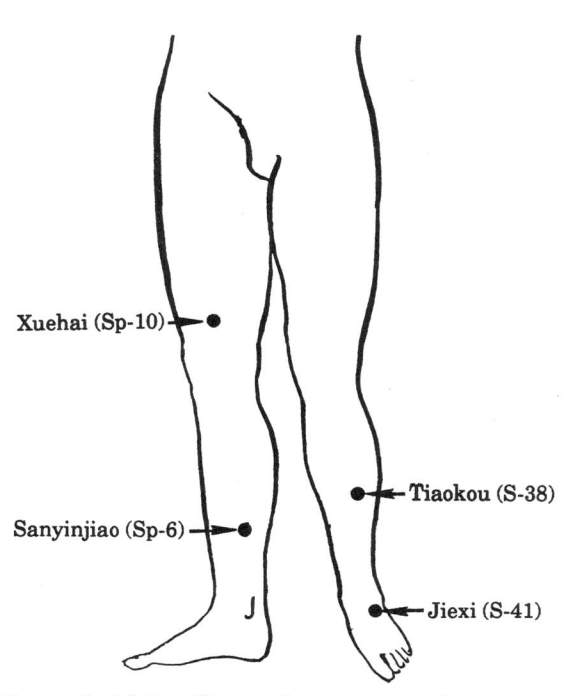

FIGURE 6-125

FIGURE 6-126. THE XUEHAI, SANYINJIAO, AND JIEXI CAVITIES.

273

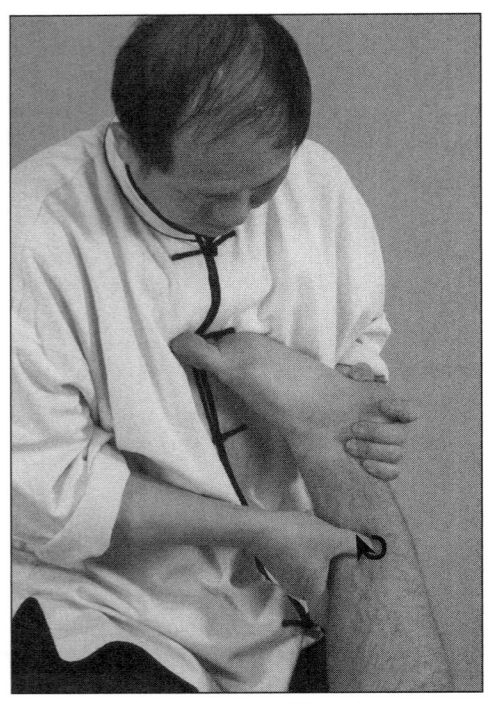

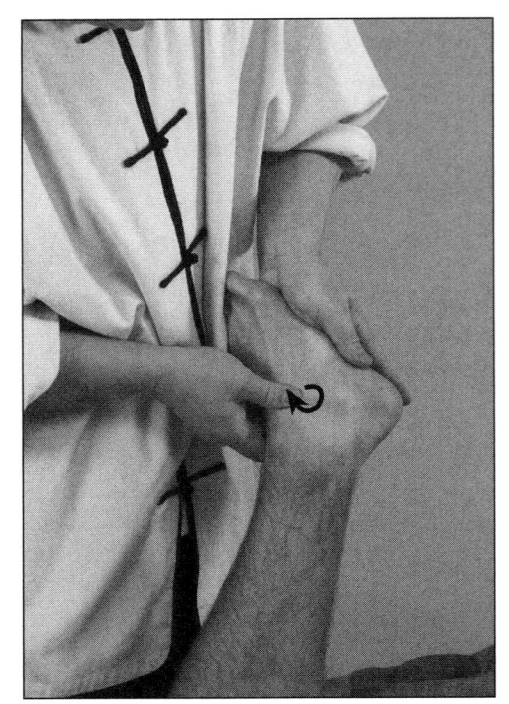

FIGURE 6-127

FIGURE 6-128

are pressed and stimulated, the Qi circulating in the inner side of the leg can be led downward.

When you massage these cavities, simply use the thumb to press in firmly and then vibrate (Figure 6-127).

Tiaokou (S-38) (條口) and Jiexi (S-41) (解溪). Tiaokou (Line's Opening) is located half-way down the chin, and Jiexi (Release Stream) is located in the middle of the crease in the front of the ankle (Figure 6-126). They both belong to the stomach channel. When Tiaokou and Jiexi are pressed and stimulated, the Qi on the front of the thigh can be led downward.

When you massage these two cavities, you may use a thumb or the second and middle fingers to press in firmly and rub around (Figure 6-128).

Yongquan (K-1) (湧泉). Yonquan (Gushing Spring) is located on the sole of the foot, one third of the way from the base of the second toe to the heel. It is the final point on the kidney channel. It is an important Qi gate which can regulate the Qi in the kidneys. Like the Laogong cavity in the hand, stimulating this cavity will lead Qi from the torso downward to the bottoms of the feet and spread it out there.

When you massage Yongquan, you can use a thumb to press in and circle firmly. When you use your right hand to circle clockwise on the right foot, you are nourishing the kidneys (Figure 6-129). However, if you use your right hand to circle clockwise on the left foot, you will release Qi.

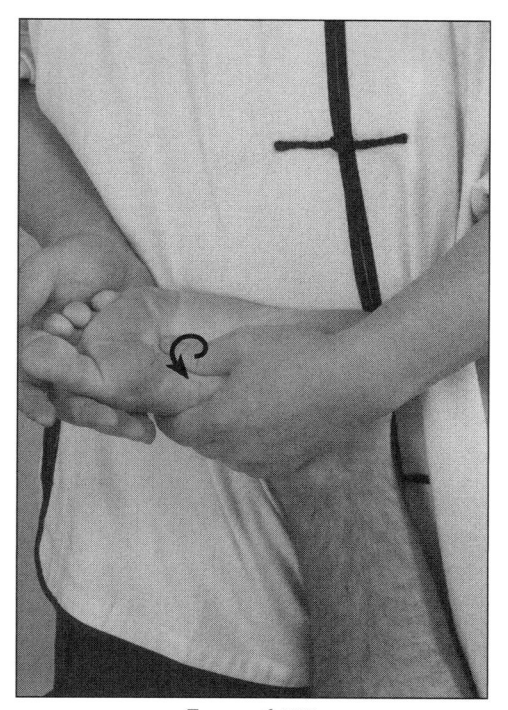

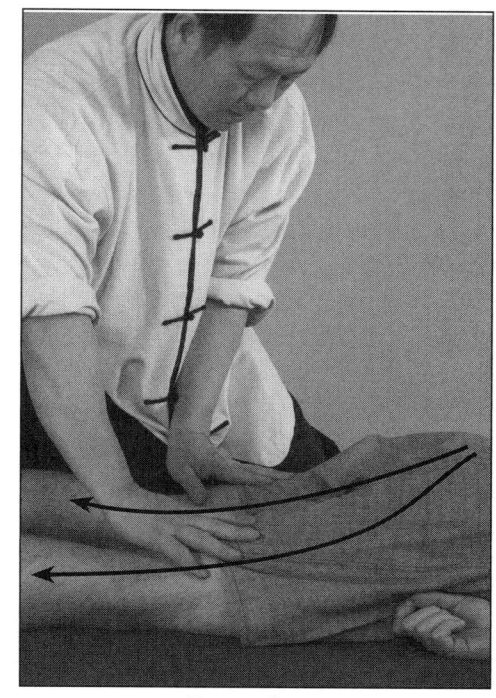

FIGURE 6-129   FIGURE 6-130

Massaging the Back of the Thighs and Legs

Before you massage the legs, first cover your partner's body with a blanket or towel to keep them warm. After a massage, the pores in the skin are wide open, and it is easy to catch a cold.

Step 1. First run your hands lightly over your partner's skin from their lower back to the bottom of their feet (Figure 6-130). Repeat several times. Next, repeat the same process on the sides of the waist, moving down along the sides of the legs to the bottom of the feet. Finally, do the same thing from the sacrum down the insides of the legs to the bottom of the feet. This will help your partner to relax, and also bring their mind back to their legs, which will help to lead the Qi there.

Step 2. Next, massage and open the gates on the buttocks and upper legs. Before you do this, however, you should massage the lower back to loosen up the lower spine and the trunk muscles in the lower back.

Qigong Massage

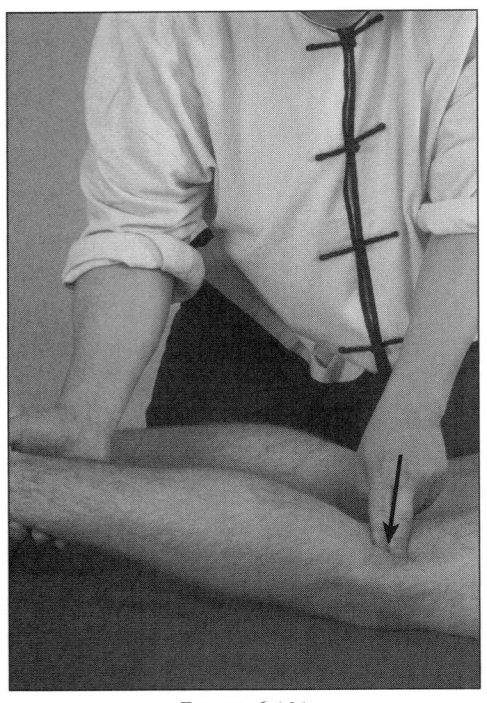

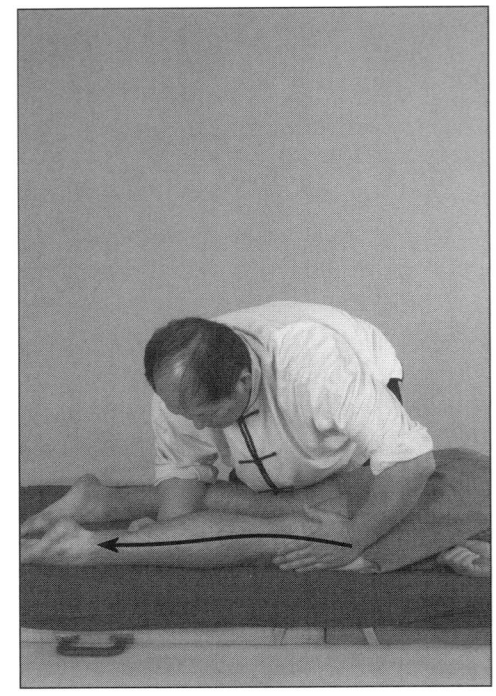

FIGURE 6-131

FIGURE 6-132

Then, massage and stimulate the gates on the back of the hips (Zhongkong, Zhibian, and Yinmen) and the back of the knees and calves (Weizhong, and Chengshan) (Figure 6-131). Finally massage the Yongquan on the bottom of the feet.

After you have opened up the back of the thighs and calves, stimulate and massage the gates on the outsides of the thighs and calves. These gates include Jiankua and Huantiao on the thigh, and Fengshi on the side of the thigh. After this, use your palm to push downward gently from the side of the thigh to the foot (Figure 6-132), and finally massage the Yongquan cavity.

Next, stimulate and massage the gates on the inside of the legs. First massage Huiyin, and then Xuehai, Sanyinjiao, and finally Yongquan. Again, use your hands to brush downward on the inside of the thighs to the bottoms of the feet.

Finally, stimulate and massage the cavities on the front of the calf: Tiaokou, Jiexi, and Yongquan. When you massage these gates, bend your partner's leg to make it easier for you.

Step 3. After you have stimulated and massaged the gates, you want to bring the accumulated Qi and blood to the surface. In order to do this, you first use the base or the edge of your palm to massage the lower back and sacrum for a few minutes. Next, use the base of your palms to press on the hips and then circle (Figure 6-133). If the circle moves up near the center and then to the sides, you are spreading the Qi and blood to the sides. This motion will also lead the Qi and blood upward. Therefore, circling in this direction is good for nourishing but not for releasing. However, if you circle in the

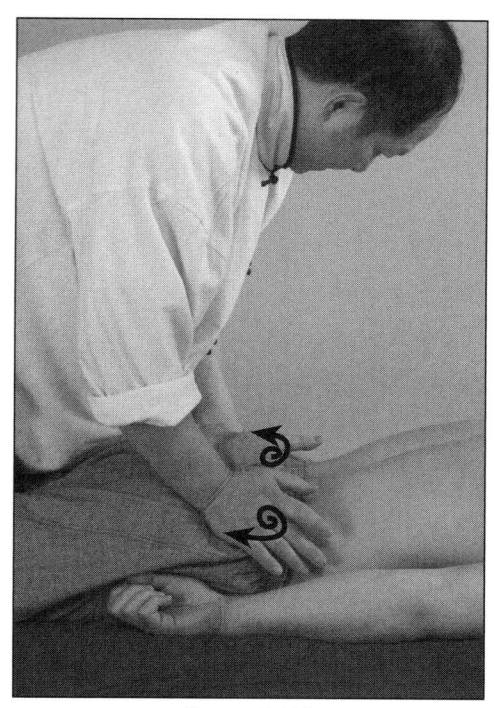

FIGURE 6-133

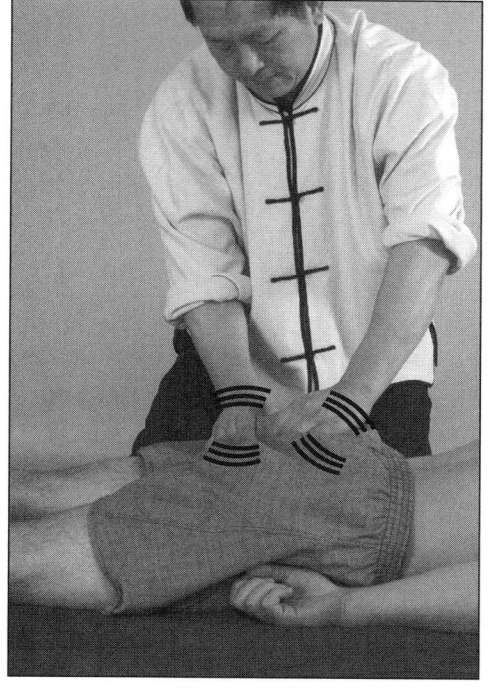

FIGURE 6-134

other direction, you will lead the Qi and blood down. This will release the Qi and relax your partner. When you massage the hips, first do the entire back of the hips from the top to the bottom, and then the outsides of the hips, again from the top to the bottom.

Finally, grab the muscles on the back of the hips with your fingers and rub them (Figure 6-134). Remember, when you massage you do not want to cause any pain or uneasiness in your partner, since this will cause tension and hinder the massage.

If you have weak hands, you may use your knees (Figure 6-135) or foot to press the hip and then circle around. Your knees and feet can generate much more power than your hands, so you must be very careful when you use them.

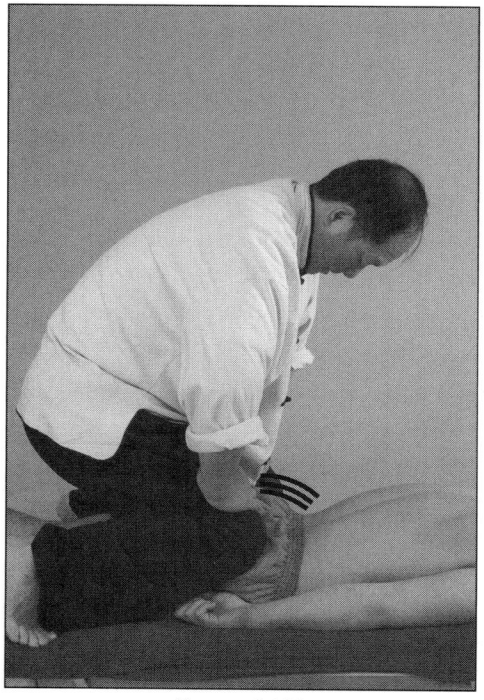

FIGURE 6-135

Qigong Massage

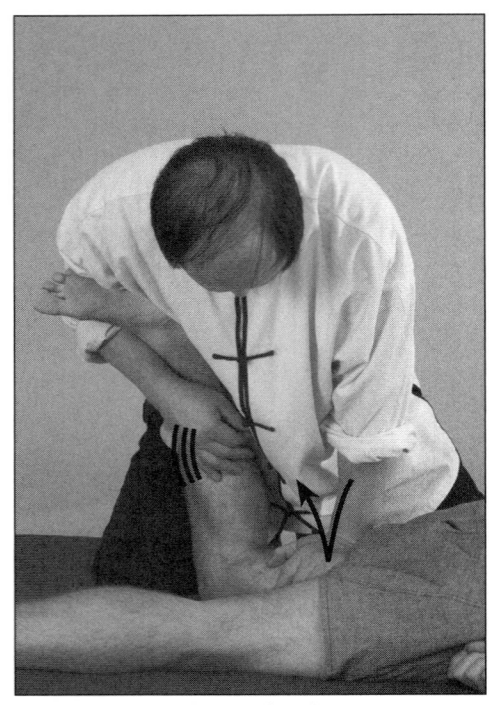

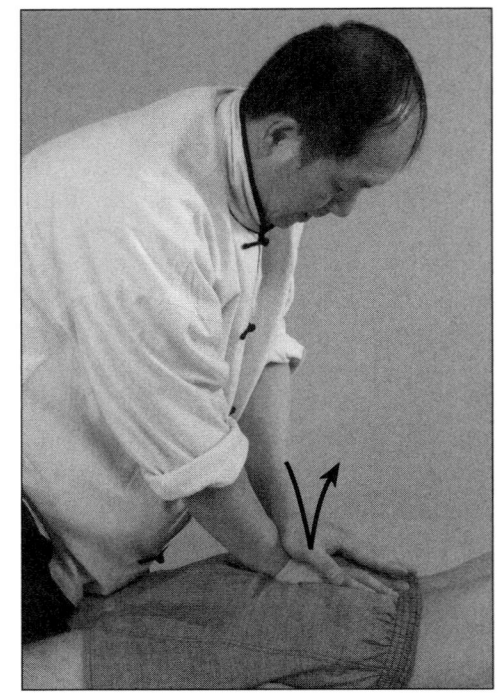

FIGURE 6-136   FIGURE 6-137

Step 4. After finishing the hips, raise the foot up to relax the thigh and calf muscles for an easier massage. Next, press down firmly with the base of your palm and then release on the back of the thighs from the top to the knees (Figure 6-136). If you find that you cannot generate enough penetrating power with one hand, you may use two hands (Figure 6-137). Repeat several times.

Next, use the base of both palms to press inward and circle evenly on the sides of the thighs downward to the knees (Figure 6-138). Repeat several times. When you do this, pay attention to the inside of the thighs. The inside of the thigh is tender and can be injured easily if you use power incorrectly. Also be careful that you do not rub the skin.

Next, grab the back of the thigh muscles with you fingers and rub from the top of the thigh to the knee (Figure 6-139). In order to prevent injuring the inside of the thighs, keep your thumbs on the outside and the other four fingers on the inside of the thighs. Repeat the entire process several times.

Next, use the sides of your palms to gently hit the back and side of the hips and thighs and from the hips down to the knees (Figure 6-140). This will bring the accumulated Qi and blood to the surface. Repeat the procedure several times.

If your hands are too weak to massage the thigh muscles, you may use one or both feet instead (Figure 6-141). When you use the feet to massage, your foot should be as relaxed as possible. Simply place your foot on the thigh, and generate the motion with your knee or hip.

Chapter 6: General Massage

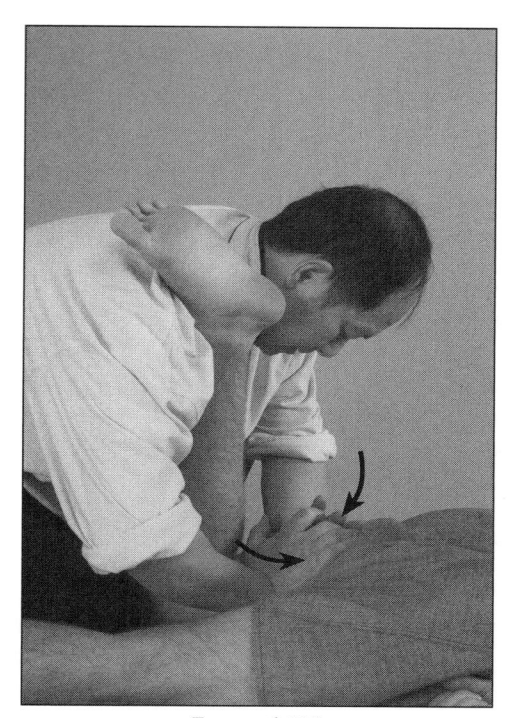

FIGURE 6-138

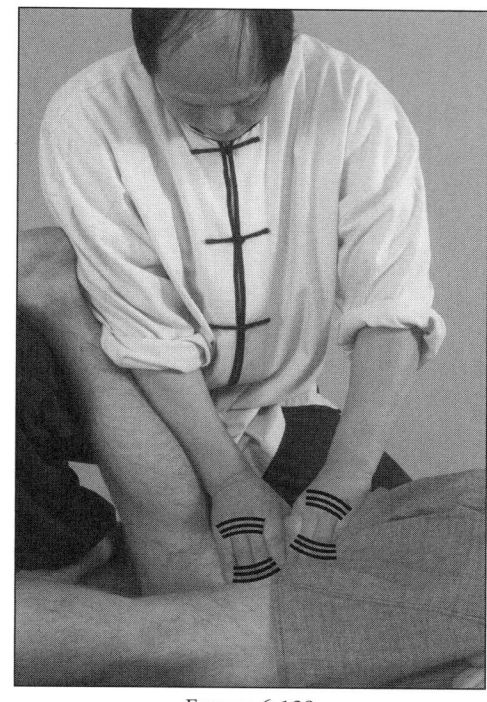

FIGURE 6-139

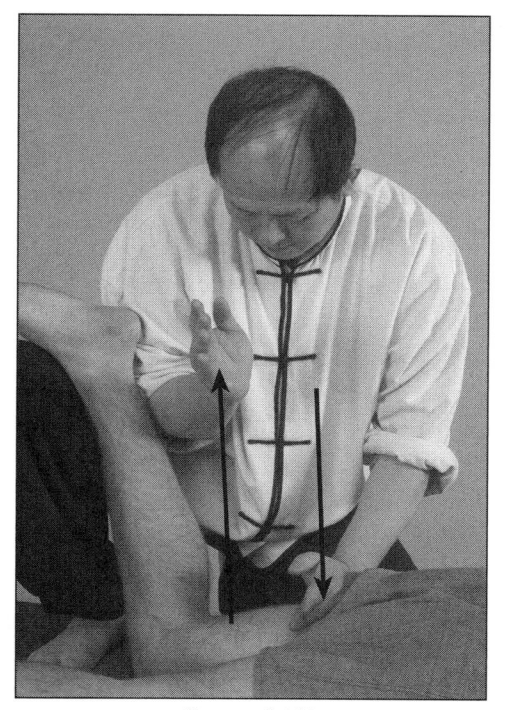

FIGURE 6-140

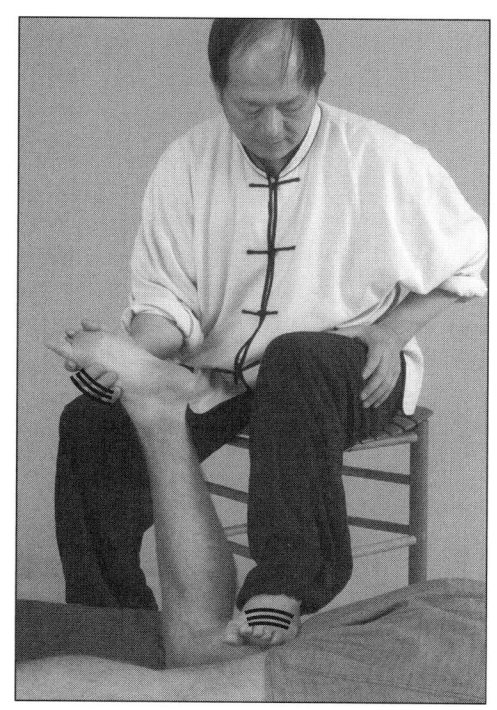

FIGURE 6-141

279

Qigong Massage

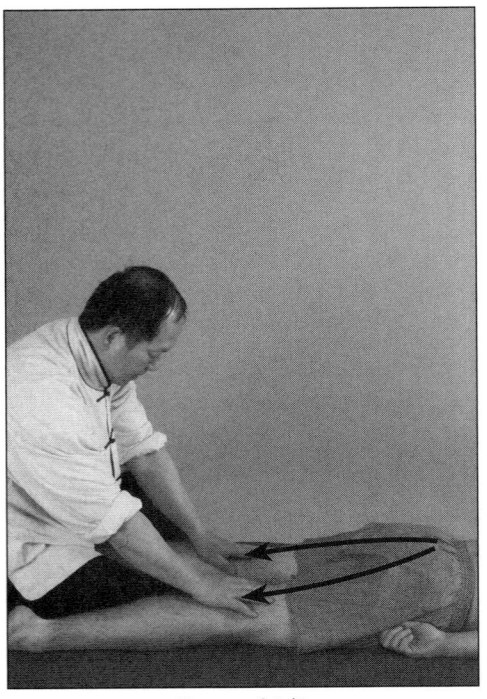

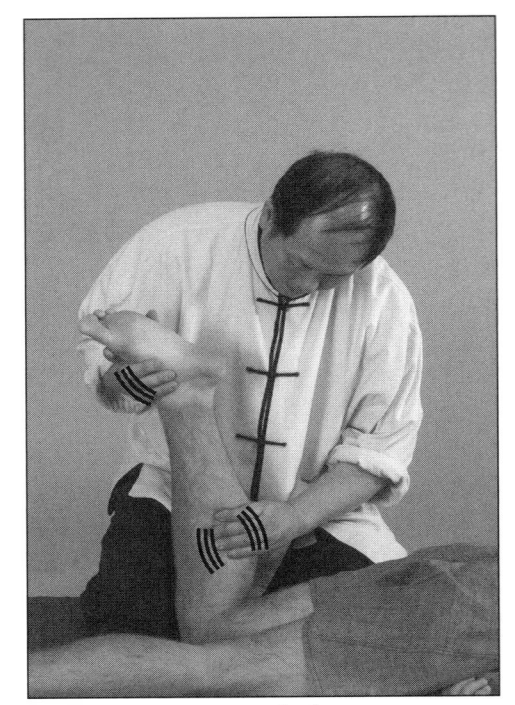

FIGURE 6-142

FIGURE 6-143

After you have completed this massage, brush downward several times with your hands on the backs, insides, and outsides of the hips and thighs from the hips to the knees (Figure 6-142).

Step 5. Next, massage the calves. When you massage the calf, you may again keep your partner's feet in the raised position to relax the calf muscles. You may also place your partner's foot on your chest while you are massaging the calf.

Again, the inside of the calf is tender and can be injured easily if you are not careful. Grab the muscles on the back and sides of the calf and rub downward from the knee to the ankle (Figure 6-143). Alternatively, you may also use the side of a palm to press and rub from the knee to the ankle (Figure 6-144).

Next, use both palms to press in gently and rub around from the knee to the ankle (Figure 6-145). Repeat the process several times.

Step 6. Next, massage the ankle and foot. First, gently rub the skin on the ankle and foot for a few minutes (Figure 6-146). Then, hold the lower calf firmly but gently with one hand, and move the foot in a circle (Figure 6-147). Circle slowly and smoothly about twenty times in each direction.

Chapter 6: General Massage

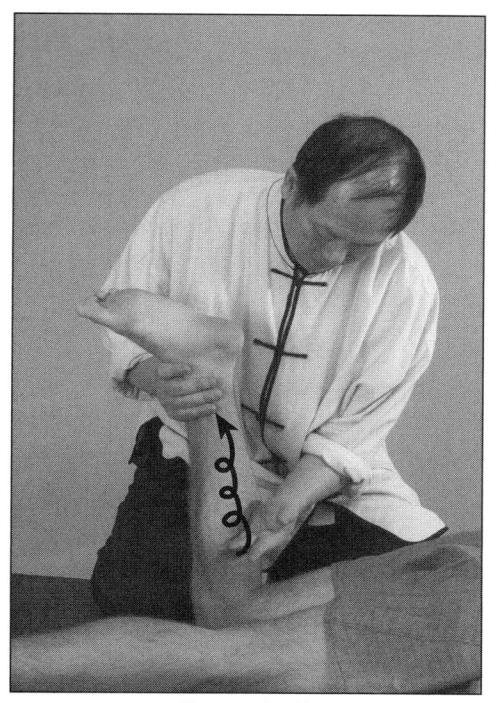

FIGURE 6-144

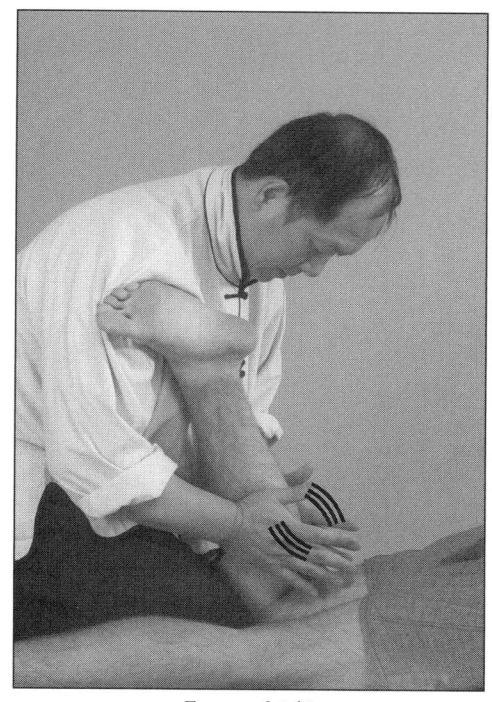

FIGURE 6-145

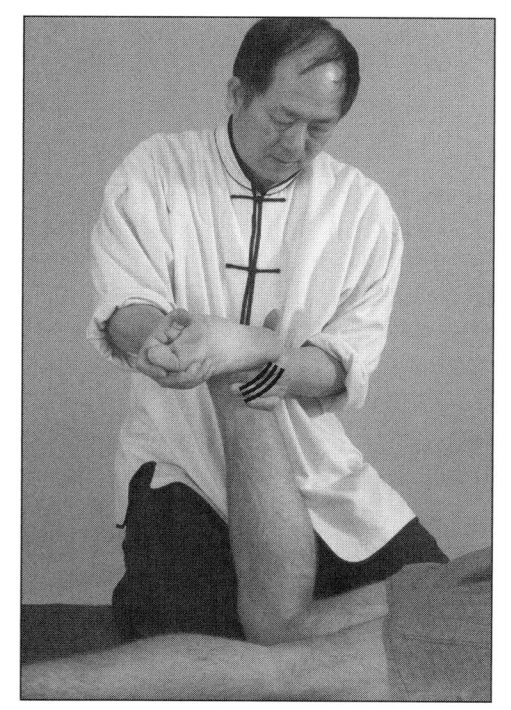

FIGURE 6-146

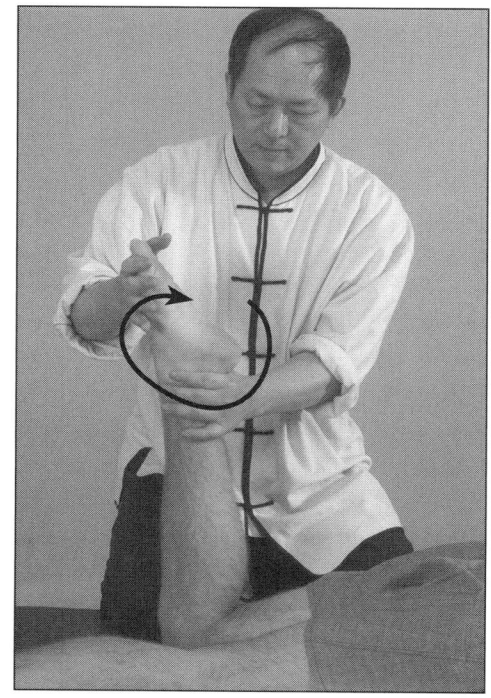

FIGURE 6-147

281

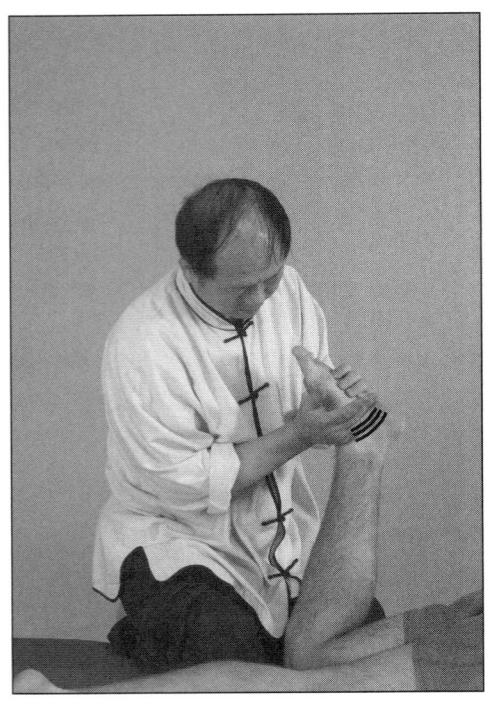

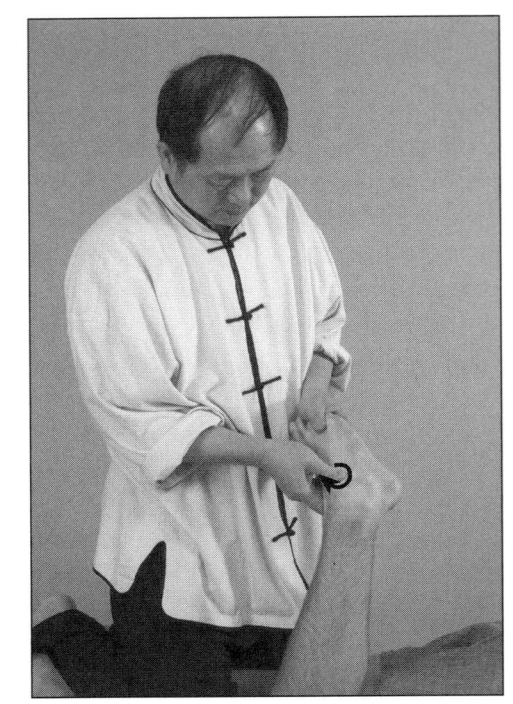

FIGURE 6-148

FIGURE 6-149

Massage the ankle area with your fingers or the edge of your palm (Figure 6-148). Then press inward gently with your thumb and massage the entire ankle joint (Figure 6-149).

Next, use a thumb to massage the entire foot, especially the bottom of the foot, from the ankle to the toes (Figure 6-150). Repeat several times. Finally, grab every toe with your thumb and second finger and gently pull several times. You do not need to pop the joints.

Step 7. After finishing the above massage, grab the foot or the lower section of the calf with both hands and lift up slightly. Pull gently and move the whole leg in a circle (Figure 6-151). Again, brush the entire leg from the hip downward to the bottom of the foot a few times to complete the leg massage.

During the course of the leg massage, you may repeatedly massage the gates whenever you are in the area; this will keep them open as you massage.

Chapter 6: General Massage

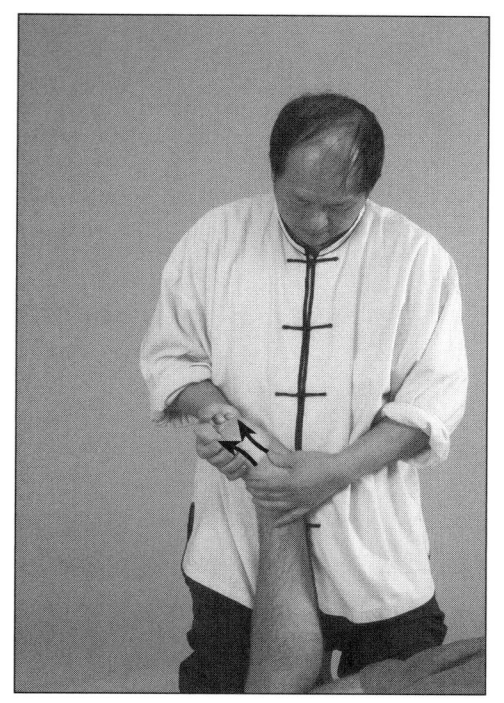

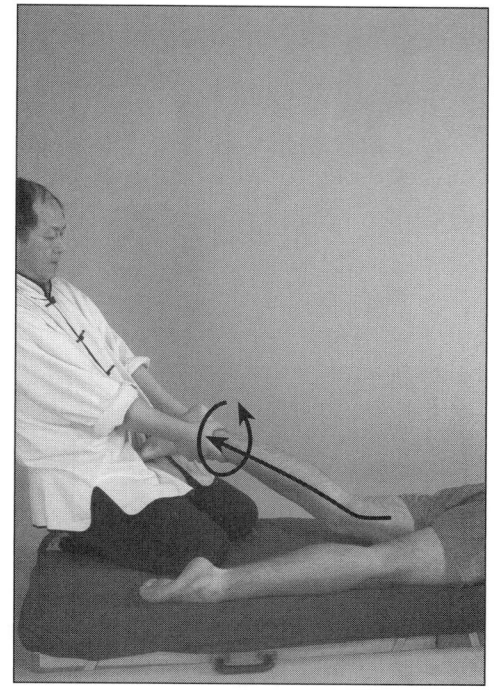

FIGURE 6-150

FIGURE 6-151

Massaging the Back of the Upper Arms, Forearms, and Hands

Before massaging the arms, you should cover your partner's legs with a towel or blanket to keep them warm. However, this may not be needed if the room is warm enough.

Anatomical Structure of the Arm and Its Circulatory Systems. Just beneath the skin on the back of the arm is muscle, some nerves extending from the shoulder down to the hand, and some veins on the back and inside of the arm (Figure 6-152).

Once all the muscles are removed, you can see the main nerve and artery coming down from the shoulder to the hand (Figure 6-153). You can also see some of the arteries and nerves extending from under the shoulder blade to the top of the shoulder.

Finally, you can see the front and the back of the hands (Figures 6-154 and 6-155). You can see in these two pictures that most of the blood circulatory system and the nerves are hidden in the gaps between the bones of the palm.

283

Qigong Massage

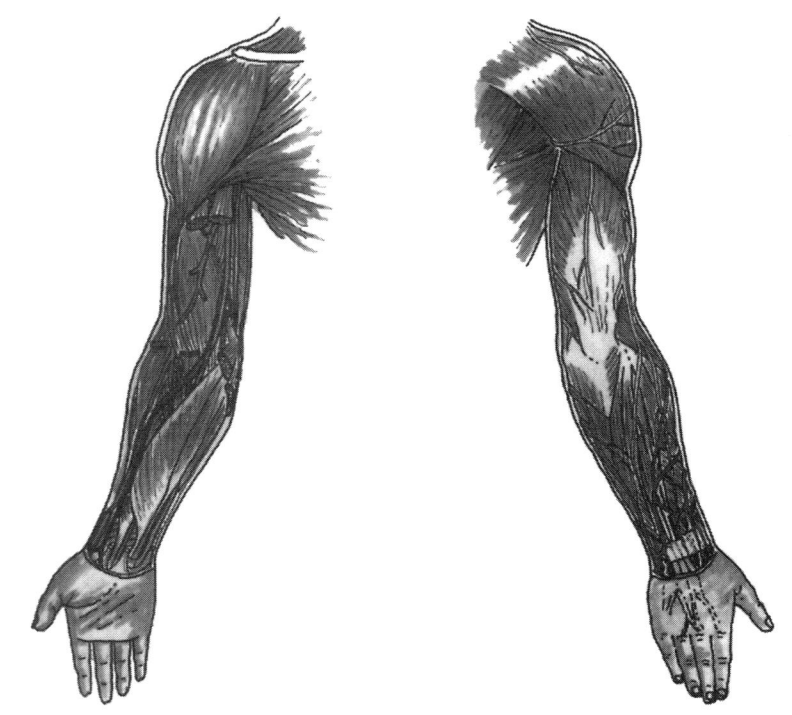

FIGURE 6-152. SUPERFICIAL ANATOMICAL STRUCTURE OF THE POSTERIOR ASPECT OF THE ARM.

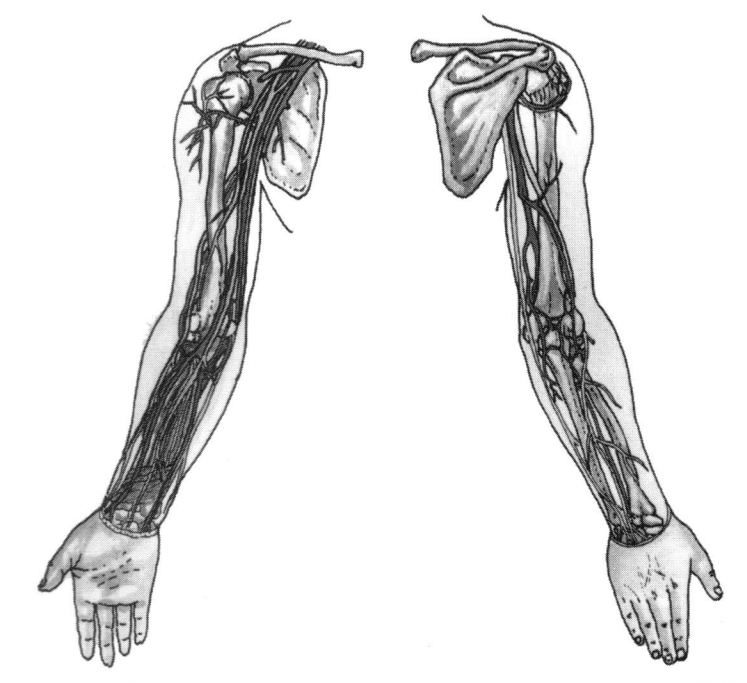

FIGURE 6-153. DEEP ANATOMICAL STRUCTURE OF THE POSTERIOR ASPECT OF THE ARM.

Chapter 6: General Massage

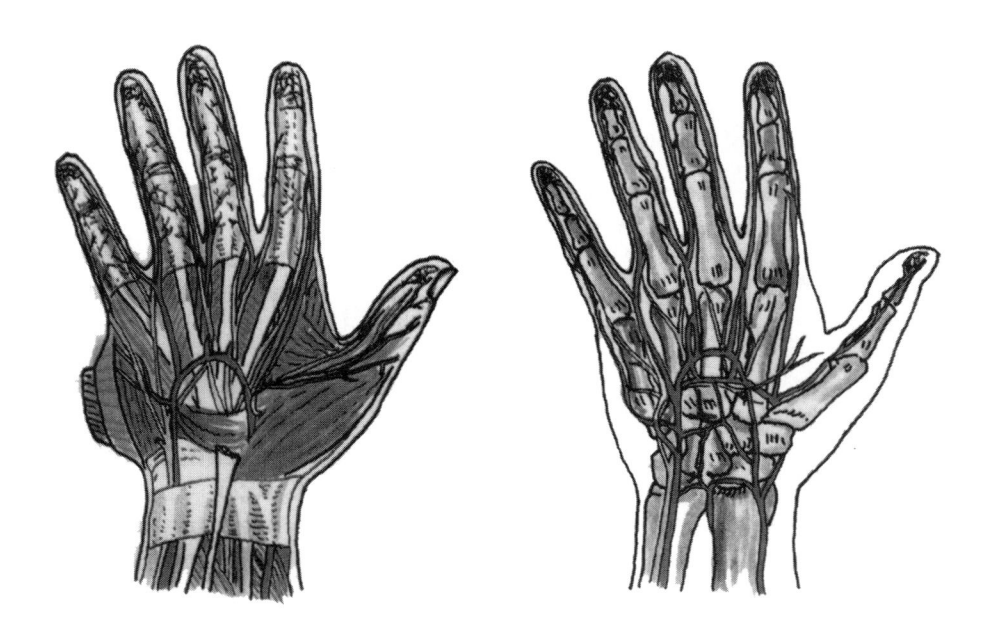

FIGURE 6-154. ANATOMICAL STRUCTURE OF THE POSTERIOR ASPECT OF THE HAND (FRONT VIEW).

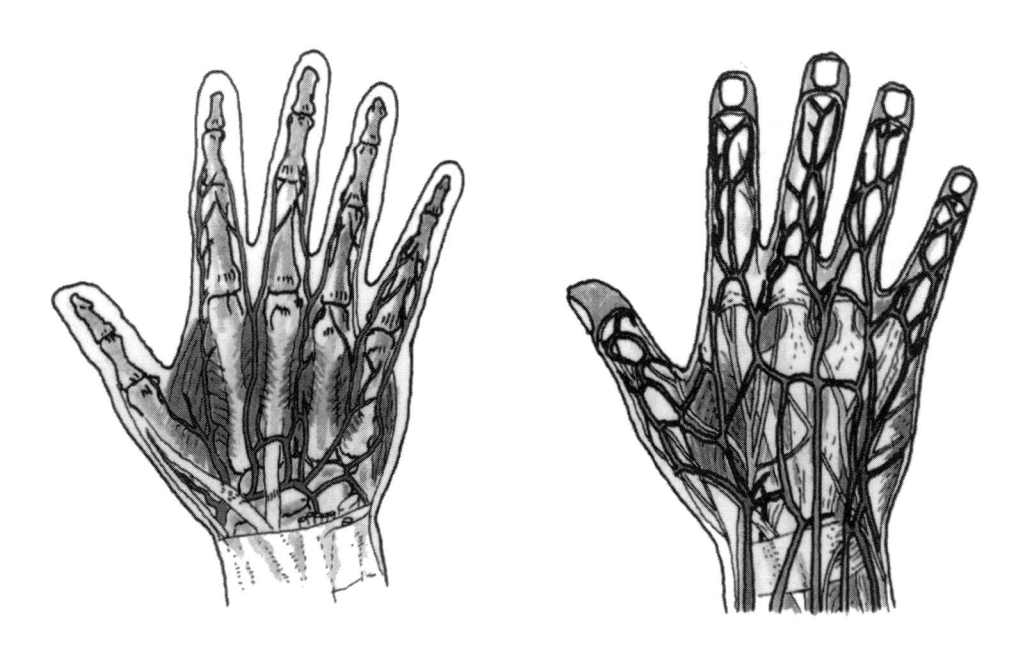

FIGURE 6-155. DEEP ANATOMICAL STRUCTURE OF THE POSTERIOR ASPECT OF THE HAND (BACK VIEW).

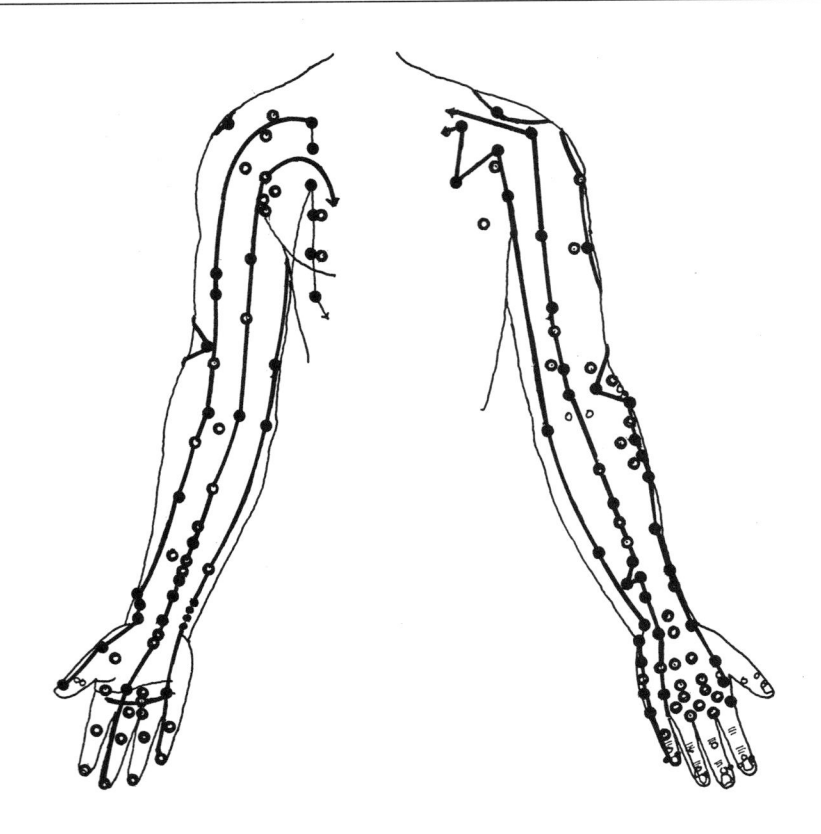

FIGURE 6-156. PROMARY QI CHANNELS AND ACUPUNCTURE CAVITIES ON THE ARMS.

Theory. After you have finished the legs, massage the arms to complete the massage of the back of the body. Like the legs, there are six primary Qi channels connected to the arms. Because of these channels, the arms are important in general massage, although they are not considered quite as important as the legs. This is because the muscles in the arms are not as large as those in the legs, and so there is less accumulation of Qi and blood in the arms, and it is more easily removed. In Tui Na (推拿) massage, however, the arms are the most important area to massage for healing.

Like the legs, there are three Yin channels on the inside and three Yang channels on the outside of the arm. Therefore, the inside of the arm is more tender than the outside, and you should be gentler and more careful with your power.

The basic idea of arm massage is to lead the Qi accumulated in the upper body to the hands and finally release it from the body. We will next introduce the important gates on the back of the upper arm, forearm, and the hand, and then go on to discuss massage techniques. But first, please review the Qi circulatory system of the arms (Figure 6-156).

Chapter 6: General Massage

FIGURE 6-157. THE JIANYU, JIANLIAO, BIANO, QUCHI, AND HEGU CAVITIES.

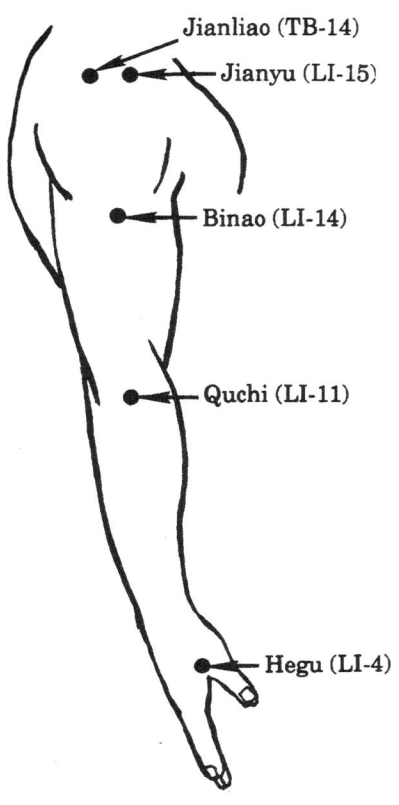

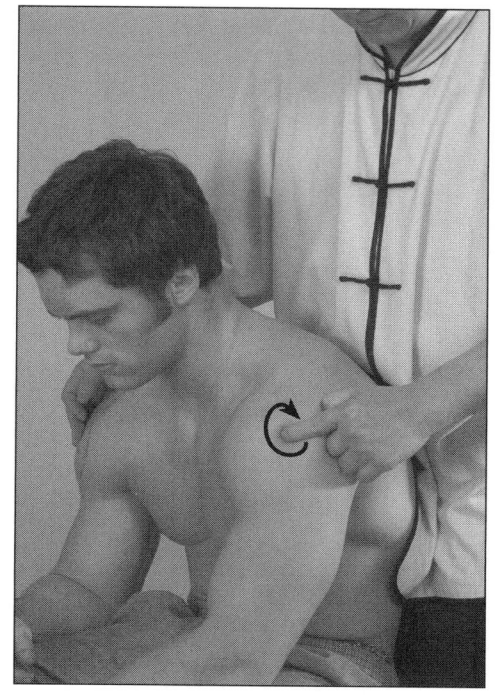

FIGURE 6-158

Gates

Jianliao (TB-14) (肩髎) **and Jianyu (LI-15)** (肩髃). Jianliao (Shoulder Seam) and Jianyu (Shoulder Bone) are located in the shoulder area (Figure 6-157). When these two cavities are massaged and stimulated, Qi in the upper body can be led to the upper arms.

To massage these two gates, you may use your thumb, second, or the middle finger to press on the cavity. If you are using the right hand on the right shoulder, you should circle in a counterclockwise direction (Figure 6-158). Naturally, if you are using the left hand on the left shoulder, you should circle in a clockwise direction.

287

FIGURE 6-159. THE NAOHUI AND SIDU CAVITIES.

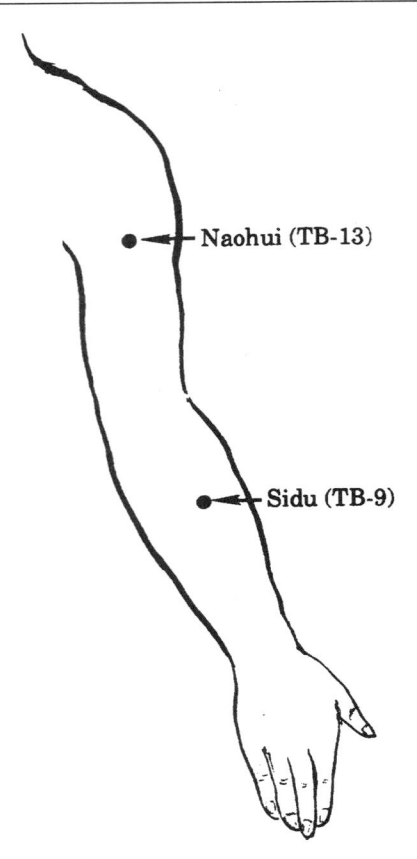

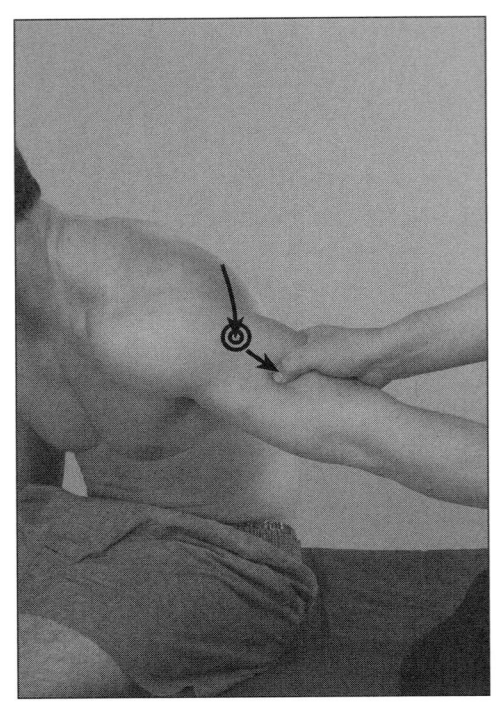

FIGURE 6-160

Naohui (TB-13) (臑會) **and Binao (LI-14)** (臂臑). Naohui (Shoulder's Meeting) and Binao (Arm and Scapula) are located on the outside of the upper arm (Figures 6-157 and 6-159). When these two cavities are massaged and stimulated, the Qi in the shoulders can be led to the arms.

To massage these two gates, you may use the thumb, the second and the middle fingers, or the middle finger to press on the cavity and then rub in a counterclockwise circle if you are using your right hand (Figure 6-160), or clockwise if you are using your left hand.

Quchi (LI-11) (曲池) **and Chize (L-5)** (尺澤). Quchi (Crooked Pool) and Chize (Cubit Marsh) are located near the elbow (Figures 6-157 and 6-161). When they are massaged and stimulated, Qi in the upper arm can be led downward to the elbow.

To massage these two gates, you may use your thumb or the middle finger to press on the cavity and then rub in a counterclockwise circle if you are using your right hand. If you are using your left hand, you should circle in a clockwise direction (Figure 6-162).

Chapter 6: General Massage

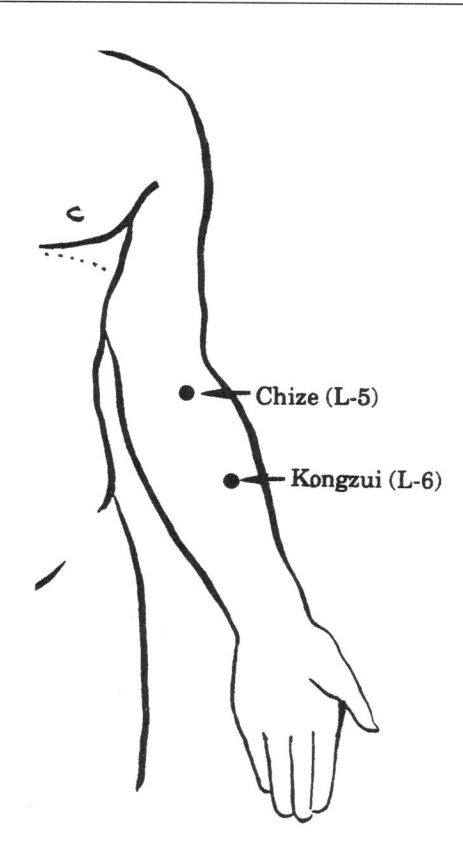

FIGURE 6-161. THE CHIZE AND KONGZUI CAVITIES.

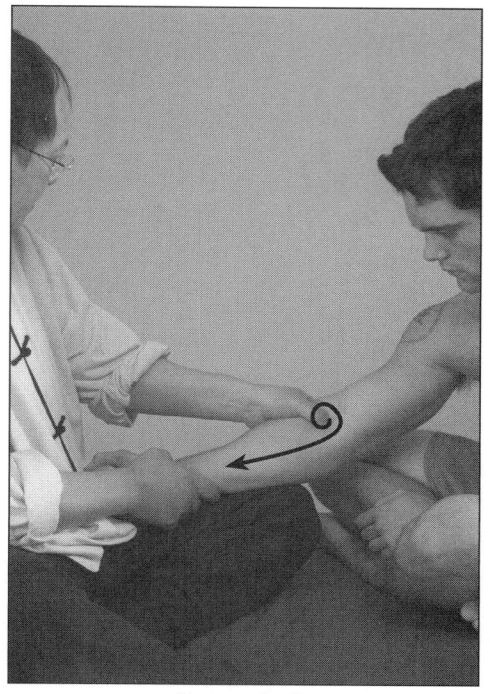

FIGURE 6-162

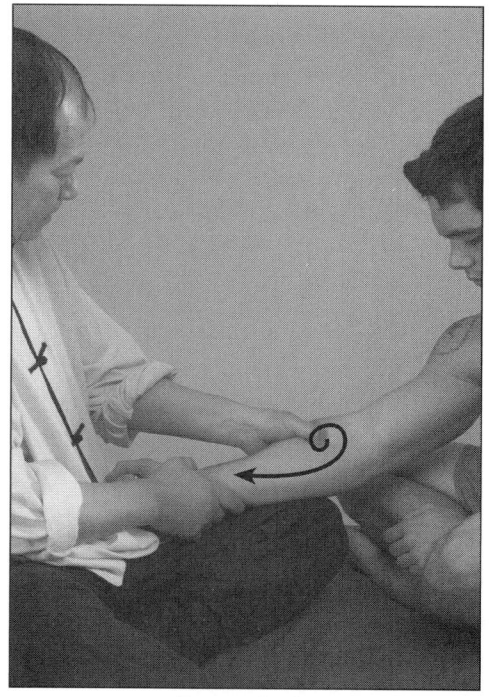

FIGURE 6-163

Kongzui (L-6) (孔最) and Sidu (TB-9) (四瀆). Kongzui (Opening Maximum) is located on the inside of the forearm, while Sidu (Four Ditch) is located on the outside (Figures 6-159 and 6-161), When they are massaged and stimulated, Qi in the upper arm can be led downward to the forearm.

To massage these two gates, you may use your thumb or middle finger to press on the cavity and rub in a counterclockwise circle if you are using your right hand, and clockwise if you are using your left hand (Figure 6-163).

289

Qigong Massage

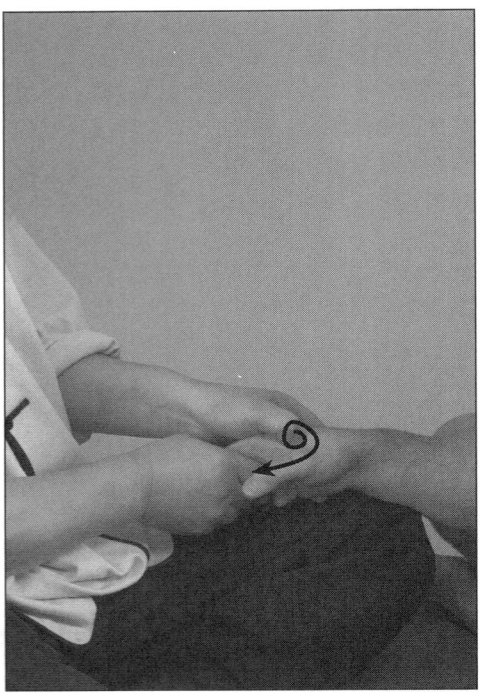

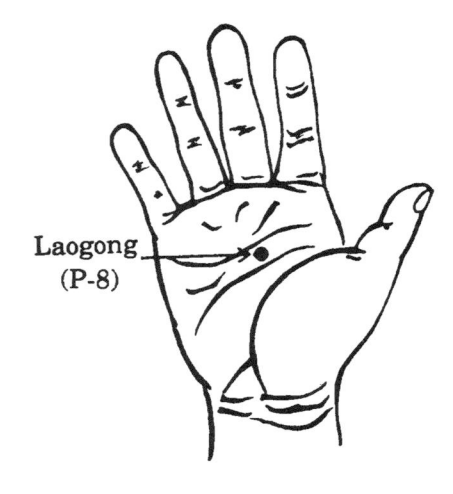

FIGURE 6-164

FIGURE 6-165. THE LAOGONG CAVITY.

Hegu (LI-4) (合谷). Hegu (Adjoining Valleys) is located on the base of the thumb and the second finger (Figure 6-157). When this cavity is massaged and stimulated, Qi in the back of the arm can be led to the hand.

To massage these two gates, you may use your thumb to press on the cavity and then rub in a counterclockwise direction if you are using your right hand (Figure 6-164), and in a clockwise direction if you are using your left hand.

Laogong (P-8) (勞宮). Laogong (Labor's Palace) is located in the center of the palm (Figure 6-165). The exact point is where the tip of the middle finger touches the palm. The two Laogong cavities are two of the four main gates on the limbs from which Qi inside the body can communicate with the Qi outside of the body. When the Laogong is massaged and stimulated, Qi can be led to the palms.

To massage Laogong, you may use your right thumb to press on the cavity and rub in a counterclockwise direction (Figure 6-166). If you circle in the other direction, you will be nourishing the Qi instead of releasing it.

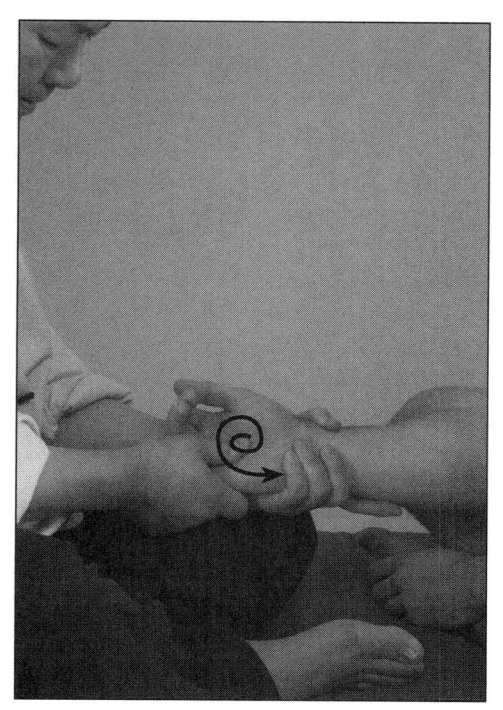

FIGURE 6-166

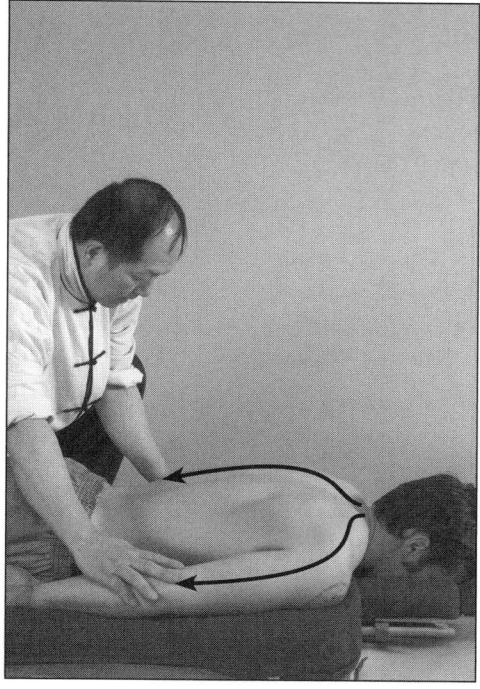

FIGURE 6-167

Massaging the Back of the Upper Arms, Forearms, and Hands

Step 1. First, brush your hands lightly over your partner's skin from their shoulders to their hands (Figure 6-167). Repeat several times. This will help them relax, and also bring their mind to their arms, which will bring a significant amount of Qi from their upper body to the arms.

Next, place your partner's arm behind their back and use both your hands to raise the shoulder gently and move it in a circle (Figure 6-168). When you circle the right arm, move it in a clockwise direction, and when you circle the left arm move it in a counterclockwise direction. This circular motion can relax the entire shoulder and can also help your partner to lead Qi to the arm.

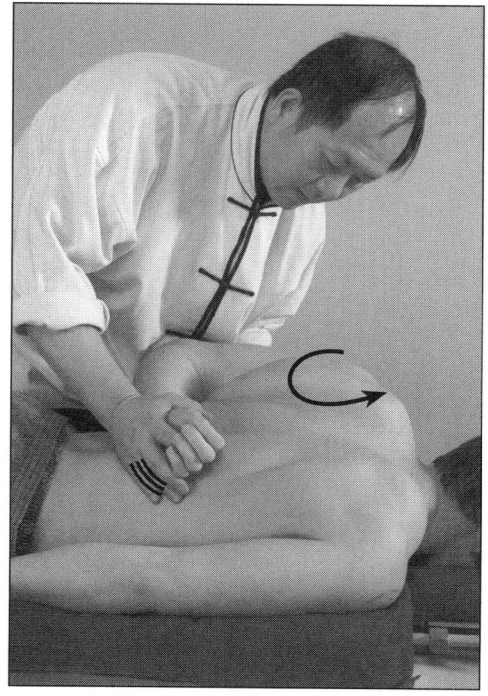

FIGURE 6-168

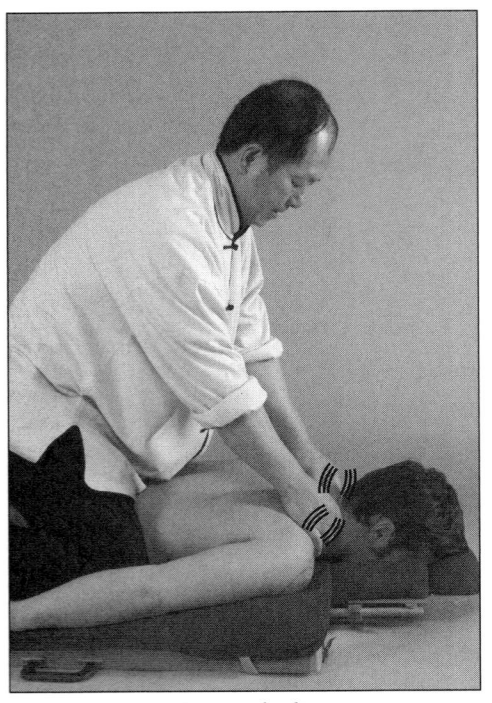

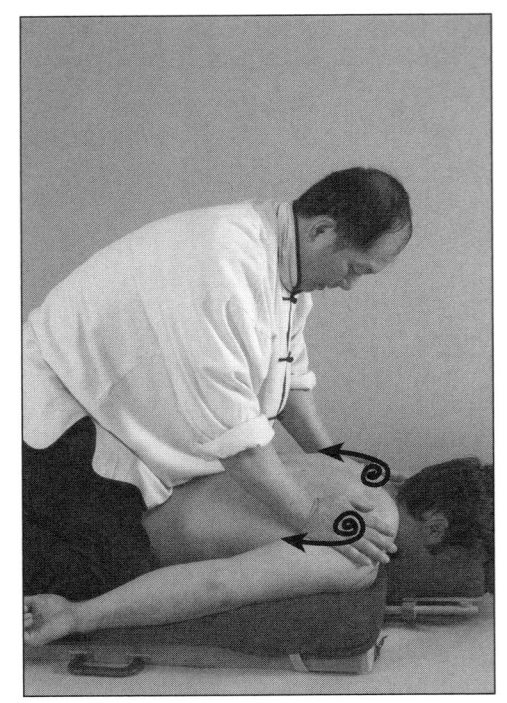

FIGURE 6-169

FIGURE 6-170

Step 2. Next, massage and open the gates on the shoulders and arms. Before you do this, you should massage the upper back again and relax the upper body. Then again stimulate the Jianjing (GB-21) (肩井) cavity located between the neck and the shoulder (Figure 6-169). You should also massage the Tianzong (SI-11) (天宗) cavity in the center of the shoulder blade (Figure 6-170).

After you have loosened up the upper body and the shoulders, use the massage techniques introduced earlier to massage and stimulate all of the gates located on the shoulders and arms. You should start from the shoulder and move down to the hand. Repeat the process several times.

Step 3. Next, use the base of your palms to sandwich the arm, gently squeezing and rubbing it around (Figure 6-171). Start at the shoulder and move down to the forearm. Repeat several times.

Step 4. Next, use your thumb and fingers to grab and rub the muscles from the shoulders to the forearms (Figure 6-172). Repeat several times.

Step 5. Next, gently slap the entire arm from the shoulder to the forearm (Figure 6-173). This will lead the Qi underneath to the surface of the skin. Finally, use a hand to brush from the shoulder to the forearm several times.

Step 6. Finally, hold your partner's hand with one hand and the forearm with the other and move the wrist around several times (Figure 6-174). Then, use a thumb to

Chapter 6: General Massage

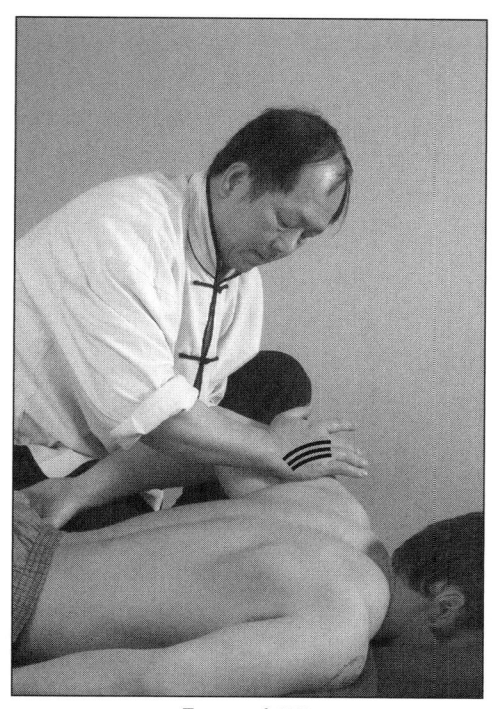

FIGURE 6-171

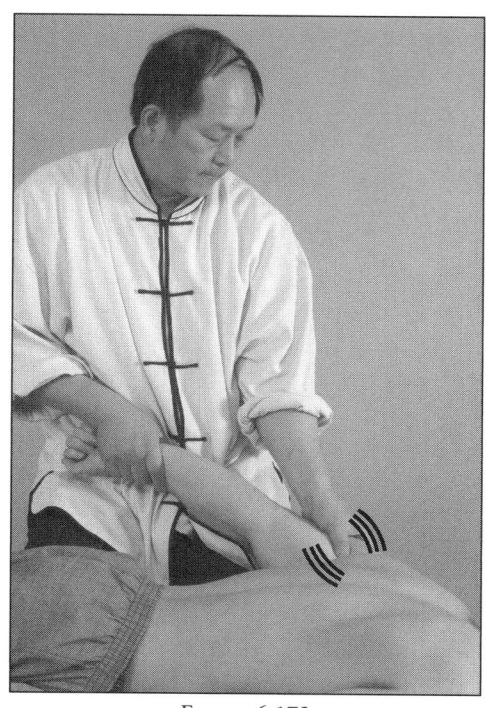

FIGURE 6-172

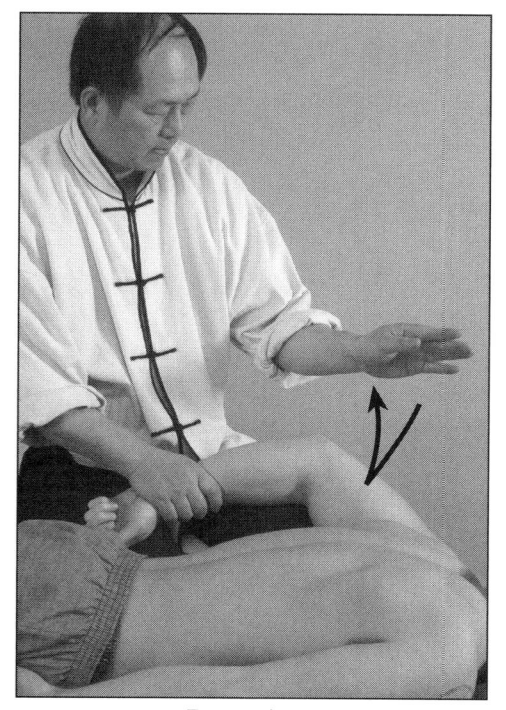

FIGURE 6-173

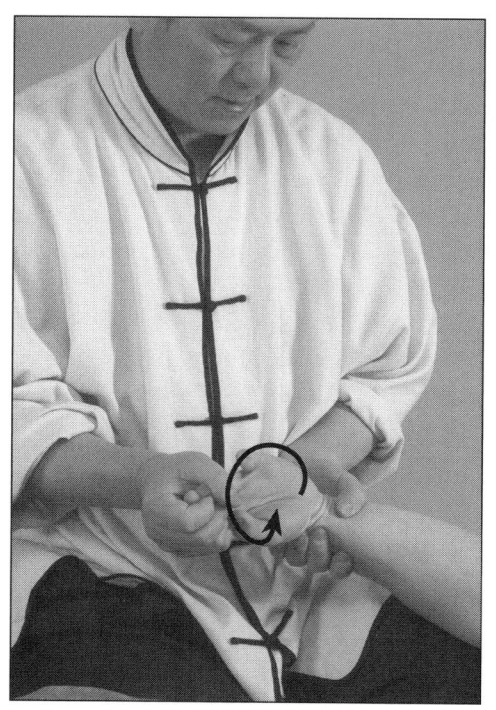

FIGURE 6-174

293

Qigong Massage

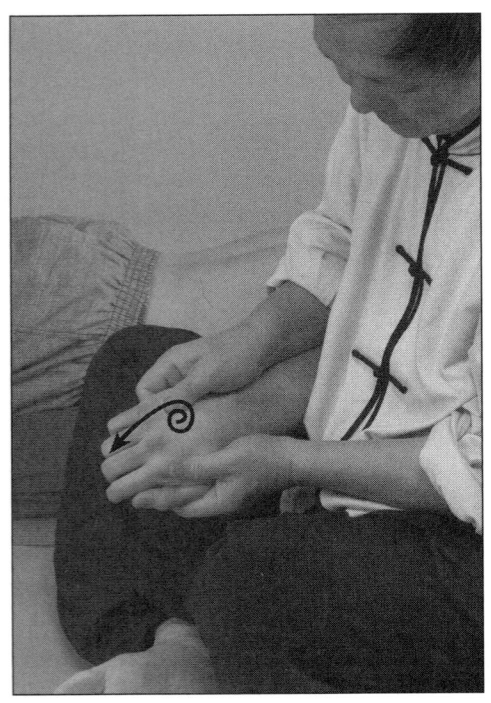

FIGURE 6-175

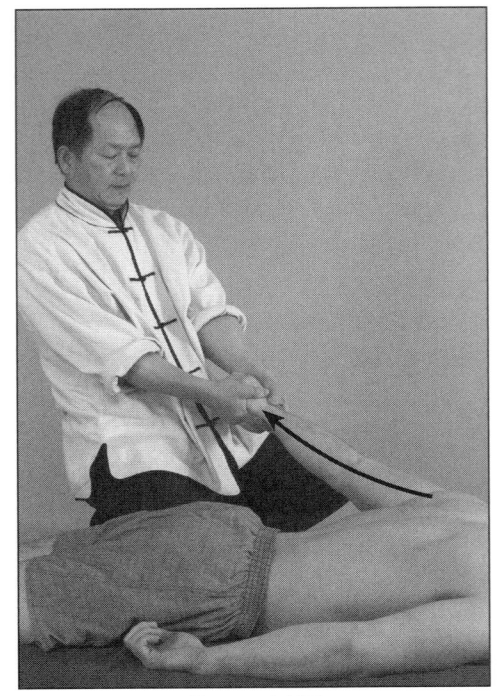

FIGURE 6-176

rub the entire hand from the wrist down to every fingertip (Figure 6-175). Next, grab the forearm with both hands and gently pull the entire arm once (Figure 6-176). and then grab each finger and pull gently (Figure 6-177). When you pull the fingers, you do not have to pop the joints.

During the course of the arm massage, you may repeatedly massage the gates whenever you are in the area. This will keep them open.

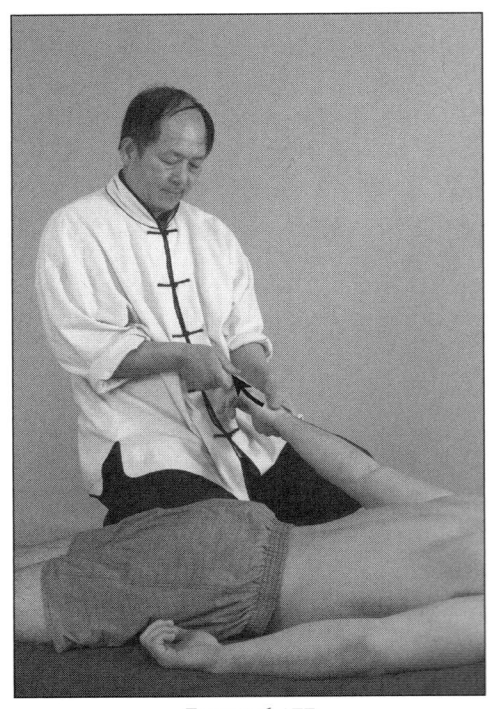

FIGURE 6-177

FIGURE 6-178. SUPERFICIAL ANATOMICAL STRUCTURE OF THE ANTERIOR ASPECT OF THE TRUNK.

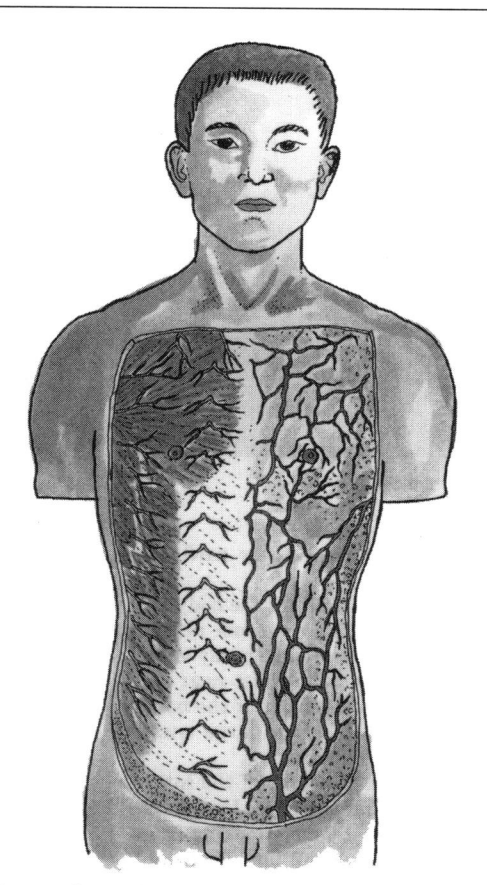

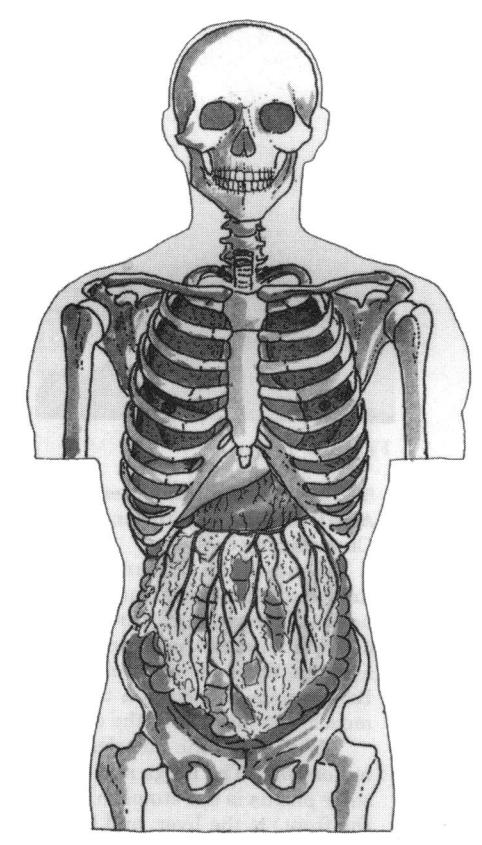

FIGURE 6-179. DEEP ANATOMICAL STRUCTURE OF THE ANTERIOR ASPECT OF THE TRUNK.

6-6. Massaging the Chest and Abdomen 胸部與腹部之按摩

Anatomical Structure of the Front of the Body and Its Circulatory Systems

Beneath the skin and the layer of fat on the front of the body, we first see the muscles, and many nerves spreading out from underneath the muscles (Figure 6-178). In addition, there are many veins distributed over the entire area. Other than on the chest near the armpits, there is not too much thick muscle on the front of the body. Beneath the muscles on the ribs, there are two sets of large trunk muscles running from the chest down to the groin area.

With all of the muscles removed, you can see some of the internal organs. The lungs and the heart are behind the ribs. Under the solar plexus is the stomach. On the left of the stomach (looking from the front is the liver, and behind the liver is the gall bladder; while on the right is the spleen. Under these organs are the large and small intestines as well as, in women, the uterus and ovaries, and finally, below the intestines is the urinary bladder (Figure 6-179).

Theory. Neither China nor the West place much emphasis upon massaging the front of the body. This is due primarily to the fact that most people feel more tension in the back of their bodies, but also because most people are more ticklish in the front, and they are more likely to become uneasy and tense if improper massaging techniques are employed. In addition, the sexual areas are in the front of the body, and massaging near them would make many people feel uncomfortable, especially in the ancient, conservative societies. For these reasons, more massage techniques have been developed for the back than for the front of the body.

From the purely physical point of view, the trunk muscles in the back are usually more tense when a person is tired or fatigued. Since the center of the body's nervous system is in the spine, massaging the back can easily bring the entire body into a relaxed state. However, from the point of view of Chinese medicine and Qigong, massaging the front of the body is at least as important as massaging the back.

First, according to Chinese medicine, the Conception Vessel (Ren Mai, 任脈) runs down the center of the front of the body. This is a Yin vessel, and it is responsible for regulating the Qi level in the six Yin primary Qi channels. In order for it to do this effectively, the center of the front of the body must be relaxed.

Second, most of the internal organs are located in the front of the body, and in giving a massage you reach them through the front of the body. The internal organs are right behind the front trunk muscles. We already know that problems in the internal organs are the cause of most illnesses. The internal organs are like machines in the production line of life. Whenever one of them malfunctions, life can be threatened. Because of this, maintaining smooth Qi circulation in and among the internal organs is a very important part of Chinese Qigong massage. The way to improve Qi circulation in the internal organs is to relax the muscles which surround them. This is why the goal of massaging the front of the body in Chinese Qigong massage is to relax the front trunk muscles.

Furthermore, according to Chinese medicine and Qigong, the lower abdomen is the site of the Lower Dan Tian (Xia Dan Tian, 下丹田), which is the residence of Original Qi (Yuan Qi, 元氣). Original Qi is the source of life energy, so increasing the flow of this Qi from its residence is an important part of massage.

Normally, after you have finished massaging the back and start massaging the front of the body, you again begin at the head and lead the Qi downward to the chest area. After massaging the chest and abdomen, you continue on to the front of the legs to lead the Qi further downward. Finish your massage with the arms. In order to know the Qi gates on the front of the body, you need to be familiar with the Qi circulatory system. Figure 6-180 shows the Conception Vessel and all of the primary channels located on the front of the body. Next, we will introduce the gates on the front of the body, and then follow this discussion with some massage techniques.

Chapter 6: General Massage

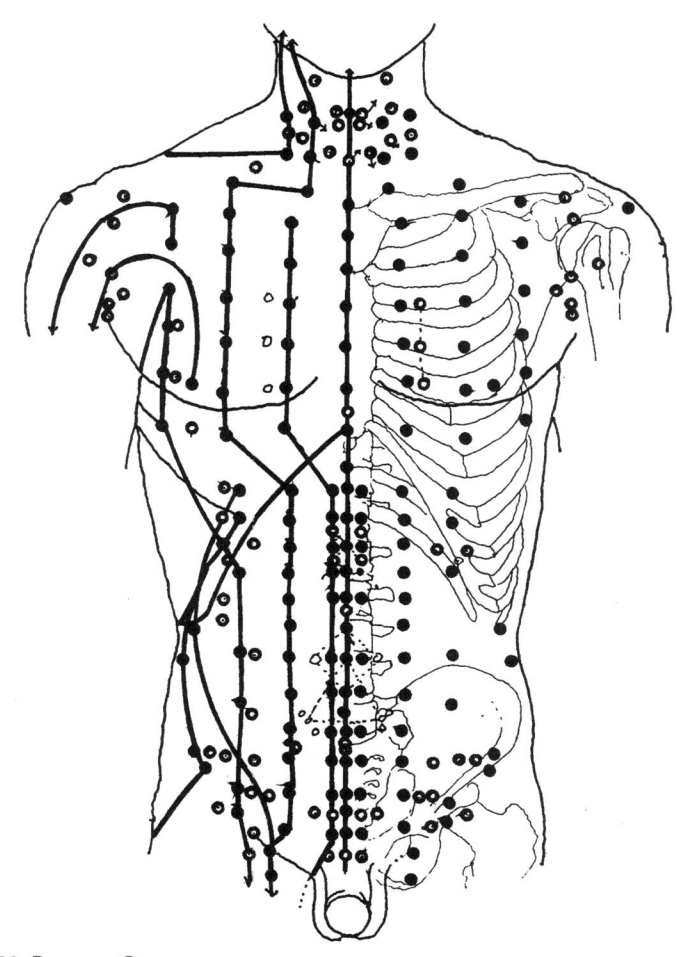

FIGURE 6-180. PRIMARY QI CHANNELS AND ACUPUNCTURE CAVITIES ON THE FRONT OF THE BODY.

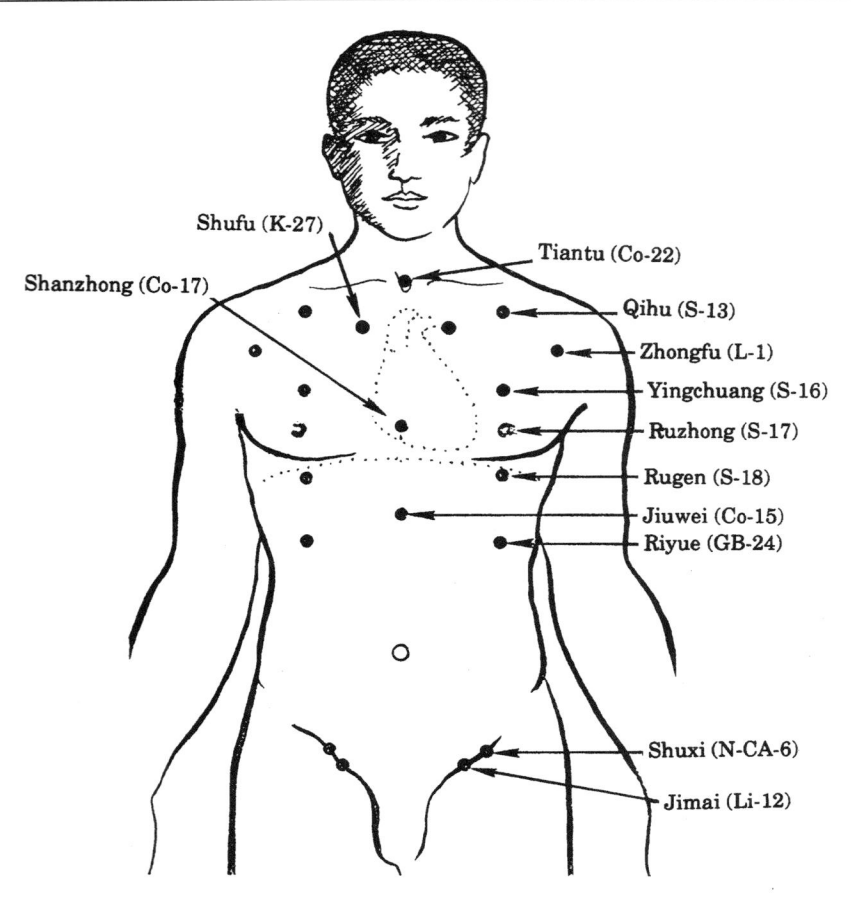

FIGURE 6-181. THE TIANTU, QIHU, SHUFU, ZHONGFU, YINCHUANG, SHANZONG, RUZHONG, RUGEN, JIUWEI, SHIUXI, AND JIMAI CAVITIES.

Gates

Tiantu (Co-22) (天突). Tiantu (Heaven's Prominence) is located on the base of the throat and is the junction of the neck and the chest (Figure 6-181). In acupuncture, the function of this cavity is to facilitate and regulate the movement of lung Qi in order to cool the throat and to clear the voice. When this gate is relaxed and wide open, the Qi communication between the throat and the chest can be smooth.

When you massage this gate, you must be very gentle. Start from the side of the gate and follow the bone, using the fingers of both hands to push toward the Tiantu cavity a few times (Figure 6-182). Next, use your thumb or the second and third fingers to rub the cavity very gently with a circular motion (Figure 6-183). Circle in a counterclockwise direction and lead the Qi downward to the chest.

Shufu (K-27) (俞府) **and Qihu (S-13)** (氣戶). Shufu (Hollow Residence) and Qihu (Qi's Household) are located above the nipples (Figure 6-181). Shufu belongs to the kidney channel. The kidneys have a primary role in water metabolism and controlling

Chapter 6: General Massage

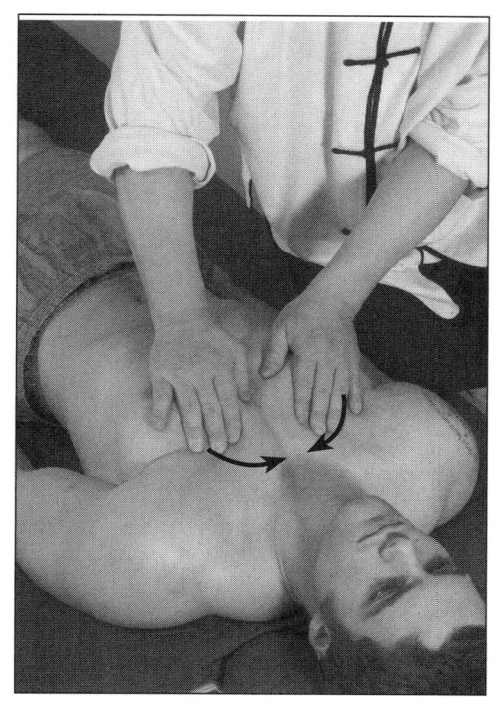

FIGURE 6-182

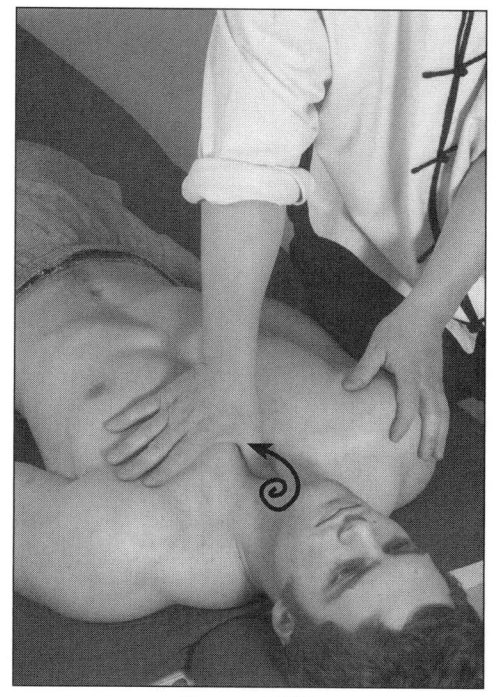

FIGURE 6-183

the body's liquids. When the Shufu cavity is massaged and stimulated, the water in the body can be led upward to the lungs. In Chinese medicine, this cavity is related to bronchitis, asthma, chest pain, vomiting, and abdominal distension.

When Qihu is massaged and stimulated, the Qi accumulated in the center of the lungs can be spread to the sides of the lungs, which will relax the chest, In addition, massaging Qihu will lead the Qi accumulated in the neck downward to the chest. In Chinese medicine, Qihu is related to such illnesses as bronchitis, asthma, hiccups, and intercostal neuralgia

When you massage these two cavities, rub in a circle with your second and middle fingers. Circle to the center and then up, and finally to the sides of the chest and out the arms (Figure 6-184).

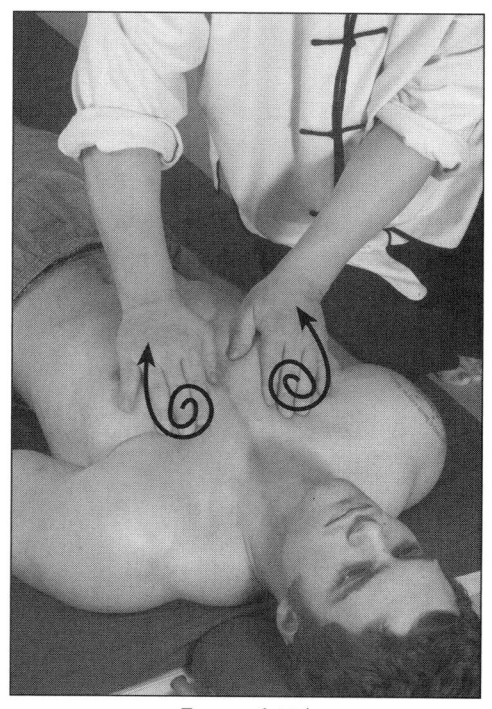

FIGURE 6-184

299

Qigong Massage

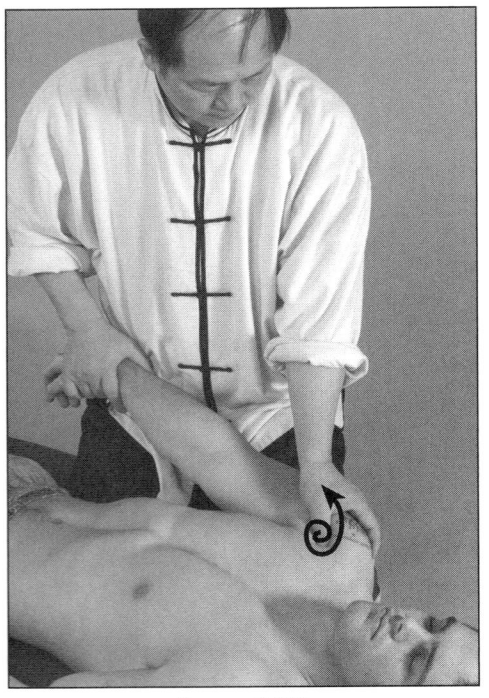

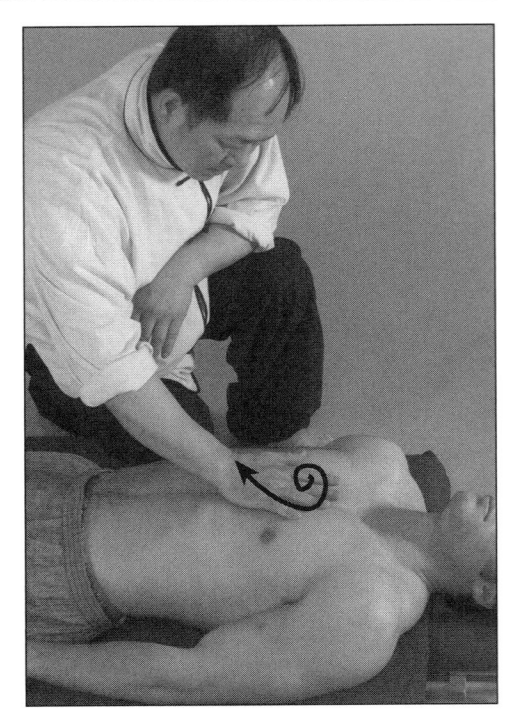

FIGURE 6-185

FIGURE 6-186

Zhongfu (L-1) (中府). Zhongfu (Central Residence) is located in the upper chest near the shoulder joint (Figure 6-181). According to Chinese medicine, this cavity is connected to the throat area, as well as to the lungs, and stomach. This cavity is the junction of the throat and upper chest with the arms. Therefore, massage will lead the Qi accumulated on the front of the neck and upper chest out to the shoulders and finally to the hands, where it can be dissipated. In Chinese medicine, this cavity is related to coughing and wheezing, coughing blood and pus, throat blockage, nasal congestion, excessive sweating, tumors and nodular growths on the neck.

When you massage this cavity, simply use the thumb or the second and middle fingers to press in and circle a few times, and then brush with your hands out to the arms (Figure 6-185). When you massage, circle toward the center and then upward and finally to the side. This will lead the Qi to the arms.

Shanzhong (Co-17) (膻中). Shanzhong (Penetrating Odor) is located directly between the nipples (Figure 6-181). When Shanzhong is massaged correctly, the Qi accumulated in the center of the chest can be spread outward. This can significantly regulate the Fire Qi (Huo Qi, 火氣) which has accumulated in the solar plexus (Middle Dan Tian; Zhong Dan Tian, 中丹田). This will release pressure and tension in the front of the body. In Chinese medicine, treating this cavity can regulate and suppress rebellious Qi, and expand the chest to benefit the diaphragm.

To massage this cavity, use the base of a palm to gently press the cavity and rub in

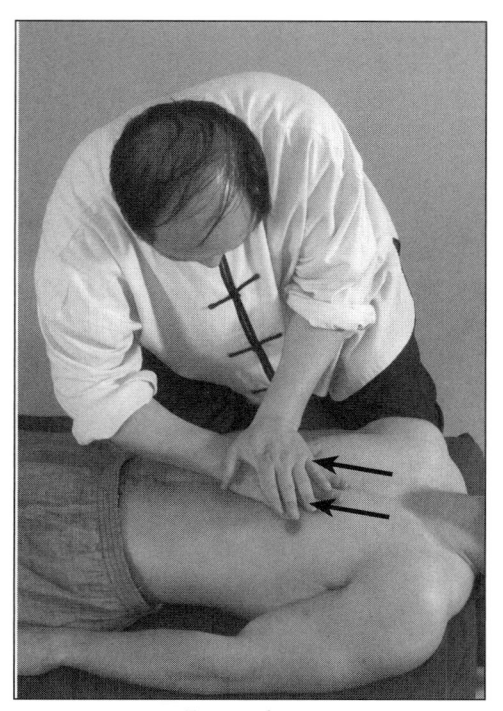

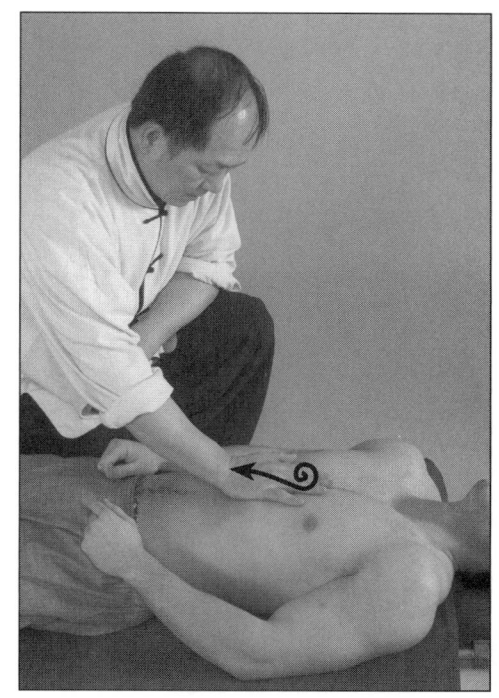

FIGURE 6-187

FIGURE 6-188

a circle a few times, then lead the Qi to the sides and away from the solar plexus (Figure 6-186). Use your right hand to circle clockwise, then spread to the side of the chest a few times, and then circle with your left hand in a counterclockwise direction the same number of times. Finally, use the palms to push downward to the abdominal area (Figure 6-187). In order to avoid leading Qi to the solar plexus, do not stop your pushing at the solar plexus area.

Jiuwei (Co-15) (鳩尾). Jiuwei (Wild Pigeon's Tail) is called the solar plexus in the West, and the Middle Dan Tian in Chinese Qigong. The Middle Dan Tian is the residence of Fire Qi or Post-birth Qi, which is converted from air and food. Physically, this place is the junction between the lungs and the stomach, which is beneath the diaphragm. Whenever too much Qi accumulates in this area, you will feel uncomfortable and experience tension or heartburn in your chest. Because of the excess Yang you will feel tired. One of the practices of Chinese Qigong is to lead the Qi accumulated here downward to the Lower Dan Tian. In Chinese medicine, this cavity is related to such illnesses as angina pectoris, seizures, hiccups, mental illness, and asthma.

Massaging Jiuwei correctly will loosen the area so that the Qi can be moved easily and spread either to the sides or downward to the lower body. The method of massaging this cavity is very simple. Gently rub the cavity in a clockwise circular motion with the base of your right palm, and then lead the Qi to the side (Figure 6-188). Repeat several times. Then change to the left hand and repeat the same massage, only now use a

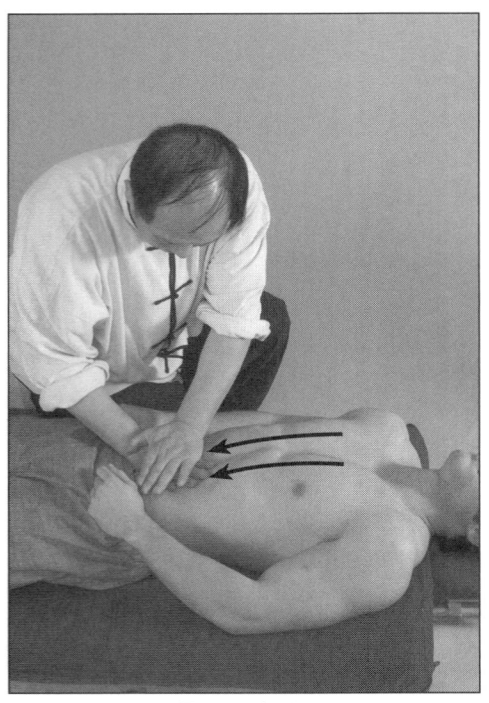

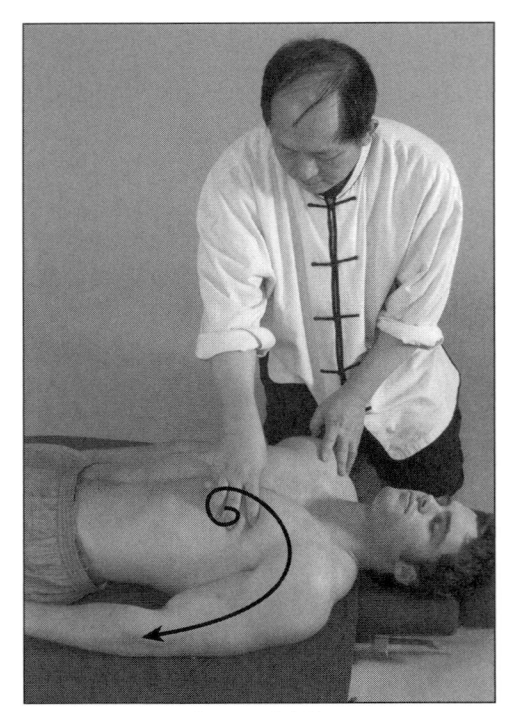

FIGURE 6-189

FIGURE 6-190

counterclockwise motion and lead the Qi down. Finally, use the palms to push downward to the abdomen (Figure 6-189).

Yingchuang (S-16) (膺窗), **Ruzhong (S-17)** (乳中), **and Rugen (S-18)** (乳根). Yingchuang (Breast's Window), Ruzhong (Middle of Breast), and Rugen (Breast's Root) are located above the nipple, in the middle of the nipple, and under the nipple (Figure 6-181). These three cavities are usually treated as one in Qigong massage. They are related to bronchitis, mastitis, asthma, intercostal neuralgia, intestinal noises and diarrhea.

Beneath these cavities is a large section of muscle which extends out to the front of the shoulder. When these muscles are relaxed, the Qi can be led easily to the sides of the chest and also to the front of the shoulder. When you massage these three cavities, first place your index, middle, and ring fingers on all three cavities at the same time, and move your fingers in circles (Figure 6-190). In order to avoid leading Qi toward the solar plexus, you should lead the Qi to the sides of the chest and shoulders.

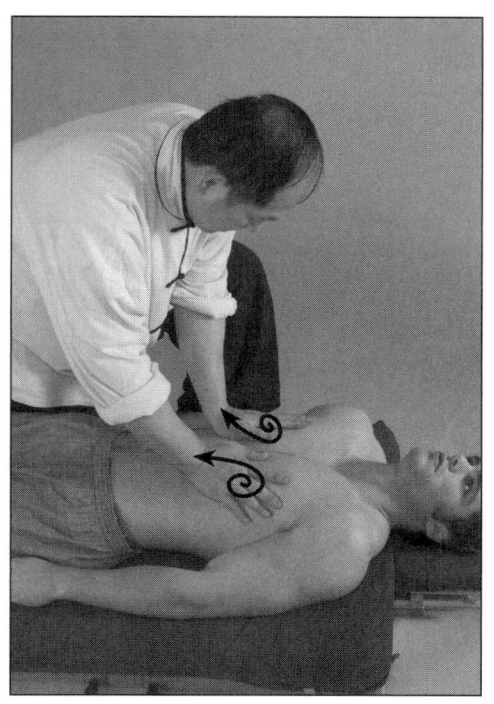

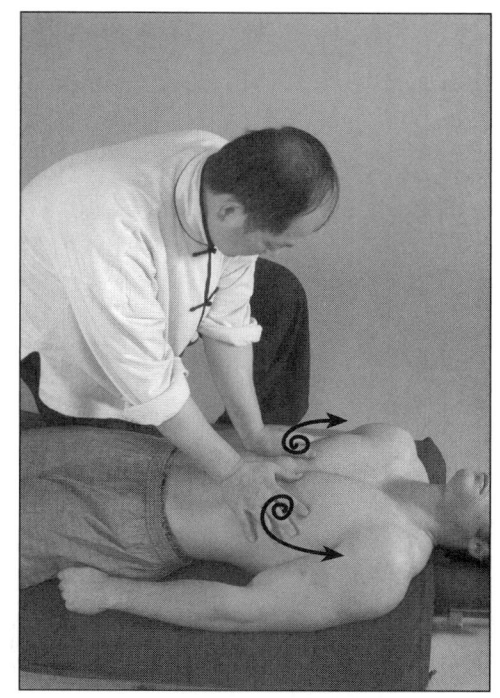

FIGURE 6-191

FIGURE 6-192

Riyue (GB-24) (日月). Riyue (Sun Moon) is located below the ribs in front of the liver and spleen (Figure 6-181). When there is an abnormal Qi condition in the liver and spleen, these two cavities may be tense, which will cause tension in the stomach and abdomen. In Qigong massage, in order to relax the internal organs below the diaphragm you need to relax these cavities. In Chinese medicine, this cavity is related to intercostal neuralgia, cholecystitis, acute and chronic hepatitis, peptic ulcer, and hiccups.

To massage these cavities, use the base of your palms to gently press the cavities and rub in a circle a few times, and then lead the motion to the center and move downward (Figure 6-191). When you massage, the right hand should circle counterclockwise and the left hand clockwise. You should also massage in the opposite direction and follow the ribs to lead the Qi to the sides (Figure 6-192).

Qigong Massage

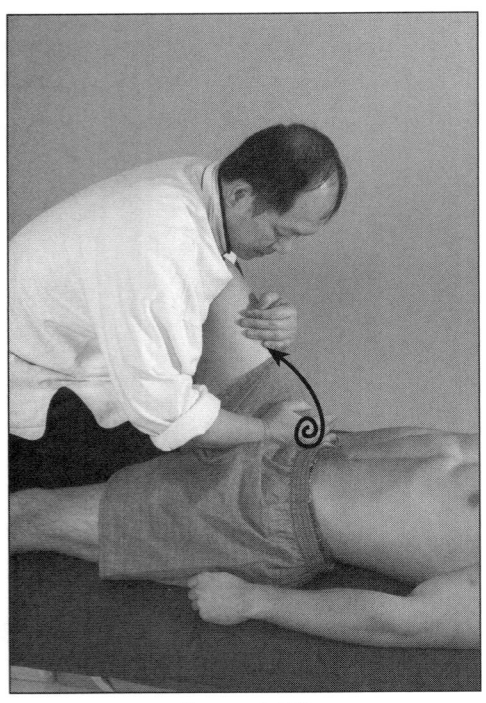

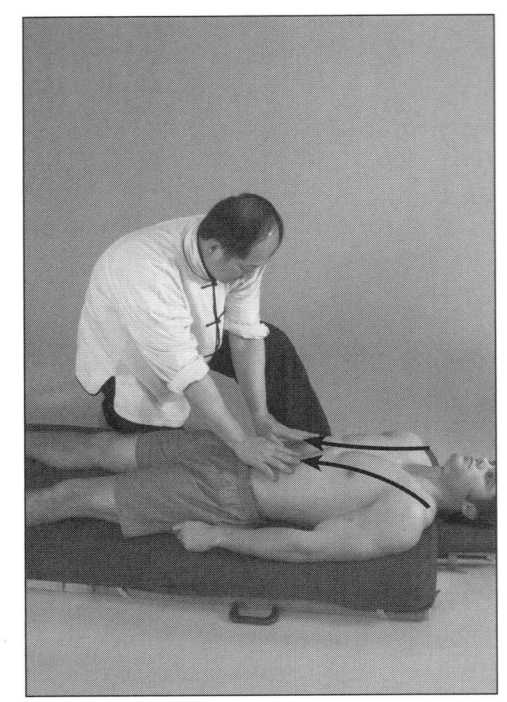

FIGURE 6-193

FIGURE 6-194

Shuxi (N-CA-6) (鼠蹊) **and Jimai (Li-12)** (急脈). Shuxi (Mouse Path) and Jimai (Urgent Pulse) are located in the crease between the thigh and abdomen (Figure 6-181). These two cavities are the junctions of the Qi circulation from the body to the legs in the front of the body. In Chinese medicine, Shuxi is related to tuberculosis of the inguinal lymph glands, and weakness of leg adductors. Jimai is related to prolapsed uterus, pain of hernia, and pain in the penis.

When you massage these two cavities, simply use the edge of our palm to press in and circle (Figure 6-193) while raising your partners thigh to relax the area.

Massaging the Chest and Abdomen

Step 1. First, use your hands to lightly and slowly brush from the face down over the chest, and finally down to the legs and the bottoms of the feet (Figure 6-194). Repeat five times, Then repeat the same process again, now brushing from the face, over the shoulders and finally down to the hands (Figure 6-195). Repeat five times.

Chapter 6: General Massage

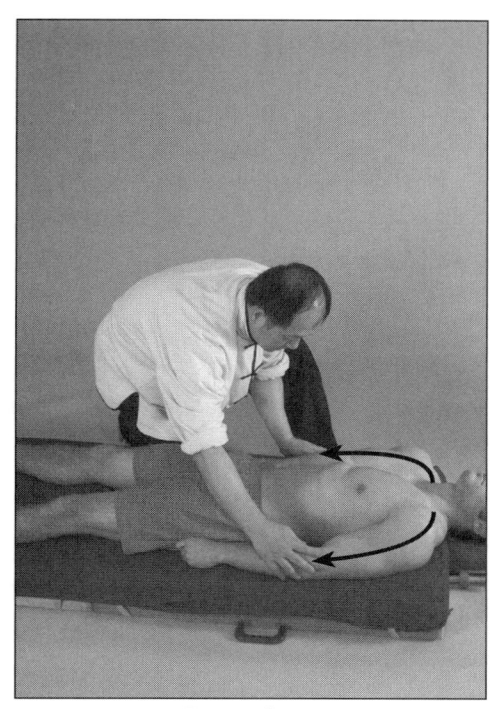

FIGURE 6-195

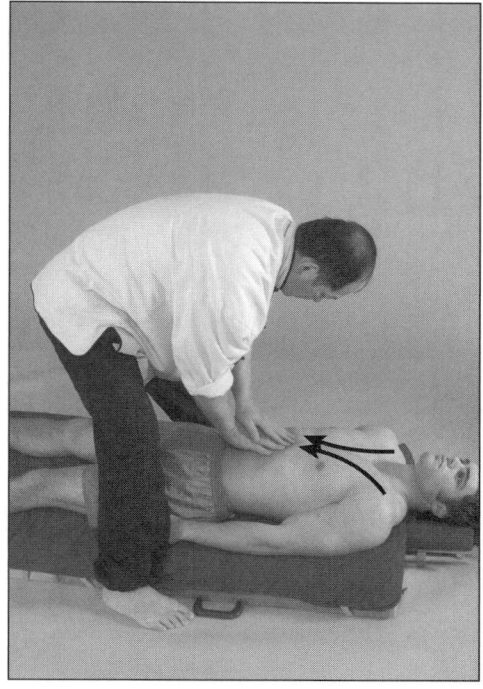

FIGURE 6-196

Step 2. Next, gently stimulate and massage the gates discussed above. Massage the top gates first, and move downward to the abdomen. This will make it easier for the Qi and blood to circulate. Frequently your partner will be ticklish and will tense up. If this happens, change your techniques so that they can relax again. For example, if you started using your fingers, you may switch to using your palms.

Step 3. Next, massage the centerline on the front of the body, leading the Qi downward. To do this, stroke downward with both hands from the back of the neck to the upper chest, and then follow the centerline downward to the abdomen (Figure 6-196). Repeat five times. Then use both hands to gently press the center of the chest from the upper chest to the solar plexus (Figure 6-197).

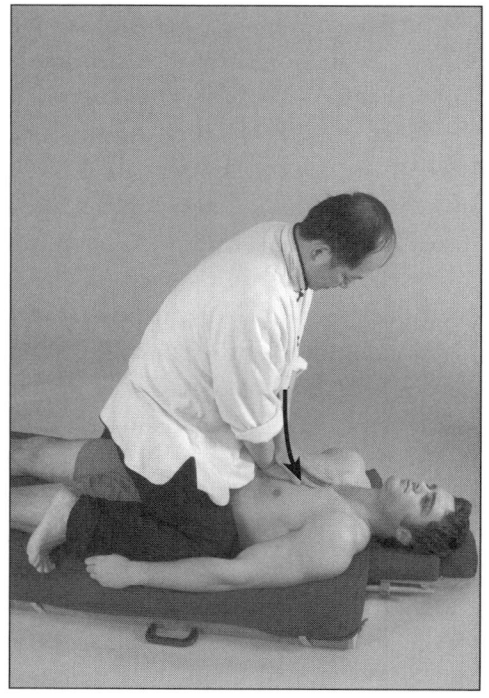

FIGURE 6-197

305

Qigong Massage

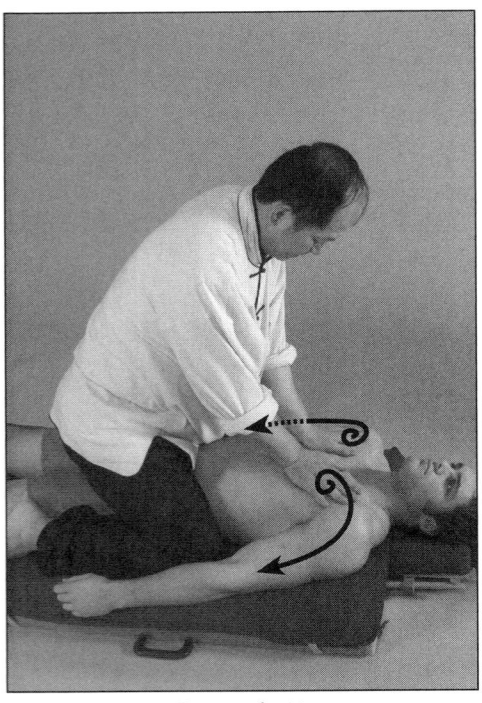

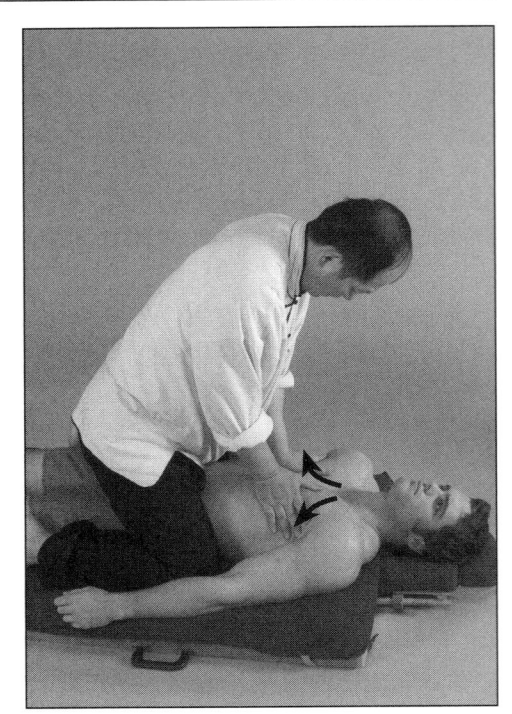

FIGURE 6-198

FIGURE 6-199

Step 4. Use the second and middle fingers of both hands to gently massage the areas above the nipples and under the shoulders for one minute. If your partner is ticklish, switch to your palms (Figure 6-198). This will lead kidney Qi and water upward to moisten the lungs.

Next, place both palms on the center of the upper chest and push the palms to the sides of the upper chest (Figure 6-199). When you do this, you should push along the ribs with your fingers between the ribs. Again, if your partner is ticklish, use your palms instead. This will spread the Qi and moisture which were led upward to the sides of the lungs. Repeat five times.

Finally, repeat the same process, however, start from the solar plexus area and move to the sides from of the chest (Figure 6-200). Repeat five times.

Step 5. Using the base or the edge of both palms, rub from the top of the chest to the diaphragm area with a circular motion (Figure 6-201). Repeat five times. The direction of the circle is very important. When your right hand is circling counterclockwise while your left hand is circling clockwise, you are leading the Qi downward, which will cool down the body. If you reverse the direction, you are leading the Qi upward. This is not desirable in general massage, because it can lead the Qi to the head and make the body too Yang.

Step 6. Next, use your thumb and fingers to grab and rub the tendons in the front of the armpits (Figure 6-202). Continue the grabbing and rubbing downward to the area of the nipples, and then use your palm to smooth and lead Qi down from the armpit (Figure 6-203). Repeat the same procedure about five times. If your partner is

Chapter 6: General Massage

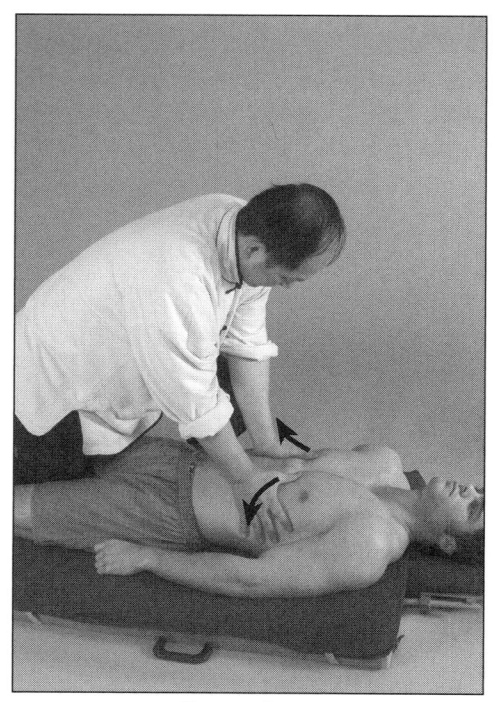

FIGURE 6-200

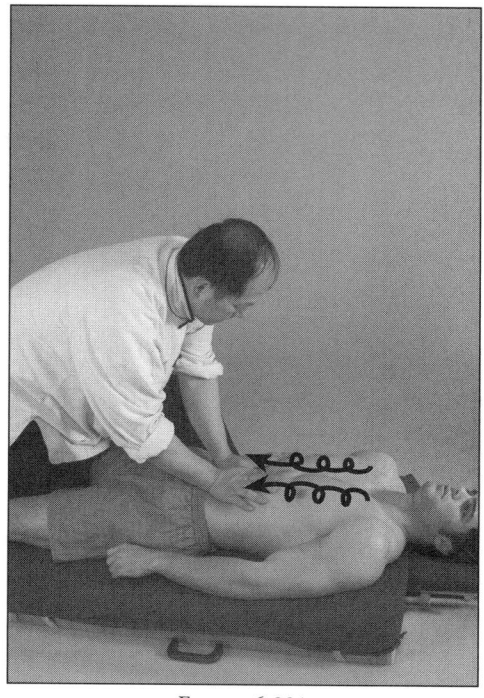

FIGURE 6-201

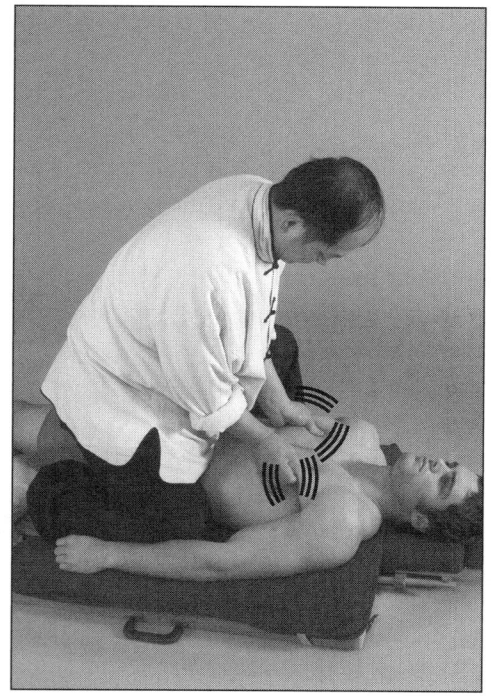

FIGURE 6-202

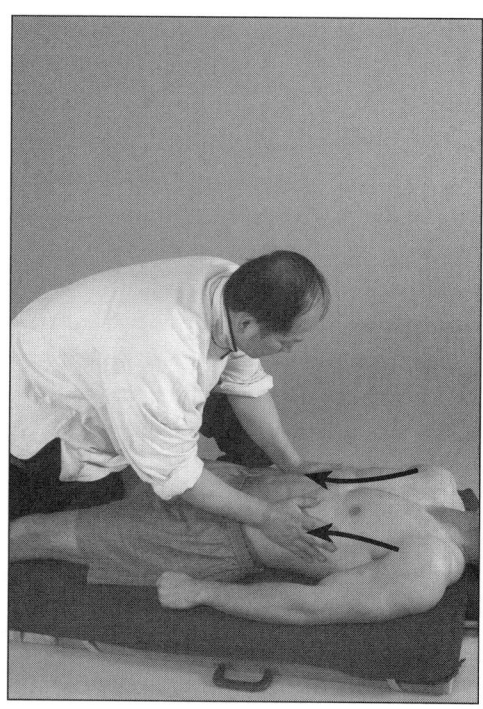

FIGURE 6-203

307

Qigong Massage

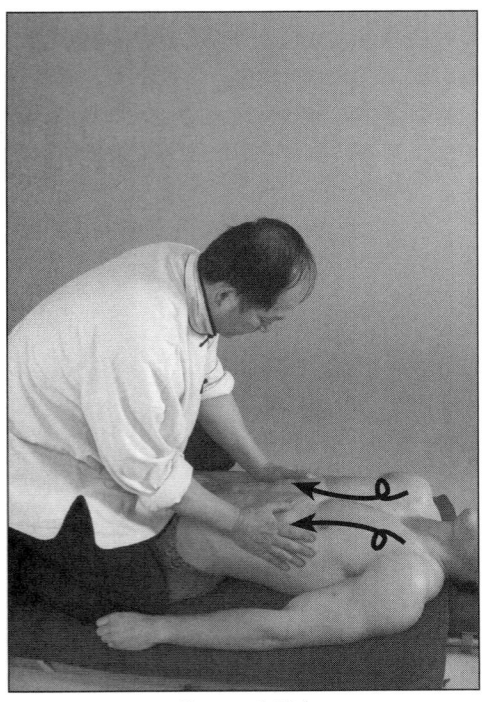

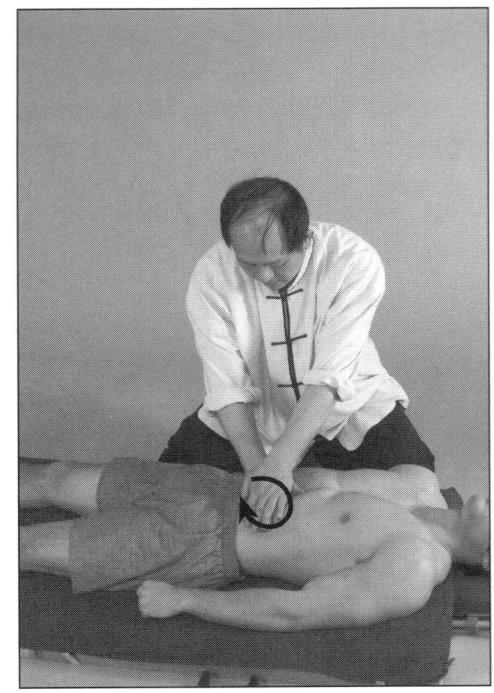

FIGURE 6-204

FIGURE 6-205

very ticklish, simply use your palms to rub in circles downward (Figure 6-204).

Step 7. After you have finished the chest massage, move downward to massage the stomach, abdomen, and waist. First, place both hands on your partner's stomach and circle gently in a clockwise direction (Figure 6-205). Circle about ten to twenty times. While circling your hands, your mind should be very calm and relaxed, and you should be paying attention to where the stomach is located inside the body. Then repeat the same process on the abdomen.

Step 8. Place your hands on both sides of the centerline at the level of your partner's diaphragm. Ask your partner to inhale and then exhale deeply. While they are exhaling, brush both hands downward to the groin area (Figure 6-206).

Then bend one of your partner's legs. With one hand holding the leg in place, massage the area around the front of the hip joint (Figure 6-207). After rubbing in a circle a few times, stroke your hand to the thigh. Repeat a few times. Repeat the same process on the other side.

Finally, spread your partner's legs a comfortable distance apart, and use your middle finger to gently massage the Huiyin (Co-1) (會陰) cavity (Figure 6-208). As mentioned before, this cavity is very important in Chinese Qigong practice.

Step 9. The last step in massaging the front of the body is the waist area. First, use both hands to massage the muscles on the sides of the waist a few times (Figure 6-209).

Chapter 6: General Massage

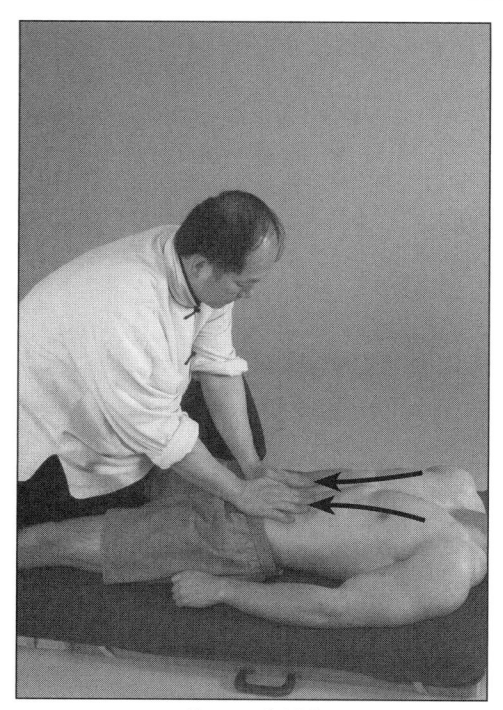

FIGURE 6-206

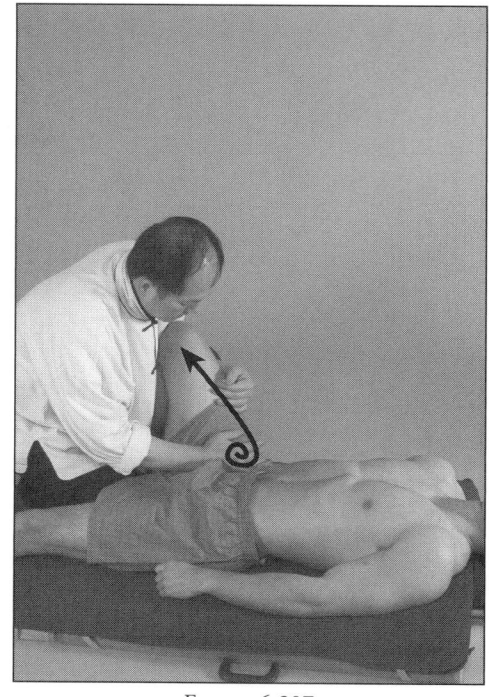

FIGURE 6-207

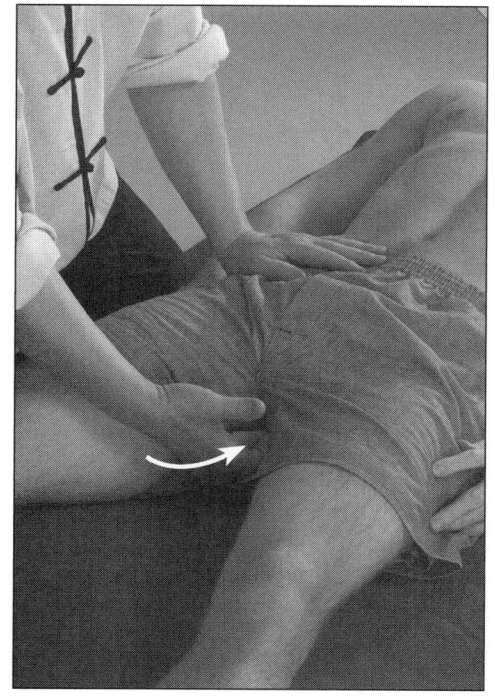

FIGURE 6-208

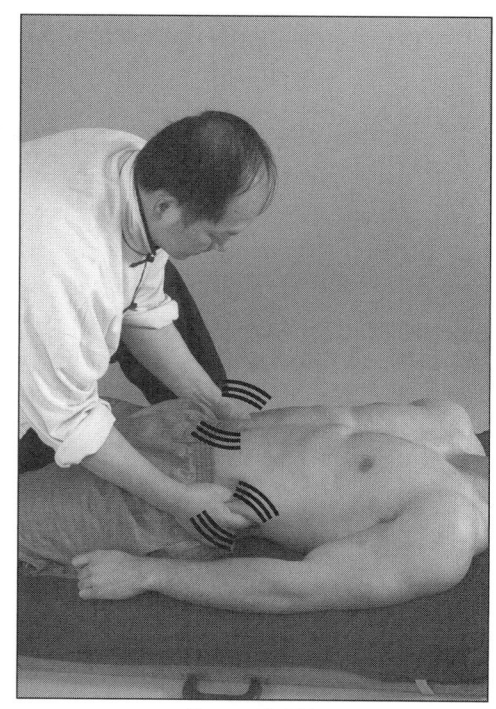

FIGURE 6-209

309

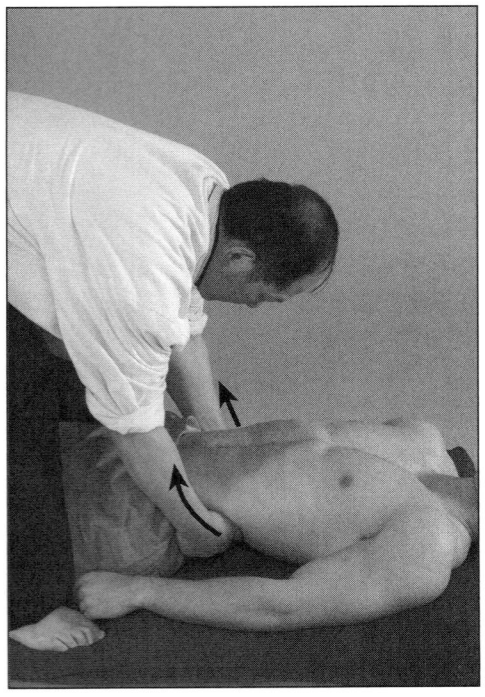

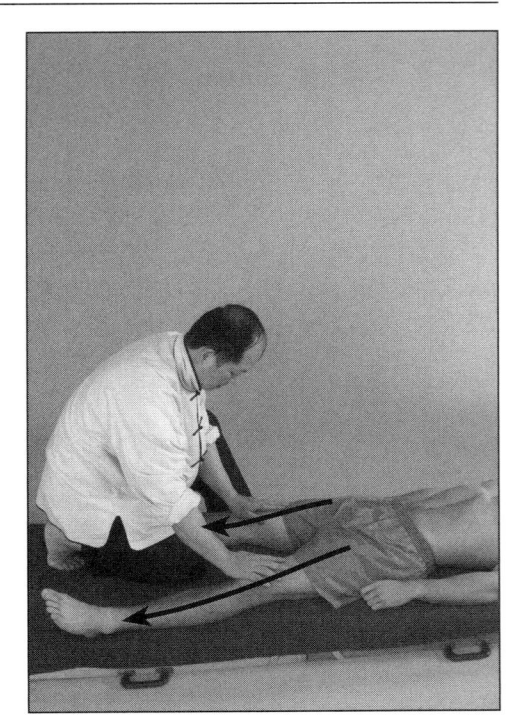

FIGURE 6-210

FIGURE 6-211

Then gently raise up the waist area and release it a couple of times (Figure 6-210). Finally, brush your hands from the waist to the front of the legs a few times (Figure 6-211).

6-7. Massaging the Front of the Limbs 四肢前部之按摩

We have already discussed the basic theory of massage when we discussed the massage of the back of the arms and legs, and we have introduced the gates on the back and sides of the thighs, upper arms, calves, feet, forearms, and hands. It is recommended that you go over the section about the massage of the back of the limbs before beginning this section.

In the previous section we discussed the structure of the arms and legs, now we will begin by introducing the gates of the thighs and upper arms. Next, we will discuss massage techniques for massaging the limbs when your partner is lying on his/her back.

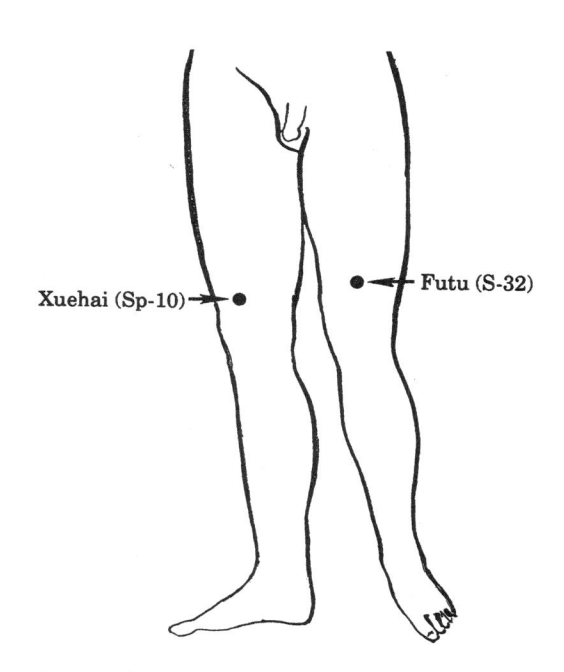

FIGURE 6-212. THE XUEHAI AND FUTU CAVITIES.

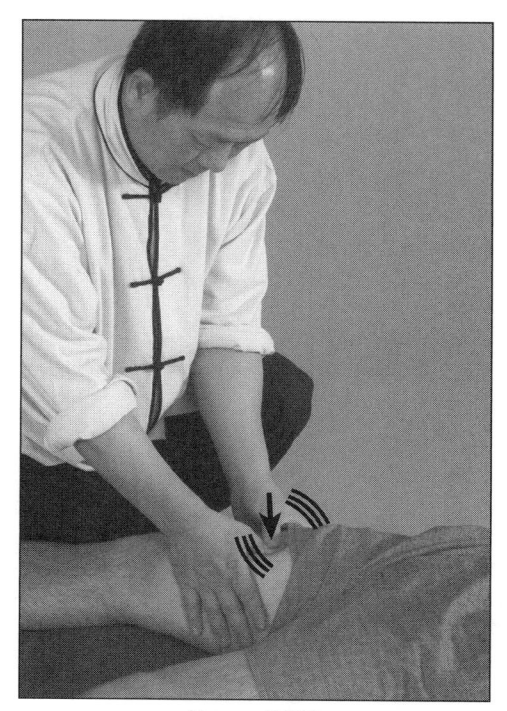

FIGURE 6-213

Gates on the Front of the Thigh

Futu (S-32) (伏兔). Futu (Hidden Rabbit) is located on the lower section of the front of the thigh (Figure 6-212). When the Qi circulation in this cavity is stagnant, the lower limb can be paralyzed. Blockage of the Qi in this cavity can cause pain in the waist and the groin area. Futu is frequently used for treating arthritis in the knees.

When this cavity is stimulated properly, the Qi in the lower body can be led downward. To stimulate this cavity, the thumb is generally used to press down on the cavity and then vibrate (Figure 6-213). However, the elbow is sometimes used to generate a more penetrating power (Figure 6-214). Normally, right after stimulation, the side or the base of the palm is used to rub downward to the knee.

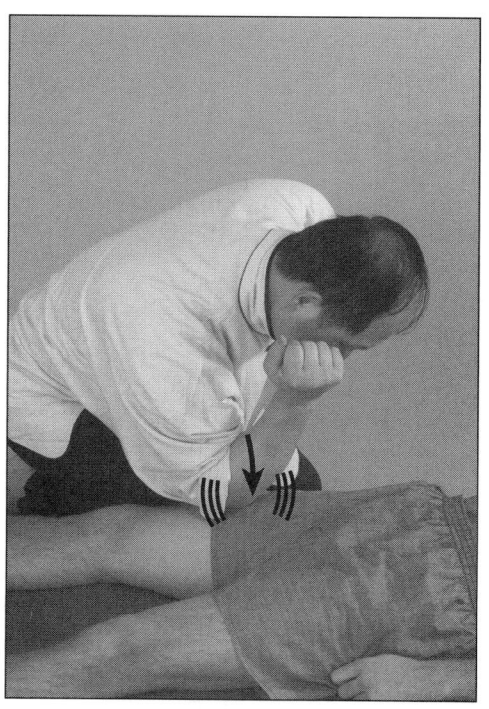

FIGURE 6-214

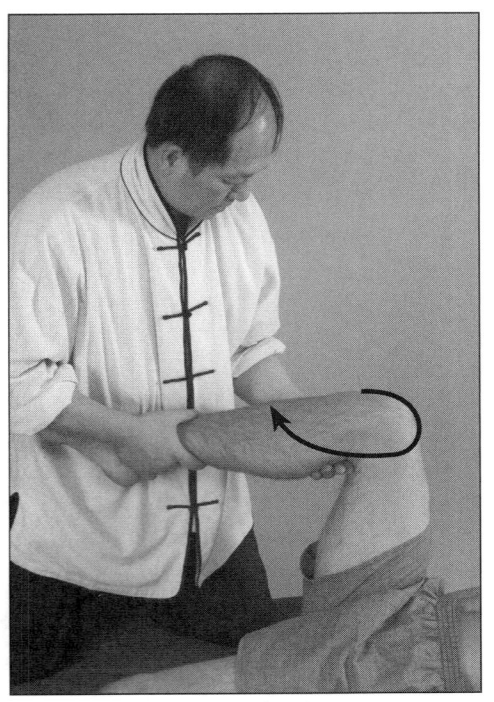

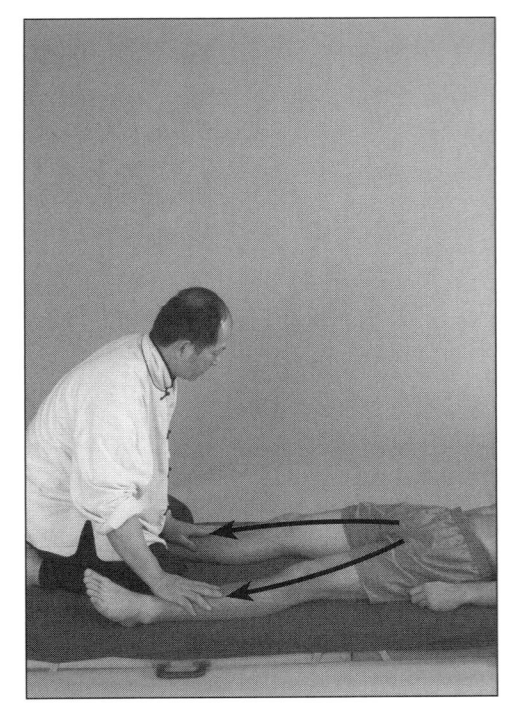

FIGURE 6-215

FIGURE 6-216

Xuehai (Sp-10) (血海). This cavity was covered in the section on massage of the back of the leg.

Massaging the Legs

Step 1. First, hold one knee with both hands and rotate the leg in the hip joint about five times in both directions (Figure 6-215), and then repeat the same process for the other leg. This will loosen up the area of the hip joint.

Next, lightly brush downward with your hands a few times from the hips to the bottom of the feet, covering the front and both sides of the legs (Figure 6-216). This will relax the leg muscles.

Step 2. Starting at the hip area, rub with the base of your palms from the hip joints down to the knees on the front of the thighs (Figure 6-217). There are three main paths on the front of the thighs: the center and the two sides.

Next, grab and rub the muscles on the top of the thighs, moving from the hips down to the knees (Figure 6-218). Then rub with the base or the edge of your palms from the hips down the outside of the thighs (Figure 6-219), and from the groin down the inside of the legs to the knees (Figure 6-220).

Chapter 6: General Massage

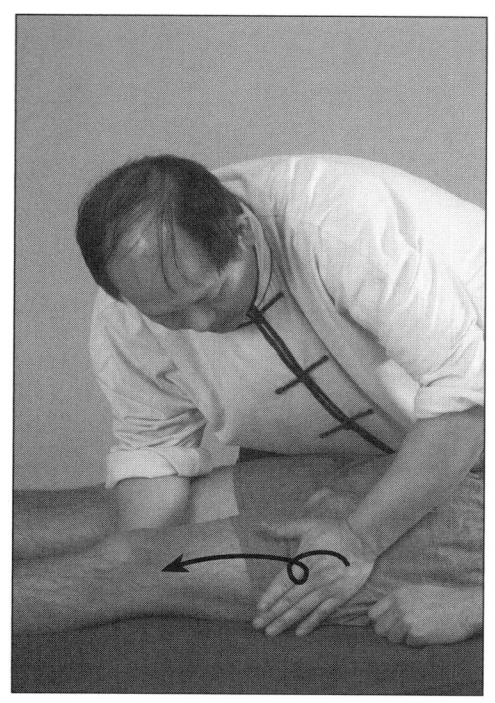

Figure 6-217

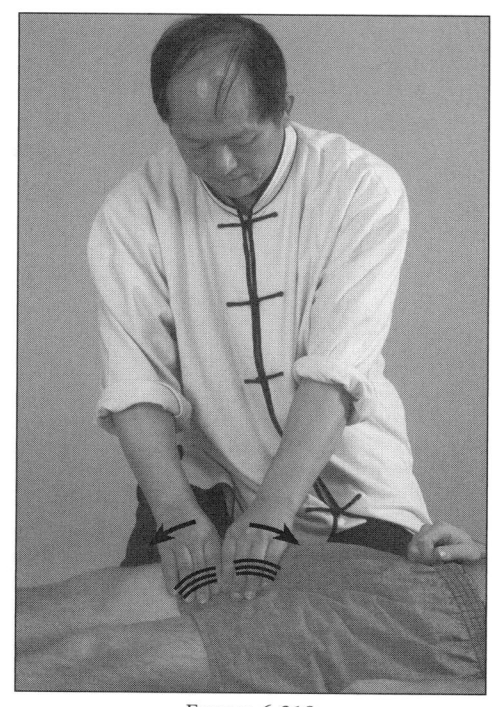

Figure 6-218

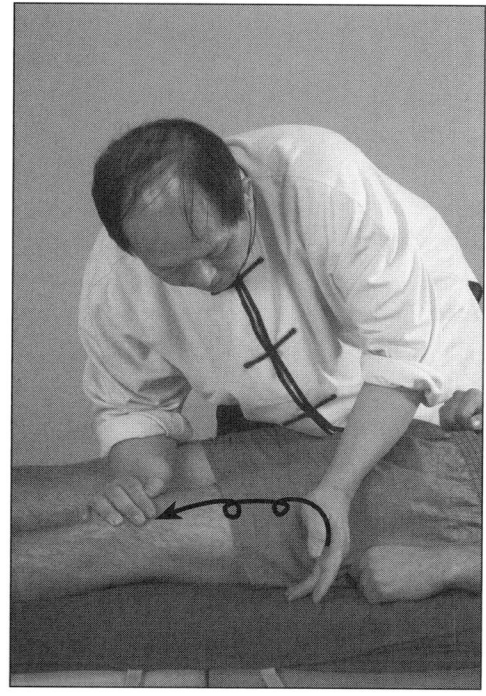

Figure 6-219

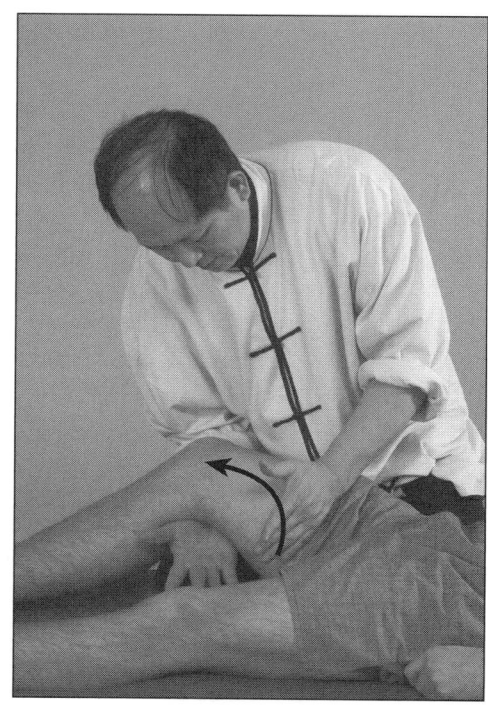

Figure 6-220

313

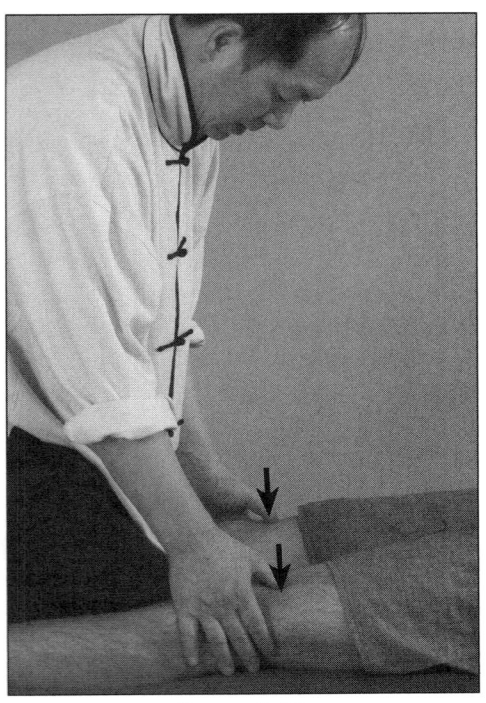

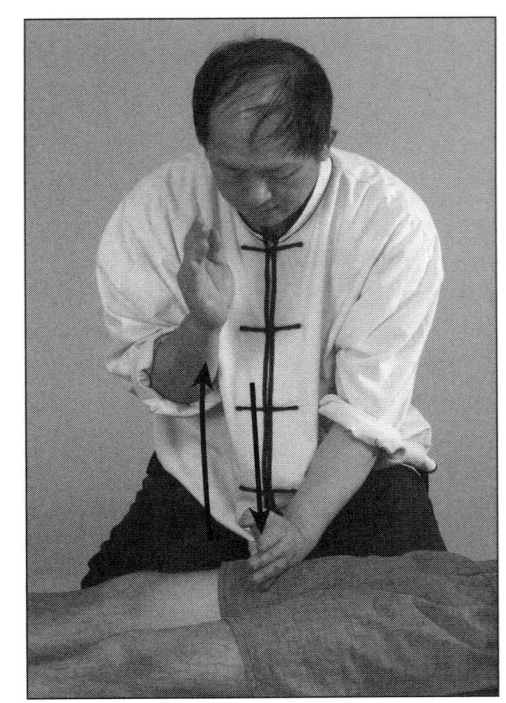

FIGURE 6-221

FIGURE 6-222

Step 3. Use your thumb, index finger, and/or middle finger (whichever is easier and more convenient) to press and vibrate the gates in the thighs (Figure 6-221). This will stimulate the cavities and enhance the Qi circulation in the primary channels. When you stimulate these cavities, start at the hips and work downward.

Step 4. Use the edge of your palms to hit the front of the thighs gently from the top to the knee a few times (Figure 6-222). Repeat the same process for the external and internal sides. When you have finished, brush downward with your hands from the hips to the feet (Figure 6-223). Repeat several times.

Step 5. Again massage the calves and feet. Since we have discussed them before, we will not cover them again. However, before you massage the feet, you should add an extra process: hold each ankle with both hands and move it in a circle a few times, and then gently pull the leg a few times (Figure 6-224).

Gates on the Front of the Upper Arm

Jubi (N-UE-10) (舉臂). Jubi (Raise Arm) is located on the front of the upper arm near the shoulder joint (Figure 6-225). When the Qi circulation in this cavity is blocked or stagnant, the arm will become numb.

Chapter 6: General Massage

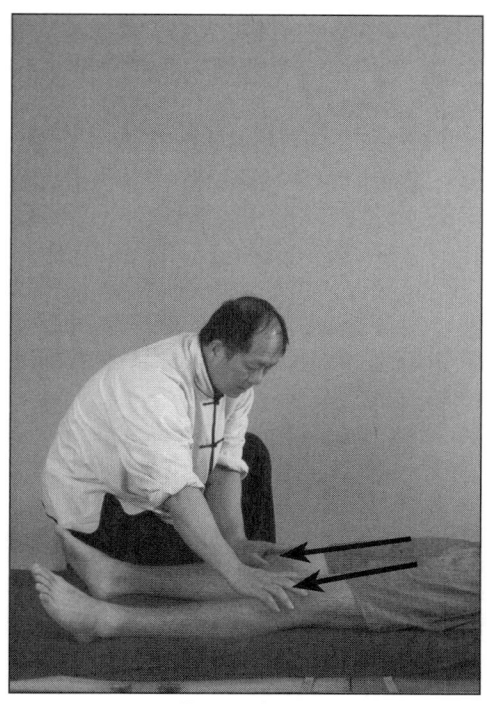

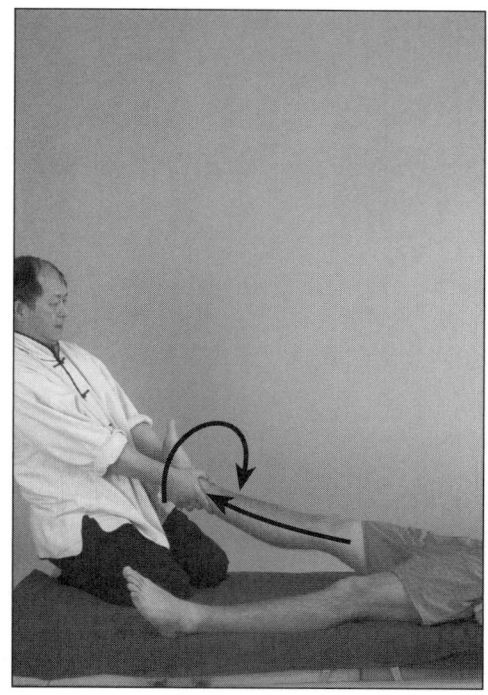

FIGURE 6-223

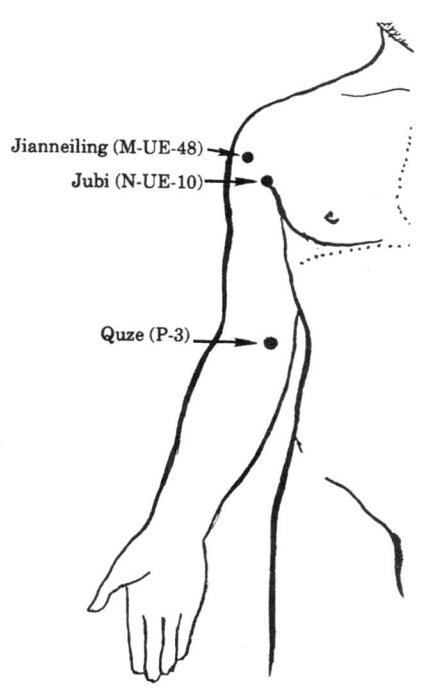

FIGURE 6-224

FIGURE 6-225. THE JIANEILING, JUBI, AND QUZE CAVITIES.

Jianneiling (M-UE-48)
Jubi (N-UE-10)
Quze (P-3)

315

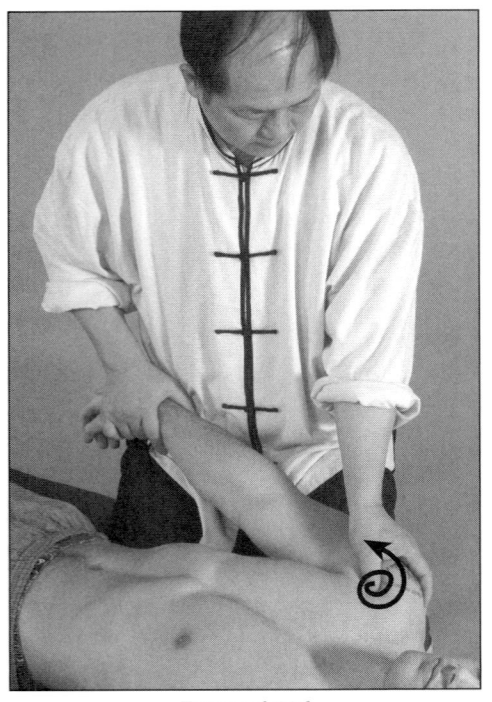

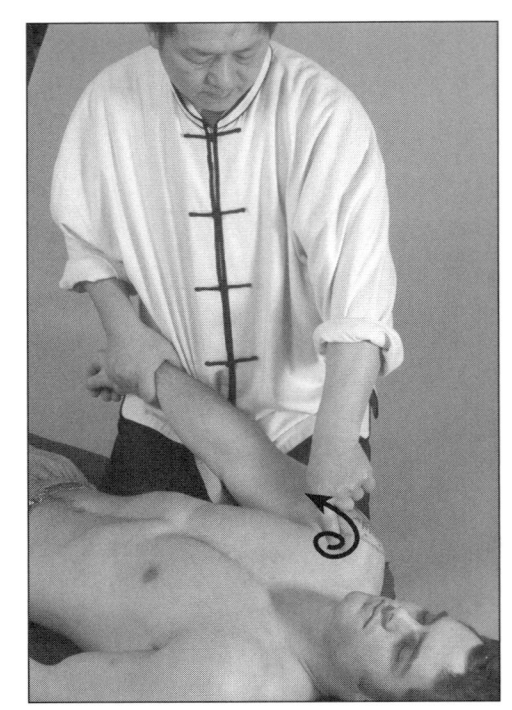

FIGURE 6-226

FIGURE 6-227

To massage this cavity, simply rub the cavity with your thumb in a circular motion (Figure 6-226). Many people also use a thumb or index finger to press on the cavity and then release it a few times.

Jianneiling (M-UE-48) (肩內陵). Jianneiling (Shoulder's Inner Tomb) is also located on the front near the shoulder joint (Figure 6-225). Like Jubi, when the Qi circulation in this cavity is blocked or stagnant, the arm will become numb. This cavity and Jubi are frequently used in the treatment of arthritis in the shoulders.

To massage this cavity, simply rub the cavity with a circular motion with your thumb or index finger (Figure 6-227).

Quze (P-3) (曲澤). Quze (Crooked Marsh) is located near the elbow joint (Figure 6-225). Its functions are opening the heart Qi, draining heat from the blood, and regulating the intestines.

When the Qi circulation is blocked or stagnant, chest pain can be experienced. This cavity is also known to be related to emotions such as fright. In addition, it is significantly related to heat exhaustion, diarrhea with vomiting (acute gastroenteritis), fever, irritability, and fullness in the body.

To massage this cavity, use the thumb to press on the cavity and rub in little circles (Figure 6-228).

Chapter 6: General Massage

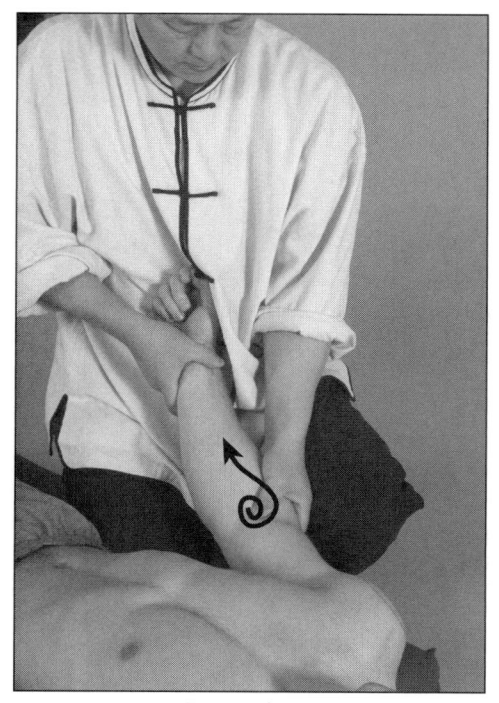

FIGURE 6-228

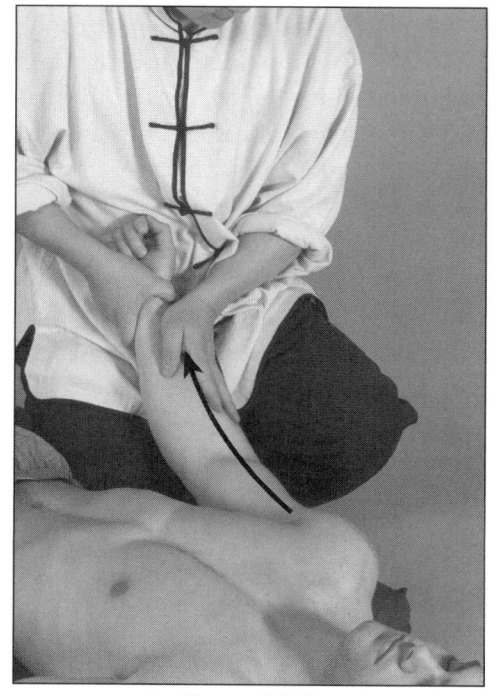

FIGURE 6-229

Massaging the Arms, Forearms, and Hands

Step 1. First, lightly brush your hands over your partner's skin from their shoulders to their hands (Figure 6-229). Repeat several times. This will help them relax, and also bring their mind to the arms, which will lead a significant amount of Qi from the upper body to the arms.

Step 2. Massage and open the gates on the shoulders and arms. Before you do this, you should massage the upper chest again to relax the upper body. Then again stimulate the Jianjing cavity, which is located between the neck and the shoulder (Figure 6-230).

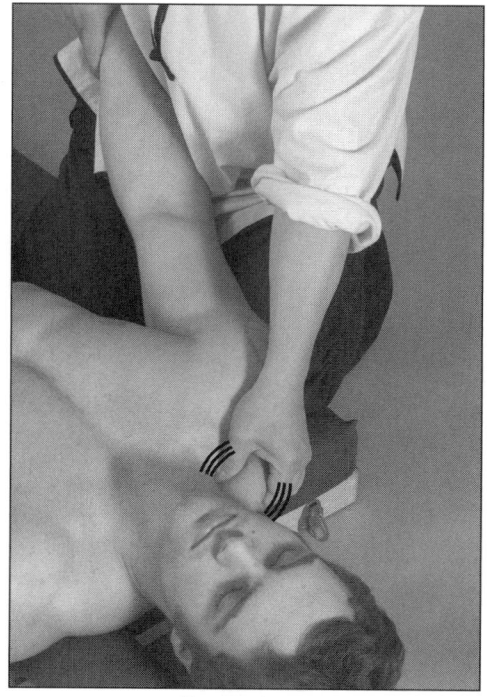

FIGURE 6-230

317

Qigong Massage

After you have loosened up the upper body and the shoulders, use the massage techniques introduced earlier to massage and stimulate all of the gates located on the shoulders and arms. You should start from the shoulders and move down to the hands. Repeat the same process several times.

Step 3. Next, grab the muscles with your thumb and all four fingers and rub in a circular motion from the shoulder to the forearm (Figure 6-231). Repeat several times. Finally, repeat the massage procedures for the forearm and hands which were discussed earlier.

During the course of massaging the arms you may massage the gates again whenever you are near them; this will keep them open as you massage.

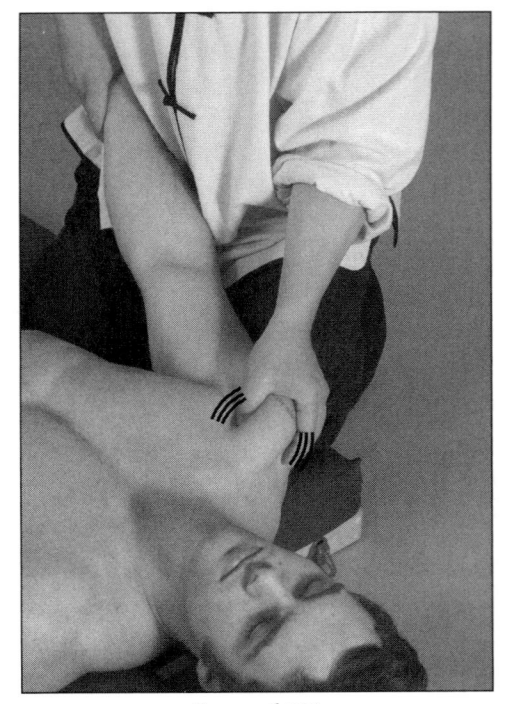

FIGURE 6-231

CHAPTER 7

General Self-Massage
普通自我按摩

7-1. GENERAL CONCEPTS 一般概念

Self-massage is a natural, human instinct to soothe the mind/spirit and ease discomfort in the body. There are many examples of this. If you accidentally get hit with a hard object, you naturally rub the hurt place to lessen the pain and also to keep a bruise from forming. When you sprain an ankle or injure any other joint, you automatically stroke the joint with your hands. Also, when an arm or leg has fallen asleep, you will sometimes hit it gently with a fist to restore feeling. And finally, when you feel discomfort in your stomach or any other internal organ, you rub it gently with your hand, and soon the discomfort goes away. All of these are examples of using self-massage to improve the Qi and blood circulation in an area where pain or discomfort is felt, in order to lessen the discomfort.

Now, let us consider some other examples. When your neck or back is stiff what is your natural reaction? In the case of your neck, you will move your head in a circle or side to side to relax it. Similarly, when your back is stiff, you flex your back, twist it from side to side, or stretch it by bending forward. What do you do when you feel discomfort in the area of your solar plexus—or tension in any other internal organ—caused by being in an improper posture for a long time, such as sitting in front of a computer? Your natural reaction is to stand up and stretch your arms while taking a few deep breaths, and sometimes you will move your body around or move your waist in a circle a few times. All of these actions release tension and let you feel comfortable again.

If you understand these natural, human reactions, then you can easily understand what self-massage is. We can therefore define self-massage as *using the hands to rub the body, or using body movement, to release tension in the body or internal organs by improving the Qi and blood circulation.*

The highest level of massage is Chinese Qigong massage, which uses Qi manipulation rather than purely physical massage. However, this cannot be done unless you have had Qigong training. In Qi self-massage, the Qigong practitioner is able to use their mind to release the tension or pressure in tensed areas. He or she can also use the mind to circulate Qi in that area in order to speed up the healing process. The theory behind this is very simple. Your entire body (which includes both your Qi body and your physical body) is governed by your mind. Originally, we were able to use our minds to lead Qi to every part of the body to cause it to move. However, through the many years of 'civilized' living we have gradually lost the instinct for this mind-body control, which most other animals still have. Through proper practice, we can regain this mind-body correspondence. In fact, this is the basic theory of all Chinese Qigong practice returning to the natural way (Dao, 道).

In this chapter, we will first review the goals of self-massage and also list the advantages and disadvantages of self-massage compared to massage by a partner. Next, in section 7-2, we will introduce self-massage using the hands. Then, in section 7-3, we will introduce two methods of internal organ self-massage: using the hands and using movement.

Goals of Self-Massage

Although many of the purposes of self-massage are obvious, from the viewpoint of Chinese Qigong its functions are both wider and more profound. In this section we would like to review these purposes so that you will have a clearer understanding of the "why" of this practice.

1. To remove any stagnation of Qi and blood and to increase their circulation. We have explained this goal already in our discussion of massage. One of the main goals of self-massage is improving the Qi and blood circulation in the whole body especially the head, eyes, ears, and scalp.

2. To lessen pain and discomfort due to injury, and also to speed up the healing process. This refers to injuries where there is no break in the skin, such as bruises caused by being struck, and swollen joints caused by improper posture during sports or exercise. When this kind of injury occurs, blood cells accumulate at the site of the injury and create a bruise. In addition, the injury causes over stimulation of the area. This, in turn, results in the accumulation of a great amount of Qi, and a localized increase in temperature. These effects are all part of our body's natural, automatic reactions, and serve to keep out invading bacteria. However, the over stimulation of the area causes pain and discomfort. This can be reduced by quickly smoothing out the Qi and blood circulation. This will also insure that the cells receive the proper amount of fresh blood and Qi which they need to make repairs. Of course, you have to make sure that you do the massage very carefully. For example, if a bone has been cracked or broken, you must make sure that the massage does not interfere with the healing process. This will be discussed more extensively in the section in the next volume on Tui Na (推拿) massage, which specializes in treating physical injuries.

3. To maintain and to improve smooth Qi and blood circulation in the internal organs. This is one of the main purposes of self-massage. When the internal organs fail, people get sick and even die. Therefore, keeping the internal organs healthy and functioning properly is one of the major subjects of Chinese Qigong. The key to doing this is maintaining the smooth circulation of Qi and blood. Self-massage accomplishes this in two ways: using the hands to massage the internal organs, and using body movement to exercise the internal organs. In fact, internal organ massage (Nei Zang An Mo, 內臟按摩) has proven to be very effective in treating almost every type of internal organ problem.

4. To help you understand your Qi body and physical body better. People usually get sick because of their unhealthy lifestyle and bad habits. It is very easy for the mind to ignore the body when it complains. In fact, most of the time our minds and bodies are acting independently, and they do not communicate and cooperate with each other smoothly and harmoniously. To be effective in self-massage, you must first learn to understand your body, and you must learn to use your mind to move your body in the most efficient way. Furthermore, you must learn to use your mind to feel the Qi in your body and to lead it. When your Qi body and your physical body are unified, they will be able to act together as one body.

5. To help you learn how to diagnose yourself. After you have unified your Qi and physical bodies, you will know yourself better, and you will be able to feel or even see any problem in your body. If you can feel or see a problem, then you will know how to correct it. Self-massage gradually teaches you how to see within your body and diagnose yourself.

6. To teach you how to massage others. Massage is done through feeling and mutual mental-correspondence between you and your partner. In Qigong An Mo, you merge with your partner so that you feel what he/she is feeling. Through physical touch and mutual Qi correspondence, the Qi is re-balanced. Self-massage teaches you how to regulate your mind and breathing, and also teaches you how to use your mind to lead the Qi to nourish your own body.

For example, when you feel uncomfortable somewhere in your body, you may massage the area either with your hands or with certain body movements. In order to make the massage effective, you must also use your mind to deeply relax the massaged area, which will allow the Qi to circulate smoothly and deeply. In addition, you can also use your mind to lead the Qi to the massaged area. Only when you combine both the external massage of your hands or body movements, and the internal massage of your concentrated mind, can the massage be truly effective. This means that when you practice self-massage, not only are you training the physical massage techniques, but, more importantly, you are also practicing how to use your mind to feel inside your body and make the massage more efficient. Once you have mastered the techniques of self massage and are familiar with how Qi feels then you will be able to communicate with other peoples bodies with your mind and your feeling for Qi, and massage them effectively. Massaging yourself is the best way to gain experience before massaging others.

You can see that there are two sides to self-massage: the ability to sense what is going on inside and move the Qi there, and the physical techniques. The internal side is Yin and the external side is Yang. When the Yin participates the external Yang massage can reach deep and be effective. Without the Yin, the massage will remain superficial.

Advantages and Disadvantages of Self-Massage

In this subsection, we will summarize the advantages and the disadvantages of self-massage when compared to massage by a partner.

Advantages of Self-Massage

1. Self-massage gives you a better understanding of your Qi and physical bodies. It increases your sensitivity, and improves the communications between your Qi body and your physical body, which is the foundation of self-diagnosis. In Chinese Qigong, accurate self-diagnosis is one of the most important keys to regulating Qi disorders before any physical damage occurs. When you massage someone else, your attention is on their body, and you usually tend to ignore your own body. It is like the physician who constantly tells his patients how to prevent sickness, but gets sick himself because he fails to pay more attention to himself. Feeling inside yourself is the key to maintaining health.

2. Self-massage improves your mind-body coordination. When someone else is massaging you, you have to coordinate your mind with their mind and techniques. Similarly, when you massage someone else, you have to have their full mental cooperation in order to be effective. This is difficult to achieve when you have just met and aren't fully comfortable with each other yet. This problem does not arise when you massage yourself, and it is much easier for you to correct Qi irregularities in your own body. With self-massage, your mind can coordinate with and control the power of the techniques. This enables you to avoid the pain and bruises that sometimes occur in cavity press massage when the minds and feelings of the masseur and patient are not in communication.

3. Self-massage is convenient. Since you do not need a partner, it can be done anytime and anyplace.

Disadvantages of Self-Massage

1. A general, massage is more relaxing and more enjoyable when someone else massages you. When massage is used for relaxation and improving the general Qi and blood circulation, rather than for healing, concentrating your mind is not so important. When someone is massaging you, you can simply relax as much as possible and enjoy the experience. Self-massage is not as satisfying, because it is not possible to completely relax.

2. It is very easy to be lazy and let your emotional mind dominate you. Even though you know that you should massage yourself; it is very easy to skip the massage. However, if you have a regular time when someone else massages you, or you massage each other, it is much harder to break the pattern. Most people usually do not take self-massage seriously until they are really sick. They forget that regular self-massage is the best way to maintain their health. It is very easy to find excuses for not massaging oneself. A common one is when people have bruises, and they complain that massaging around a bruise can hurt. It is often hard for us to discipline ourselves and do what is best.

3. It is impossible to massage some parts of your own body. The spine is a vital part of both the Qi circulatory system and the nervous system, and it is very important to massage it. Unfortunately, the only way you can massage your own spine is through certain movements, and this is not as effective as using the hands. Other areas that are difficult to massage yourself are the shoulders, the back of the neck, and the back of the thighs.

4. When you massage yourself, you miss the opportunity to share your feelings with another person. Also, with mutual massage it is often easier to regulate and balance each other's Qi. One of the practices of Qigong is to obtain a better Qi balance through Qi communication with a partner.

These advantages and disadvantages are only summarized for your reference. A good Qigong masseur should practice both self-massage and mutual massage with a partner. A high level of Qigong massage can be achieved only through a lot of practice. Practice is the best way to accumulate experience.

7-2. SELF-MASSAGE 自我按摩

In this section we will introduce the various ways of using the hands to massage the body and smooth out the Qi circulation. The methods introduced in this and the next section are mainly used for maintaining health, improving the functioning of the body, and slowing down the aging process.

Generally speaking, whether you are massaging yourself or a partner, you follow the same routine. That is, when you are massaging for relaxation and to improve Qi and blood circulation you want to lead the Qi from the center out to the limbs, and from the top of the head down to the bottom of the feet. You therefore begin your massage with the head and neck.

The head is the center of your entire being. When you massage your head, you are starting to relax your mental body, which has to relax before your physical body can start to relax. Massaging the head also improves Qi and blood circulation there, which keeps the eyes and ears healthy. Vision and hearing are usually the first senses to start deteriorating as you age. This can be avoided or postponed by leading Qi to the head to nourish these organs. The first and crucial step in this is loosening up the neck, which is the passageway for the Qi and blood.

Once you have massaged your head and neck, you massage your chest and lead the Qi downward to the stomach. After you have finished massaging your chest and abdomen, you massage your limbs to improve the Qi circulation between them and the trunk of your body.

Although you use the same massage pathways when you massage yourself as when you are massaging someone else, there are a few significant differences and disadvantages. For example, we already know that massaging the spine is more important than massaging the chest, therefore it should be done first. However, when you massage yourself, it is impossible for your hands to reach your own spine. In order to remedy this, many people learn how to move the spine to loosen it. This will be discussed in the section on self-massage through movement. Another example is that it is very difficult to massage your own hips and the backs of your own thighs, which are the junctions of the Qi and blood between the body and the legs.

Self-Massage

Head and Neck

First Path. Use your middle fingers to massage the bridge of your nose with a circular motion about five times (Figure 7-1). Then rub the fingers upward to the center of your forehead. Finally, gently stroke your hands to the top of your head, down the back of your neck, and out to your sides (Figure 7-2). Do this five to ten times. This path smoothes out the superficial Qi and blood circulation on your head.

Second Path. Again circle your middle fingers on the bridge of your nose about five times and rub them upward to your forehead. Then brush with your middle and index fingers to the sides of your forehead, circle the temples a few times, and brush down to the jaws and chin (Figure 7-3). When you do this movement you may place your thumbs on the jaw to steady your hands. Repeat the procedure five to ten times. This path improves Qi and blood circulation in your face.

Third Path. Again start at the bridge of your nose. Circle your middle fingers on the bridge of your nose five times, and then use your index and middle fingers to gently circle your eyes about five times (Figure 7-4). Finally, rub to the sides of your eyes

Chapter 7: General Self-Massage

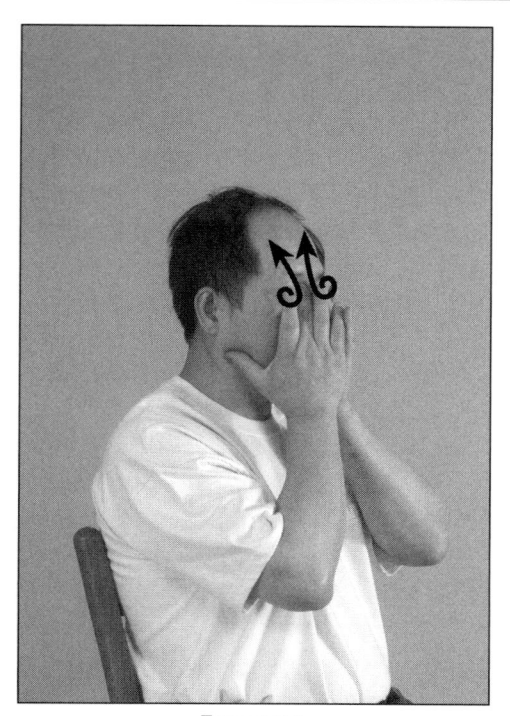

Figure 7-1

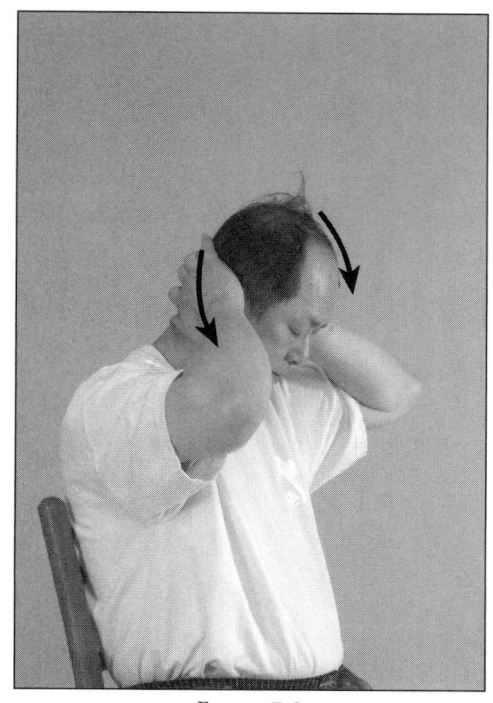

Figure 7-2

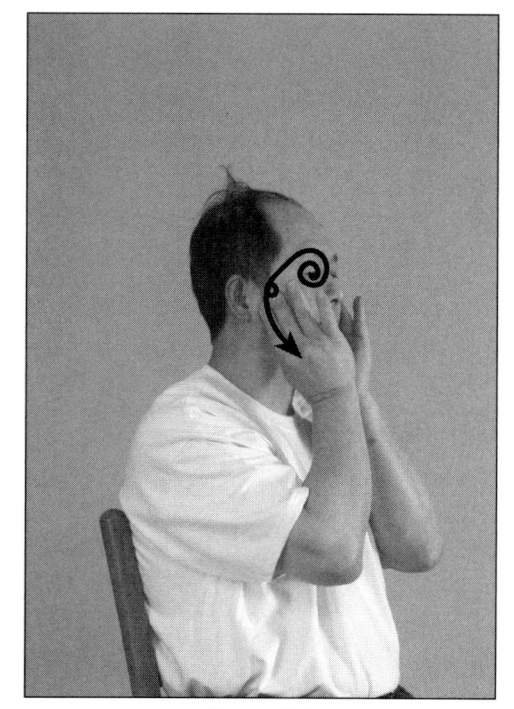

Figure 7-3

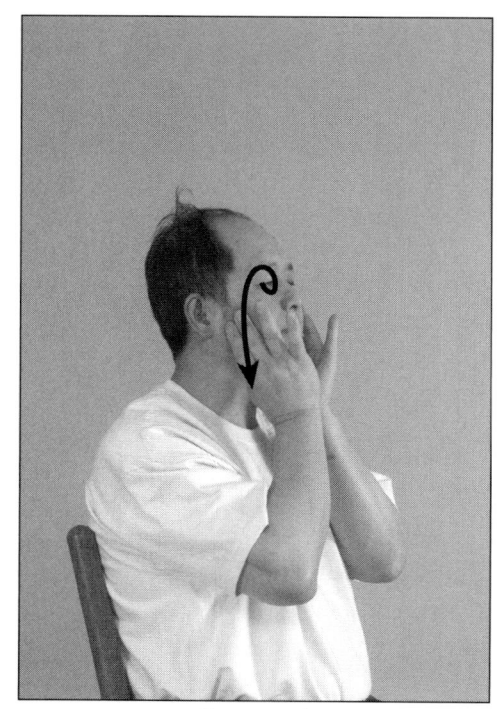

Figure 7-4

FIGURE 7-5

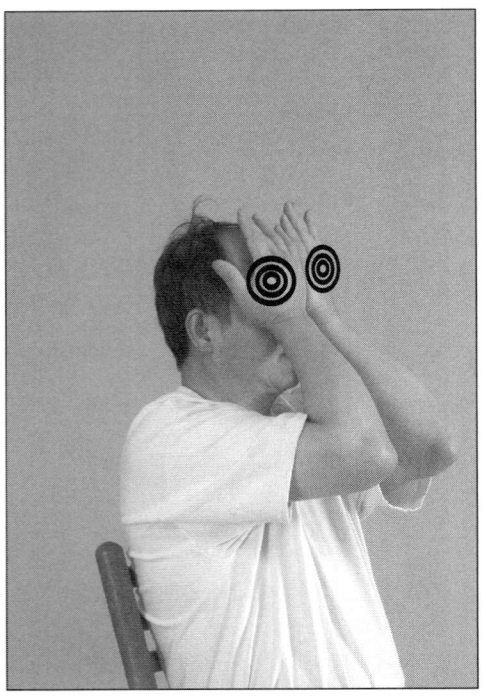

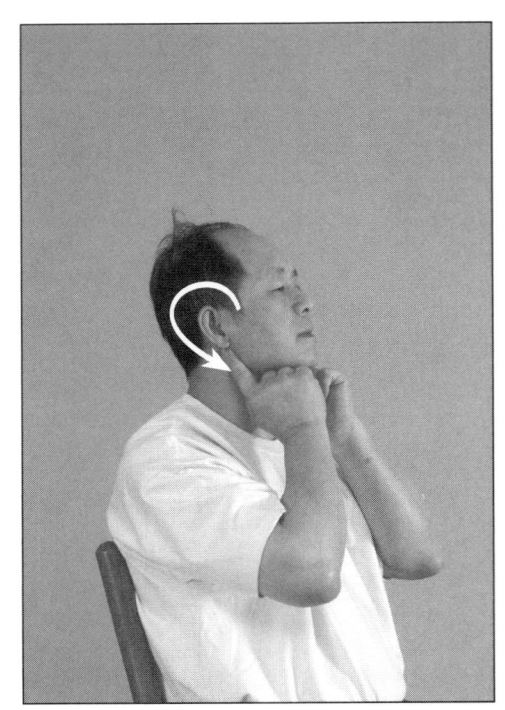

FIGURE 7-6

and downward to the jaw. You may again use your thumbs to stabilize the massaging fingers. Repeat the procedure about five to ten times. Then rub your hands together until they are warm, and gently place the bases of your palms on your eyes to nourish them with the Qi from the palms (Figure 7-5). This is called ironing the eyes (Tang Yan, 燙眼). This path improves the Qi and blood circulation around the eyes and slows the deterioration of the eyes.

Fourth Path. Gently press your index fingers in front of your ears, and rub lightly up and around the ears and finally down to the sides of the neck (Figure 7-6). Do this about five times. Next, cover your ears tightly with your hands and move your hands in a circle five times in one direction, and then five times in the other direction (Figure 7-7); finally, press your ears with your palms and then release to pop the ears five times (Figure 7-8). This path keeps the ears functioning properly.

Fifth Path. This path leads the Qi and blood downward from the back of the neck. When you massage this path, lean your head slightly backward to relax the muscles in the back of your neck. Starting at the base of your skull, press and push with your thumbs down along the neck muscles on both sides of the spine (Figure 7-9). Repeat ten times. Then use your right hand to grab and rub the back of your neck ten times, and do the same thing with your left hand (Figure 7-10). This loosens up the neck, and allows the Qi and blood to pass through the neck more smoothly. However, you also need to lead any excess Qi down out of your head so that it doesn't stagnate there. The

Chapter 7: General Self-Massage

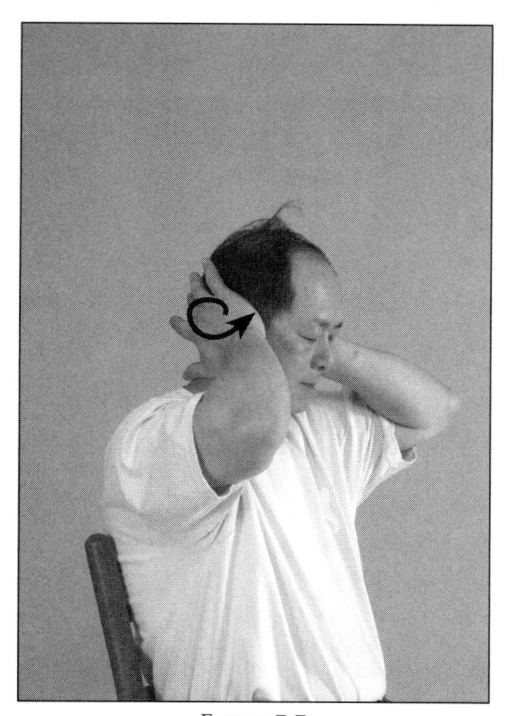

FIGURE 7-7

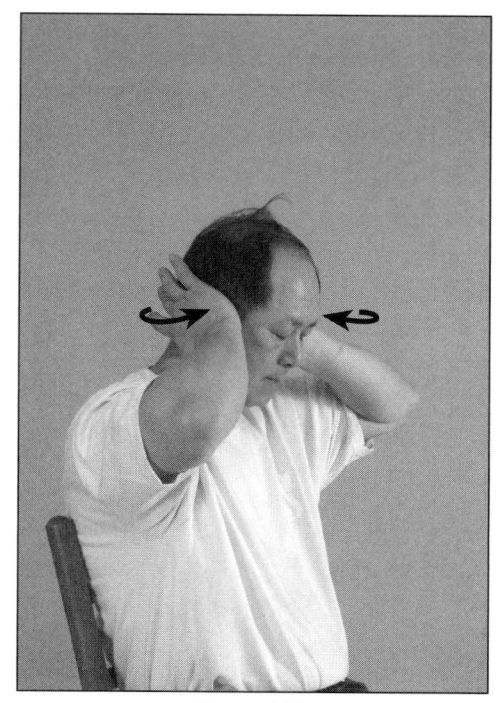

FIGURE 7-8

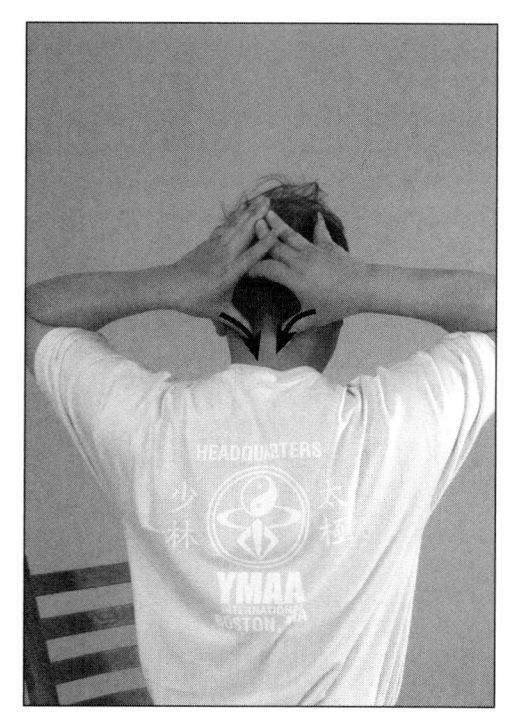

FIGURE 7-9

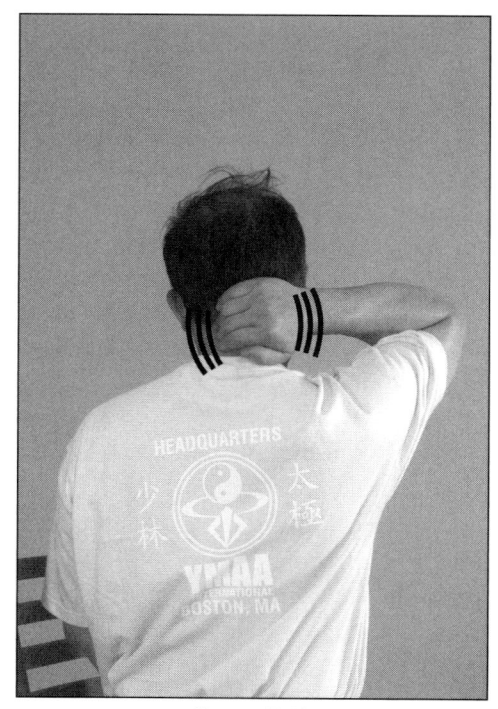

FIGURE 7-10

327

Qigong Massage

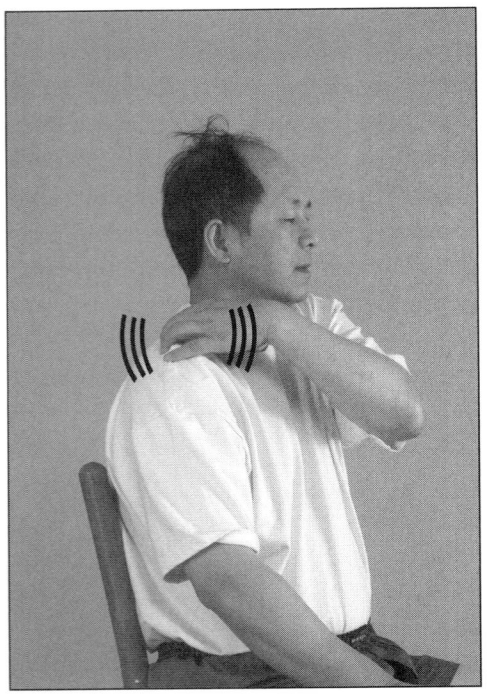

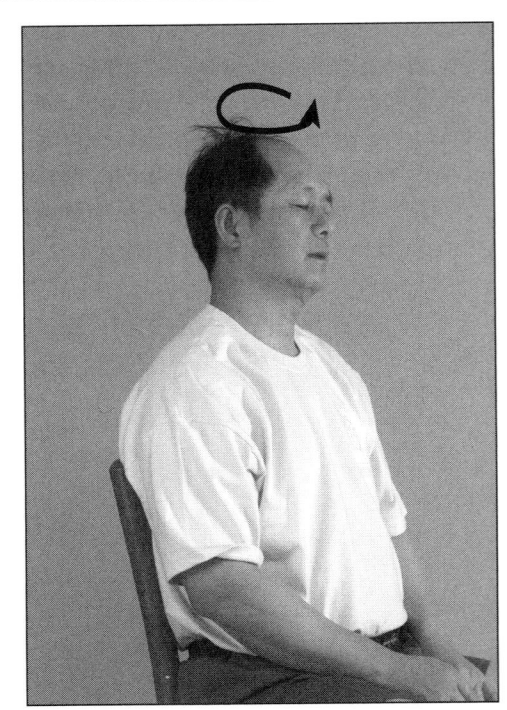

FIGURE 7-11

FIGURE 7-12

procedure is very simple: simply grab and massage your shoulder muscles on both sides with our fingers (Figure 7-11).

After you have massaged your head, you may slowly and gently move your head in a small circle ten times in each direction to help the neck muscles relax even more (Figure 7-12). Do not tilt your head all the way back, because this puts too much stress on the discs between the vertebrae.

Chest

First Path. Brush with both hands from the back of your neck to the upper chest, and then follow the centerline downward to your abdomen (Figure 7-13). When your hands are on the back of your neck, inhale deeply, and when they are moving downward in front of your chest, exhale deeply while at the same time relaxing the inside of your chest. Repeat ten times.

Second Path. This path starts under your throat. First place both of your hands under your throat (Figure 7-14), inhale deeply while staying relaxed, then exhale and at the same time brush your hands over both sides of your chest down to the bottom of your ribs (Figure 7-15). Repeat five times.

Third Path. First, use the second and middle fingers of your left hand to gently massage the area just above your right nipple for one minute (Figure 7-16). Then use the

Chapter 7: General Self-Massage

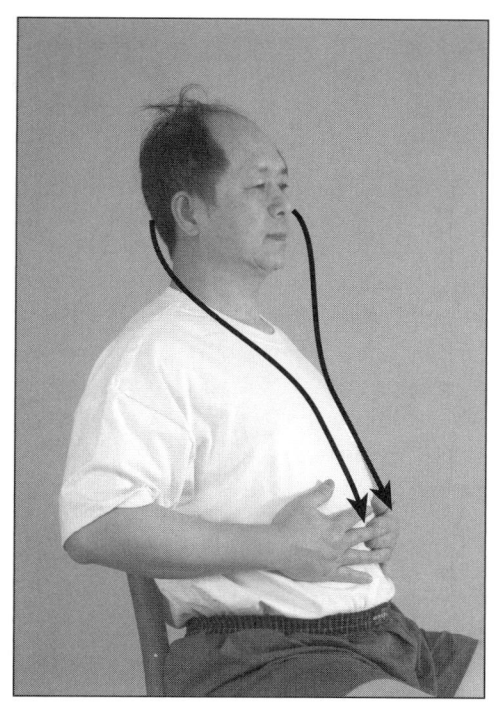

FIGURE 7-13

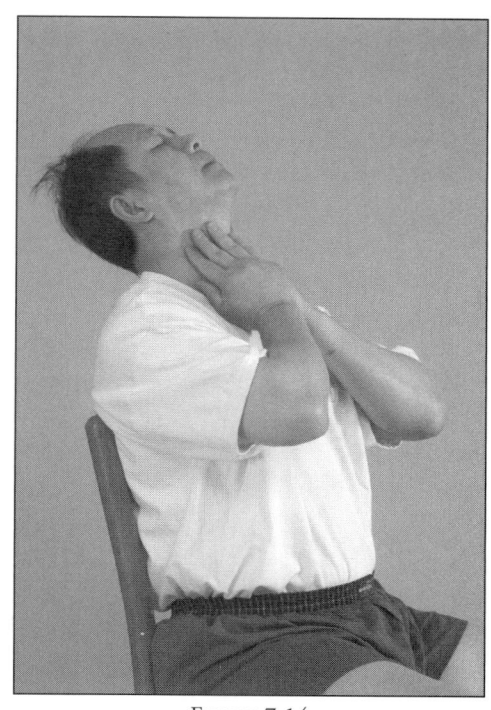

FIGURE 7-14

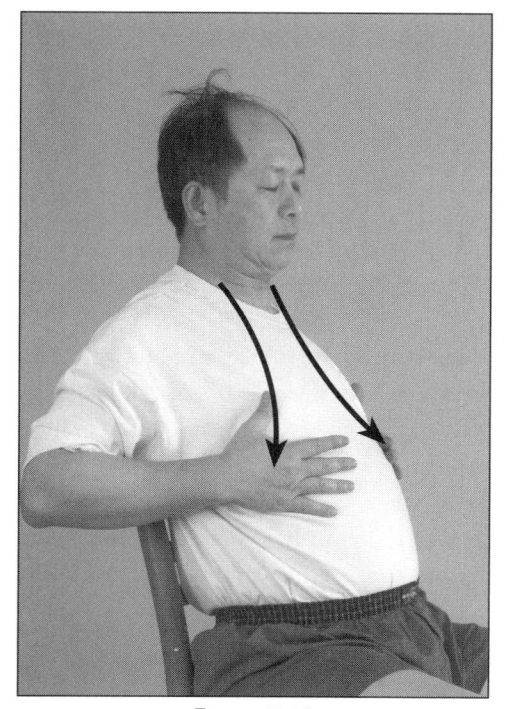

FIGURE 7-15

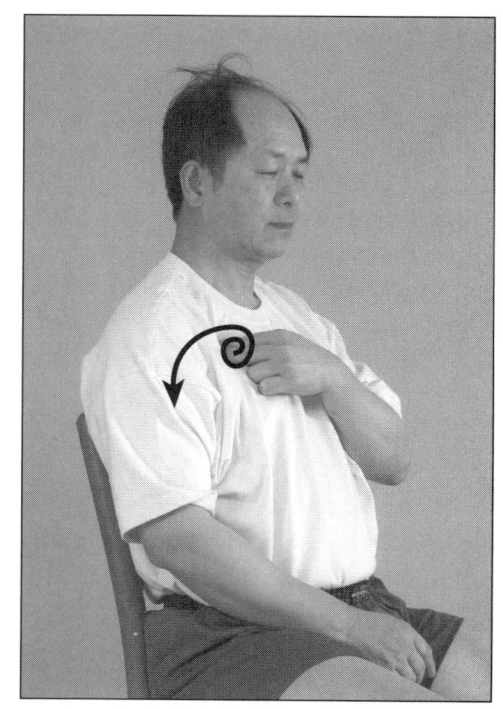

FIGURE 7-16

329

Qigong Massage

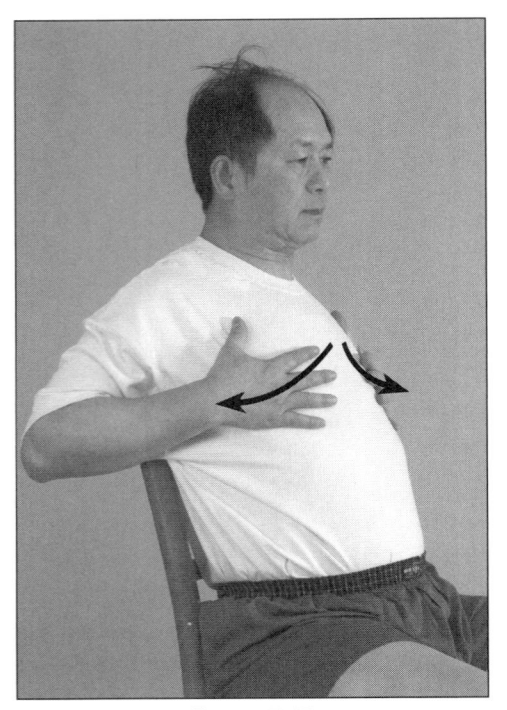

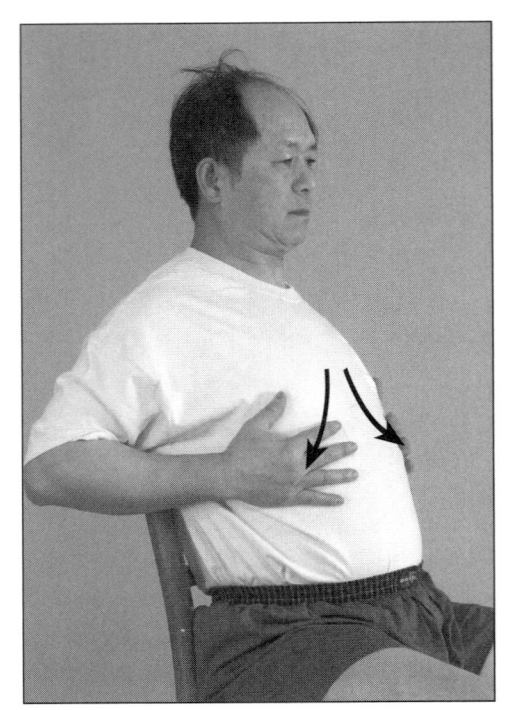

FIGURE 7-17

FIGURE 7-18

second and middle fingers of your right hand to massage the area just above your left nipple. This will lead the kidney Qi and water upward to moisten your lungs.

Next, place both palms on the center of your upper chest, inhale deeply, and then exhale and gently expand your chest as you move your palms to the sides of your upper chest (Figure 7-17). This will spread the Qi and moisture which was led upward to the sides of the lungs. Repeat five times.

Finally, place your palms on your solar plexus while inhaling, and then exhale and gently expand your chest while moving your palms to the sides of the middle of your chest (Figure 7-18). Repeat five times.

Fourth Path. Rub the upper right side of your chest with the fingers of your left hand in a circular motion, and gradually move the motion downward to your lower ribs (Figure 7-19). Repeat five times. The direction of your circling is very important. When your left hand is circling clockwise (from the point of view of someone looking at you from the front), you are leading the Qi downward, which will cool down your body. If you reverse the direction, you are leading the Qi upward to your head, which is not desirable. Repeat the same movements with your left palm another five times (Figure 7-20).

Chapter 7: General Self-Massage

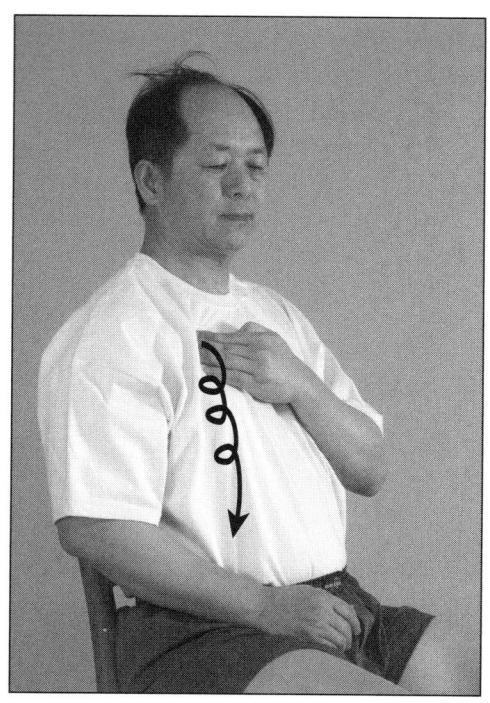

FIGURE 7-19

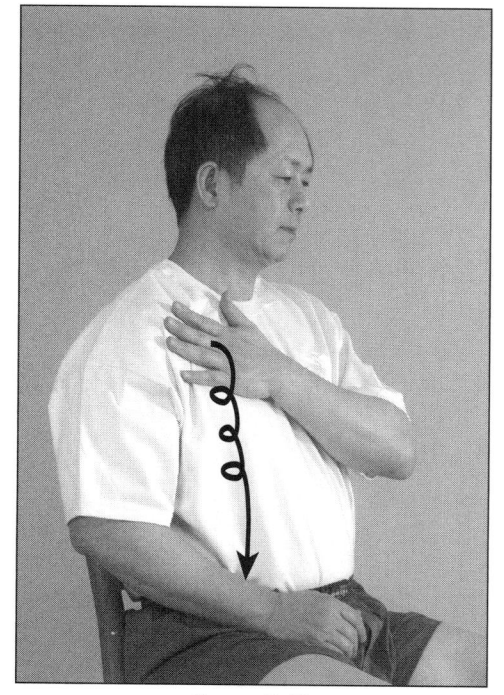

FIGURE 7-20

Finally, massage the left side of your chest with your right hand, first with your fingertips, and then with your palm. Make sure that your are now circling counter-clockwise so that you are leading the Qi down the center of your body.

Fifth Path. Use your right thumb and fingers to grab and rub the tendons in front of your left armpit (Figure 7-21). Continue the grabbing and rubbing downward to the

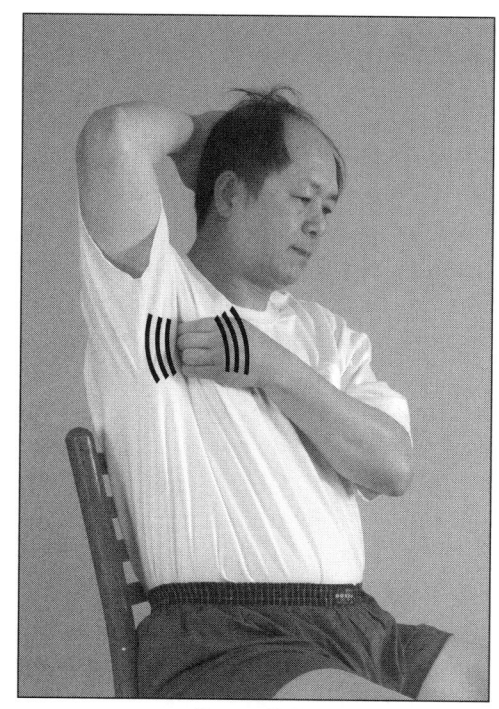

FIGURE 7-21

331

Qigong Massage

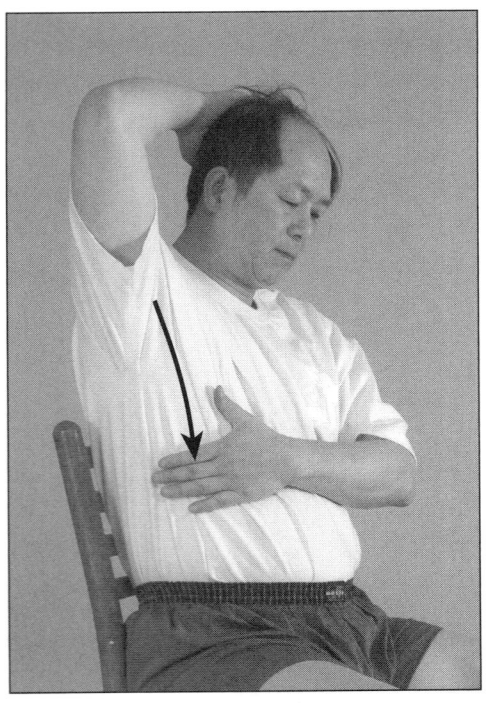

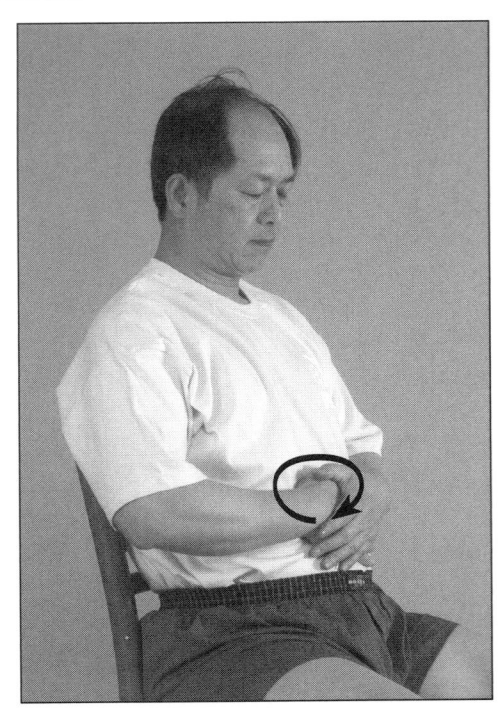

FIGURE 7-22

FIGURE 7-23

area of the nipple, and then use your palm to smooth and lead Qi down from your armpit (Figure 7-22). Repeat the same procedure about five times, and then do the other side.

Stomach, Abdomen, and Lower Back

First Path. First, place both hands on your stomach, and circle to the left and downward, continuing up the right side to the center of your stomach (Figure 7-23). Circle from ten to thirty times. While circling your hands, your mind should be very calm and relaxed. The more you relax deeply into your body, the more you can lead the Qi inside, and the more benefit you will receive.

Second Path. Place your hands on either side of the centerline of your body at the level of your diaphragm. Inhale and then exhale deeply, while at the same time brushing both hands downward to the groin area (Figure 7-24).

Third Path. Gently grab the tendons on the side of your waist and rub them for a few minutes (Figure 7-25), then use your palms to push down to the front of your thighs (Figure 7-26).

Fourth Path. Close your hands into fists, and place the thumb-sides over your kidneys (Figure 7-27). Circle your fists for a few minutes. In the wintertime, circle your fists in toward the spine and down, and in the summertime, reverse the direction. When you finish circling, use the back of your fists to lightly strike your kidneys, sacrum, and the

Chapter 7: General Self-Massage

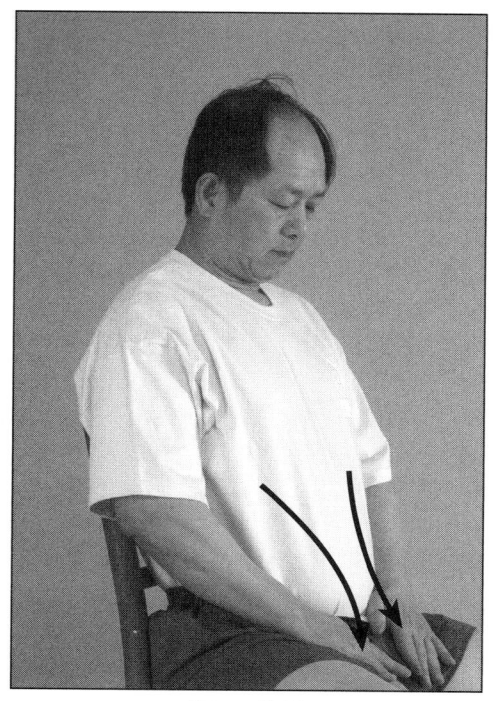

FIGURE 7-24

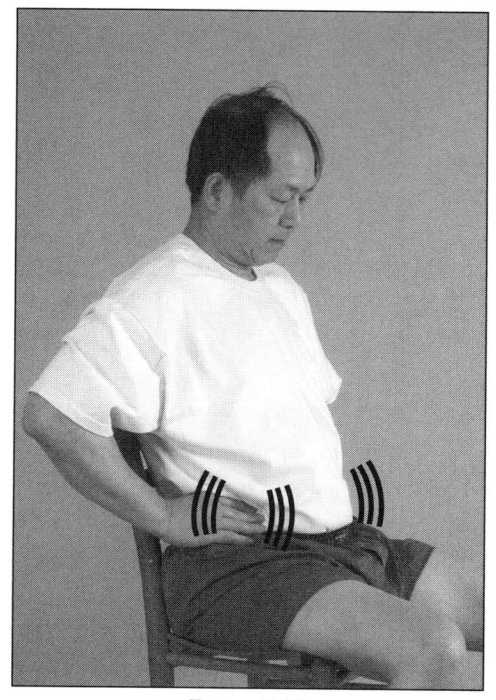

FIGURE 7-25

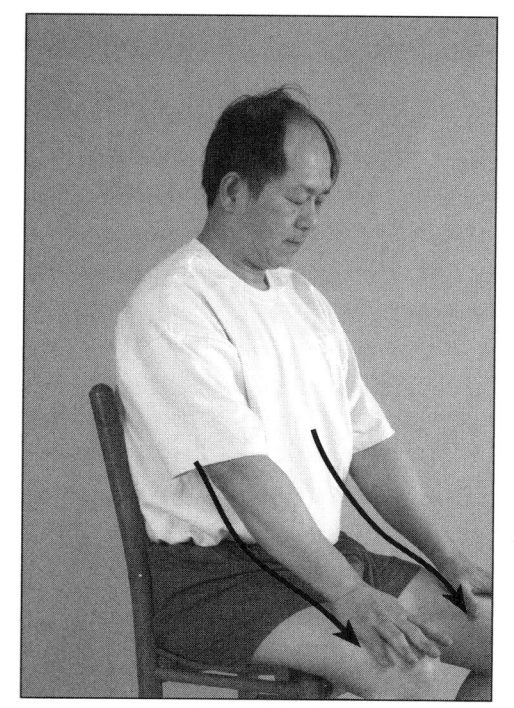

FIGURE 7-26

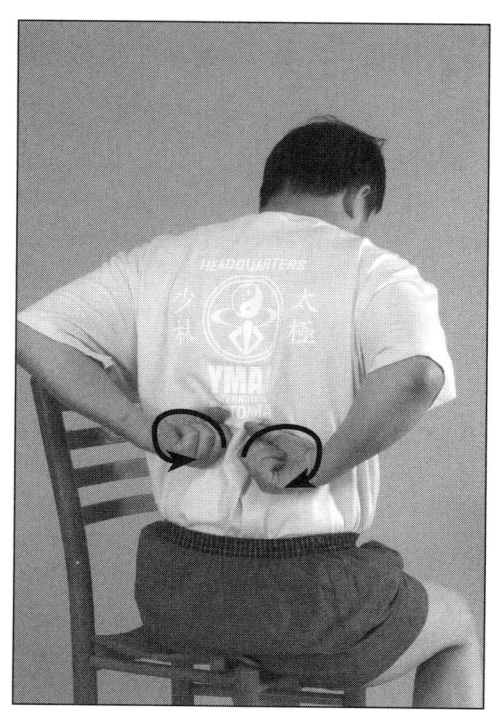

FIGURE 7-27

Qigong Massage

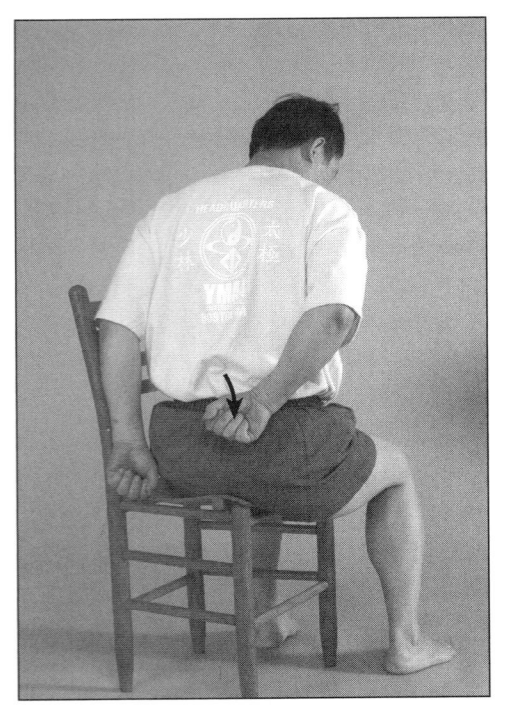

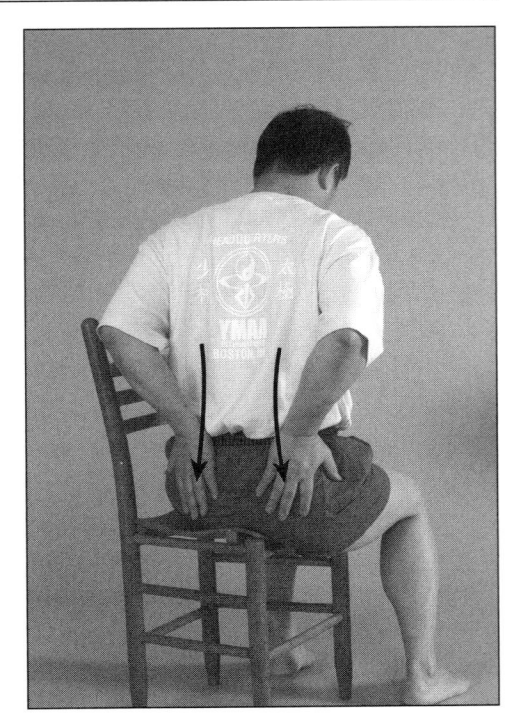

FIGURE 7-28

FIGURE 7-29

top portion of our hips for a few minutes (Figure 7-28). This will bring the stagnant Qi to the surface of the skin. Finally, starting in the area of the kidneys, brush downward with your hands past your hips and down to the back of your thighs (Figure 7-29).

Legs

Starting at your hip, use the base of your palms to rub and move from the hip joints down the front of your thighs to your knees (Figure 7-30). There are three main paths on the front of the thighs the center and the two sides. Next, grab and rub the muscles on the top of the thighs, moving from the hips down to your knees on each of the three pathways (Figure 7-31).

Next, use the base or the edge of your palms to rub and move from your hips down the outside of the thighs (Figure 7-32), and from your groin down the inside of your legs to the knees (Figure 7-33). Then grab and rub the muscles on the sides and back of

Chapter 7: General Self-Massage

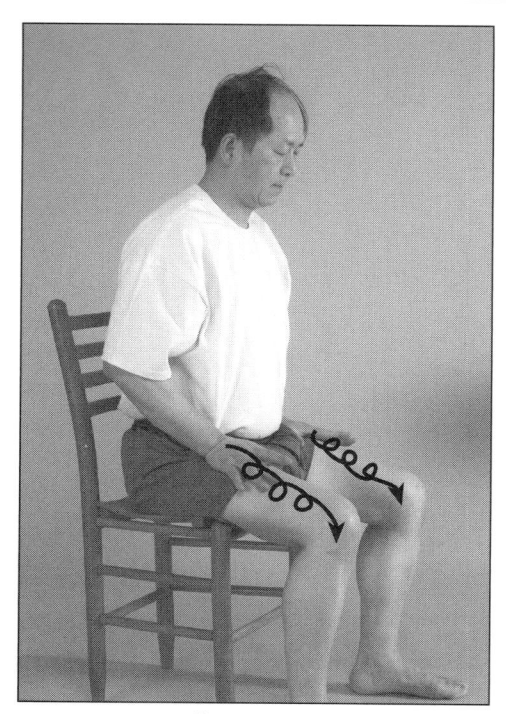

FIGURE 7-30

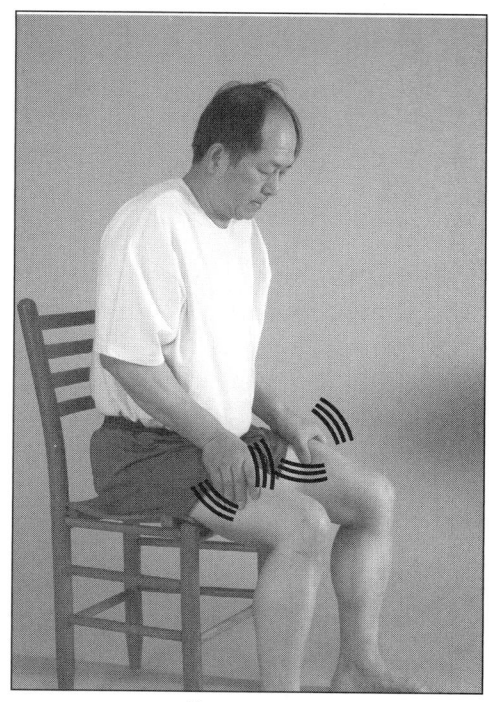

FIGURE 7-31

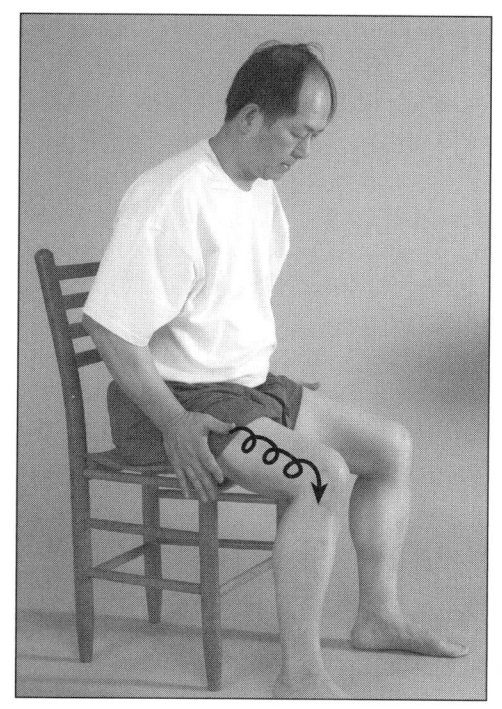

FIGURE 7-32

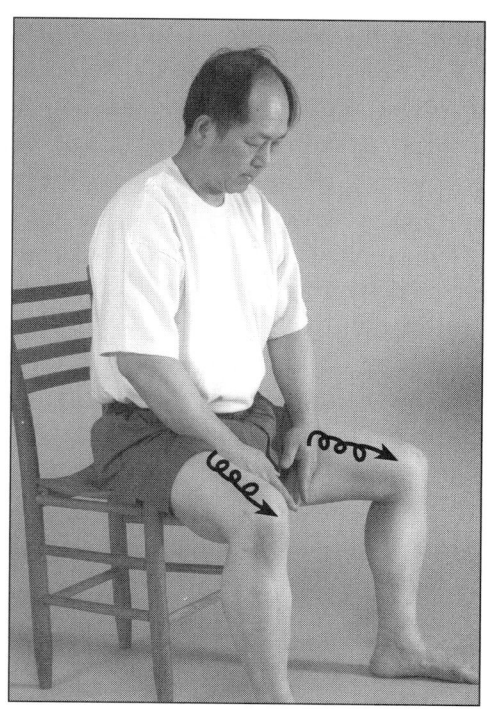

FIGURE 7-33

335

Qigong Massage

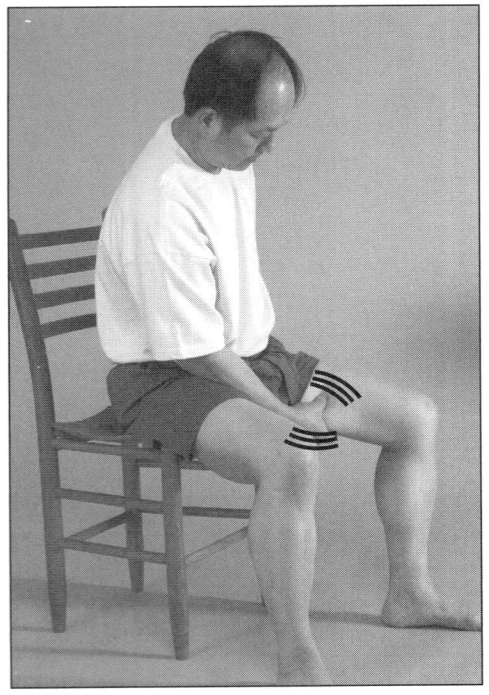

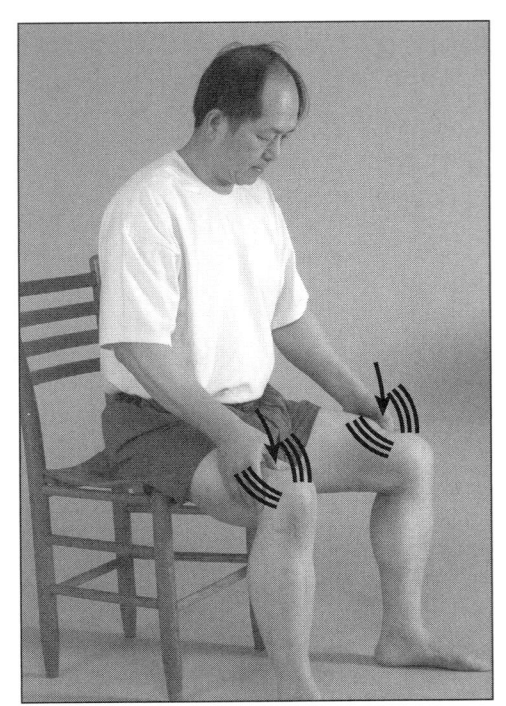

FIGURE 7-34

FIGURE 7-35

your thighs (Figure 7-34). When you massage the inside of your thighs, it is better to use the right hand to massage the left thigh, and vice versa.

Next, use your thumb, second finger, and/or the middle finger (whichever is easier) to press and vibrate some of the acupuncture cavities in your thighs (Figure 7-35). You should refer to the last chapter for the locations of the cavities in the legs. This will stimulate the cavities and enhance the Qi circulation in the primary channels. When you stimulate the cavities, start on the hips and work downward. When you have finished, brush downward with your hands from your hips to your knees (Figure 7-36). Repeat ten times.

Next, massage your knees and calves. First, use the base or the edge of your palms to massage your knees (Figure 7-37). Then use the base or the edge of your palms to press and rub downward from your knees to your ankles (Figure 7-38). After this, grab and rub the calf muscles (Figure 7-39). Then, stimulate the cavities in the calves (Figure 7-40).

Chapter 7: General Self-Massage

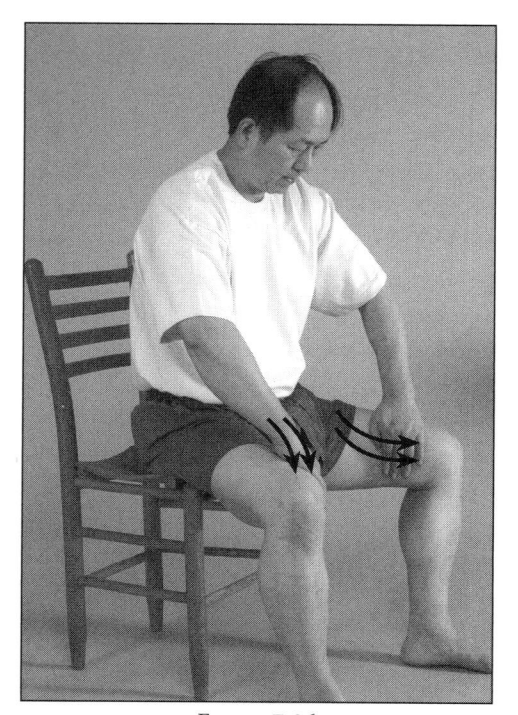

FIGURE 7-36

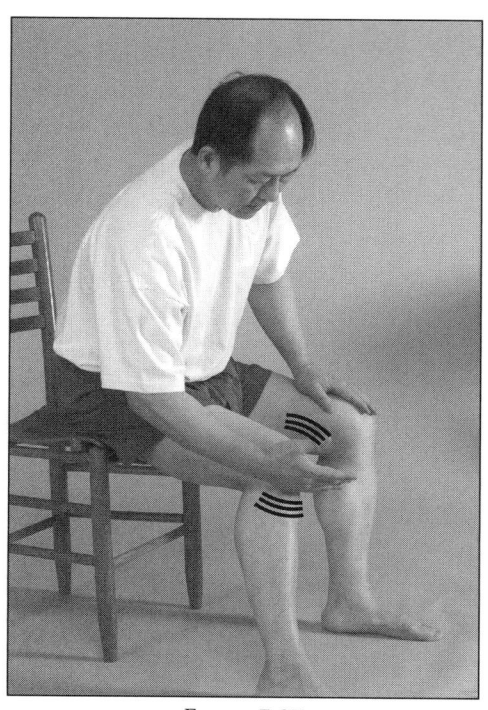

FIGURE 7-37

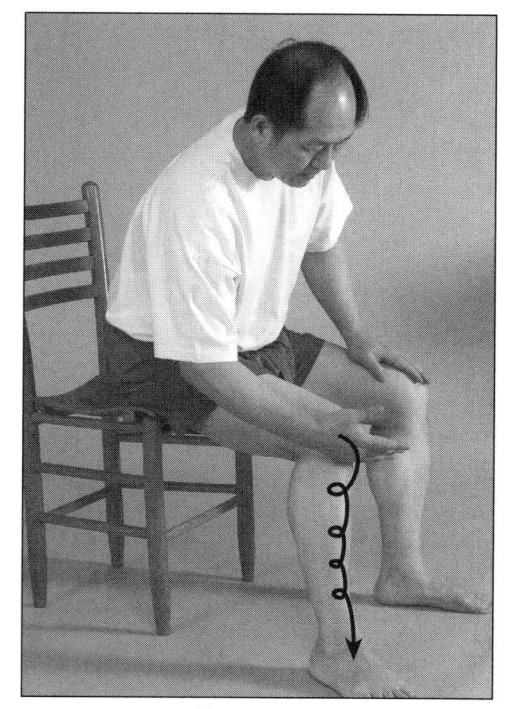

FIGURE 7-38

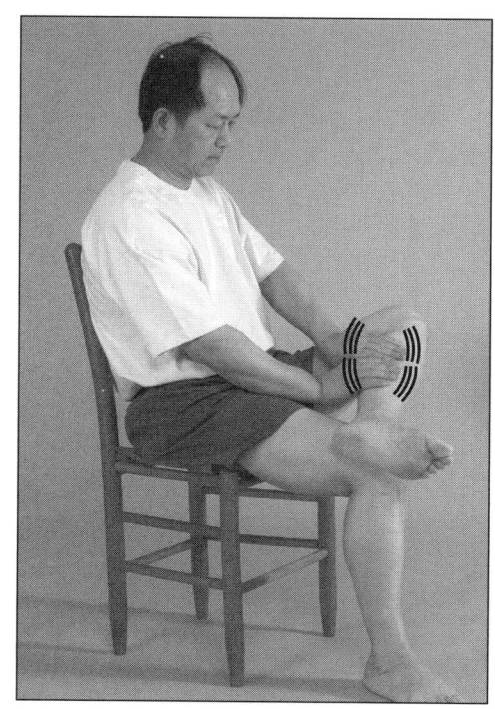

FIGURE 7-39

337

Qigong Massage

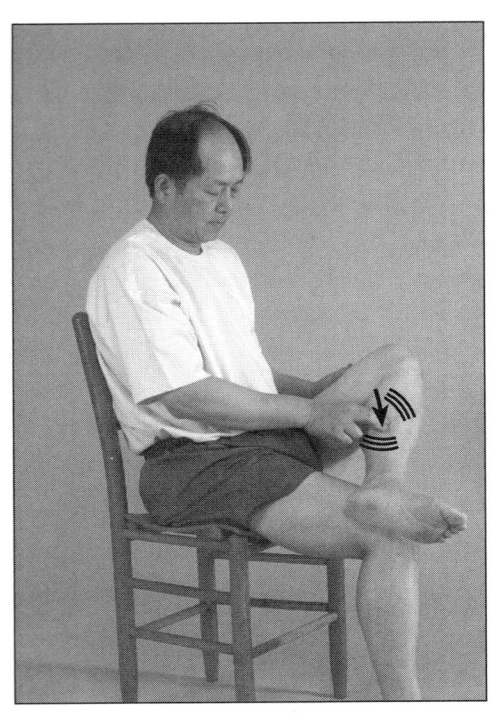

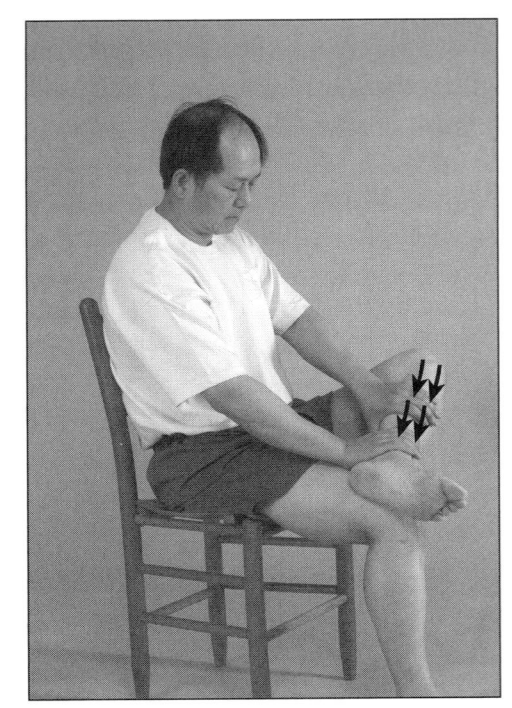

FIGURE 7-40

FIGURE 7-41

Finally, use your hands to brush downward to lead the Qi to your feet (Figure 7-41).

Feet

We know from Chinese medicine that the hands and feet are actually connected and closely related to the internal organs. Six primary Qi channels end in the fingers, and six in the toes (Table 7-1). There are many other zones on the hands and feet which are related to internal organs or even other parts of the body (Figure 7-42). Stimulating these channels and zones can improve the functioning of the related organs or parts of the body. This kind of stimulation of the hands and feet is now commonly called reflexology (Fan She An Mo, 反射按摩). We recommend that, when you finish the following general hand and foot massage, you devote some time to hone reflexology.

Chapter 7: General Self-Massage

Order of Chi Circulation

From	To	Channel	Name	Time Period
Top of Chest	Outside of Thumb	Hand *Taiyin*	Lung	3 to 5 A.M.
Tip of Index Finger	Side of Nose	Hand *Yangming*	Large Intestine	5 to 7 A.M.
Under the Eye	Second Toe	Foot *Yangming*	Stomach	7 to 9 A.M.
Big Toe	Top of Chest	Foot *Taiyin*	Spleen	9 to 11 A.M.
Armpit	Little Finger	Hand *Shaoyin*	Heart	11 to 1 P.M.
Little Finger	Front of Ear	Hand *Taiyang*	Small Intestine	1 to 3 P.M.
Inner Corner of Eye	Little Toe	Foot *Taiyang*	Bladder	3 to 5 P.M.
Little Toe	Collarbone	Foot *Shaoyin*	Kidney	5 to 7 P.M.
Chest	Middle Finger	Hand *Jueyin*	Pericardium	7 to 9 P.M.
Ring Finger	Outside of Eyebrow	Hand *Shaoyang*	Triple Burner	9 to 11 P.M.
Outside Corner of the Eye	Fourth Toe	Foot *Shaoyang*	Gall Bladder	11 to 1 A.M.
Outside of Big Toe	Side of Nipple	Foot *Jueyin*	Liver	1 to 3 A.M.

TABLE 7-1. QI CIRCULATION IN THE TWELVE PRIMARY CHANNELS.

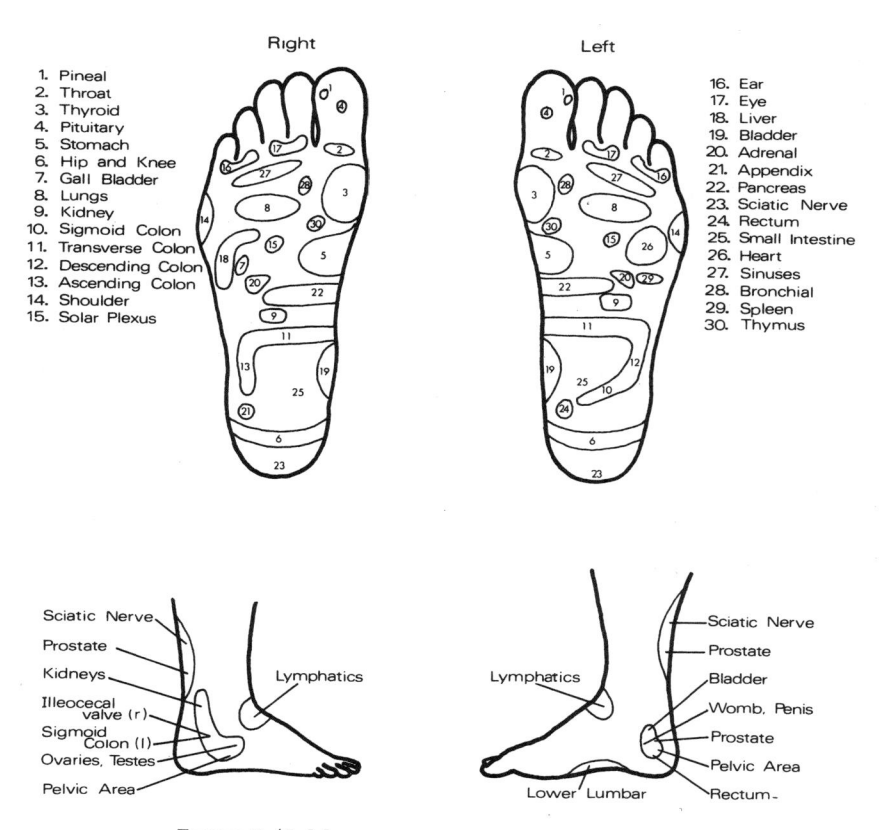

Right

1. Pineal
2. Throat
3. Thyroid
4. Pituitary
5. Stomach
6. Hip and Knee
7. Gall Bladder
8. Lungs
9. Kidney
10. Sigmoid Colon
11. Transverse Colon
12. Descending Colon
13. Ascending Colon
14. Shoulder
15. Solar Plexus

Left

16. Ear
17. Eye
18. Liver
19. Bladder
20. Adrenal
21. Appendix
22. Pancreas
23. Sciatic Nerve
24. Rectum
25. Small Intestine
26. Heart
27. Sinuses
28. Bronchial
29. Spleen
30. Thymus

Sciatic Nerve
Prostate
Kidneys
Illeocecal valve (r)
Sigmoid Colon (l)
Ovaries, Testes
Pelvic Area
Lymphatics

Lymphatics
Sciatic Nerve
Prostate
Bladder
Womb, Penis
Prostate
Pelvic Area
Lower Lumbar
Rectum

FIGURE 7-42. MASSAGE ZONES FOR FOOT REFLEXOLOGY.

Qigong Massage

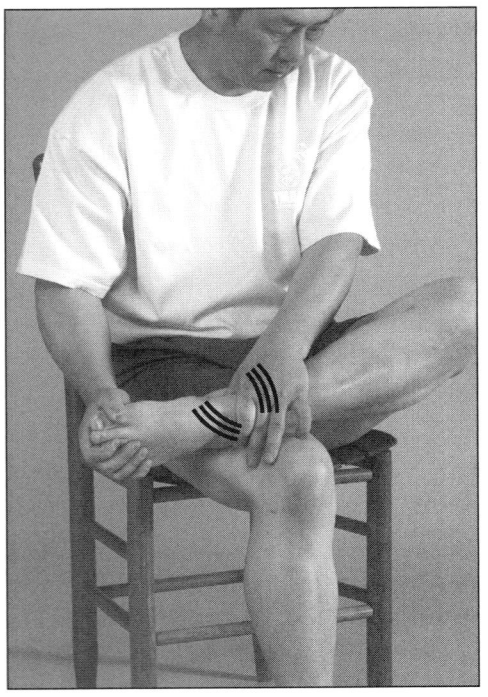

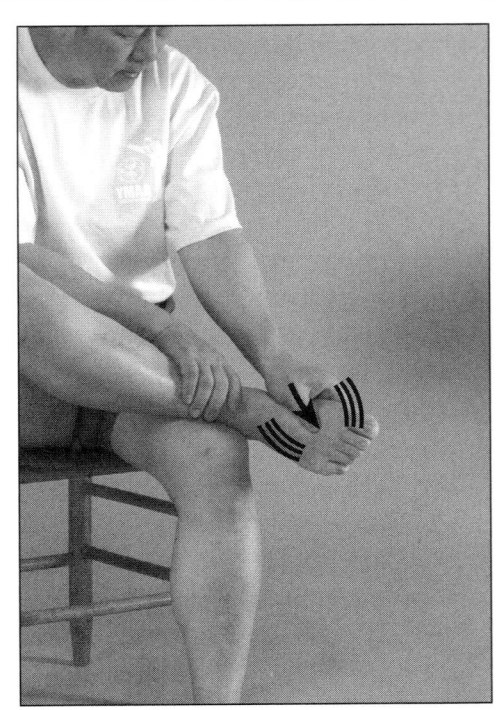

FIGURE 7-43

FIGURE 7-44

To massage your feet, first hold your foot and move it in a circle about twenty times in each direction (Figure 7-43). Then rub every portion of your feet with your thumb, using the other four fingers to stabilize the thumb and help regulate the power. Start with the back of the feet and toes (Figure 7-44). Pay special attention to the spaces between the bones. Next, press your thumb into the gaps between the bones, and drag or push from the ankle to the base of the toes (Figure 7-45). This will stimulate deep inside the foot. It will also remove any Qi and blood stagnation between the bones, which can interfere with the functioning of the foot and even cause arthritis.

Repeat the massage on the bottoms of the feet (Figure 7-46), then press in with the thumbs between the bones and press or drag from the heel to the toes (Figure 7-47). Finally, grab the last section of each toe and gently pull and shake it (Figure 7-48).

After you have massaged your feet, stimulate the zones of the feet (Figure 7-42). To do this, press your thumb on each zone and rub in a circle.

Chapter 7: General Self-Massage

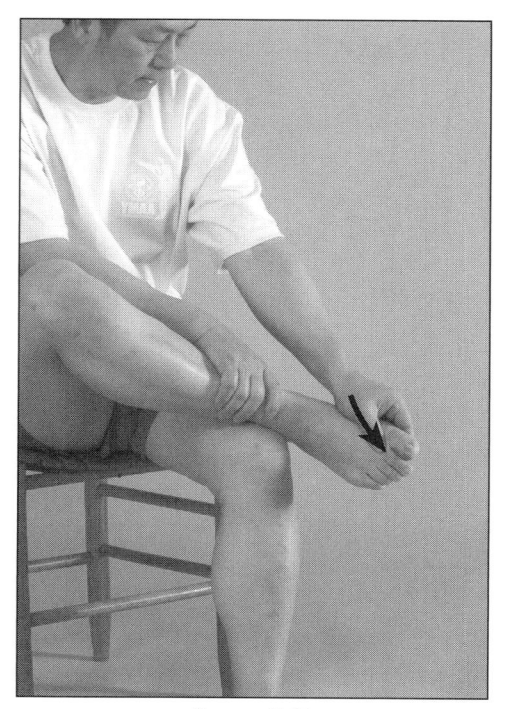

FIGURE 7-45

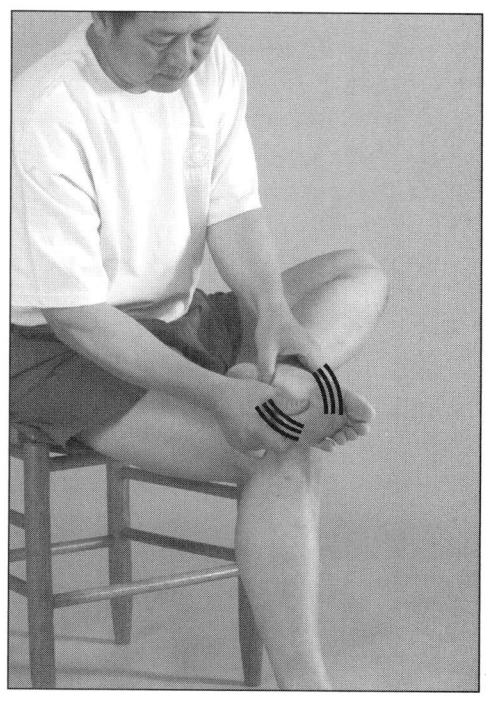

FIGURE 7-46

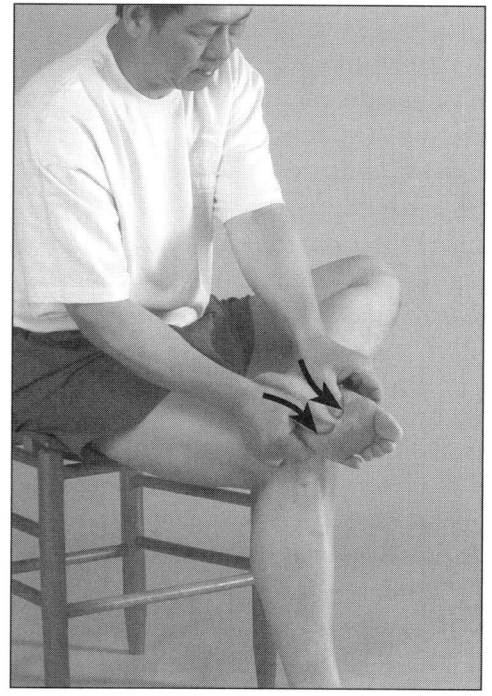

FIGURE 7-47

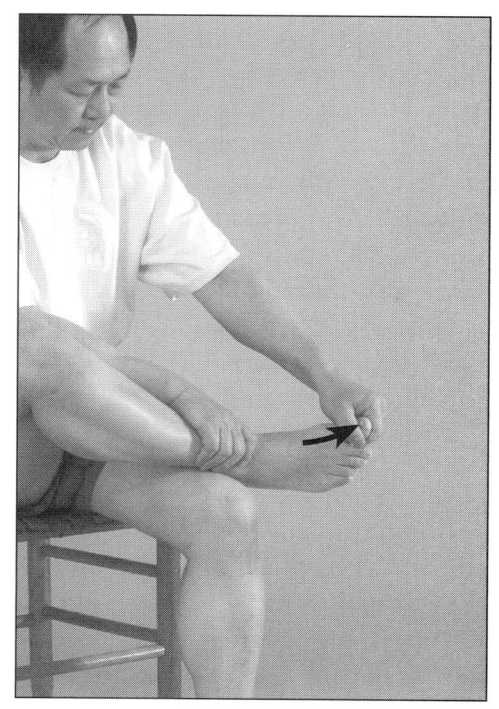

FIGURE 7-48

341

Qigong Massage

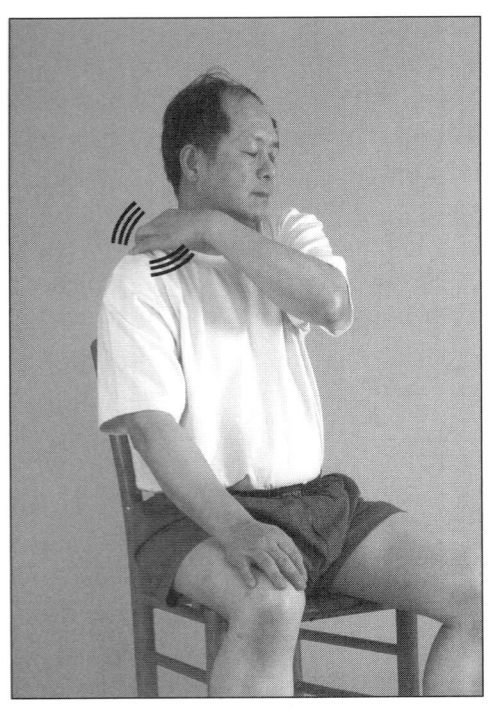

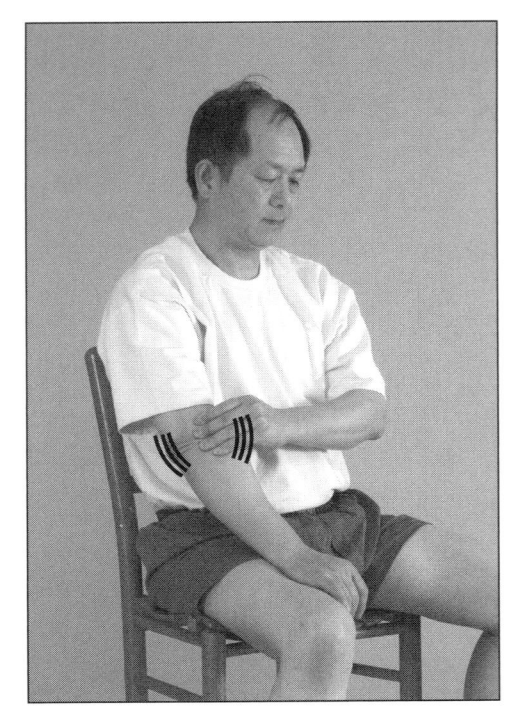

FIGURE 7-49

FIGURE 7-50

Testicles

Massaging the testicles increases the production of hormones. According to Chinese Muscle/Tendon Changing and Marrow/Brain Washing Qigong (Yi Jin Jing and Xi Sui Jing; 易筋經、洗髓經), massaging the testicles correctly will increase hormone production and increase the amount of Qi led upward to the brain. Other effects are increasing the amount of Qi stored in the body and strengthening the immune system. There are many ways to massage the testicles. For example, you may hold the testicles gently between your palms and move your hands in a circle. You may also simply hold them in your hand and gently press and rub them. This subject is discussed in more detail in the YMAA book: *Qigong—The Secret of Youth*.

Arms

After you have finished massaging your legs, you finally massage your arms and hands. When you massage your arms, start with the muscles and tendons between the neck and the shoulders. Use the grabbing techniques to grab the muscles and rub around (Figure 7-49). Gradually move from your shoulders down to your hands to loosen up the muscles in your arms (Figure 7-50). Then use your thumb and your index and/or middle finger (depending on which is easier) to press and vibrate some of the acupuncture cavities in your arms (Figure 7-51). This will stimulate the cavities and enhance the Qi circulation in the primary channels. Please refer to the previous chapter for the locations

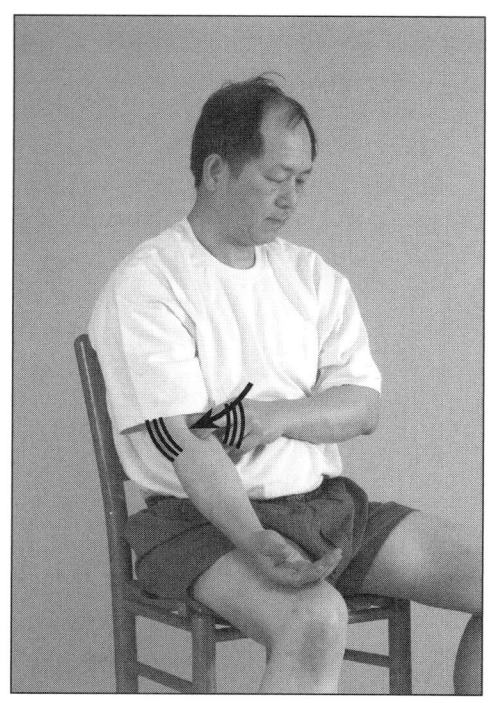

FIGURE 7-51

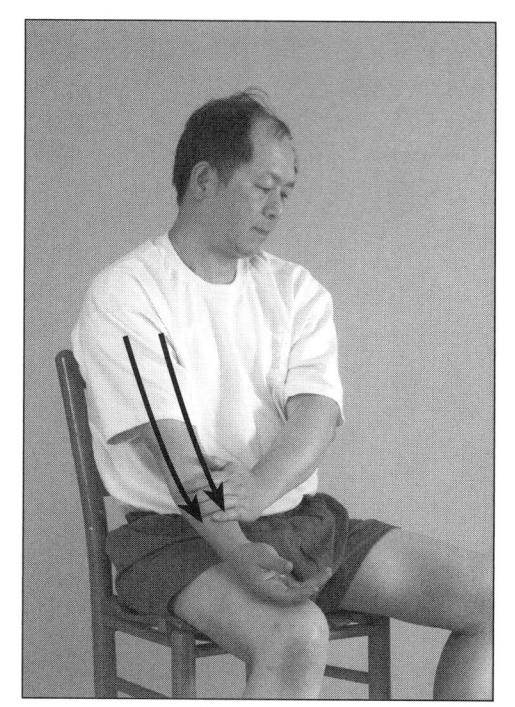

FIGURE 7-52

of the cavities in the arms. When you stimulate the cavities, start at your shoulders and work downward. Repeat several times. After you finish the cavity press, brush downward with a hand from your shoulder to your hand (Figure 7-52). Repeat ten times.

Hands

First, use your thumb to rub every portion of your wrist, hand, and fingers, starting on the back of the hand. Use the other four fingers to stabilize your thumb and help to regulate the power (Figure 7-53). Pay special attention to the spaces between the bones. Next, press your thumb into the spaces between the bones in the hand, and drag or push from your wrist to the base of the fingers (Figure 7-54). This will help to stimulate the deeper places in your hand, and remove any Qi and blood stagnation between the bones

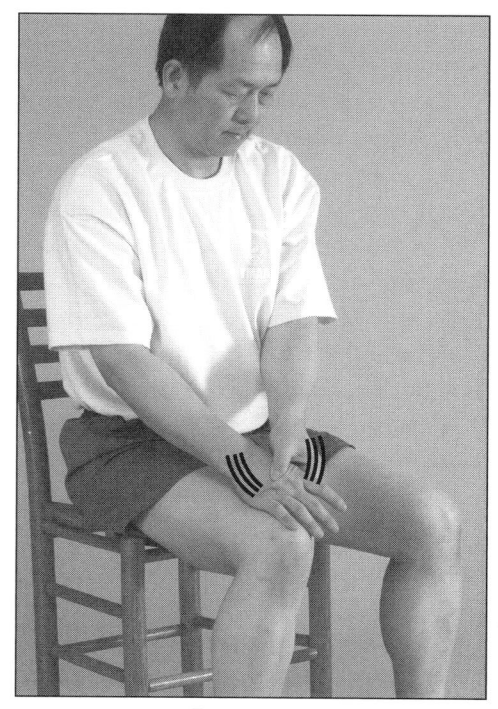

FIGURE 7-53

Qigong Massage

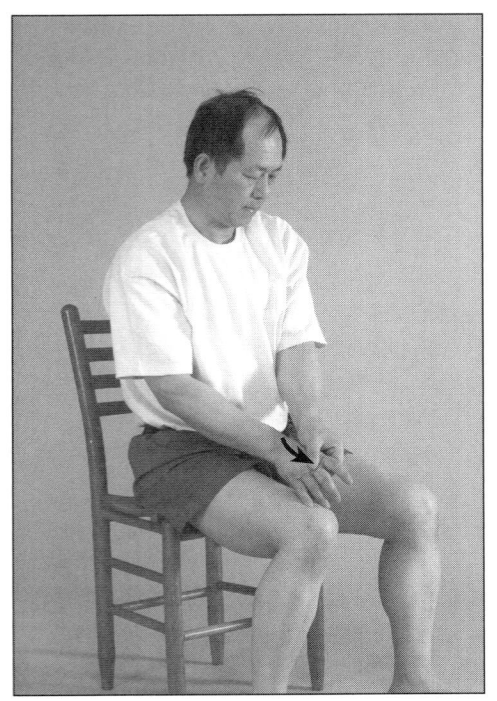

FIGURE 7-54

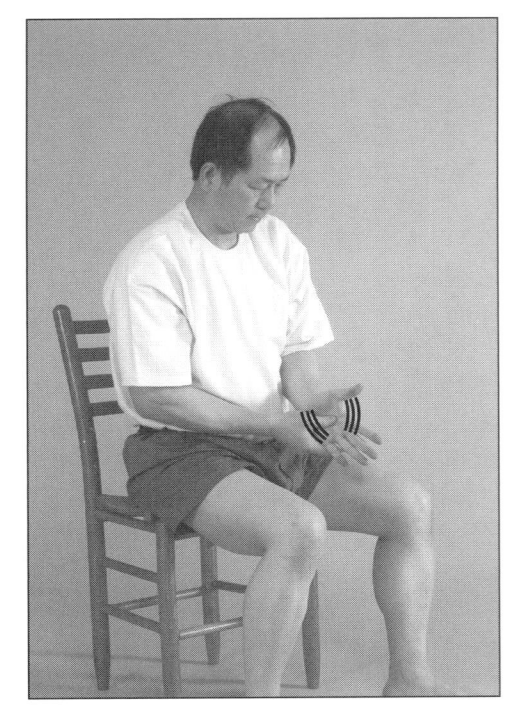

FIGURE 7-55

which can hinder the functioning of the hands or even cause arthritis.

Repeat the rubbing massage on the palm side of your hand (Figure 7-55), and press in while dragging or pushing from your wrist to the base of the fingers (Figure 7-56).

Grab one finger at a time and pull lightly, letting the finger slip out of your grasp (Figure 7-57). Do each finger three times. This will lead the Qi to the fingertips. Finally, grab the last section of each finger and gently pull and shake it a few times (Figure 7-58).

When you have finished one hand, repeat the same process on the other one, then stimulate the zones mentioned earlier (Figure 7-59). To do this, simply press on the zone with your thumb and rub in a circle. Again, use the other four fingers to stabilize the thumb and control the power.

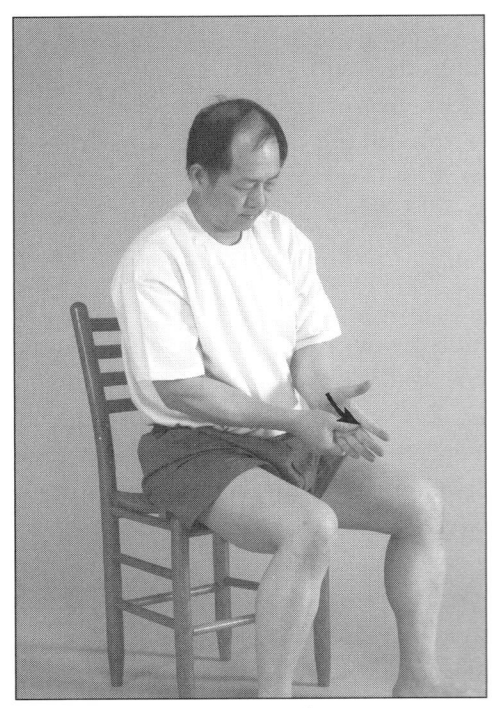

FIGURE 7-56

Chapter 7: General Self-Massage

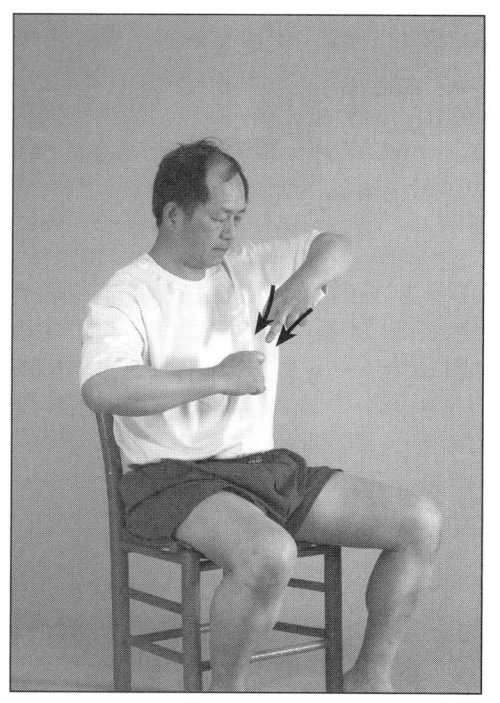

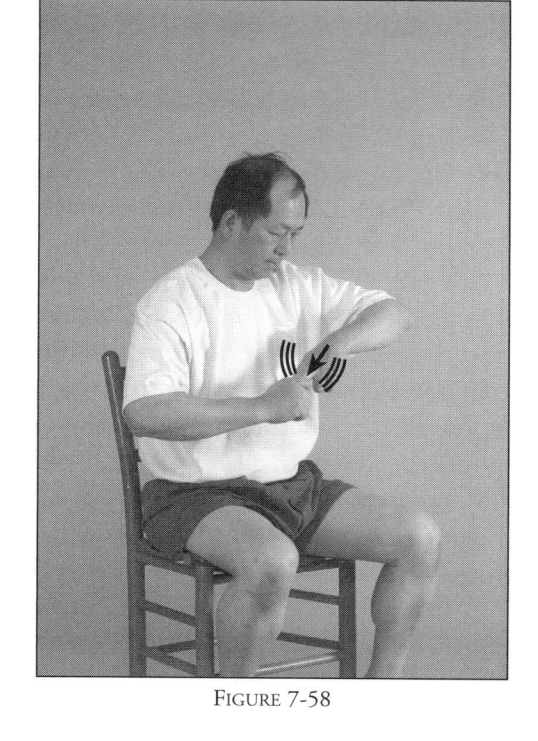

FIGURE 7-57

FIGURE 7-58

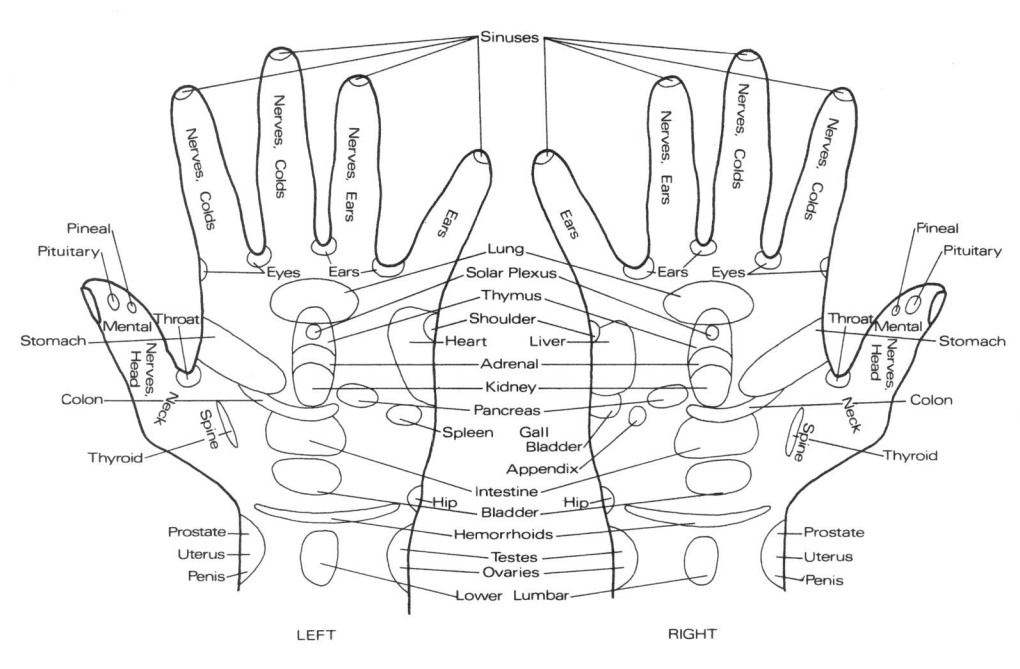

FIGURE 7-59. MASSAGE ZONES FOR HAND REFLEXOLOGY.

345

7-3. Self-Massage of the Internal Organs 內臟自我按摩

In this section we would like to introduce two types of Qigong massage which are commonly used to improve Qi circulation around the internal organs. The first type of massage is for improving the Qi circulation around the internal organs by massaging either directly over the organs or on acupuncture cavities which are connected to the organs. The second type of practice is massaging the internal organs by moving the muscles inside the torso.

Your internal organs are the foundation of your health. Most deaths are due to malfunction or failure of the internal organs. In order to be healthy and avoid degeneration, your organs need to have the correct amount of Qi circulating smoothly through them. The internal organs manage the energy in our bodies, and carry out a variety of physical processes. When any organ starts to malfunction, the Qi circulation in the body will be disrupted, and the production of hormones will be affected. This state can result in a variety of disorders. Therefore, to maintain your health, you must first learn how to maintain the healthy functioning of your internal organs. To reach this goal, you have to learn how to keep the Qi and blood circulating smoothly in your organs.

Using the hands to massage the internal organs is a natural human instinct, and we do it whenever we feel pain or Qi stagnation in or near an organ. For example, if you have diarrhea and feel pain in your abdomen, you naturally massage yourself with your hands, and if you overeat, you automatically stroke or rub your stomach with your palms to ease the pain.

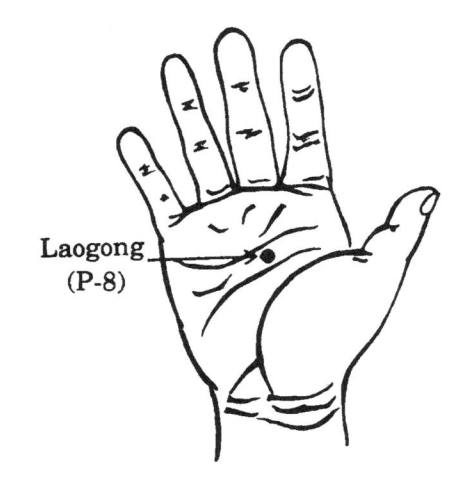

FIGURE 7-60. THE LAOGONG CAVITY.

There are two methods of using the hands to massage the internal organs. The first method uses gentle rubbing to loosen and relax the muscles around the internal organs. In the second method, the hands are placed on the afflicted area, and Qi is released from the centers of the palms to remove Qi and blood stagnation around the internal organs. As you can probably guess, in the second method the Qi does the actual healing.

We mentioned earlier that in the center of each palm is a cavity or gate called the Laogong (P-8) (勞宮) (Figure 7-60) which is used to regulate the Qi of the heart whenever the Qi flow is too strong. Unless you are sick, the Qi in the heart is normally more positive than is necessary, especially in the summertime. When you are excited or nervous, even more Qi accumulates around the heart. When this happens, the centers of your palms will feel warm and will often sweat.

Since the Qi in the center of the palm is always strong, you can use this Qi to help stagnant Qi in an organ to flow smoothly. Chinese physicians and Qigong practitioners have developed a number of ways of using the hands to improve the Qi circulation in the internal organs. In this section we will first introduce a few common methods for using the hands to massage the internal organs, and then we will explain how to use body movements to attain the same goal. These techniques can be practiced easily by anyone.

Massaging your Internal Organs with your Hands

Some of the techniques for massaging your internal organs are similar or identical to those discussed previously for massaging the waist. Since keeping the internal organs functioning properly is a goal shared by both general self-massage and self-massage of the organs, they both follow the same theory and use the same or similar techniques. However, regulating the Qi in the internal organs requires that the mind be in a more meditative and concentrated state so that you can reach deeply inside your body. You also need to build up your Qi so that it will be stronger and more penetrating. This takes more time than when you are only giving yourself a general self-massage.

We recommend that you compare the theory and techniques discussed in this section with those introduced in the previous one. This will give you a deeper understanding of the techniques.

Large and Small Intestines

To massage your abdomen and regulate the Qi circulation in your large and small intestines, place one hand on top of the other on your lower abdomen. If you are right-handed, it is better if you place your right hand on the bottom and the left hand on the top, and if you are left-handed, place your left hand on the bottom. The reason for this is quite simple. The Qi is strongest in the hand you use most often, and it is easier for you to lead the Qi from it.

When you massage your abdomen, it is best if you lie down so that your lower body is relaxed and the Qi can circulate more easily and smoothly. Hold your hand lightly against the skin and gently circle your hands clockwise, which is the direction of movement within the large intestine (Figure 7-61). Circling in the other direction would hinder the natural movements of peristalsis. Massage until you feel warm and comfortable deep inside your body.

As you massage, your breathing should be relaxed, deep, and comfortable. Place your mind a few inches under your palms. The mind will then be able to lead the Qi inward to smooth out Qi and blood stagnation.

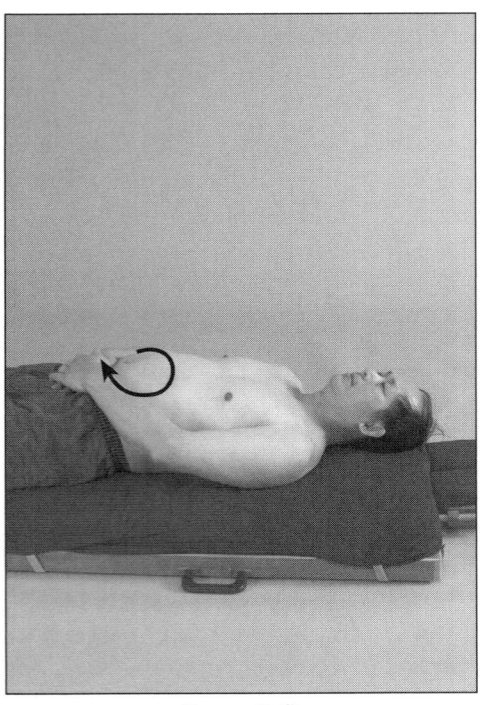

FIGURE 7-61

FIGURE 7-62

Liver, Stomach, Spleen, and Gall Bladder

In Qigong massage for the internal organs, the liver, stomach, spleen, and gall bladder are usually included in the same techniques because they are all located in the middle of the front of the body. Maintaining healthy Qi circulation in an organ requires not only that the circulation in the organ itself be smooth, but also that the circulation between the organs be smooth. Therefore, when you massage these four internal organs, you should treat them as one instead of four.

Hold your hands as you did when massaging the lower abdomen, only now place them above the navel. Experience has shown that clockwise is again more effective than counterclockwise (Figure 7-62). It is also easiest to do this massage when you are lying down. Massage until you feel warm inside.

Kidneys

Chinese medicine considers the kidneys one of the most important internal organs. The kidneys affect how the other organs function, so almost all forms of Qigong place heavy emphasis on keeping them healthy.

To massage your own kidneys, close your hands into fists and place the thumb/index finger sides on your kidneys. Gently circle both fists until the kidneys are warm. In the summer, when your kidneys are normally too Yang, it is desirable to dissipate some of the Qi. This can be done by circling your right hand clockwise and your

Chapter 7: General Self-Massage

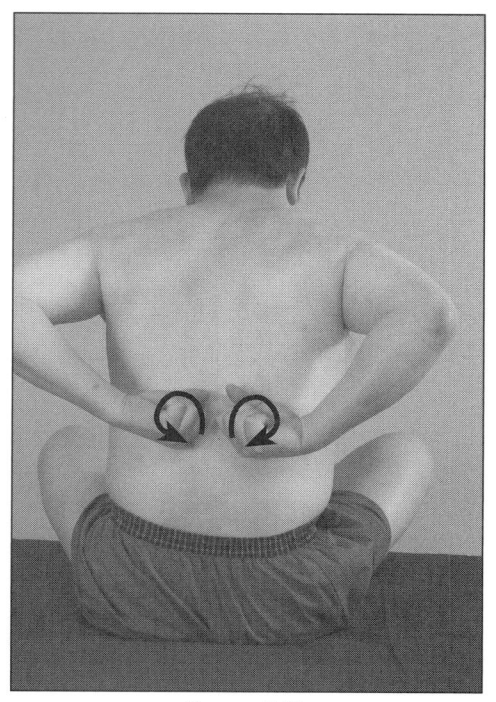

FIGURE 7-63

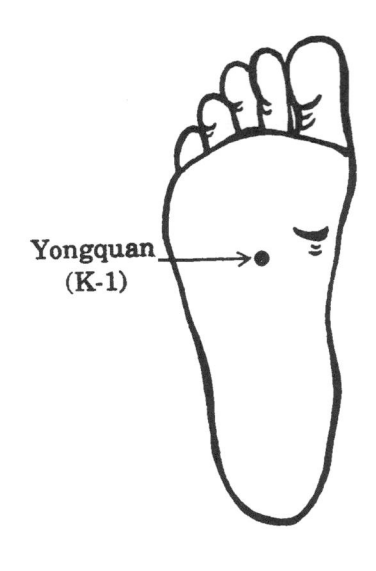

FIGURE 7-64. THE YONGQUAN CAVITY.

left hand counterclockwise (Figure 7-63). This leads the Qi to the sides of your body. However, when you massage your kidneys in the wintertime, when the kidney Qi is normally deficient, then you should reverse the direction and lead the Qi to the center of your back to nourish the kidneys. As usual, the breathing and the mind are important keys to successful practice.

There are other methods of improving the Qi circulation in the kidneys. The most common of which is to massage the bottoms of your feet. There is a Qi gate in the front center of each sole which is called Yongquan (K-1) (湧泉) (Gushing Spring) (Figure 7-64). Massaging these two cavities will stimulate the Qi circulation in the kidneys and help to regulate them (Figure 7-65).

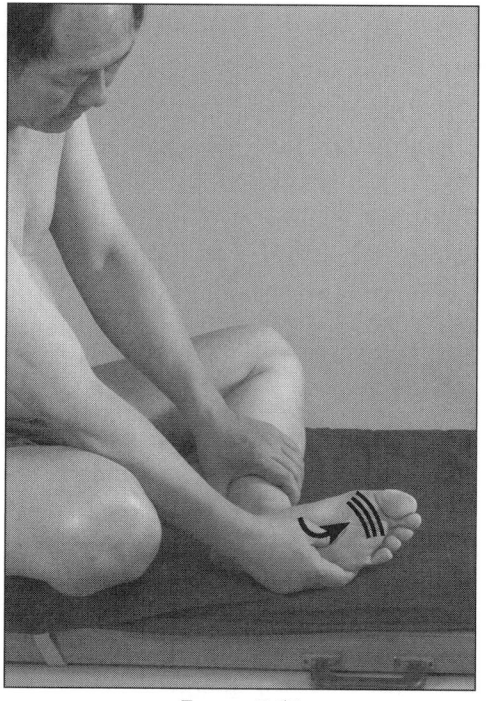

FIGURE 7-65

Lungs

According to the five elements theory, the lungs belong to Metal (Jin, 金) while the heart belongs to Fire (Huo, 火). According to this theory, the Metal lungs can be used to regulate the heart Fire just as metal can absorb heat. If you pay attention carefully you will notice that when you feel heat around your heart because of excitement, you will normally thrust out your chest and greatly expand your lungs while inhaling. Doing this a few times reduces the pressure and the feeling of heat in the heart.

To do Qigong massage for your lungs, place both hands on the center of your chest just above the solar plexus (Figure 7-66). Inhale deeply, and then exhale while lightly pushing both hands to the sides (Figure 7-67). Do this until your lungs feel relaxed and comfortable. This massage is also good for the heart.

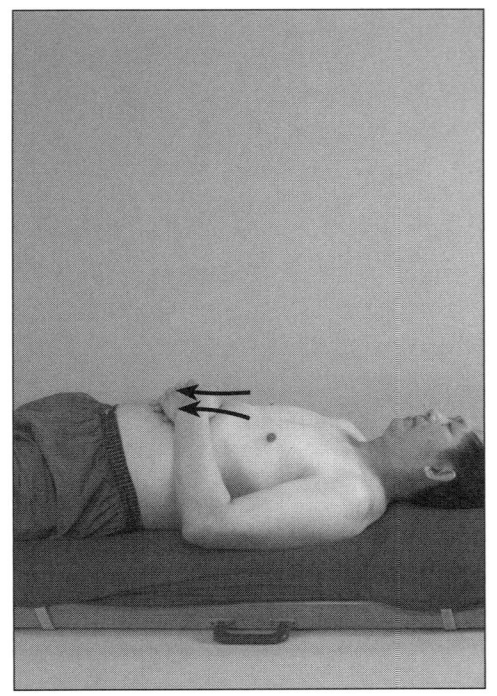

FIGURE 7-66

Heart

Qigong teachers do not normally encourage students to massage their own hearts unless they are fairly advanced in skill. The heart is the most vital organ, and if you mistreat it you are in big trouble.

When you massage your heart, unlike all the other internal organs, you cannot place your mind on it. If you do place your mind on your heart you will lead more Qi to it and make it even more positive. You may have noticed that when your heart is beating fast after exercising, if you pay attention to your heartbeat it will start beating even faster. A person who is prone to heart attacks can possibly bring one on by paying too much attention to his heart. If your heart is beating too hard, the best thing is to pay attention to your lungs and breathe deeply and gently. After only a few breaths your heart will slow down and regain its regular pace.

Therefore, when you massage your heart, your mind should not be on your heart. Instead, keep your mind on the movement of your hands. To massage your heart, place your right hand over your heart at least three inches above your chest. Move your hand in a small clockwise circle, and gradually increase the size of the circle. This takes the Qi in the heart and spreads it out around the chest. Finally, lead the Qi past the liver and down the right leg (Figure 7-68).

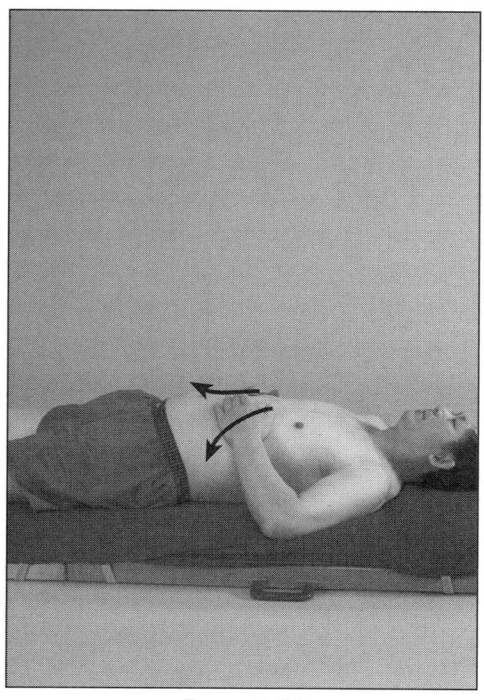

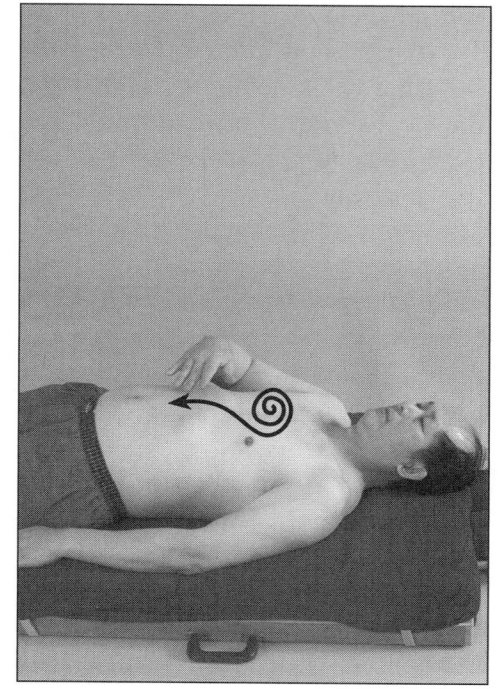

FIGURE 7-67   FIGURE 7-68

Massaging the Internal Organs with Movement

In this section we will introduce methods for massaging the internal organs through body movements both when you are standing and also when you are sitting. This type of massage has been practiced in China for more than one thousand years. The Eight Pieces of Brocade (Ba Duan Jin, 八段錦) is a very well known set of exercises that exemplifies this type of massage. If you would like to learn more about The Eight Pieces of Brocade, please refer to the YMAA book: *Eight Simple Qigong Exercises for Health.*

The internal organs are surrounded by muscles, but, except for some of the trunk muscles which we use constantly throughout the day, most of these muscles are ignored. According to Qigong theory, if you can bring your Yi (意) (mind) to a muscle, you can lead Qi to energize it and move it. For example, if you decide you want to be able to wiggle your ears, if you keep trying, you will eventually be able to. It's the same with the internal muscles. This means that if you practice becoming very calm and bringing your attention deeper and deeper into the center of your body, you will soon be able to feel and sense the structure and condition of the inside of your body. Once this happens, you can use your mind to move the internal muscles and massage the internal organs.

The way to gain control of the muscles inside your body is to start using your trunk muscles to make the movements. After you have practiced for a while, your mind will be able to reach deeper and feel other muscles as well. Once you are able to feel these muscles, you will be able to move them. With a bit more practice you will be able to

Qigong Massage

control them while keeping them relaxed, and the movements will become natural, easy, and comfortable. Remember that the muscles have to be relaxed before the organs can be relaxed and before the Qi can circulate smoothly.

In this subsection we will introduce the beginning steps of internal organ massage through trunk movement. After you are able to do these exercises easily and smoothly, you should continue to lead your mind deeper and deeper into your body until you can sense your organs.

It is a good idea to loosen up your trunk before starting these massaging movements. This will let you move more naturally and comfortably. The following stretching and warming up exercises can be used for both standing and sitting internal organ massage.

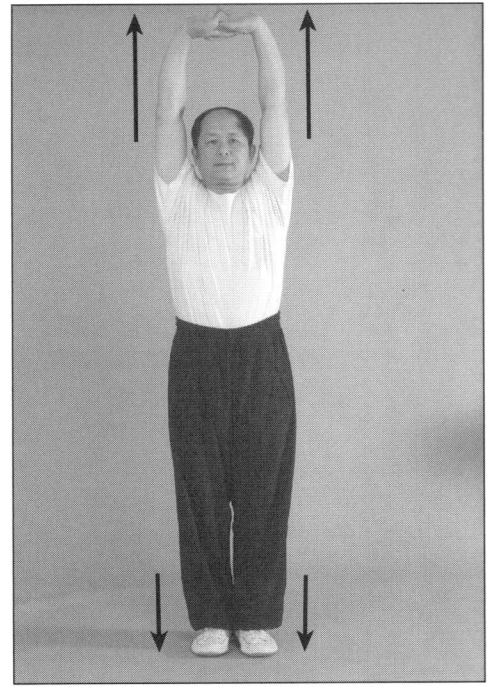

FIGURE 7-69

Loosening the Trunk Muscles

The trunk is the center of the whole body, and it contains the muscles which control the trunk and also surround the internal organs. When the trunk muscles are tense, the whole body will be tense and the internal organs will be compressed. This causes stagnation of the Qi circulation in the body and especially in the organs. For this reason, the trunk muscles should be stretched and loosened up before any moving Qigong practice.

First, interlock your fingers and lift your hands up over your head while imagining that you are pushing upward with your hands and pushing downward with your feet (Figure 7-69). Do not tense your muscles, because this will constrict your body and prevent you from stretching. If you do this stretch correctly, you will feel the muscles in your waist area tensing slightly because they are being pulled simultaneously from the top and the bottom.

Next, use your mind to relax even more, and stretch out a little bit more. After you have stretched for about ten seconds, turn your upper body to one side to twist the trunk muscles (Figure 7-70). Stay to the side for three to five seconds, turn your body to face forward and then turn to the other side. Stay there for three to five seconds. Repeat the upper body twisting three times, then tilt your upper body to the side and stay there for about three seconds (Figure 7-71), then tilt to the other side. Next, bend forward and touch your hands to the floor (Figure 7-72) and stay there for three to five seconds. Finally, squat down with your feet flat on the floor to stretch your ankles (Figure 7-73),

Chapter 7: General Self-Massage

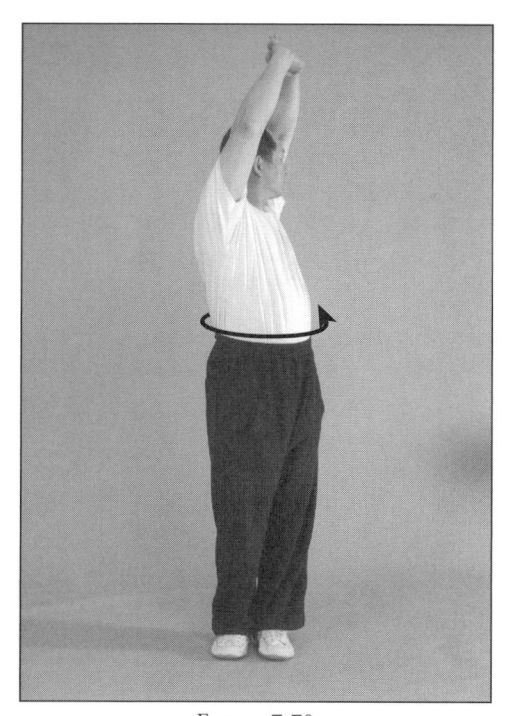

FIGURE 7-70

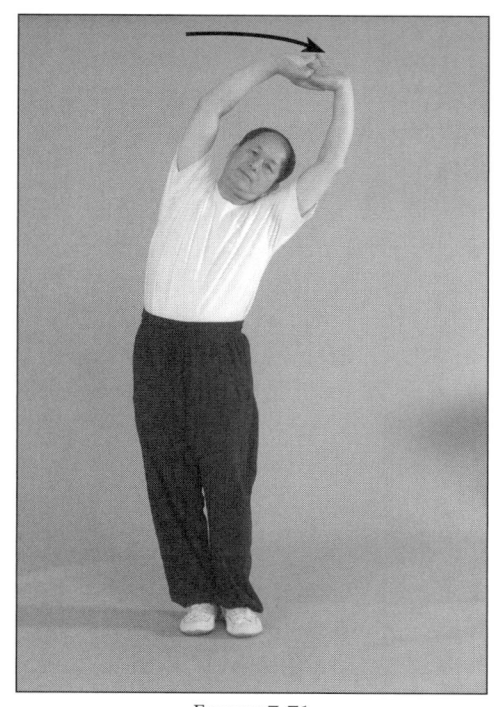

FIGURE 7-71

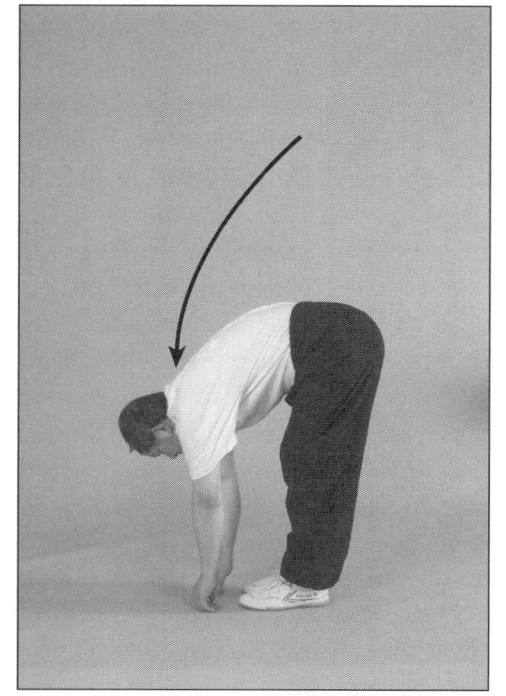

FIGURE 7-72

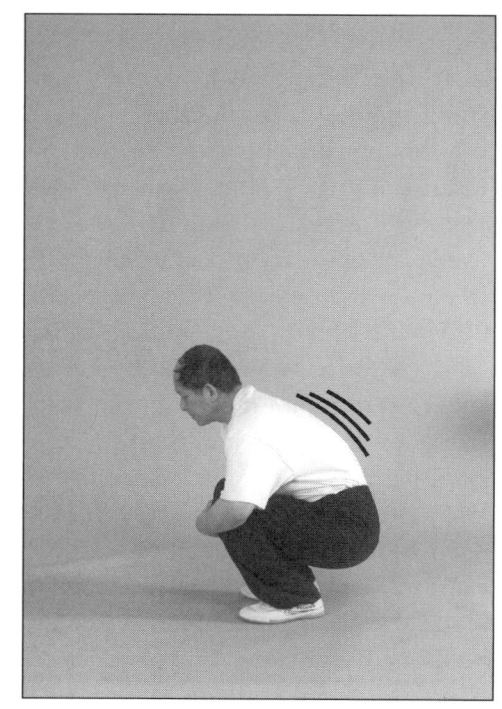

FIGURE 7-73

353

and then lift your heels up to stretch the toes (Figure 7-74). Repeat the entire process ten times. After you finish, the inside of your body should feel very comfortable and warm.

The torso is supported by the spine and the trunk muscles. Once you have stretched your trunk muscles, you can loosen up the torso. This also moves the muscles inside your body around, which moves and relaxes your internal organs. This, in turn, makes it possible for the Qi to circulate smoothly inside your body.

Massaging the Internal Organs While Standing

Massaging the Large Intestine, Small Intestine, Urinary Bladder, and Kidneys. This exercise helps you to regain conscious control of the muscles in your abdomen. There are four major benefits to this abdominal exercise. First, when your Lower Dan Tian (Xia Dan Tian, 下丹田) area is loose, the Qi can flow in and out easily. The Lower Dan Tian is the main residence of your Original Qi (Yuan Qi, 元氣). The Qi in your Dan Tian can be led easily only when your abdomen is loose and relaxed. Second, when the abdominal area is loose, the Qi circulation in the large and small intestines will be smooth, and they will be able to absorb nutrients and eliminate waste efficiently. If your body does not eliminate effectively, the absorption of nutrients will be hindered, and you may become sick. Third, when the abdominal area is loose, the Qi in the kidneys will circulate smoothly and the Original Essence (Yuan Jing, 元精) stored there can be converted more efficiently into Qi. In addition, when the kidney area is loosened, the kidney Qi can be led downward and upward to nourish the entire body. Fourth, these exercises eliminate Qi stagnation in the lower back, healing and preventing lower back pain.

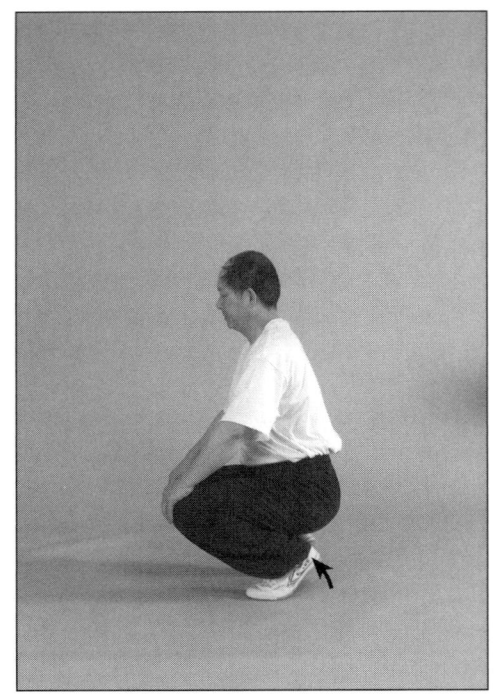

FIGURE 7-74

To practice this exercise, stand with your feet a comfortable distance apart and your knees slightly bent. As you get more used to this exercise and your legs become stronger, bend your knees a little bit more. Without moving your thighs or upper body, use the waist muscles to move the abdomen around in a horizontal circle (Figure 7-75). Circle in one direction about ten times, and then in the other direction about ten times. If you hold one hand over your Lower Dan Tian and the other on your sacrum, you may be able to focus your attention better on the area you want to control.

In the beginning, you may have difficulty making your body move the way you

Chapter 7: General Self-Massage

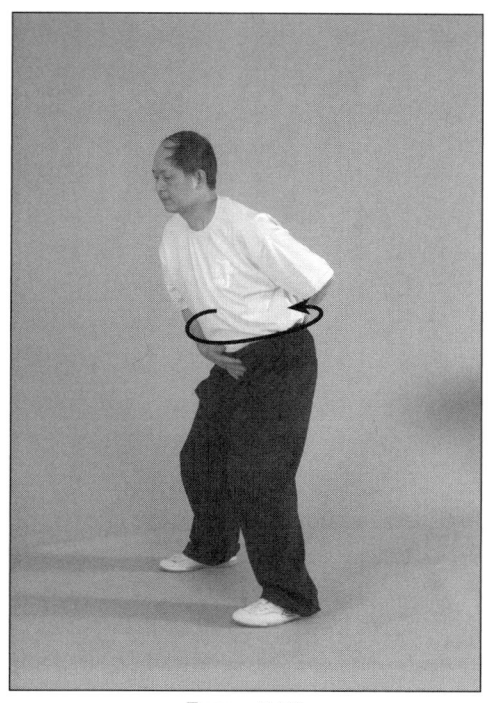

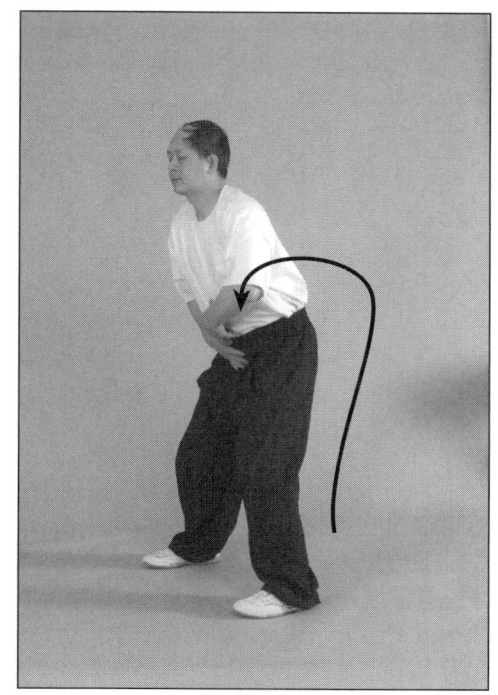

FIGURE 7-75

FIGURE 7-76

want it to, but if you keep practicing you will quickly learn how to do it. Once you can do the movement comfortably, make the circles larger and larger. Naturally, this will cause the muscles to tense somewhat and inhibit the Qi flow, but the more you practice the sooner you will be able to relax again. After you have practiced for a while and can control your waist muscles easily, start making the circles smaller, and also start using your Yi to lead the Qi from the Dan Tian to move in these circles. The final goal is to have only a slight physical movement, but a strong movement of Qi.

When you practice, concentrate your mind on your abdomen and inhale and exhale deeply and smoothly. Remember that breathing deep does not mean breathing heavily. When you breathe deep, keep the muscles controlling the lungs and diaphragm relaxed. Inhale to lead the Qi into the center of the body and exhale to lead the Qi out from the skin.

Massaging the Stomach, Liver, Spleen, Gall Bladder, and Kidneys. Beneath your diaphragm is your stomach, on its right are your liver and gall bladder, on its left is your spleen, and in the back are the kidneys. Once you can comfortably do the movement in your lower abdomen, change the movement from horizontal to vertical, and extend it up to your diaphragm. The easiest way to loosen the area around the diaphragm is to use a wave-like motion between the perineum and the diaphragm (Figure 7-76). You may find it helpful when you practice this to place one hand on your Lower Dan Tian and your other hand above it with the thumb on the solar plexus. Use a forward and

355

Qigong Massage

backward wave-like motion, flowing up to the diaphragm and down to the perineum and back. While you do this, inhale deeply when the motion is starting at the perineum and exhale as it reaches the diaphragm. Practice ten times.

Next, continue the movement while turning your body slowly to one side and then to the other (Figure 7-77). This will slightly tense the muscles on one side and loosen them on the other, which will massage the internal organs. Repeat ten times.

This exercise loosens the muscles around the stomach, liver, gall bladder, spleen, and kidneys, and therefore improves the Qi circulation there. It also trains you in using your mind to lead Qi from your Lower Dan Tian upward to the solar plexus area.

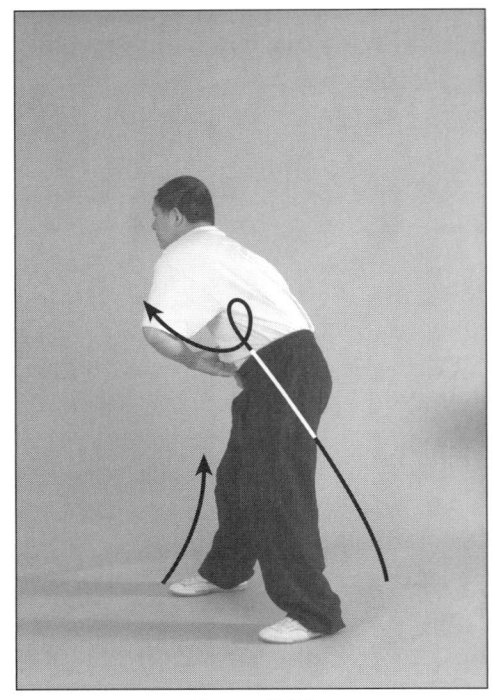

FIGURE 7-77

Massaging the Lungs and Heart. This exercise loosens up the chest and helps to regulate and improve the Qi circulation in the lungs. According to the theory of the five phases (Wu Xing, 五行) in Chinese medicine, the lungs belong to the element Metal (Jin, 金) while the heart belongs to the element Fire (Huo, 火). Metal is able to cool down Fire, and the lungs are able to regulate the Qi of the heart. The heart is the most vital organ, and its condition is closely related to our life and death. If there is too much Qi in the heart (when it is too Yang), you speed up its degeneration and become prone to heart attacks. For this reason, Qigong places great emphasis on using the lungs to regulate the Qi in the heart. If we know how to relax the lungs and keep the Qi circulating in them smoothly, they will be able to regulate the heart more efficiently.

After loosening up the center portion of your body, extend the movement up to your chest. The wave-like movement starts in the abdomen, moves through the stomach and up to the chest. You may find it easier to feel the movement if you hold one hand on your abdomen and the other lightly touching your chest (Figure 7-78). After you have done the movement ten times, extend the movement to your shoulders (Figure 7-79). Inhale when you move your shoulders backward and exhale when you move them forward. The inhalation and exhalation should be as deep as comfortably possible, and the entire chest should be very loose. Repeat the motion ten times.

Chapter 7: General Self-Massage

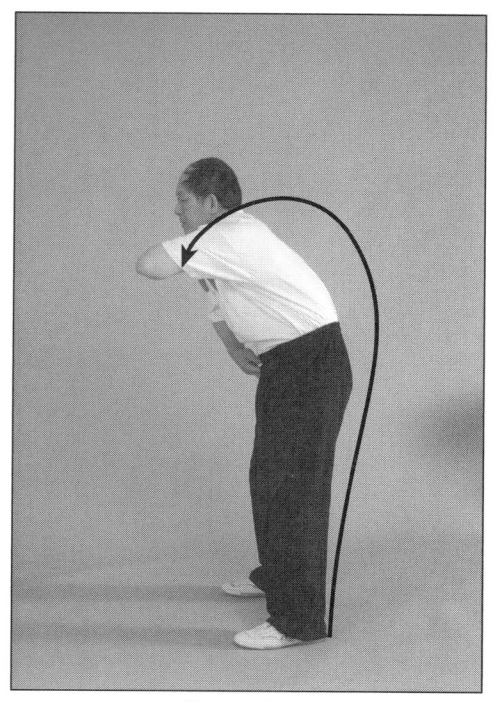

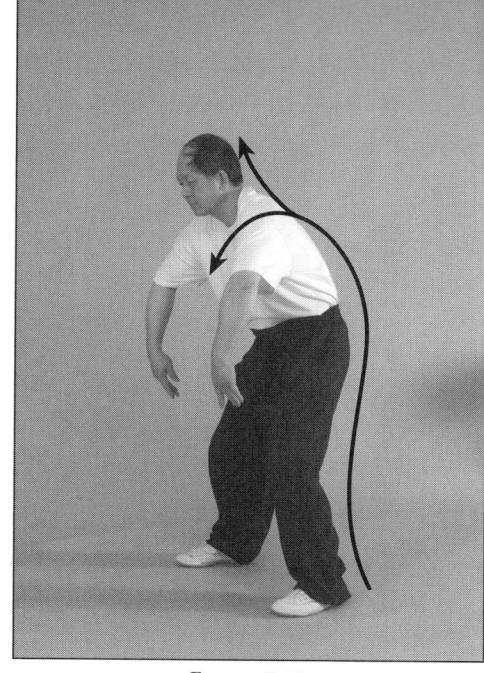

FIGURE 7-78

FIGURE 7-79

Massaging the Internal Organs While Sitting

The theory of self-massage of the internal organs with movement is the same whether you are standing or sitting. The only difference is that when you are sitting, the internal organs in the lower part of body such as the urinary bladder, large intestine, and small intestine cannot be massaged as easily as when you are standing.

Self-massage of the organs with movement is not as easy or convenient to do when you are sitting, but it can still be very valuable for people who have difficulty standing. As a matter of fact, since ancient times many Chinese have practiced these movements right after awakening in the morning. The Sitting Eight Pieces of Brocade (Zuo Shi Ba Duan Jin, 坐勢八段錦) is a popular set of exercises that was created for this purpose. If you are interested in this set, you may refer to the YMAA publication: *Eight Simple Qigong Exercises for Health*.

I believe that many people today will find the sitting self-massage of the organs to be more useful than the standing exercises. Many jobs require long hours sitting in front of a computer terminal or in a car, and uncomfortable feelings in the internal organs are a common experience. The sitting exercises are just the thing to relieve tension in the internal organs, improve Qi and blood circulation, and keep the organs healthy.

Loosening Up the Spine and Trunk Muscles. Before you massage your internal organs with movement, you should first loosen up your spine and trunk muscles. First, starting at your sacrum, move your spine in a wave-like motion upward to your neck

Qigong Massage

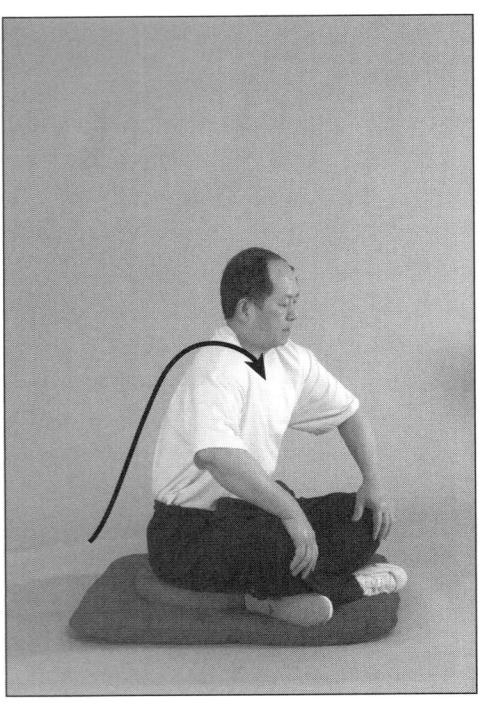

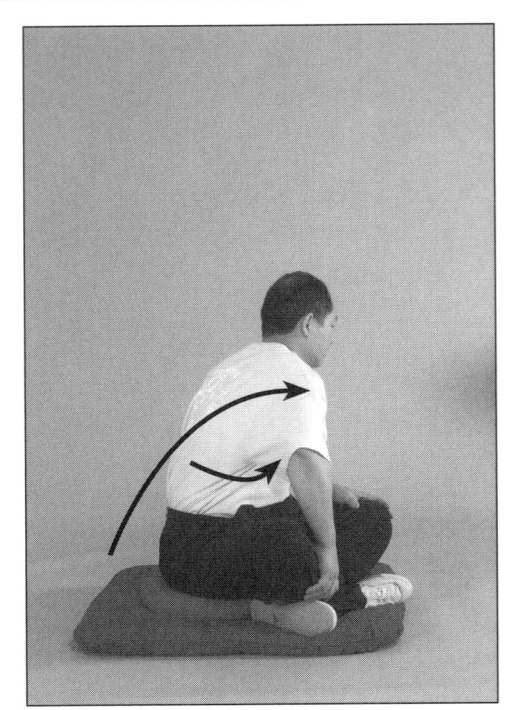

FIGURE 7-80

FIGURE 7-81

(Figure 7-80). Keep your body as relaxed as possible, especially your trunk muscles. Repeat about ten times. Then, continue the same motion while slowly turning your body to the sides (Figure 7-81). Finally, turn your body slowly to one side and then the other as much as you can to stretch the trunk muscles (Figure 7-82). Do this about five times to each side.

1. **Massaging the Large and Small Intestines and the Urinary Bladder.** First learn how to move the muscles in your lower abdomen. Inhale deeply and slowly while expanding your abdomen and gently pushing your anus and Huiyin cavity out (Figure 7-83). Then, exhale deeply and slowly while withdrawing your abdomen and gently pulling in your anus and Huiyin cavity. Keep your mind calm and natural, and your body centered and relaxed. Repeat about ten to twenty times. This up and down movement massages the organs in the lower abdomen.

   Interlock your fingers and place them behind your head. Continue inhaling and exhaling deeply. As you exhale, slowly bend your body forward, and as you inhale, straighten up (Figure 7-84). Repeat ten times.

Chapter 7: General Self-Massage

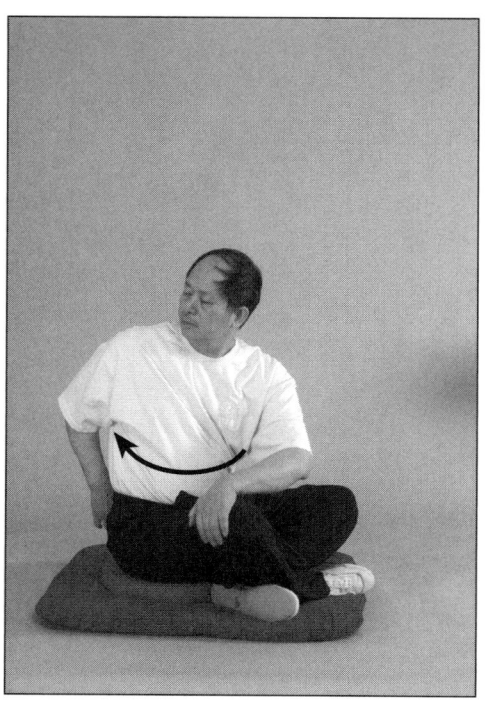

FIGURE 7-82

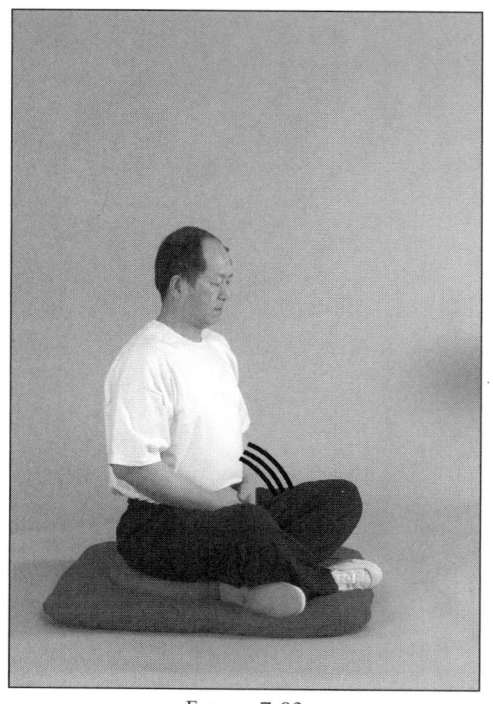

FIGURE 7-83

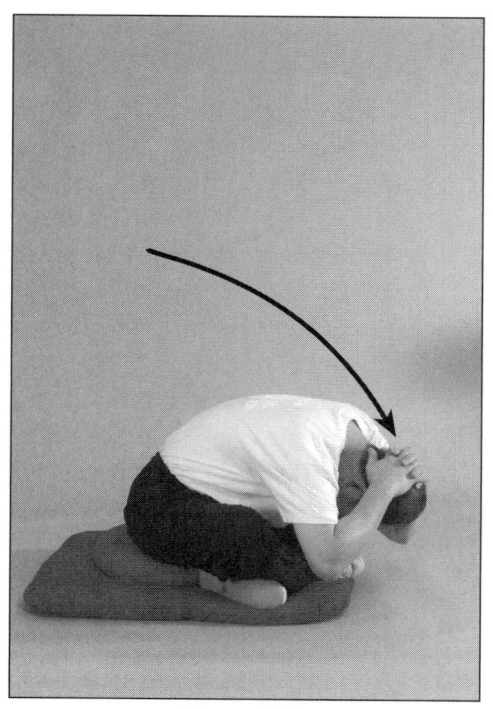

FIGURE 7-84

359

Qigong Massage

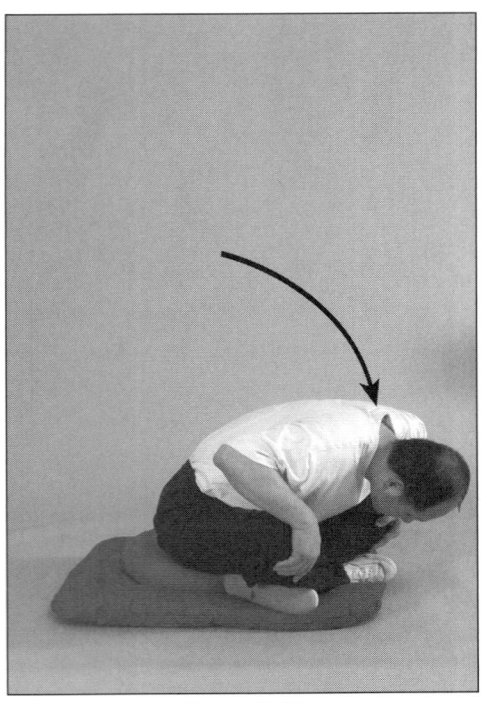

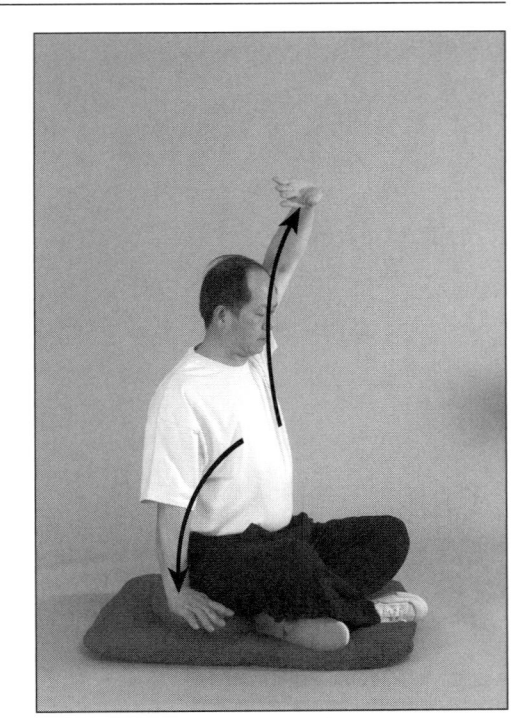

FIGURE 7-85

FIGURE 7-86

Finally, place your hands on your knees and repeat the same movements (Figure 7-85). With your hands on your knees your trunk muscles can relax more, and the movements can reach deeper into the body.

2. **Massaging the Liver, Gall Bladder, Stomach, Spleen, and Kidneys.** As you did in the preceding section, bend forward and straighten up in coordination with your breathing. Now, however, keep your attention on the middle of your body, at the level of your lower ribs, rather than on your stomach. This will focus the movement there, and massage the liver and other organs there. Next, inhale deeply, and raise your left hand and press down your right hand as you exhale (Figure 7-86). As you inhale, lower your left arm. Then raise your right hand and press down your left hand as you exhale, and lower it as your inhale. Remember that deep and relaxed breathing is the key to massaging the internal organs in the middle of the body. When you breathe correctly, your diaphragm moves up and down, alternately applying and releasing pressure on the organs. Raise and lower each arm at least five times.

Next, continue raising and lowering your arms in coordination with your breathing, only now start turning your body from side to side (Figure 7-87). As you raise your right hand, turn to your left, and as you raise your left hand, turn to your right. Repeat ten times.

Chapter 7: General Self-Massage

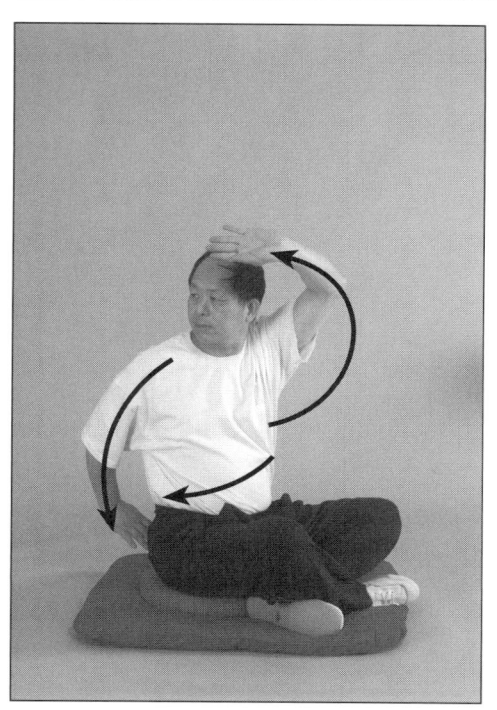

FIGURE 7-87

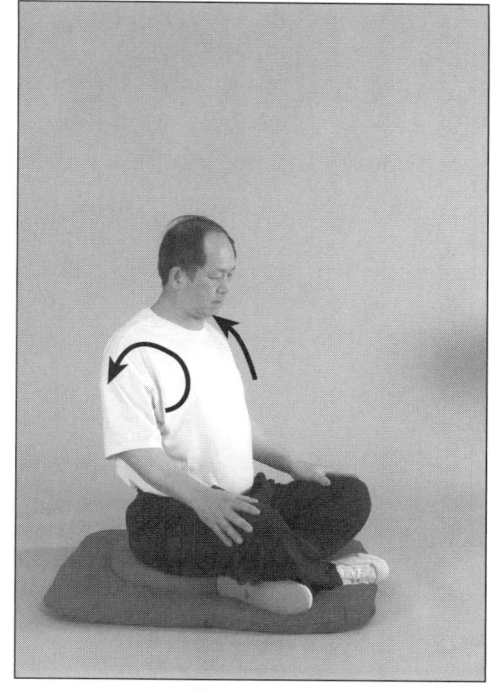

FIGURE 7-88

When you are through, still your mind and breathe deeply for a few minutes.

3. **Massaging the Lungs and Heart.** Continue normal abdominal breathing. As you inhale, gently circle your shoulders to the rear, and as you exhale, circle them forward (Figure 7-88). Repeat the motion ten times, and then do ten more repetitions circling in the other direction.

Finally, raise your hands in front of your chest while inhaling (Figure 7-89), and circle them forward, to the sides, and then down to your waist as you exhale (Figure 7-90). Repeat ten times.

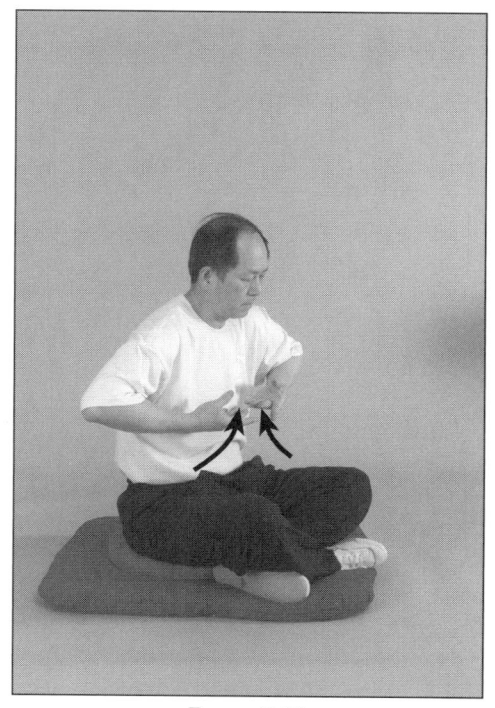

FIGURE 7-89

We have introduced you to only a few of the many techniques for massaging your internal organs. We hope that it is enough to serve you as an adequate introduction. Once you understand the theory and have accumulated some experience, you should be able to discover other movements and techniques which are also beneficial.

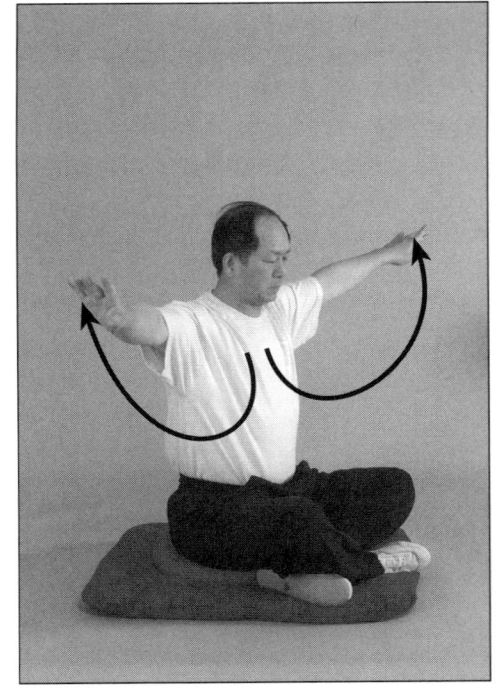

FIGURE 7-90

CHAPTER 8

Conclusion 結論

Now that you have read this book, the next step is to practice self-massage by yourself and to also find a partner with whom you can practice general massage. Always remember that knowledge is only the Yin side of study. To become proficient you also need to manifest the Yang side through action.

During the course of your study, you should refer to the many other books about massage that are available. The more you read and study, the better you will be, and the more your knowledge will increase. If you can gather the opinions of many authors and learn through them the correct path, then you will surely be a wise practitioner.

You should also understand that this book is only the first part of an entire series of Chinese Qigong massage. The massage in this book is limited to maintaining health. If, after finishing this book, you wish to go on and enter the field of Qigong massage for healing, you should read the next volume in this series.

APPENDIX A

Translation and Glossary of Chinese Terms
中文術語之翻譯與解釋

An 按 Press. A major technique of Chinese massage.
An Mo 按摩 Literally: press rub. Together they mean massage.
Ba 八 Means "eight."
Ba 拔 Uprooting.
Ba Duan Jin 八段錦 The Eight Pieces of Brocade. An ancient External Elixir (Wai Dan, 外丹) medical Qigong created by Marshal Yue, Fei (岳飛) during Chinese Song dynasty (960-1280 A.D.) (宋朝).
Ba Mai 八脈 Eight vessels and means "Eight Extraordinary Vessels."
Bagua 八卦 Literally: Eight Divinations. Also called the Eight Trigrams. In Chinese philosophy, the eight basic variations; shown in the Yi *Jing* (易經) (i.e. *Book of Changes*) as groups of single and broken lines.
Bai He 少林白鶴 White Crane. A style of Chinese martial arts.
Baihui (Gv-20) 百會 Literally "hundred meetings." An important acupuncture cavity located on the top of the head. The Baihui cavity belongs to the Governing Vessel. Baihui is called "Tianlingai" (天靈蓋) in the Chinese martial arts and "Niwangong" (泥丸宮) in Daoist society.
Ban 扳 Twisting, one of the massage techniques.
Bei 背 Carrying on the back. One of the massage techniques.
Bi Qi 閉氣 Seal the breath. One of the Chinese Qin Na (擒拿) categories.
Bian 砭 Stone probes.
Bian Shi 砭石 Stone Probe. Bian Shi were used to stimulate acupuncture cavities in the treatment of illnesses during the Yellow Emperor era (2690-2590 B.C.) (黃帝) before metal needles became available. Bian Shi is also called Shi Zhen (石針) which means "stone needle."
Bin Ru Gaohuang 病入膏肓 Means "the sickness has reached the Gaohuang" which implies the sickness has become serious or hopeless.
Bu 補 Means "to nourish."

365

Ca 擦 Wiping. One of the massage techniques.

Cao Jie 操接 Cao means "to operate or to manipulate" and Jie means "to connect." Cao Jie is a common name bone connection in Fujian (福建) and Taiwan (臺灣). Cao Jie is commonly done by martial artists.

Chan 纏 Reeling. One of the massage techniques.

Chang 長 Long.

Changquan (Chang Chuan) 長拳 Chang (長) means "long," and Quan (拳) means "fist, style, or sequence." A style of Northern Chinese Gongfu which specializes in kicking and long range fighting. Changquan has also been used to refer to Taijiquan (太極拳).

Che 扯 Quick pull. One of the massage techniques.

Cheng Fo 成佛 Buddhist term. When one has achieved the Buddhahood they are called Cheng Fo.

Cheng, Gin-Gsao (1911-1976 A.D.) 曾金灶 Dr. Yang, Jwing-Ming's White Crane master.

Chin Na (Qin Na) 擒拿 Literally, grab control. A type of Chinese Gongfu (功夫) which emphasizes grabbing techniques to control the opponent's joints in conjunction with attacking certain acupuncture cavities.

Chong Mai 衝脈 Thrusting Vessel. One of the eight extraordinary vessels.

Chun Qiu 春秋 Spring and Autumn Period. One of the Chinese warring periods (722-484 B.C.).

Cuo 搓 Filing. One of the massage techniques.

Da 打 Striking. One of the massage techniques.

Dai Mai 帶脈 The Girdle Vessel. One of the eight extraordinary vessels.

Dan Tian 丹田 Literally: Field of Elixir. Locations in the body which are able to store and generate Qi (elixir) in the body. The Upper, Middle, and Lower Dan Tian are located respectively between the eyebrows, at the solar plexus, and a few inches below the navel.

Dao 搗 Threshing. One of the massage techniques.

Dao (Tao) 道 The way. The 'natural' way of everything.

Dao Jia Hu Xi 道家呼吸 Daoist breathing, also called Reverse Abdominal Breathing (Ni Fu Hu Xi, 逆腹呼吸).

Di 地 The Earth. Earth, Heaven (Tian, 天), and Man (Ren, 人) are the Three Natural Powers (San Cai, 三才).

Di Li Shi 地理師 Geomancy teachers. Di Li means "geomancy" and Shi means "teacher." Therefore Di Li Shi means a teacher or master who analyzes geographic locations according to formulas in the *Yi Jing* (易經) (*Book of Changes*) and the energy distributions in the Earth.

Di Qi 地氣 Earth Qi.

Dian 點 Pointing. One of the Chinese massage techniques.

Dian Da 點打 Point striking. One of the Chinese massage techniques.

Dian Qi 電氣 Dian means electricity, and so Dian Qi means "electrical energy" (electricity). In China, a word is often placed before "Qi" to identify the different kinds of energy.

Dian Xue 點穴 Dian means "to point and exert pressure" and Xue means "the cavities." In Chinese martial arts society, Dian Xue refers to those Qin Na (擒拿) techniques which specialize in attacking acupuncture cavities to immobilize or kill an opponent.

Dian Xue An Mo 點穴按摩 Dian Xue (cavity press) massage for illnesses. One of main massage categories in Chinese massage.

Die 迭 Folding. A Chinese massage technique.

Die Da 跌打 Die means 'fallen' and Da means "struck" which reflect the fact that it specializes in treating injuries caused by falling and being struck.

Ding 頂 Supporting. A Chinese massage technique.

Dou 抖 Waving. A Chinese massage technique.

Du Mai 督脈 Usually translated Governing Vessel. One of the eight extraordinary vessels.

Duan 端 Holding. A Chinese massage technique.

Fan Fu Hu Xi 反腹呼吸 Reverse abdominal breathing, also called Daoist Breathing (Dao Jia Hu Xi, 道家呼吸).

Fan She An Mo 反射按摩 Reflexology. A Chinese massage category that emphasizes massaging the hands and feet. From massaging these extensions, abnormal Qi circulation in the body can be regulated.

Fen 分 Dividing. A Chinese massage technique.

Feng Shui 風水 "Wind-Water." Implies geomancy.

Feng Shui Shi 風水師 Literally: wind water teacher. Teacher or master of geomancy. Geomancy is the art or science of analyzing the natural energy relationships in a location, especially the interrelationships between 'wind' and 'water,' hence the name. Also called Di Li Shi (地理師).

Feng Yang Men 鳳陽門 Phoenix Sun Style. A Daoist martial art and meditation system which also specializes in Qigong massage.

Fo Jia Hu Xi 佛家呼吸 Buddhist Breathing, also called Normal Abdominal Breathing (Zheng Fu Hu Xi, 正腹呼吸).

Fu 腑 The bowels. The Yang organs: the Gall Bladder, Small Intestine, Large Intestine, Stomach, Bladder, and Triple Burner.

Fu 膚息 Skin breathing, also called 'body' (Ti Xi, 體息). A Chinese Qigong breathing technique that leads the Qi to the surface of skin to enhance the Guardian Qi (Wei Qi, 衛氣).

Fujian 福建 A province located in the southeast corner of China.

Gao, Tao 高濤 Dr. Yang, Jwing-Ming's first Taijiquan teacher, from 1962-1965.

Gong 功 Abbreviation of "Gongfu," which means energy-time. Any study, learning, or practice that requires a lot of patience, energy, and time to complete. Since practicing Chinese martial arts requires a great deal of time and energy, Chinese martial arts are commonly called Gongfu (功夫).

Gongfu (Kung Fu) 功夫 Literally: energy-time. Any study, learning, or practice which requires a lot of patience, energy, and time to complete. Since practicing Chinese martial arts requires a great deal of time and energy, Chinese martial arts are commonly called Gongfu.

Gu Zhen 骨針 Bone needle. An acupuncture needle made from animal bone. Gu Zhen were used for acupuncture before metal needles were introduced.

Gua 刮 Scraping. A Chinese massage technique.

Guan 貫 Pounding. A Chinese massage technique.

Guan Jie Hu Xi 關節呼吸 Joint breathing. A Chinese Qigong practice in which the mind is used to lead the Qi to the center of the joints and then lead out with the coordination of the breath.

Gui Qi 鬼氣 Ghost Qi. The Qi residue of a dead person. It is believed by the Chinese Buddhists and Daoists that this Qi residue is a so called ghost (Gui, 鬼).

Gun 滾 Rolling. A Chinese massage technique.

Guoshu 國術 Literally: national techniques. Another name for Chinese martial arts. First used by President Chiang, Kai-Shek (蔣介石) in 1928 at the founding of the Nanking Central Guoshu Institute (南京中央國術館).

Ha 哈 The sound of laughing. This sound is commonly used to lead the Qi outward to strengthen Guardian Qi (Wei Qi, 衛氣).

Han dynasty (206 B.C.-221 A.D.) 漢朝 One of the Chinese dynasties.

Han, Ching-Tang 韓慶堂 Dr. Yang, Jwing-Ming's Shaolin Long Fist grandmaster. Master Li, Mao-Ching's teacher.

He 合 Combining. A Chinese massage technique.

Hegu (LI-4) 合谷 An acupuncture cavity located between the bases of the thumb and the second finger. Hegu is also commonly called Hukou (虎口) (tiger mouth).

Hen 哼 The sound of crying or sighing. This sound is commonly used to lead the Qi to the bone marrow to nourish it.

Hou Tian Qi 後天氣 Post-Birth Qi or Post-Heaven Qi, converted from the Jing of the food and air we take consume.

Hsing Yi Chuan (Xingyiquan) 形意拳 Literally: Shape-mind Fist. An internal style of Gongfu in which the mind or thinking determines the shape or movement of the body. Creation of the style is attributed to Marshal Yue, Fei (岳飛).

Huan 緩 Slow.

Huan Jing Bu Nao 還精補腦 Literally, to return the Essence to nourish the brain. A Daoist Qigong training process wherein Qi which has been converted from Essence (Jing, 精) is lead to the brain to nourish it.

Appendix A: Translation and Glossary of Chinese Terms

Huang 晃 Swaying. A Chinese massage technique.

Hukou 虎口 Tiger mouth. An acupuncture cavity located between the bases of the thumb and the second finger. Tiger mouth is called Hegu (LI-4) (合谷) in Chinese medicine.

Huo 火 Fire.

Huo Qi 火氣 Fire Qi. Excess Qi manifestation in the body which sets the body on fire (i.e. too Yang) is called Fire Qi. "Fire Qi" also commonly means the Qi converted from food and air (i.e. Post-Heaven Essence).

Huo Qi 活氣 Vital Qi. The Qi in living things.

Ji 擠 Squeezing. A Chinese massage technique.

Jia Gu Wen 甲骨文 Oracle-Bone Scripture. Earliest evidence of the Chinese use of the written word. Found on pieces of turtle shell and animal bone from the Shang dynasty (1766-1154 B.C.) (商朝). Most of the information recorded was of a religious nature.

Jiao Hui Dian 交會點 Junctions. Means the junctions of Qi meridians or vessels.

Jie 接 Connect. A Chinese massage technique.

Jie 結 Knot or junction. Usually located on the junctions of blood or Qi vessels.

Jie Gu Ke 接骨科 Connect bone category. A medical training during the Chinese Ming dynasty (1368-1644 A.D.) (明朝).

Jin 金 Metal. One of the Five Elements (Wu Xing, 五行).

Jin dynasty (265-420 A.D.) 晉朝 A dynasty in Chinese history.

Jin, Shao-Feng 金紹峰 Dr. Yang, Jwing-Ming's White Crane grand-master.

Jin 勁 A power in Chinese martial arts which is derived from muscles which have been energized by Qi to their maximum potential.

Jing 經 Channel. Sometimes translated meridian. Refers to the twelve organ-related 'rivers' which circulate Qi throughout the body.

Jing 靜 Calmness.

Jing 精 Essence. The most refined part of anything.

Jing Qi 精氣 Essence Qi. The Qi which has been converted from Original Essence.

Jing Qi 經氣 Channel Qi. This Qi is responsible for the transportive and moving functions of the channels.

Jing Zi 精子 Means "Essence of the Son." Sperm.

Jueyin 厥陰 Absolute Yin. One of the six classifications in Chinese acupuncture of the Qi state in the Qi primary channels.

Kan 坎 A phase of the eight trigrams representing water.

Kan-Li 坎離 Water-fire. The methods of adjusting the body's Yin and Yang condition.

Kong Qi 空氣 Literally, space energy which means "air."

Kong Zi (551-479 B.C.) 孔子 Confucius. A Chinese scholar during the Spring and Autumn Period (722-484 B.C.) (Chun Qiu, 春秋), whose philosophy has significantly influenced Chinese culture.

Kou 叩 Cupping. A Chinese massage technique.

369

Kung Fu (Gongfu) 功夫 Literally "energy-time." Any study, learning, or practice which requires a lot of patience, energy, and time to complete. Since practicing Chinese martial arts requires a great deal of time and energy, Chinese martial arts are commonly called Gongfu.

La 拉 Pulling. A Chinese massage technique.

Lao Zi (604-531 B.C.) 老子 The creator of Daoism, also called Li Er (李耳) or Lao Dan (老聃), or by his nickname, Bo Yang (伯陽).

Laogong (P-8) 勞宮 "Labor's Palace." Cavity name. On the Pericardium Primary Qi Channel in the center of the palm.

Le 勒 Reining. A Chinese massage technique.

Li 離 One of the Eight Trigrams (Bagua, 八卦). Corresponds to Fire.

Li, Mao-Ching 李茂清 Dr. Yang, Jwing-Ming's Long Fist master.

Lian Jing Hua Qi 練精化氣 To refine the Essence and convert it into Qi. One of the Qigong training processes through which you convert Essence into Qi.

Lian Qi Hua Shen 練氣化神 To refine the Qi to nourish the spirit. Part of the Qigong training process in which you learn how to lead Qi to the head to nourish the brain and Shen (神) (spirit).

Lu 戮 Jabbing. A Chinese massage technique.

Luo 絡 Qi channels or Qi branches, often compared to streams. The small Qi channels that branch out from the primary Qi channels and are connected to the skin and to the bone marrow.

Mai 脈 Means "Qi vessels."

Men 門 Means "gate" or "door."

Mi Zong 秘宗 Secret style. A Tibetan Buddhist society which specializes in meditation and martial arts.

Mian 綿 Soft. One of the goals in regulating the breathing.

Ming dynasty (1368-1644 A.D.) 明朝 A dynasty in Chinese history.

Mo 摸 Touching or caressing. A Chinese massage technique.

Mo 摩 Rub. A major technique of Chinese Qigong massage.

Mu 木 Wood. One of the Five Elements (Wu Xing, 五行).

Na 拿 Grab. A major technique of Chinese Tui Na Qigong massage.

Nan Jing 難經 *Classic on Disorders.* Name of an ancient medical book written by a well-known physician, Bian Que (扁鵲) during the Chinese Qin and Han Dynasties (255 B.C.-220 A.D., 秦・漢).

Nei Dan 內丹 Literally: internal elixir. A form of Qigong in which Qi (the elixir) is built up in the body and spread out to the limbs.

Nei Jing 內經 *Internal Classic.* The name of the oldest Chinese medical book. It contains two major parts: *Su Wen* (素問) and *Ling Shu* (靈樞).

Nei Shi Gongfu 內視功夫 Nei Shi means "to look internally," so Nei Shi Gongfu refers to the art of looking inside yourself to read the state of your health and the condition of your Qi. Since it will take a lot of practice and experience to reach a profound level, it is called Gongfu (功夫).

Nei Zang An Mo 內臟按摩 Internal organ massage. Massage internal organs either through body movements or hand manipulations.

Ni Fu Hu Xi 逆腹呼吸 Reverse Abdominal Breathing. Also called Fan Fu Hu Xi (反腹呼吸) or Daoist Breathing (Dao Jia Hu Xi, 道家呼吸).

Nie 捏 Kneading. A Chinese massage technique.

Niwangong 泥丸宮 A Daoist name for the cavity on the top of the head. It is also called Tianlingai (天靈蓋) in the Chinese martial arts and Baihui (Gv-20) (百會) in Chinese medicine.

Nuo 挪 Shifting, slipping. A Chinese massage technique.

Pai 拍 Slapping. A Chinese massage technique.

Pi 劈 Chopping. A Chinese massage technique.

Pu Tong An Mo 普通按摩 General massage. A category of Chinese Qigong massage.

Qi 氣 The general definition of Qi is: universal energy, including heat, light, and electromagnetic energy. A narrower definition of Qi refers to the energy circulating in human or animal bodies.

Qi 奇 Means odd, strange, or mysterious.

Qi An Mo 氣按摩 Qi massage. One of the high levels of massage techniques in which a massage doctor will use his or her Qi to remove the Qi stagnation in a patient's body. Qi massage is also called "Wai Qi Liao Fa" (外氣療法) which means "healing with the external Qi."

Qi Hua Lun 氣化論 *Theory of Qi's Variation.* An ancient treatise which discusses the variations of Qi in the universe.

Qi Huo 起火 To start the fire. In Qigong practice, when you start to build up Qi at the Lower Dan Tian (Xia Dan Tian, 下丹田).

Qi Jing Ba Mai 奇經八脈 Literally: strange (odd) channels eight vessels. Usually referred to as the eight extraordinary vessels, or simply as the vessels. Called odd or strange because they are not well understood and do not all exist in pairs.

Qi Ma 氣脈 Qi vessels, often compared to reservoirs. The eight vessels involved with transporting, storing, and regulating Qi.

Qi Shi 氣勢 Energy state. Shi (勢) means the way something looks or feels. Therefore: the feeling of Qi as it expresses itself.

Qi Xue 氣穴 Qi cavities.

Qi Xue 氣血 Literally "Qi blood." According to Chinese medicine. Qi and blood cannot be separated in our body, and so the two words are commonly used together.

Qia 掐 Piercing. A Chinese massage technique.

Qian Long Men 乾龍門 The name of a Daoist society.

Qiao 敲 Knocking. A Chinese massage technique.

371

Qiao 蹻 The heel. Qiao is also a name for the Chinese massage technique which uses the feet.

Qiao Men 竅門 The secret or tricky entrance. Qiao Men is commonly used to refer to the key points which you need to know when entering into a new field of knowledge or practice.

Qie 切 Cascading. A Chinese massage technique.

Qigong (Chi Kung) 氣功 Gong (功) means Gongfu (功夫) (lit, energy-time). Therefore, Qigong means study, research, and/or practices related to Qi.

Qin Na (Chin Na) 擒拿 Literally, grab control. A type of Chinese Gongfu which emphasizes grabbing techniques to control the opponent's joints in conjunction with attacking certain acupuncture cavities.

Qing dynasty (1644-1911 A.D.) 清朝 A dynasty in Chinese history.

Qu 曲 Bending. A Chinese massage technique.

Re Qi 熱氣 Re (熱) means warmth or heat. Generally, Re Qi is used to represent heat. It is used sometimes to imply that a person or animal is still alive since the body is warm.

Ren 人 Man or mankind.

Ren Mai 任脈 Usually translated Conception Vessel. One of the eight extraordinary vessels.

Ren Qi 人氣 Human Qi.

Ren Shi 人事 Literally: human relations. Human events, activities, and relationships.

Rou 揉 Rubbing. One of the major Chinese massage techniques.

San Cai 三才 Three powers. Heaven, Earth, and Man.

San Yuan 三元 Three origins. Also called "San Bao" (三寶) (three treasures). Human Essence (Jing, 精), energy (Qi, 氣) and spirit (Shen, 神).

Sao 搔 Scratching. A Chinese massage technique.

Shang Dan Tian 上丹田 Upper Dan Tian. Located at the third eye, it is the residence of the Shen (spirit).

Shang dynasty (1766-1122 B.C.) 商朝 A dynasty in Chinese history.

Shaolin 少林 A Buddhist temple in Henan province (河南省), famous for its martial arts.

Shaoyang 少陽 Lesser Yang. One of the six classifications in Chinese acupuncture of the Qi state of Qi primary channels.

Shaoyin 少陰 Means "lesser Yin." One of the six classifications of the Qi state in Chinese acupuncture Qi primary channels.

Shen 深 Deep.

Shen 神 Spirit. According to Chinese Qigong, the Shen resides at the Upper Dan Tian (the third eye).

Shen 伸 Extending. A Chinese massage technique.

Shen Long 神龍 Spiritual Dragon, a Daoist society.

Shen Tong 神通 Spiritual Enlightenment.

Shen Xin Ping Heng 身心平衡 Body and heart (mind) balanced. This means a balance between the physical body and the mental body.

Shi Er Jing 十二經 The Twelve Primary Qi Channels in Chinese medicine.

Shi Zhen 石針 Stone needle. Stone needles were used for acupuncture before metal needles were invented. Also called Bian Shi (砭石).

Shu 梳 Combing. A Chinese massage technique.

Shu 俞 Means "allowance" or "admittance." Sometimes translated as "doors."

Shuai 摔 Swinging. A Chinese massage technique.

Shui 水 Water. One of the Five Elements (Wu Xing, 五行).

Shui Qi 水氣 Water Qi. Qi created from Original Essence, which is able to calm your body.

Si Qi 死氣 Dead Qi. The Qi remaining in a dead body. Sometimes called ghost Qi (Gui Qi, 鬼氣).

Song dynasty (960-1280 A.D.) 宋朝 A dynasty in Chinese history.

Suan Ming Shi 算命師 Literally: calculate life teacher. A fortune teller who is able to calculate your future and destiny.

Sui dynasty (605-618 A.D.) 隋朝 A dynasty in Chinese history.

Sui Xi 髓息 Sui means the marrow (Gu Sui, 骨髓) or brain (Nao Sui, 腦髓). Therefore, Sui Xi means the Qigong breathing technique which is able to lead the Qi to the bone marrow and brain.

Su Wen 素問 The first part of the medical treatise *Nei Jing* (內經). The second part is Ling Shu (靈樞).

Tai Xi 胎息 Embryo breathing. A Qigong breathing technique which can be used to store the Qi in the Real Dan Tian (Zhen Dan Tian, 真丹田).

Taijiquan (Tai Chi Chuan) 太極拳 Great Ultimate Fist. A style of Chinese internal martial arts which emphasizes the cultivation of internal Qi. The creation of Taijiquan during the Chinese Song dynasty (960-1280 A.D.) (宋朝) is credited to Zhang, San-Feng (張三豐).

Taiwan 台灣 An island to the southeast of mainland China. Also known as "Formosa."

Taiyang 太陽 Greater Yang. One of the six classifications in Chinese acupuncture of the Qi state of Qi primary channels.

Taiyin 太陰 Greater Yin. One of the six classifications in Chinese acupuncture of the Qi state of Qi primary channels.

Taizuquan 太祖拳 A style of Chinese martial arts which is said to have been created by Song Taizu (宋太祖), founder of the Song dynasty (960-1280 A.D.) (宋朝).

Tan 彈 Flicking. A Chinese massage technique.

Tang dynasty (618-907 A.D.) 唐朝 A dynasty in Chinese history.

Tang Yan 燙眼 Ironing the eyes. A Qigong technique that can be used to maintain healthy eyes.

Tao Dredging. A Chinese massage technique.

Tao (Dao) 道 The way. The 'natural' way of everything.

Ti 提 Raising or lifting. A Chinese massage technique.

Ti Xi 體息 "Body Breathing." Also called Fu Xi (膚息), which means "skin breathing." This is a Qigong breathing technique which allows you to use your mind to lead the Qi to the skin surface, to strengthen the guardian Qi.

Tian 天 Heaven or sky. In ancient China, people believed that heaven was the most powerful natural energy in this universe.

Tian Qi 天氣 Heaven Qi. It is now commonly used to mean the weather, since weather is governed by heaven Qi.

Tian Shi 天時 Heavenly timing. The repeated natural cycles generated by the heavens such as: seasons, months, days, and hours.

Tianlingai 天靈蓋 Heavenly spiritual cover. A term used in the Chinese martial arts for the cavity on the top of the head. Tianlingai is also called Niwangong (泥丸宮) in Daoist society and Baihui (Gv-20) (百會) in Chinese medicine.

Tiao 調 A gradual regulating process resulting in that which is regulated achieving harmony with others.

Tiao Qi 調氣 To regulate the Qi.

Tiao Shen 調神 To regulate the spirit.

Tiao Shen 調身 To regulate the body.

Tiao Xi 調息 To regulate the breathing.

Tiao Xin 調心 To regulate the emotional mind.

Tie Bu Shan 鐵布衫 Iron shirt. Gongfu training which toughens the body externally and internally.

Tong Men 通門 Gates.

Tu 土 Earth. One of the Five Elements (Wu Xing, 五行).

Tui 推 Push. A major technique in Chinese Tui Na Qigong massage.

Tui Na 推拿 Literally: push grab. Tui Na is one of the traditional Chinese massage styles which specializes in using pushing and grabbing to adjust abnormal Qi circulation and cure sicknesses.

Wai Dan 外丹 External elixir. External Qigong exercises in which a practitioner will build up his Qi in his limbs and then lead it into the center of the body for nourishment.

Wai Qi Liao Fa 外氣療法 Wai Qi (外氣) means "external Qi" and Liao Fa (療法) means "techniques for healing." Wai Qi Liao Fa is a Qigong healing method which uses Qi emitted by the healer.

Wei Qi 衛氣 Protective Qi or Guardian Qi. The Qi at the surface of the body which generates a shield to protect the body from negative external influences such as colds.

Weilu 尾閭 Coccyx. This place is called Changqiang (Gv-1) (長強) (Long Strength) in Chinese medical society.

Wu Xing 五行 Five phases. Also called the five elements. Metal, wood, water, fire, and earth, representing the five phases of any process.

Wudang Mountain 武當山 Located in Hubei province (湖北) in China.

Wuji 無極 "No extremities," which means no polarities.

Wushu 武術 Literally: martial techniques. A common name for the Chinese martial arts. Many other terms are used, including: Wuyi (武藝) (martial arts), Wugong (武功) (martial Gongfu), Guoshu (國術) (national techniques), and Gongfu (功夫) (energy-time). Because Wushu has been modified in mainland China over the past forty years into gymnastic martial performance, many traditional Chinese martial artist have given up this name in order to avoid confusing modern Wushu with traditional Wushu. Recently, mainland China has attempted to bring modern Wushu back toward its traditional training and practice.

Xi 細 Slender. One of the key goals of regulating the breathing.

Xi Sui Jing 洗髓經 Literally: *Washing Marrow Classic*, usually translated *Marrow Washing Classic*. A Qigong training which specializes in leading Qi to the marrow to cleanse it. It is believed that Xi Sui Jing training is the key to longevity and reaching spiritual enlightenment.

Xi Sui Qigong 洗髓氣功 Gongfu of marrow and brain washing Qigong practice.

Xia Dan Tian 下丹田 Lower Dan Tian. Located in the lower abdomen, it is believed to be the residence of water Qi (Original Qi).

Xia dynasty (2205-1766 B.C.) 夏朝 A dynasty in Chinese history.

Xian Gu 仙骨 Immortal bone which implies "the sacrum."

Xian Tian Qi 先天氣 Pre-Birth Qi or Pre-Heaven Qi. Also called Dan Tian Qi (丹田氣). The Qi which is converted from Original Essence (Yuan Jing, 元精) and is stored in the Lower Dan Tian (Xia Dan Tian, 下丹田). Considered to be "water Qi," it is able to calm the body.

Xiao Zhou Tian 小周天 "Small Cyclic Heaven" or "Small Circulation Meditation." This is also commonly known as Microcosmic Meditation in Yoga or Turning the Wheel of Natural Law (Zhuan Fa Lun, 轉法輪) by Buddhist society. A Nei Dan Qigong (內丹氣功) training in which Qi is generated at the Dan Tian (丹田), and then moved in a circle through the Conception and Governing Vessels (Ren, Du Mai, 任・督脈).

Xie 洩 Releasing. Means to release the Qi to lower the Qi level.

Xie Qi 邪氣 Evil Qi, which means the abdominal Qi circulation or storage in the body.

Xin 心 Literally: Heart. Refers to the emotional mind.

Xin Xi Xiang Yi 心息相依 A famous proverb in Chinese Qigong society which means "heart (mind) and breathing (are) mutually dependent."

Xing 行 Means "to walk or to move"; probably more pertinent, it means "a process."

Xingyiquan (Hsing Yi Chuan) 形意拳 Literally: Shape-mind Fist. An internal style of Gongfu in which the mind or thinking determines the shape or movement of the body. Creation of the style is attributed to Marshal Yue, Fei (岳飛) during Chinese Song dynasty (960-1280 A.D.) (宋朝).

Xinzhu Xian 新竹縣 Birthplace of Dr. Yang, Jwing-Ming in Taiwan.

Xuan 旋 Rotating. A Chinese massage technique.

Xue 穴 Literally: cave or hole. An acupuncture cavity.

Yan 言 Means "speaking or talking."

Yang 陽 In Chinese philosophy, the active, positive, masculine polarity. In Chinese medicine, Yang means excessive, overactive, overheated. The Yang or outer organs are the Gall Bladder, Small Intestine, Large Intestine, Stomach, Bladder, and Triple Burner.

Yang, Jwing-Ming, Ph.D. 楊俊敏博士 Author of this book.

Yangming 陽明 Yang brightness. One of the six classifications in Chinese acupuncture of the Qi state of Qi primary channels.

Yangqiao Mai 陽蹻脈 Yang Heel Vessel. One of the eight extraordinary vessels.

Yangwei Mai 陽維脈 Yang Linking Vessel. One of the eight extraordinary vessels.

Yao 搖 Shaking. A Chinese massage technique.

Yi 意 Mind. Specifically, the mind which is generated by clear thinking and judgement, and which is able to make you calm, peaceful, and wise.

Yi Jin Jing 易筋經 Literally: changing muscle/tendon classic, usually called *The Muscle/Tendon Changing Classic*. Credited to Da Mo (達摩) around 550 A.D. This work discusses Wai Dan Qigong (外丹氣功) training for strengthening the physical body.

Yi Jing 易經 *Book of Changes*. A book of divination written during the Zhou dynasty (1122-255 B.C.) (周朝).

Yi Shou Dan Tian 意守丹田 A famous proverb in Qigong society that means "to keep the Mind on the Dan Tian."

Yi Yi Yin Qi 以意引氣 A famous proverb in Qigong society that means "using your Yi (意) (Mind) to lead your Qi."

Yin 陰 In Chinese philosophy, the passive, negative, feminine polarity In Chinese medicine, Yin means deficient. The Yin (internal) organs are the Heart, Lungs, Liver, Kidneys, Spleen, and Pericardium.

Yin Qi 陰氣 The Qi state which is weaker than normal.

Yin Xu 殷墟 A burial ground in An Yang, Henan province (河南・安陽), used during the Shang dynasty (1766-1154 B.C.) (商朝).

Ying Qi 營氣
Managing Qi or Nourishing Qi. The Qi which manages the functioning of the organs and the body.

Ying Zhua Men 鷹爪門 Eagle claw style. A style of Chinese martial arts.

Yinqiao Mai 陰蹻脈 Yin Heel Vessel. One of the eight extraordinary vessels.

Yinwei Mai 陰維脈 Yin Linking Vessel. One of the eight extraordinary vessels.

You 悠 Continuous. One of the goals of regulating the breathing is to keep the breathing uniform.

Yuan dynasty (1206-1368 A.D.) 元朝 A dynasty in Chinese history.

Yuan Jing 元精 Original Essence. The fundamental, original substance inherited from your parents, it is converted into Original Qi (Yuan Qi, 元氣).

Yuan Qi 元氣 Original Qi. Created from the Original Essence (Yuan Jing, 元精) inherited from your parents.

Yun 勻 Uniform. One of the goals of regulating the breathing is to keep the breathing uniform.

Yun 運 Transporting. A Chinese massage technique.

Zan Fu Zhi Qi 臟腑之氣 Organ Qi. The Qi in organs that keeps the organ functioning.

Zang 臟 Viscera. The six Yin organs. Five of these are considered the core of the entire human system: the Liver, Heart, Spleen, Lungs, and Kidneys. Usually, when a discussion involves the channels and all the Organs, the Pericardium is added, otherwise it is treated as an adjunct of the Heart.

Zhang, Xiang-San 張祥三 A well-known martial artist in Taiwan during the 1960s.

Zhen Shi 箴石 Stone needle. Same as Shi Zhen (石針).

Zhen Xia Dan Tian 真下丹田 Real Lower Dan Tian, which is the main Qi reservoir or bioelectric battery in our body.

Zhen Zhan 震顫 Vibrating. A Chinese massage technique.

Zheng Fu Hu Xi 正腹呼吸 Formal Abdominal Breathing or Normal Abdominal Breathing. More commonly called Buddhist Breathing (Fo Jia Hu Xi, 佛家呼吸).

Zheng Gu Ke 正骨科 Align bone category. A medical training category in the Yuan dynasty (1206-1368 A.D.) (元朝).

Zheng Qi 正氣 Righteous Qi or Normal Qi. When a person is righteous, it is said that he has righteous Qi which evil Qi cannot overcome.

Zhong Dan Tian 中丹田 Middle Dan Tian. Located in the area of the solar plexus, it is the residence of fire Qi.

Zhong Jiao 中焦 Middle Triple Burner. The section of the Triple Burner which is located between the diaphragm and the navel.

Zhou 周 Means "to be complete," "to be perfect," or "to be round."

Zhou Dynasty (1122-255 B.C.) 周朝 A dynasty in Chinese history.

Zhua Long 抓龍 Zhua means "to grab," and Long means "dragon" and refers to the tendons and muscles. Zhua Long is a common name for general massage in Taiwan.

Zhuo 啄 Pecking. A Chinese massage technique.

Zong Qi 宗氣 Ancestral Qi.

Zuo Shi Ba Duan Jin 坐勢八段錦 The sitting Eight Pieces of Brocade. Eight Pieces of Brocade is a Wai Dan Qigong (外丹氣功) practice that is said to have been created by Marshal Yue, Fei (岳飛) during the Southern Song Dynasty (1127-1280 A.D.) (南宋). This medical Qigong practice includes two sets, a sitting set and a standing set.

Index

abdomen 202
acupuncture 12, 20, 96-97
aging 18-19
air 16
anus 95
arms 201, 202
back 201
Bagua 9
Baihuanshu (B-30) 64, 268
Baihui (Gv-20) 62, 81, 97, 221, 365, 371, 374
battery 112
Bending (Qu) 178
Biliang 219
Binao (LI-14) 52, 288
bioelectricity 13, 15-16, 33
bioelectromagnetic energy 12
blood 36, 45-46, 206
blood, stagnant 193
bone marrow 198
Book of Changes 8-9
brain 16, 217, 218
breathing 51, 107, 113, 116, 131, 132, 134
Caressing (Mo) 162
Carrying On the Back (Bei) 174
Cascading (Qie) 186
cavities 20, 48-49, 96-97
cavity press massage 20-21
Changqiang (Gv-1) 81, 252, 374
channels 47-48
channels, Yang 49
channels, Yin 49
Chengshan (B-57) 64, 269, 271
chest 202
Chize (L-5) 49, 288
Chopping (Pi) 174
clergy 24
clothing 101
Combing (Shu) 182
Combining (He) 172
concentration 135
Conception Vessel 82-84
conditioning 124
Cupping (Kou) 186
Dan Tian 53, 60, 111, 112, 130, 213
Dao 10
Dian Xue massage 143, 146
Dividing (Fen) 172
Dredging (Tao) 186
ears 95
eight vessels 10-11, 15, 77-78
elbow 153
emotion 67-68, 92-93, 107
enjoyment 19

enthusiasm 140
environment 101-102
Ermen (TB-21) 70, 222, 224
exercise 16-17
Extending (Shen) 177
eyes 94-95
fasciae 35, 196
fat 35
fatigue 18
feet 154
Fengshi (GB-31) 74, 270, 272
Filing (Cuo) 170
fingers 126, 144, 148
fingertips 143
Five Elements 47-48
Five Phases 47
Flicking (Tan) 170
Folding (Die) 172
food 16, 67-68
forearm 153
Futu (S-32) 53, 55, 311
gall bladder 72-74, 348, 355, 360
Gall Bladder Channel of Foot 72-74
Gaohuang (B-38) 228, 248, 254
gates 34, 93, 200, 226
Girdle Vessel 86
Governing Vessel 80-82
Grabbing (Na) 162
head 201, 214
heart 58-60, 350, 356, 361
Heart Channel of Hand 58-60
Hegu (LI-4) 51, 290, 368, 369
Holding (Duan) 164
hormone production 111
hormones 194, 200
Huang Di Nei Jing 25-26
Huantiao (GB-30) 74, 270, 272
Huiyin (Co-1) 81, 82, 85, 86, 100, 131, 132, 197, 270, 308
illness 18
immune system 194, 200
injuries 19-20
Internal Classic of the Yellow Emperor 25-26
internal organs 197
intestine 62, 347, 354
Jabbing (Lu) 184
Jianjing (GB-21) 70, 74, 89, 227, 246, 254, 292
Jiankua (N-LE-55) 270, 272
Jianliao (TB-14) 70, 254, 287
Jianneiling (M-UE-48) 316
Jianyu (LI-15) 52, 87, 287
Jiexi (S-41) 55, 272, 274
Jimai (Li-12) 76, 304
Jing 109, 110

Index

Jiuwei (Co-15) 301
joint injuries 156
joints 97-98, 128, 197
Jubi (N-UE-10) 314
junctions 34, 93-94, 98-100
Kan and Li 105
kidney 64-65
Kidney Channel of Foot 65-68
kidneys 66-68, 348, 354, 355, 360
Kneading (Nie) 166
knees 154
knuckles 150
Kongzui (L-6) 49, 289
Laogong (P-8) 21, 68, 93, 97, 152, 262, 290, 346, 370
Laogong cavity 21-22, 94, 97, 262
Large Intestine Channel of Hand 51-53
legs 201, 202
light 101-102
Lingtai (Gv-l0) 249
liver 76-77, 348, 355, 360
Liver Channel of Foot 74-79
lower back 128
Lung Channel of Hand 49-51
lungs 51, 350, 356, 361
lymph organs 38-39
martial artists 23-24
massage,
    cavity press 20
    Chinese vs. Western 5
    general 17-18, 192, 209
    history 22, 24-29, 103
    pathways 202, 204, 205
    purposes 103-105, 192-194
    push grab 19
    Qi 21
    Qigong 30
    table 101, 210, 211
massaging the back 242-260
massaging the backs of the limbs 261-294
massaging the front of the limbs 310-318
massaging the head 226-240
mental body 194, 212
mental processes 90-93
mental tension 192
Mingmen (Gv-4) 81, 97, 250
mouth 94-95
muscles 196
Naohu (Gv-17) 62, 81, 97, 225, 226
Naohui (TB-13) 70, 288
neck 201, 242
nerve endings 195
nerve junctions 206
nerves 98
nervous system 34, 39-42, 42-43, 193
noise 102

Normal Abdominal Breathing 131, 134
nose 95
Oracle-Bone Scripture 25
organs 46-47
palms 150, 152
pathways 202
Pecking (Zhuo) 182
Pericardium Channel of Hand 68-69
physical body 3, 33, 34
physicians 22-23
Piercing (Qia) 176
Pinyin vi
pituitary gland 111
Point Striking or Knocking (Dian Da, Qiao) 164
Pointing (Dian) 176
pores 95
Pounding (Guan) 184
power 207
Pressing (An) 159
Pulling (La) 166
Pushing (Tui) 160
Qi,
    body 3, 33, 43-45, 199
    channels 47-48, 49
    circulation 136, 245
    endings 199
    recovery 138
    balance 107
    definition 6, 7, 11, 14
    Earth 9-10
    flow 11, 14-15, 35, 109
    Heaven 9
    Human 9-10
    leading 204
    stagnant 193
    types of 45
Qigong, definition 8, 10-11
Qihu (S-13) 55, 298
Qubin (GB-7) 73, 222, 223
Quchi (LI-11) 288
Quick Pull (Che) 177
Quze (P-3) 68, 316
Raising or Lifting (Ti) 166
Reeling (Chan) 184
regulating the body 113, 114, 138
regulating the breathing 113, 116, 131
regulating the mind 113, 118, 135, 140
regulating the Qi 113, 122, 138
regulating the spirit 113, 123, 140
Reining (Le) 179
relaxation 18, 114
Renzhong (Gv-26) 26, 51, 53, 81, 100, 214, 221
reservoirs 48
Reverse Abdominal Breathing 133, 135
Riyue (GB-24) 57, 74, 303
Rolling (Gun) 172

379

rooting 115
Rotating (Xuan) 182
Rubbing (Rou or Mo) 156
Rugen (S-18) 55, 302
Ruzhong (S-17) 55, 302
Sacrum (Jian Gu) 250
Sanyinjiao (Sp-6) 57, 74, 272
Scraping (Gua) 184
Scratching (Sao) 182
self-massage 319
sensory organs 196
Shaking (Yao) 168
Shanzhong (Co-17) 70, 82, 300
Shen 109, 111
Shenshu (B-23) 64, 246, 250
Shiatsu massage 5
Shifting, Slipping (Nuo) 178
Shufu (K-27) 65, 298
Shuxi (N-CA-6) 304
sickness 11
Sidu (TB-9) 70, 289
skin conductivity 96
skin contact 21-22
Slapping (Pai) 170
Small Intestine Channel of Hand 60-62
spine 196, 201, 243
spiritual center 214
Spiritual Embryo 112
spleen 55, 348, 355, 360
Spleen Channel of Foot 56-58
Squeezing (Ji) 180
stomach 55-56, 348, 355, 360
Stomach Channel of Foot 53-55
Striking (Da) 178
Supporting (Ding) 168
Swaying (Huang) 182
Swinging (Shuai) 170
Taiyang (M-HN-9) 222
temperature 101
three treasures 109
Threshing (Dao) 180
Thrusting Vessel 84-86
Tiantu (Co-22) 82, 90, 298
Tianzhu (B-10) 64, 224
Tianzong (SI-11) 61, 248, 254, 258, 292
Tiaokou (S-38) 55, 274
Tong Men 34
traditional Chinese medicine (TCM) 4
Transporting (Yun) 176
Triple Burner Channel of Hand 70-72
Tui Na massage 19, 143, 144
twelve major channels 10-11
Twisting (Ban) 180
Uprooting (Ba) 180
urethra 95
urinary bladder 64-65, 354

Urinary Bladder Channel of Foot 62-64, 246
Vibrating (Zhen Zhan) 164
Wade-Giles vi
Wai Dan Qigong 263
Waving (Dou) 174
Weizhong (B-54) 64, 269, 271
Western medicine xvii, 33
Wiping (Ca) 186
wrists 124
Wuji 109
Xiaguan (S-7) 55, 72, 224
Xuehai (Sp-10) 57, 271, 272, 312
Yale vi
Yang 15
Yang body 3
Yang Heel Vessel 86-88
Yang Linking Vessel 89-90
Yi Jing 8-9
Yifeng (TB-17) 70, 72, 222, 224
Yin 15
Yin and Yang 105
Yin and Yang balance 33, 106
Yin body 3
Yin Conception Vessel 100
Yin Linking Vessel 90-226
Yingchuang (S-16) 55, 302
Yinmen (B-51) 64, 269, 271
Yongquan (K-1) 65, 69, 97, 262-263, 268-269, 272, 274, 349
Zhibian (B-49) 64, 268
Zhongfu (L-1) 49, 57, 300
Zhongkong (M-BW-26) 268

BOOKS FROM YMAA

Title	Code
6 HEALING MOVEMENTS	B906
101 REFLECTIONS ON TAI CHI CHUAN	B868
108 INSIGHTS INTO TAI CHI CHUAN — A STRING OF PEARLS	B582
A WOMAN'S QIGONG GUIDE	B833
ADVANCING IN TAE KWON DO	B072X
ANCIENT CHINESE WEAPONS	B671
ANALYSIS OF SHAOLIN CHIN NA 2ND ED.	B0002
ARTHRITIS RELIEF — CHINESE QIGONG FOR HEALING & PREVENTION, 3RD ED.	B0339
BACK PAIN RELIEF — CHINESE QIGONG FOR HEALING & PREVENTION 2ND ED	B0258
BAGUAZHANG	B300
CARDIO KICKBOXING ELITE	B922
CHIN NA IN GROUND FIGHTING	B663
CHINESE FAST WRESTLING — THE ART OF SAN SHOU KUAI JIAO	B493
CHINESE FITNESS — A MIND / BODY APPROACH	B37X
CHINESE TUI NA MASSAGE	B043
COMPREHENSIVE APPLICATIONS OF SHAOLIN CHIN NA	B36X
DR. WU'S HEAD MASSAGE—ANTI-AGING AND HOLISTIC HEALING THERAPY	B0576
EIGHT SIMPLE QIGONG EXERCISES FOR HEALTH, 2ND ED.	B523
ESSENCE OF SHAOLIN WHITE CRANE	B353
ESSENCE OF TAIJI QIGONG, 2ND ED.	B639
EXPLORING TAI CHI	B424
FIGHTING ARTS	B213
INSIDE TAI CHI	B108
KATA AND THE TRANSMISSION OF KNOWLEDGE	B0266
LIUHEBAFA FIVE CHARACTER SECRETS	B728
MARTIAL ARTS ATHLETE	B655
MARTIAL ARTS INSTRUCTION	B024X
MARTIAL WAY AND ITS VIRTUES	B698
MEDITATIONS ON VIOLENCE	B1187
NATURAL HEALING WITH QIGONG — THERAPEUTIC QIGONG	B0010
NORTHERN SHAOLIN SWORD, 2ND ED.	B85X
OKINAWA'S COMPLETE KARATE SYSTEM — ISSHIN RYU	B914
PRINCIPLES OF TRADITIONAL CHINESE MEDICINE	B99X
QIGONG FOR HEALTH & MARTIAL ARTS 2ND ED.	B574
QIGONG FOR LIVING	B116
QIGONG FOR TREATING COMMON AILMENTS	B701
QIGONG MASSAGE —FUND. TECHNIQUES FOR HEALTH AND RELAXATION 2ND ED.	B0487
QIGONG MEDITATION — EMBRYONIC BREATHING	B736
QIGONG MEDITATION—SMALL CIRCULATION	B0673
QIGONG, THE SECRET OF YOUTH	B841
QUIET TEACHER	B1170
ROOT OF CHINESE QIGONG, 2ND ED.	B507
SHIHAN TE — THE BUNKAI OF KATA	B884
SUNRISE TAI CHI	B0838
SURVIVING ARMED ASSAULTS	B0711
TAEKWONDO — ANCIENT WISDOM FOR THE MODERN WARRIOR	B930
TAE KWON DO — THE KOREAN MARTIAL ART	B0869
TAEKWONDO — SPIRIT AND PRACTICE	B221
TAI CHI BOOK	B647
TAI CHI CHUAN — 24 & 48 POSTURES	B337
TAI CHI CHUAN MARTIAL APPLICATIONS, 2ND ED.	B442
TAI CHI CONNECTIONS	B0320
TAI CHI DYNAMICS	B1163
TAI CHI SECRETS OF THE ANCIENT MASTERS	B71X
TAI CHI SECRETS OF THE WU & LI STYLES	B981
TAI CHI SECRETS OF THE WU STYLE	B175
TAI CHI SECRETS OF THE YANG STYLE	B094
TAI CHI THEORY & MARTIAL POWER, 2ND ED.	B434
TAI CHI WALKING	B23X
TAIJI CHIN NA	B378
TAIJI SWORD, CLASSICAL YANG STYLE	B744
TAIJIQUAN, CLASSICAL YANG STYLE	B68X
TAIJIQUAN THEORY OF DR. YANG, JWING-MING	B432
THE CROCODILE AND THE CRANE	B0876
THE CUTTING SEASON	B0821
THE WAY OF KATA—A COMPREHENSIVE GUIDE TO DECIPHERING MARTIAL APPS.	B0584
THE WAY OF KENDO AND KENJITSU	B0029
THE WAY OF SANCHIN KATA	B0845
THE WAY TO BLACK BELT	B0852
TRADITIONAL CHINESE HEALTH SECRETS	B892
TRADITIONAL TAEKWONDO—CORE TECHNIQUES, HISTORY, AND PHILOSOPHY	B0665
WILD GOOSE QIGONG	B787
XINGYIQUAN, 2ND ED.	B416

more products available from...

YMAA Publication Center, Inc. 楊氏東方文化出版中心
1-800-669-8892 • ymaa@aol.com • www.ymaa.com

VIDEOS FROM YMAA

ADVANCED PRACTICAL CHIN NA — 1	T0061
ADVANCED PRACTICAL CHIN NA — 2	T007X
COMP. APPLICATIONS OF SHAOLIN CHIN NA 1	T386
COMP. APPLICATIONS OF SHAOLIN CHIN NA 2	T394
EIGHT SIMPLE QIGONG EXERCISES FOR HEALTH 2ND ED.	T54X
NORTHERN SHAOLIN SWORD — SAN CAI JIAN & ITS APPLICATIONS	T051
NORTHERN SHAOLIN SWORD — KUN WU JIAN & ITS APPLICATIONS	T06X
NORTHERN SHAOLIN SWORD — QI MEN JIAN & ITS APPLICATIONS	T078
QIGONG: 15 MINUTES TO HEALTH	T140
SHAOLIN LONG FIST KUNG FU — YI LU MEI FU & ER LU MAI FU	T256
SHAOLIN LONG FIST KUNG FU — SHI ZI TANG	T264
SHAOLIN LONG FIST KUNG FU — XIAO HU YAN	T604
SHAOLIN WHITE CRANE GONG FU — BASIC TRAINING 3	T0185
SIMPLIFIED TAI CHI CHUAN — 24 & 48	T329
SUN STYLE TAIJIQUAN	T469
TAI CHI CHUAN & APPLICATIONS — 24 & 4	T485
TAIJI CHIN NA IN DEPTH — 1	T0282
TAIJI CHIN NA IN DEPTH — 2	T0290
TAIJI CHIN NA IN DEPTH — 3	T0304
TAIJI CHIN NA IN DEPTH — 4	T0312
TAIJI WRESTLING — 1	T0371
TAIJI WRESTLING — 2	T038X
TAIJI YIN & YANG SYMBOL STICKING HANDS–YANG TAIJI TRAINING	T580
TAIJI YIN & YANG SYMBOL STICKING HANDS–YIN TAIJI TRAINING	T0177
WILD GOOSE QIGONG	T949
WU STYLE TAIJIQUAN	T477
XINGYIQUAN — 12 ANIMAL FORM	T310

DVDS FROM YMAA

ANALYSIS OF SHAOLIN CHIN NA	D0231
BAGUAZHANG 1,2, & 3 —EMEI BAGUAZHANG	D0649
CHEN STYLE TAIJIQUAN	D0819
CHIN NA IN DEPTH COURSES 1 — 4	D602
CHIN NA IN DEPTH COURSES 5 — 8	D610
CHIN NA IN DEPTH COURSES 9 — 12	D629
EIGHT SIMPLE QIGONG EXERCISES FOR HEALTH	D0037
FIVE ANIMAL SPORTS	D1106
THE ESSENCE OF TAIJI QIGONG	D0215
QIGONG MASSAGE—FUNDAMENTAL TECHNIQUES FOR HEALTH AND RELAXATION	D0592
SHAOLIN KUNG FU FUNDAMENTAL TRAINING 1&2	D0436
SHAOLIN LONG FIST KUNG FU — BASIC SEQUENCES	D661
SHAOLIN SABER — BASIC SEQUENCES	D0616
SHAOLIN STAFF — BASIC SEQUENCES	D0920
SHAOLIN WHITE CRANE GONG FU BASIC TRAINING 1&2	D599
SIMPLE QIGONG EXERCISES FOR ARTHRITIS RELIEF	D0890
SIMPLE QIGONG EXERCISES FOR BACK PAIN RELIEF	D0883
SIMPLIFIED TAI CHI CHUAN	D0630
SUNRISE TAI CHI	D0274
SUNSET TAI CHI	D0760
TAI CHI CONNECTIONS	D0444
TAI CHI ENERGY PATTERNS	D0525
TAI CHI FIGHTING SET—TWO PERSON MATCHING SET	D0509
TAIJI BALL QIGONG COURSES 1&2—16 CIRCLING AND 16 ROTATING PATTERNS	D0517
TAIJI BALL QIGONG COURSES 3&4—16 PATTERNS OF WRAP-COILING & APPLICATIONS	D0777
TAIJI MARTIAL APPLICATIONS — 37 POSTURES	D1057
TAIJI PUSHING HANDS 1&2—YANG STYLE SINGLE AND DOUBLE PUSHING HANDS	D0495
TAIJI PUSHING HANDS 3&4—MOVING SINGLE AND DOUBLE PUSHING HANDS	D0681
TAIJI SABER — THE COMPLETE FORM, QIGONG & APPLICATIONS	D1026
TAIJI & SHAOLIN STAFF - FUNDAMENTAL TRAINING	D0906
TAIJI YIN YANG STICKING HANDS	D1040
TAIJIQUAN CLASSICAL YANG STYLE	D645
TAIJI SWORD, CLASSICAL YANG STYLE	D0452
UNDERSTANDING QIGONG 1 — WHAT IS QI? • HUMAN QI CIRCULATORY SYSTEM	D069X
UNDERSTANDING QIGONG 2 — KEY POINTS • QIGONG BREATHING	D0418
UNDERSTANDING QIGONG 3 — EMBRYONIC BREATHING	D0555
UNDERSTANDING QIGONG 4 — FOUR SEASONS QIGONG	D0562
UNDERSTANDING QIGONG 5 — SMALL CIRCULATION	D0753
UNDERSTANDING QIGONG 6 — MARTIAL QIGONG BREATHING	D0913
WHITE CRANE HARD & SOFT QIGONG	D637

more products available from...
YMAA Publication Center, Inc. 楊氏東方文化出版中心
1-800-669-8892 • ymaa@aol.com • www.ymaa.com

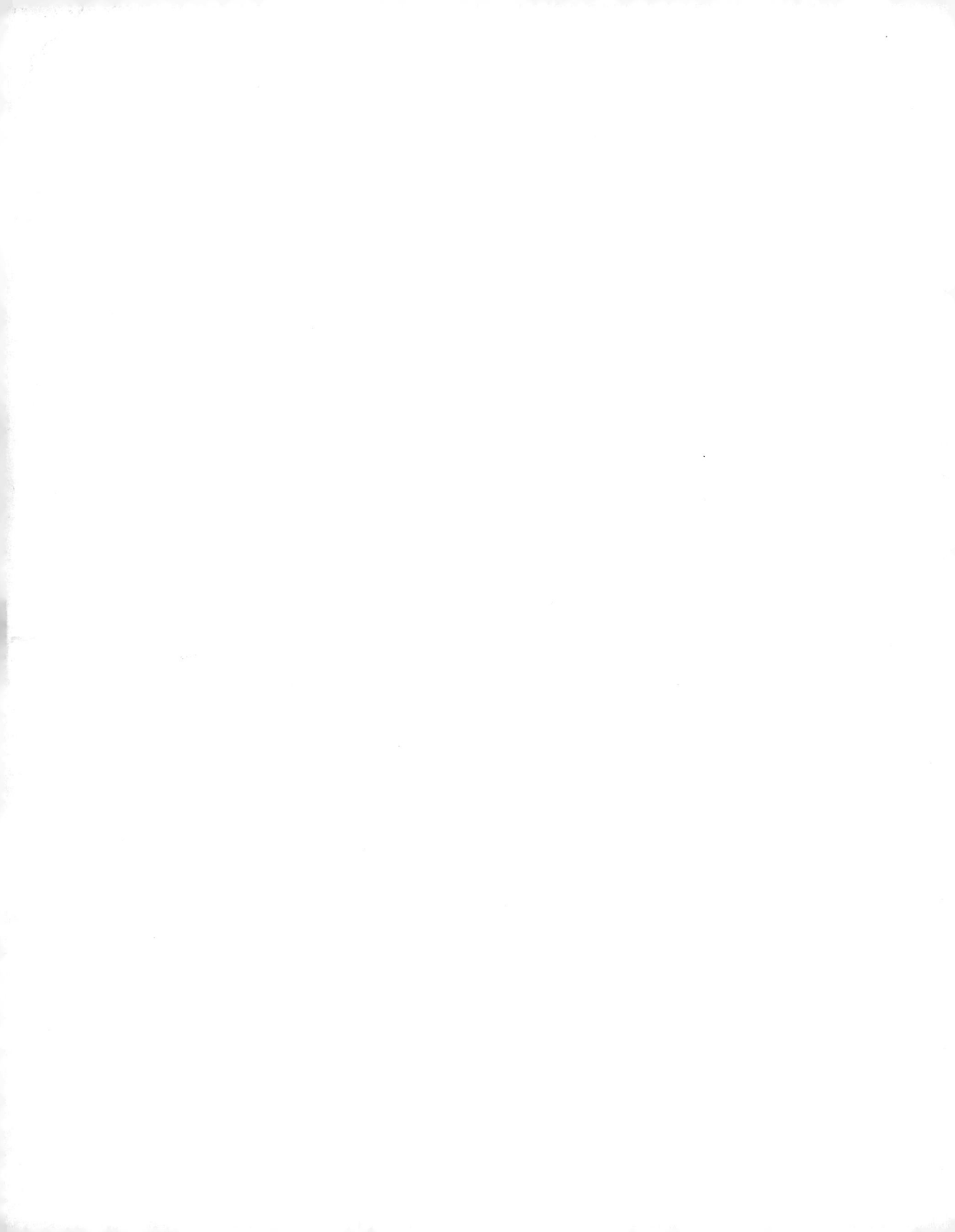